Arthroscopic and Endoscopic Spinal Surgery

Arthroscopic and Endoscopic Spinal Surgery

Text and Atlas, Second Edition

Edited by

Parviz Kambin, MD

Professor of Orthopedic Surgery and Endowed Chair of Spinal Surgery, Drexel University College of Medicine, Philadelphia, PA

HUMANA PRESS ✳ TOTOWA, NEW JERSEY

999 Riverview Drive, Suite 208
Totowa, NJ 07512

www.humanapress.com

Production Editor: Tracy Catanese

Cover design by Patricia F. Cleary

Cover Illustrations: Figures 38A and 35B from Chapter 4, "Herniated Lumbar Disc and Lumbar Radiculopathy," and Figures 7A and 12B from Chapter 5, "Management of Discogenic Pain and Spinal Instability Using Minimally Invasive Surgical Techniques," by Parviz Kambin.

For additional copies, pricing for bulk purchases, and/or information about other Humana titles, contact Humana at the above address or at any of the following numbers: Tel.: 973-256-1699; Fax: 973-256-8341; E-mail: orders@humanapr.com or visit our website: http://humanapress.com

This publication is printed on acid-free paper. ∞
ANSI Z39.48-1984 (American National Standards Institute) Permanence of Paper for Printed Library Materials.

Printed in the United States of America. 10 9 8 7 6 5 4 3 2 1

e-ISBN: 1-59259-904-4

Library of Congress Cataloging-in-Publication Data
Arthroscopic and endoscopic spinal surgery : text and atlas / edited by Parviz Kambin.
p. ; cm.
Includes bibliographical references and index.
ISBN 1-58829-522-2 (alk. paper)
1. Spine--Endoscopic surgery. 2. Spine--Endoscopic surgery--Atlases.
[DNLM: 1. Spine--surgery--Atlases. 2. Arthroscopy--methods--Atlases. 3. Endoscopy--methods--Atlases. 4. Surgical Procedures, Minimally Invasive--methods--Atlases. WE 17 A7875 2005] I. Kambin, Parviz.
RD533.A785 2005
617.5'60597--dc22

2004026633

Dedication

The authors wish to dedicate this text and atlas to their families, colleagues, and students of minimally invasive spinal surgery.

Preface

The term "minimally invasive spinal surgery" was coined in early 1990 following publication of the first edition of this text entitled *Arthroscopic Microdiscectomy: Minimal Intervention in Spinal Surgery*, and subsequent establishment of the International Society for Minimal Intervention in Spinal Surgery (ISMISS) under the auspices of the International Society of Orthopaedic Surgery and Traumatology (SICOT) in April 1990.

The orthopedic and neurological surgeons who participated in lectures and hands-on workshops both in Philadelphia and abroad have witnessed the evolution of minimally invasive spinal surgery from blind nucleotomy to endoscopic fragmentectomy, decompression of lateral recess stenosis, foraminoplasty, and spinal stabilization.

In *Arthroscopic and Endoscopic Spinal Surgery: Text and Atlas, Second Edition*, experts describe and illustrate various techniques and approaches that are currently used in this field. In addition, the ongoing research for the betterment of spine care via minimally invasive approaches is briefly reviewed.

I would like to express my sincere appreciation to so many of my colleagues who supported my efforts in the field of minimally invasive spinal surgery throughout the years. Many of them participated in our teaching symposiums and have provided valuable contributions to this text.

Parviz Kambin, MD

Contents

Contributors

JOHN C. CHIU, DSc, MD • *Director, Neurospine Surgery Department, California Spine Institute Medical Center Inc., Park, CA*

TERRY P. CORBIN, BS • *Clinical Outcomes Research Center, University of Minnesota, Maple Grove, MN*

RICHARD G. FESSLER, MD, PhD • *Professor and Chief, Section of Neurosurgery, University of Chicago, Chicago, IL*

LAURENCE N. FITZHENRY, MD • *Department of Orthopedic Surgery, Thomas Jefferson University and the Rothman Institute, Philadelphia, PA*

ROBERT D. FRASER, MD • *Alamo Bone and Joint Clinic, San Antonio, TX*

IOANNIS GAITANIS • *Orthopaedic Surgeon, University of Crete, Crete, Greece*

RICHARD D. GUYER, MD • *Associate Clinical Professor, Department of Orthopaedic Surgery, UT Southwestern Medical School, Dallas, and Research Founder and Chairman of the Board, Texas Back Institute, Plano, TX*

ALEXANDER G. HADJIPAVLOU, MD • *Professor of Orthopaedics-Traumatology, University of Crete, Crete, Greece*

PARVIZ KAMBIN, MD • *Professor of Orthopaedic Surgery, Drexel University College of Medicine, Philadelphia, PA*

ANDREW KARDUNA, PhD • *Department of Physical Therapy, University of Oregon, Eugene, OR*

GARRETT KINE, MD • *Anesthesiologist, SpineCare Medical Group, Daly City, CA*

GEORGE M. KONTAKIS, MD • *Assistant Professor of Orthopaedics-Traumatology, University of Crete, Crete, Greece*

ISADOR H. LIEBERMAN, MD, MBA, FRCS (C) • *Center Director and Director of Minimally Invasive Surgery, Center for Advanced Skills Training; Department of Orthopaedic Surgery and Spine Institute, The Cleveland Clinic Foundation, Cleveland, OH*

ANTHONY LOWMAN, PhD • *Assistant Professor, Department of Chemical Engineering, Drexel University, Philadelphia, PA*

MICHELE MARCOLONGO, PhD • *Assistant Professor, Department of Materials Science and Engineering, College of Engineering, Drexel University, Philadelphia, PA*

GEOFFREY M. MCCULLEN, MD • *Orthopedic Surgeon, Neurological and Spinal Surgery, LLC, Lincoln, NE*

WESLEY W. PARKE, PhD • *Professor and Chair Emeritus, Department of Anatomy, University of South Dakota School of Medicine, Vermillion, SD*

JAMES REYNOLDS, MD • *Orthopedic Surgeon, SpineCare Medical Group, Daly City, CA*

MARTIN H. SAVITZ, MD, FACS, FICS • *Executive Director, American Academy of Minimally Invasive Spinal Medicine and Surgery, and Adjunct Professor of Bioethics, MCP-Hahnemann School of Medicine, Philadelphia, PA*

James W. Simmons, Jr., MD • *Alamo Bone and Joint Clinic, San Antonio, TX*

Kern Singh, MD • *Department of Orthopedic Surgery, Rush-Presbyterian-St. Luke's Medical Center, Chicago, IL*

Daisuke Togawa, MD, PhD • *Department of Orthopaedic Surgery and Spine Institute, The Cleveland Clinic Foundation, Cleveland, OH*

Trent L. Tredway, MD • *Assistant Professor, Department of Neurosurgery, University of Washington, Seattle, WA*

Michael Tzermiadianos • *Orthopedic Surgeon, University of Crete, Crete, Greece*

Alexander R. Vaccaro, MD • *Professor of Orthopedic Surgery, Thomas Jefferson University and the Rothman Institute, Philadelphia, PA*

Douglas Wardlaw, ChM, FRCS(Ed) • *Consultant, and Orthopaedic and Spinal Surgeon, Grampion University Hospitals Trust–Woodend Hospital, Aberdeen, Scotland*

Anthony T. Yeung, MD • *Voluntary Associate Clinical Professor, Department of Orthopaedics, University of California San Diego School of Medicine, San Diego, CA, and Arizona Institute for Minimally Invasive Spine Care, Phoenix, AZ*

Hansen A. Yuan, MD • *Professor of Orthopedic and Neurological Surgery, State University of New York Upstate Medical University, Syracuse, NY*

Color Plates

Color plates 1–39 appear in an insert following p. 144.

Companion DVD

The companion DVD to this volume contains three video segments from the editor. The DVD can be played in any "set-top" DVD player attached to an NTSC standard definition television set. The DVD may also be viewed using any computer with a DVD drive and DVD compatible playback software such as Apple DVD Player, Windows Media Player 8 or higher (Win XP), PowerDVD, or WinDVD.

1

History of Surgical Management of Herniated Lumbar Discs From Cauterization to Arthroscopic and Endoscopic Spinal Surgery

Parviz Kambin, MD

INTRODUCTION

A review of the history of the surgical management of herniated lumbar discs as a common cause of sciatica is not complete without acknowledging the efforts of many investigators and researchers who have contributed to the understanding of the anatomy and origin of the sciatic nerve and lumbar intervertebral discs. In addition, the efforts of scientists and clinicians who have participated in developing the surgical management of disc herniation in the last seven decades should be recognized.

MANAGEMENT OF BACK AND LEG PAIN IN ANCIENT MEDICINE

Low back and sciatic pain has been one of the most common and disabling spinal disorders recorded in medical history. The role of the spinal canal's contents in extremity function is well demonstrated in the Dying Lioness (Fig. 1), a ca. 650 BC. Assyrian artwork.

In the writings of Hippocrates (460–370 BC) one can find references to the anatomy of the brain, brachial plexus, and sciatic nerve. In animal dissections it appears that he had difficulty in differentiating tendons from peripheral nerves. However, he attributed the development of paresthesia, weakness of the limbs, and fecal and urinary retention to spinal cord compression *(1)*.

On the basis of his animal and human dissections, Aristotle (384–322 BC) described vertebrate anatomy *(2)*. Erasistratus (250 BC) distinguished between the role of motor and sensory nerve fibers in his findings from cadaver dissections *(3)*.

Avicenna (980–1037 AD), a Persian physician and philosopher who was born in Bokhara, also wrote extensively on human anatomy and the peripheral nerves. However, his writings make no clear reference to sciatic pain. His text *Canon of Medicine* formed the cornerstone of medical practice for ensuing centuries. Avicenna condemned the reliance on mysticism and astrology in medicine *(4)*. His writings were translated into Latin and included in the medical curriculum of European universities. Avicenna's principal method of treating spinal disorders by traction and manipulation remains an accepted practice in many centers at present (Fig. 2), *(5,6)*. A calligraphy (Fig.3), dating

From: *Arthroscopic and Endoscopic Spinal Surgery: Text and Atlas: Second Edition*
Edited by: P. Kambin © Humana Press Inc., Totowa, NJ

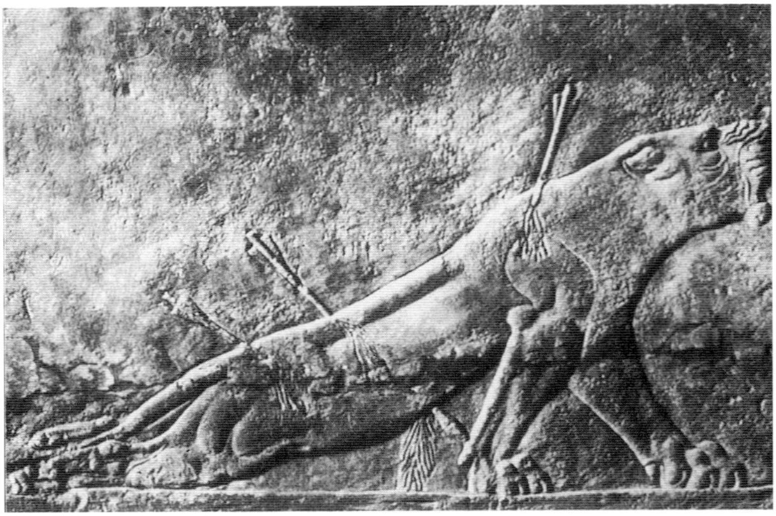

Fig. 1. The dying lioness, ca 650 BC. (Reprinted with permission from refs. *1* and *42*.)

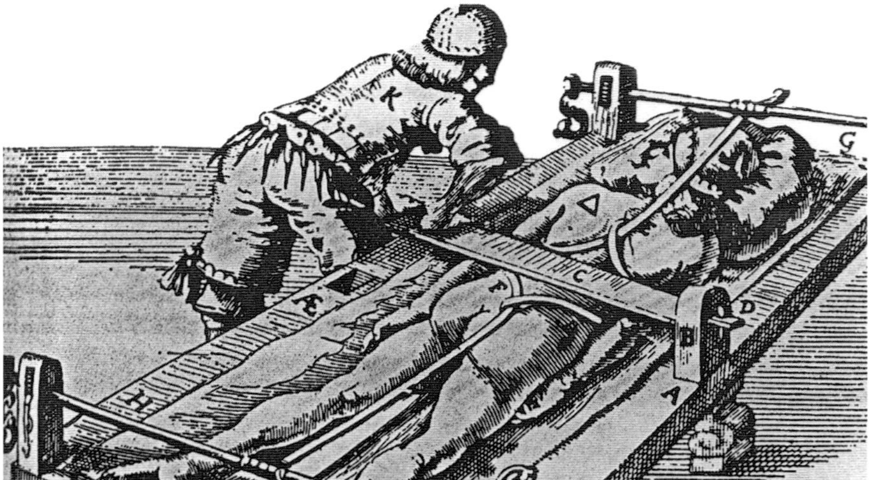

Fig. 2. Avicenna's a "Method of Treating Spinal Disorders by Traction and Manipulation." (Reprinted with permission from ref. *5*.)

to 1400 AD demonstrates the depth of curiosity of the times, and the information that was gathered from cadaver dissections. Their illustrations show the presence of 6 cervical, 12 thoracic, and 5 lumbar segments. The origins of the brachial plexus from the cervical segments, the intercostal nerves from the thoracic nerves, and the sciatic nerve

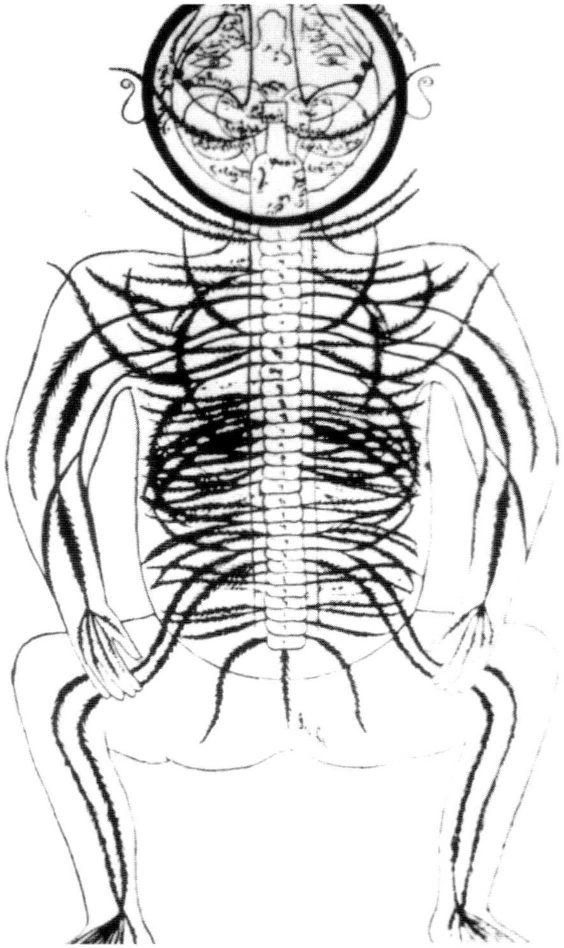

Fig. 3. Persian miniature from about 1400 AD. (Reprinted with permission refs. *1* and *42*.)

from the lumbar segments are described. In addition, the two divisions of the sciatic nerve as it extends into the lower extremities are shown.

In the ancient literature there is no reference to surgical management of sciatic pain. However, the use of traction, local cauterization (Fig. 4), cupping, bloodletting, and opioids was common in Arabic, Persian, and Islamic medicine and subsequently in European medicine. Acupuncture has been practiced in Chinese medicine for centuries.

RECOGNITION OF SCIATICA AND ITS ASSOCIATED SYMPTOMATOLOGY

Domenico Cotugno (Fig. 5), an eighteenth century Italian physician *(7)*, introduced the term sciatica into the medical vocabulary. Without having knowledge of the common etiology of this disabling spinal disorder, he described some of the signs and symptoms commonly seen in association with sciatic pain. Subsequently, Cotugno's disease as an entity gained acceptance in European medicine. Associated clinical findings of sciatica

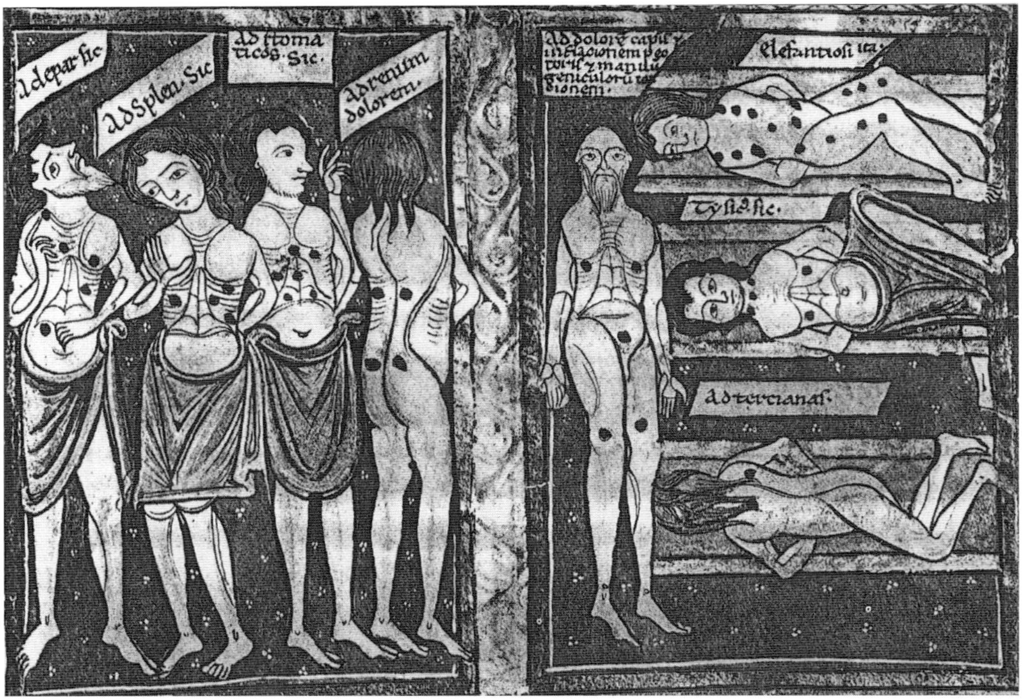

Fig. 4. Cauterization points for spine and other disorders. (Reprinted with permission from ref. *5*.)

were further detailed and documented by the writings of Putti *(8)*, Valleix *(9)*, Lasègue *(10)*, and Brissard *(11)* in later years.

IDENTIFICATION OF ANATOMICAL AND PATHOLOGICAL CONDITIONS OF THE INTERVERTEBRAL DISC

In the late nineteenth and early twentieth centuries, many investigators contributed to the understanding of intervertebral disc anatomy. In 1857, Virchow *(12)* published autopsy findings on the intervertebral disc in a patient who was injured and later expired. In 1868, von Luschka *(13)* described posterior disc protrusion in cadavers found in the course of routine autopsy procedures. Kocher *(14)* referred to his findings on intervertebral discs at L1-L2 in a patient who had a traumatic injury. Schmorl's *(15)* contribution to anatomical structures of the intervertebral disc also deserves recognition. In 1926, he reported on autopsy findings on 5000 intervertebral discs, 15 of which showed evidence of disc protrusion into the spinal canal. However, despite this significant anatomical finding, he had not yet established the causal connection between disc herniation and sciatic pain.

HISTORY OF SURGICAL MANAGEMENT OF SCIATICA

In the early twentieth century, laminectomy was being performed for the treatment of a variety of spinal disorders. In 1911, Goldthwait *(16)* described the management of a 39-yr-old male who underwent spinal manipulation, and then he developed paralysis in

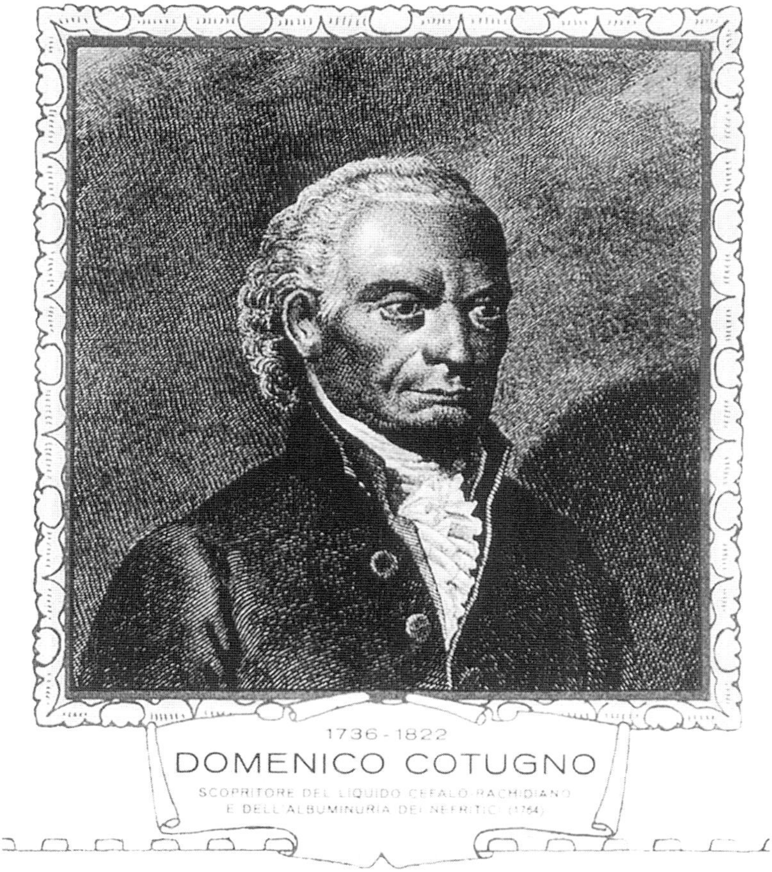

Fig. 5. Potrait of Domenico Cotugno.

the lower extremities. His conservative management included plaster immobilization and rest. The patient failed to show improvement, and 6 wk later he underwent extensive decompressive laminectomy, extending from L1 to S2. The patient responded to the operative procedure and showed improvement. Goldthwait *(16)* attributed the patient's neurological deficit to detachment and protrusion of the fibrotic annulus into the spinal canal, slippage of the articular processes, and abnormality of the transverse process of the lumbar segment.

In 1913, Dr. Elsberg of the New York Neurological Institute and Mt. Sinai Hospital, reported on his findings on 60 consecutive laminectomies. However, he did not believe disc pathology was responsible for the presenting symptomatology in any of the patients described *(17)*. In 1928, in a paper entitled a "Extradural Spinal Tumors, Primary, Seconary, Metastisis," Dr. Elsberg attributed compression of the cauda equina to the presence of cartilaginous tumors (chondromas) *(18)*.

In 1927, Putti *(8)* reported on one of his patients who underwent laminectomy and facetectomy to decompress the L5 and S1 nerve roots and relieve sciatic pain. He further elaborated on the contribution of Sicard, who performed laminectomy from L3 to the sacrum to provide relief from sciatic pain.

Other investigators, including Stookey in 1928 *(19)* and Bucy in 1930 *(20)*, also reported on the removal of chondroma-type tumors from the intervertebral discs that were causing pressure on the neural structures. Alajouanine, a neurologist residing in Paris, reported on two patients who underwent laminectomy and discectomy in 1928 *(21,22)*. A brief translation of his article is as follows:

It is a very specific type of radiculomedullary compression that we call "a fibrocartilaginous nodule of the posterior aspect of the intervertebral discs." This compression is manifested by radicular signs, more rarely medullary, most often unilateral. Surgical ablation, although sometimes laborious, like all premedullary tumors, usually results in the rapid regression of compressive disorders. Their first presentation was made in 1928 to the Surgical Society of a unilateral cauda equina syndrome due to a curious formation related to an intervertebral disc (ref. 2: Bull et Mem de la Soc nat de chir 12 Oct 1928, 54: 1452). *Now we have seen a second case, absolutely identical to the first.*

Case 1. Male, 37 years old, complained of left lumbosacral pain with root, sensory and sphincter problems for 4 years. The flow of Lipiodol was blocked below L5-S1. Ablation of fibrocartilaginous nodule from L5-S1 intervertebral disc. Rapid and complete cure.

Case 2. Female, 20 years old, had a 3-year history of pain in the left leg and while walking. There was foot drop, absence of achilles and medial plantar reflexes. Anesthesia of L4-L5 and all sacral roots. Positive Lipiodol test at L3-L4. On July 18, 1929, disc protrusion, transdural approach, removal of fibrocartilaginous nodule in comparison to the first case. Partial recovery of the foot drop but not the ankle reflex. Notes probable compression of nerve roots by rongeurs in the course of laminectomy.

These nodules are neither tumors, chondromas nor fibrochondromas and are distinctly different from chordomas. Basically, they are always related to the intervertebral disc. We have shown that these curious formations should be considered to result from herniation of the central pulp of the disc across the latter, the hernia produced either by trauma or by pathological changes in the disc; in addition, the effects of these two causes can be combined.

The use of Lipiodol is indispensable, not only with radiography but also with fluoroscopy. The prognosis depends upon surgical treatment which is midline through the dura. If the protrusion is very lateral, the dura mater should be incised laterally. There is a problem with retraction of the spinal cord in the neck and thorax, particularly evident when the nodule is calcified and embedded in the cord. Such nodules should be suspected in refractory lumbalgia and sciatica.

In 1931, Crouzon et al. (23) gave credit to the contribution of Alajouanine and further detailed and described the clinical outcome of patients who underwent laminectomy and discectomy. A translation of their publication is as follows.

This is a new example of a fibrocartilaginous nodule on the posterior aspect of the intervertebral disc, producing a very specific type of root compression that one of us, with Alajouanine, has called attention to in a recent report. [Alajouanine T, Petit-Dutaillis D. Le nodule fibrocartilageneux de la face posterieure des disques intervertebraux. Presse Medicale nos. 98 and 102 of 6 and 20 September 1930]. The favorable results obtained by surgical intervention make it possible to emphasize once more its clinical and therapeutic value in such a disorder.

[There follows a case history, summarized here.]

A brickmaker, 44 years old, was hospitalized by Dr. Crouzon for refractory sciatica that had kept him out of all work for 6 months. There was no special precipitating factor, but there was a history of an acute injury to the lumbar region 7 years earlier when he fell 4 meters onto his back and kidneys. After severe pain immobilized him for some days, he was able to go back to work, but with intermittent episodes of "lumbago" making him rest for 3 to 4 days. Only after 7 years did he begin to have (In June 1930) pains in the left leg that became increasingly severe and frequent. Examination on 20 February 1931 showed areas of pain in the lumbar region, calf and left heel. These were aggravated by the slightest movement, cough or strain. When he stood, his weight was placed on the intact right extremity. There was an antalgic spasm of the lumbar muscles, but hypotonia of the quadriceps and calf on the left side. His body was held forward when he walked with obvious pain. The spine was held flexed forward and to one side. There was some atrophy of the left thigh and calf, the latter measuring 3 cm less than the healthy calf. There was a slight decrease in strength of flexion and extension of the foot on the left side. Knee reflexes were equal, but the achilles and medial plantar reflexes were absent on the left. Sensory exam showed sharp pain on pressure all along the left sciatic nerve and sharp pain on Lasègue's maneuver.

There was pain on pressure and percussion over the spinous processes of L4 and L5. The sensory exam of the plantar aspect of the foot was consistent with anesthesia for all modalities on the plantar aspect of the foot and posterior aspect of the left calf, extending 5 cm onto the posterior of the thigh. There was also a band of sensory loss on the lateral aspect of the foot and adjacent leg, ascribed to L5, S1 and S2. There was some sphincter dysfunction with pain on defecation and difficulty in urination. Lumbar puncture on February 25, 1931 showed normal fluid and normal pressure, slight dissociation between albumin and cells (40 g albumin and 2 cells). Wasserman tests of blood and CSF were negative. X-rays showed some narrowing at L4-L5. A Lipiodol study showed temporary blockage at L4-L5 under the fluoroscope, but by the time the patient reached the radiography room, the oil had all fallen to the bottom. The temporary blockage was pronounced enough to induce Dr. Alajouanine to operate on the patient on 7 March 1931. Laminectomy of L3-L5 showed ossification of the ligamentum flavum at L4-L5; the dura was indented, and the ligament was removed. The dura was opened to show displacement of the nerve roots by a whitish nodule compressing the left L5 root. The root was compressed to a thread at the level of the intervertebral foramen, as if it had been partially destroyed by stretching. In order to free it without further damage, the dura was cut transversely. This made it possible to displace the root of L5 to the left and the rest of the roots to the right. The dura was incised anteriorly over the nodule, and a specially designed spatula was used to hold the root while the fibrocartilaginous nodule was removed. Because of the transverse cut in the dura, no attempt was made to suture it, and the wound was closed in layers with catgut and without drainage.

The postoperative course was uneventful; sutures were removed on Day 9. The outcome of surgery was very good and recovery was rapid. The day after surgery the patient said the left leg no longer hurt, and re-examination showed a return of sensation in the areas of L5, S1 and S2. He could now feel the bedsheets on his foot. Fifteen days after surgery he had no complaints and could get out of bed; 25 days after surgery he stood straight and walked normally without pain or fatigue.

Examination on April 25, 7 weeks after surgery, showed normal posture, with weight equally distributed on the two legs. Flexion and extension of the left foot were normal. Mild hypotonia persisted in the left thigh as did slight atrophy of the calf and thigh on the left. The achilles and medial plantar reflexes were still absent. There was no pain on pressure over the course of the left sciatic nerve. There was no pain on straight-leg raising. Objective examination of sensation showed a slight decrease in tactile sensation on the lateral border of the left foot. The sphincter problems had resolved, and the patient's general health was excellent.

Histological study of the specimen by Dr. I. Bertrand showed fibrocartilaginous tissue with abundant interstitial stroma containing amorphous tissue with some collagen bundles. There were only a few cells, but those seen resembled cartilage cells. An examination for Virchow's physaliferous cells was negative. There were few vessels, and in some places the absence of staining indicated some necrosis.

This case should be added to similar cases published in France by Alajouanine and Petit-Dutaillis, by Robineau and, in the foreign press, by Adson, Stookey, then Bucy and P. Bailey, and, very recently, by Katzenborn, making a total of 23 operated cases. The new case reported appears to prove that this is not a very rare condition and that the numbers will soon increase now that attention has been directed to these facts.

In view of this new case, it seems appropriate to emphasize certain points: the role of trauma is beyond doubt, even though in this case it may be dismissed, for in this case the injury occurred 7 years previously. Emphasis is placed on the occasionally long latent period before symptoms become manifest. Some temporary lumbar symptoms of an apparently common type may occur in this period, as if the lesion, only produced by the initial trauma, gradually becomes more pronounced, undoubtedly affected by repeated strains in those whose occupations are strenuous. There is a notable incidence of unilateral symptoms. The lumbar region is not the only site of pathological disc changes; the first cases dealt with those in the neck. Although Stookey initially thought these fibrocartilaginous lesions were exclusively cervical, it is clear that they may occur elsewhere, although they do appear to be rare in the thoracic region.

In addition to clinical signs and symptoms, compression is also manifested by a dissociation between albumin and cells and by a blockage of Lipiodol. The blockage of the oil may be quite temporary and be seen only on fluoroscopy. For this reason the authors emphasize the need for this diagnostic procedure as well as radiography. The absence of the disc in radiograms was similar to that in long-standing Pott's disease. However, it should be noted that there is no sign of herniation into the vertebral bodies. It seems likely that in compression phenomena of traumatic origin the compression, or even absence, of the disc might promote the development of fibrocartilaginous nodule formation.

The histological study also shows that these nodules should not be considered to be tumors (neoplasms) as has been thought to be the case by those authors who called them fibrochondromas, ecchondromas or even chondromas of the disc. These structures are an integral part of the intervertebral disc with no neoplastic characteristics, but should be considered protrusions of the disc or of the nucleus pulposus across a break in the posterior part of the intervertebral disc into the spinal canal. This interpretation (Schmorl, Andrae) seems the only logical one.

It is more painstaking to surgically remove these pathological structures than other intraspinal tumors. In the region of the cauda equina the compressed roots must be freed very gently and very slowly. Even if the size of the nodule is small, its consistency is very hard and it exerts a very firm compression. In our case the left root at L5 had already been heavily compressed and stretched. Sometimes the root may be in contact with the lamina, and care must be taken in removing the lamina to avoid injuring the root.

Dandy *(24)* independently reported on the removal of a detached fragment of cartilaginous tissue from the intervertebral disc for treatment of sciatic pain.

Mixter and Barr are credited for establishing a clear causal connection between the herniated disc and sciatica. They provided a detailed description of disc herniation and popularized laminectomy and discectomy for surgical management of herniated lumbar discs *(25)*.

Between the 1930s and 1950s, orthopedic and neurological surgeons followed the traditional teaching of Mixter and Barr that consisted of wide exposure, bilateral dissection of the paraspinal muscles, laminectomy, and extensive epidural hemostasis and coagulation in the course of extraction of herniated disc fragments.

The traditional surgery described by Mixter and Barr was later modified and became less invasive with the introduction of the microscope to the surgical field by Yasargil, a Turkish surgeon, in 1972 *(26,27)*. This concept was further advanced by other investigators *(28)*.

EMERGENCE OF THE MINIMALISTS' CONCEPT

Annular Fenestration and Reduction of Hydrostatic Pressure in the Intervertebral Disc

The earliest recorded departure from the concept of traditional laminectomy and discectomy in the treatment of a herniated lumbar disc is found in an article published by Hult *(29)* in 1950, in which he advocated an anterior retroperitoneal annular fenestration for decompression of herniated lumbar discs. The relationship between hydrostatic pressure of the intervertebral disc and the size of the annular bulge and protrusion has been a subject of interest to many investigators. Virgen *(30)* demonstrated that the height of the intervertebral disc is decreased and the annulus bulged outward when intervertebral discs were subjected to axial loading. Brown et al. *(31)* showed that the annular bulge was increased on the side on which the spine was flexed and the annulus was flattened on the opposite side. Nachemson *(32,33)* also demonstrated bulging of the annulus associated with increased intradiscal pressure under load, particularly in the sitting position and with forward bending and lifting. Kambin and colleagues reported on their in vivo evaluation of hydrostatic pressure in the intervertebral disc prior to and following annular fenestration via a 4.9-mm-outer diameter (od) trephine and partial nuclear resection. A considerable reduction of intradiscal pressure was observed when patients were instructed to extend and rotate the trunk following annular venting *(34,35)*. However, long-term patency of the annular fenestration remains highly questionable. Although Sakamoto et al. *(36)* showed that the reduction of intradiscal hydrostatic pressure may be maintained up to 21 mo postoperatively, Hampton et al. *(37)* reported healing and closure of the surgically created defect in the annulus between 3 and 12 wk after surgery. This phenomenon was also confirmed in the my own experience when a repeated surgery was required a few months following the original percutaneous arthroscopic discectomy. It was found that the original site of annular fenestration was closed with scar tissue.

Concept of Nuclear Mass Reduction

Lyman Smith should be recognized as a champion of the minimally invasive movement *(38)*. Learning from the experience of Lewis Thomas in rabbits *(39)*, he introduced the concept of dissolving the nucleus pulposus by intradiscal injection of chymopapain. The simplicity of the procedure and the fact that the operative technique did not violate the content of the spinal canal attracted the attention of many orthopaedic and neurological surgeons, both in the United States and abroad. This was followed by many presentations, hands-on seminars, and publications in the ensuing years.

Encouraged by previously reported satisfactory outcomes of chemonucleolysis, in the early 1970s, following institutional approval, Kambin (Fig. 6) initiated a feasibility study on the efficacy of mechanical nuclear debulking for the treatment of herniated lumbar discs via a Craig cannula inserted into the intervertebral disc dorsolaterally *(40,41)*.

Clinical research conducted by my colleagues and I in the ensuing years was directed toward establishing the effect of central nucleotomy on the size of the bulge or herniation. In 1973, at The Graduate Hospital of Philadelphia, we combined the central nucleotomy via a Craig biopsy cannula with laminectomy in patients who demonstrated signs, symptoms, and imaging evidence of disc herniation (Fig. 7) *(35)*. In 1973, a 60-yr-old male with myelographic and clinical evidence of disc herniation at L3-L4 and

DOCTORS HOSPITAL
1700 VINE STREET, PHILADELPHIA, PA. 19103

OFFICERS
William T. Lemmon, M. D.
President
Marcel S. Sussman, M. D.
Vice-President
Thomas B. Mervine, M. D.
Secretary
J. G. Manley, M. D.
Treasurer

MEMBERS OF
BOARD OF GOVERNORS
John W. Bransfield, M. D.
B. H. K. Miller, M. D.
J. Wallace Davis, M. D.
William DeCherney, M. D.
William A. Tomasco, M. D.
Armando Goracci, M. D.
Marvin Krane, M. D.
Cyril L. Velkoff, M. D.
Luis Vera, M. D.

ADMINISTRATOR
Estelle P. Hoag

April 15, 1969

Parviz Kambin, M.D.
1930 Chestnut Street
Philadelphia, Pennsylvania 19103

Dear Dr. Kambin:

Per your request, please be advised that you may use standard Craig instrumentation for decompression of intervertebral disc on patients who give proper consent for this procedure.

Sincerely,

William T. Lemmon, M.D.
President
Board of Governors

WTL:mpw

Fig. 6. Authorization by Board of Governors of Doctors Hospital permitting use of Craig cannula for nucleotomy in management of disc herniation.

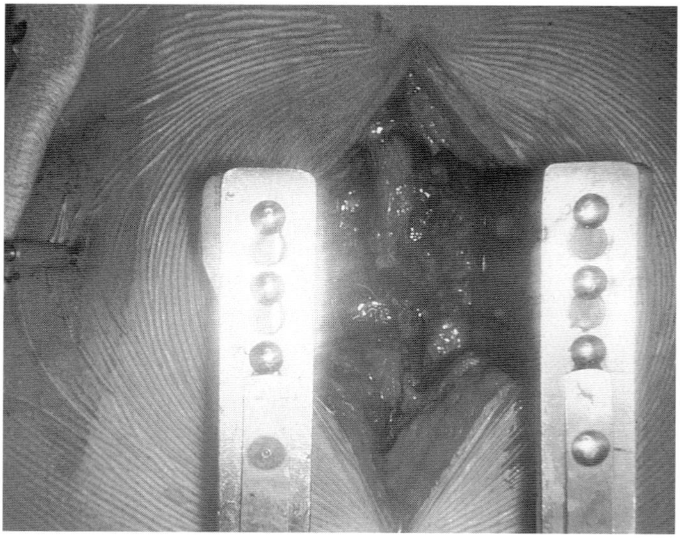

Fig. 7. Intraoperative photo demonstrating effect of nucleotomy via a Craig cannula on contour and geometry of herniated disc, which was visualized through open laminatomy.

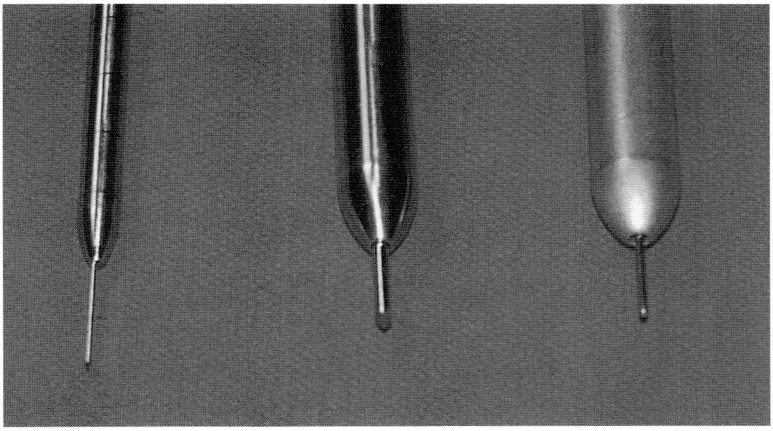

Fig. 8. Kambin cannulated spinal obturators. Blunt-end cannulated obturators for precise positioning of the instruments as shown.

L4-L5 underwent open laminectomy at both levels. The larger disc herniation at L3-L4 was removed through the laminectomy exposure. However, the smaller protrusion at L4-L5 was decompressed through the posterolaterally introduced Craig cannula. The patient had a satisfactory outcome with no complications.

In February 1974, a 52-yr-old male presented with right sciatica and was diagnosed with herniated discs at L3-L4 and L4-L5. This patient underwent a combined operative procedure. The herniated disc at L4-L5 was removed through the laminectomy site; however, the L3-L4 intervertebral disc was decompressed through the cannula that had been inserted dorsolaterally.

In April 1974, a 43-yr-old female with unremitting sciatic pain and myographic evidence of disc herniation at L4-L5 underwent percutaneous nucleotomy via a Craig cannula. This patient failed to respond to the nucleotomy procedure and subsequently required a laminectomy when a large disc herniation at the index level was identified and excised.

In June 1974, a similar combined operation was performed on a 52-yr-old male with clinical and myographic evidence of a large disc herniation at L5-S1 and a smaller protrusion at L4-L5. The L5-S1 herniation was excised through the laminectomy site, and the L4-L5 intervertebral disc was decompressed via a mechanical nucleotomy technique through the inserted cannula. Although in the ensuing years a number of patients underwent a simple mechanical nucleotomy via the inserted cannula and the combined procedure, we were unable to demonstrate an appreciable reduction in the size or shape of the herniation following a simple central nucleotomy. Therefore, our efforts were then directed toward the development of instruments and surgical techniques that would provide better access to posterolaterally dislodged disc fragments via a posterolateral approach. Newly designed instruments were developed that included a cannulated obturator (Fig. 8) for precise positioning of instruments and a 6.5-mm-od cannula that accommodated an upbiting forceps. This was followed by development of a flexible-tip forceps and a deflecting tube that permitted dorsal angulation of the inserted forceps and aided in evacuation of posterior nuclear tissue. In 1981, under the auspices of the Human Subjects Committee of The Graduate Hospital (Fig. 9), I initiated a series of preliminary

THE GRADUATE HOSPITAL
One Graduate Plaza, Philadelphia, Pa 19146 • (215) 893-2000

July 13, 1981

Dr. Parviz Kambin
Orthopaedic Surgery
2027 Pine Street
Philadelphia, Pa. 19103

Dear Doctor Kambin:

The Human Subjects Committee of the Graduate Hospital met on May 21, 1961 and approved your project/protocol entitled, "Per Cutaneous Lateral Diskectomy". The Committee also approved the consent form as drafted.

You are hereby authorized to initiate the aforementioned study in accordance with the terms and conditions as outlined in the protocol.

Sincerely yours,

Marta Lee Bussard

(Miss) Marta Lee Bussard
Coordinator, Human Subjects Committee
Office of Research Administration

MLB

Fig. 9. Permission from Human Subjects Committee of The Graduate Hospital for experimental use of 6.4-mm-od cannula, using upbiting and flexible-tip forceps in percutaneous disc surgery.

investigations on the feasibility of the use of a 6.4-mm-od cannula using upbiting and flexible-tip forceps (Figs. 10 and 11) *(34,35,40–43)*.

In 1975, Hijikata (Fig. 12) from the Toden Hospital in Japan independently experimented with mechanical nucleotomy via a 2.6-mm-od cannula that was inserted into the center of the intervertebral disc via a posterolateral access. He reported a satisfactory postoperative outcome in 64% of patients *(44)*. Following Hijikata's experience, Schreiber and Suezawa developed a series of cannulas that were telescoped one over the other and placed in the center of the intervertebral disc via a posterolateral access. The larger cannulas with a 7 to 8-mm internal diameter (id) permitted the insertion of larger forceps and more rapid evacuation of nuclear tissue *(45)*. In 1981, in the United States, Blum et al. *(46)* experimented with Hijikata's nucleotomy technique and reported their findings before the International Society of the Lumbar Spine. In 1983, Hoppenfield *(47)* also used a posterolateral approach and manual instruments for nucleotomy. Friedman and Jacobson experimented with a far lateral approach to access the lumbar intervertebral disc. These investigators passed a no. 40 French chest tube through an incision over the iliac crest and directed it toward the intervertebral disc at the index level. After annulotomy the disc fragments were evacuated with manual forceps *(48)*. In 1985, Onick promoted the concept of central nucleotomy via a mechanical tool called a nucleotomy *(49)*. The small caliber of the instruments and the simplicity of the operative procedure contributed to the popularity of the operative technique in the ensuing years (Fig. 13).

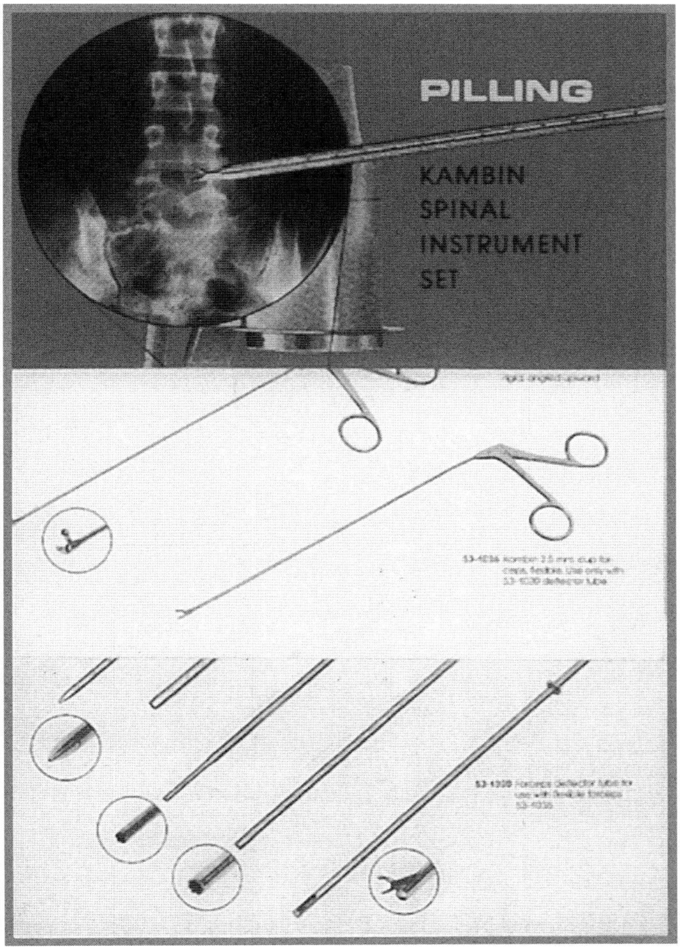

Fig. 10. Original instruments developed in early 1980s for percutaneous discectomy under X-ray control.

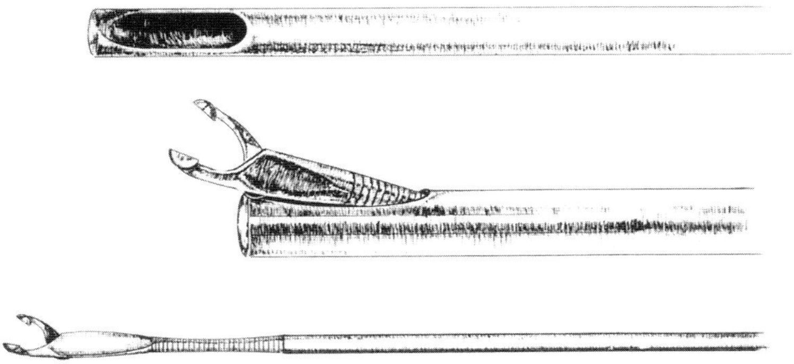

Fig. 11. Deflecting tube and flexible-tip forceps for access and removal of posteriorly lodged disc herniation and entry to L5-S1 intervertebral disc.

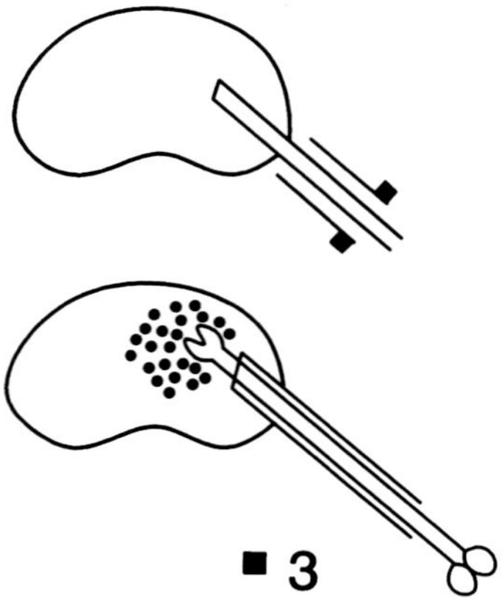

Fig. 12. Illustration from article by Hijikata showing the principle of central nucleotomy in 1975.

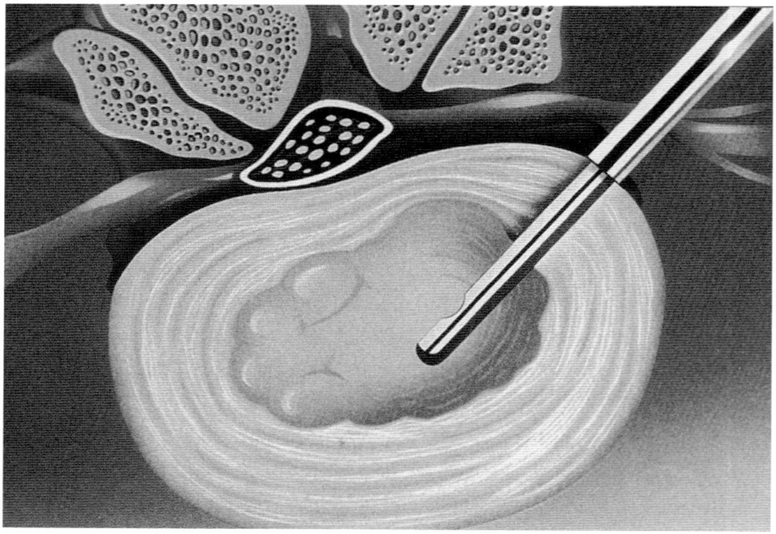

Fig. 13. Illustration demonstrating the use of nucleotome in the treatment of disc herniation.

The introduction of laser light into the surgical armamentarium opened another front in the management of lumbar disc herniation *(35–50)*. The small caliber and relative flexibility of the laser fibers was a source of encouragement and appeared to be suitable for nuclear vaporization. A variety of laser lights were introduced into the marketplace and then used by many investigators. In January 1990, with the permission of the Federal Drug Administration and Internal Review Board of The Graduate Hospital, I initiated a clinical study of the feasibility of vaporizing disc fragments with laser light under arthroscopic illumination and magnification *(51)*. It was found that the wide arc of deflection of the laser fibers and concern about injury to neural structures prevented adequate decompression and lysis of posterior herniated disc fragments.

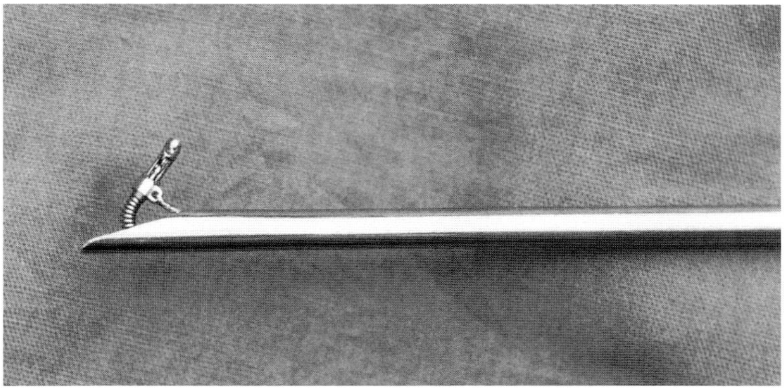

Fig. 14. Articulating suction forceps used for intradiscal access to non-migrated sequestrated disc herniation.

Striving Toward Access and Retrieval of Posterior Herniated Disc Fragments Via an Intradiscal Approach

While the advantages and safety of a small-caliber nucleotome and laser fibers for nuclear decompression were being promoted and debated in the late 1980s, my colleagues and I continued to utilize the standard 6.4-mm-od cannula for discectomy. Although our deflecting tube and flexible-tip forceps (Fig. 11) permitted posterior nucleotomy, we were unable to adequately access and retrieve subligamentous or nondisplaced extraligamentous herniations.

After a series of cadaver studies, it was determined that a high negative atmospheric pressure could be introduced into a contained intervertebral disc without any inadvertent complications. Subsequently, we introduced this technique into our clinical practice in an attempt to dislodge the herniated disc fragments and move them into the path of the inserted cannula *(34,40,41)*. However, this technique was not always successful and was therefore later abandoned. An articulating forceps (Fig. 14) was introduced whose tip deflected far enough to access posterior and posterolateral herniated disc fragments intradiscally and to decompress directly the nerve roots *(42,43,52)*.

IDENTIFICATION OF A SAFE ZONE ADJACENT TO NERVE ROOTS FOR ANCHORING OF INSTRUMENTS

Although posterolateral access to the intervertebral disc was used for biopsy of vertebral bodies *(53–55)*, discography, chemonucleolysis *(38)*, and automated nucleotomy *(49)*, the site of lodging of instruments and annular window on the annulus had not been clearly defined. The close proximity of major neurovascular structures to the posterolaterally inserted instruments necessitated the identification of a safe zone on the posterolateral surface of the annulus fibrosus for anchoring cannulas with larger diameters. After a series of cadaver dissections at The Graduate Hospital and the Anatomy Laboratory of the Hospital of the University of Pennsylvania, a triangular safe zone on the posterolateral annulus, between the traversing and exiting nerve roots, was identified. Subsequently, we positioned needles in and around the safe zone and radiographic studies were conducted. These allowed us to identify the radiographic

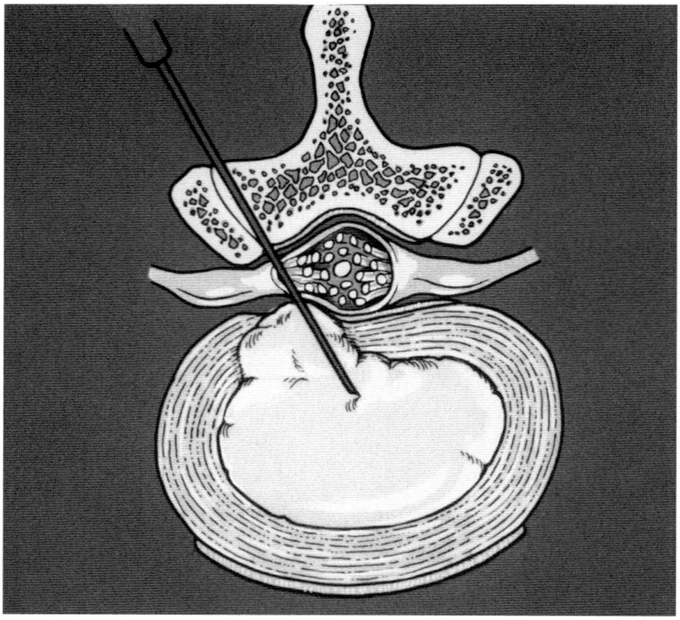

Fig. 15. Illustration demonstrating complications that may become associated with localization of needle in the center of the disc at the onset of percutaneous spine surgery. Note that the needle may pass through the ligamentum flavum dora and enter the intervertebral disc with a final satisfactory radiographic appearance in the anteropasterior and lateral projection.

landmarks of the safe zone in both the anteroposterior and lateral projections. Therefore, we began to emphasize the importance of localization of the tip of the inserted needle on the annulus at the onset of the operative procedure rather than in the center of the intervertebral disc (Fig. 15).

The triangular working zone is bordered anteriorly by the exiting root, inferiorly by the proximal plate of the lower lumbar segment, and medially by the traversing root and the dural sac. The floor of the triangular working zone is occupied by the intervertebral disc, the vertebral plate, and the posterior boundary of the adjacent vertebra (Fig. 16 A,B) *(42,43,56,57)*. This region is covered by loosely woven adipose tissue and, at times, superficial veins, which are readily observed by arthroscopic or endoscopic examination. Mirkovik and Schwartz *(58)* independently measured the dimensions of the triangular working zone and have confirmed that cannulas with larger diameters can be safely inserted between the traversing and exiting roots in the course of arthroscopic or endoscopic spinal surgery.

The description of the radiographic landmarks of the triangular working zone made it possible to lodge the instruments precisely and to monitor them fluoroscopically both anteroposteriorly and laterally. It was stipulated that a midpedicular positioning of the instruments in the anteroposterior projection is suitable for intradiscal subligamentous or intracanalicular access to the contents of the spinal canal. Lateral pedicular line positioning in the anteroposterior projection may be used for evacuation of an extraforaminal herniation *(42,43)*.

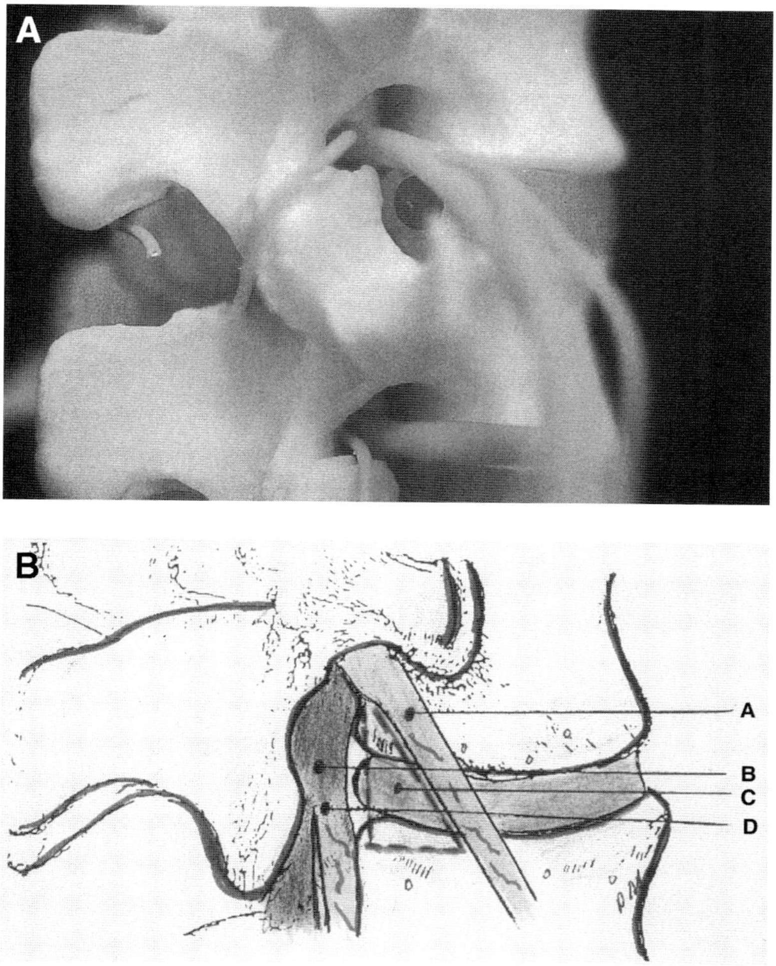

Fig. 16. **(A)** Copy of photo of triangular working zone which was published in 1988. **(B)** Illustration showing the boundaries of the triangular working zone: A, the exiting root; B, dural sac; C, intervertebral disc; D, traversing root.

History of Development of Larger-Diameter Cannulas

The oldest and most commonly used cannulas are the ones described by Ottolenghi *(54)* and Craig *(53)* that were commonly used for vertebral body biopsy. Hijikata originally suggested the use of a 2.6-mm-od cannula *(44)*. However, he later modified his technique and used larger-diameter cannulas.

Onik developed an automated nucleotome (Fig. 13) for mechanical resection of nuclear tissue *(49)*. The instrument was designed along the lines of Hijikata's instruments. At this stage of development, emphasis was placed on access and retrieval of nuclear tissue, rather than removal of herniated disc fragments and direct decompression of the nerve roots. Introduction of a large-diameter cannula in the clinical setting lead to further investigation and description of the triangular working zone on the posterolateral annulus.

My colleagues and I originally used a Craig cannula for mechanical nucleotomy. However, in the early 1980s, we began to use cannulas with a larger diameter (6.4-mm od) *(40)*. These provided a 5-mm inner working space. In addition, we introduced the concept of using a blunt-tipped cannulated obturator for precise positioning of the instruments on the annulus (Fig. 8).

We later introduced the concept of the unilateral biportal approach and oval cannulas (5×8 and 5×10 mm id) *(59–64)*, (Fig. 17 A,B) that were designed to fit within the triangular working zone. The height of the intervertebral disc in the triangular working zone prevents the insertion of larger cylindrical-shaped cannulas into the intravertebral disc without the need for undue resection of the vertebral plates and part of the vertebral bodies of the adjacent segments. Schreiber et al. *(45)* and Shepperd *(65)* have continued to use gradually dilating, telescopic cannulas up to 10 mm in diameter to enter the intervertebral disc via a posterolateral access. In our experience, overstretching of the nerve roots by the larger cannulas was associated with postoperative dysesthesia, which led to the development of oval-shaped cannulas that proved safe in our clinical practice.

As early as 1991, we used 10- to 23-mm-id cannulas for the endoscopic interlaminar approach and intracanalicular surgery *(62,63,66)* (Fig. 18A,B) and arthroscopic foraminal decompression *(60,79)* (Fig. 18C). A modified version of this technology recently has been marketed *(67)*.

Arthroscopic and Endoscopic Visualization and Birth of the Term Minimally Invasive Spinal Surgery

Bozzini, an obstetrician from Frankfurt, is credited with introducing the concept of visualizing internal organs in 1807 (Fig. 19), *(68)*. His work was originally introduced to a faculty in Vienna and was rejected. He was criticized and censored for having unreasonable curiosity. However, Bozzini's noble idea continued to flourish, and many investigators further developed, enhanced, and successfully utilized endoscopes for the diagnosis and treatment of a variety of medical disorders *(69)*.

Use of the scope for diagnosis of spinal abnormalities dates back to 1931, when Burman from the Hospital for Joint Diseases in New York City described his experience with the use of an endoscope for visualization of intracanalicular pathologies of the cauda equina in cadaver specimens. However, owing to the size of the instruments, he was unable to inspect the intrathecal structures *(70)*.

In 1938, Pool from Columbia-Presbyterian Hospital in New York developed a myeloscope for intra thecal inspection of normal and abnormal structures *(71,72)*. In recent years, other investigators have utilized rigid and flexible fiberoptics for visualization of the epidural and subarachnoid spaces *(73,74)*. However, in our experience, it is difficult to advance flexible fiberoptics, particularly on the ventral surface of the dura. Invariably, close contact with and adhesions between the ventral dura and the posterior longitudinal ligament prevent clear visualization and advancement of the fibers and may result in a dural tear.

Hausmann and Forst *(75)* used an arthroscope to inspect the contents of the intervertebral disc following open laminectomy and discectomy. Schreiber et al. *(45)* used an arthroscope via a second portal that was inserted into the intervertebral disc dorsolaterally from the opposite side in order to inspect and resect nuclear tissue under direct visualization.

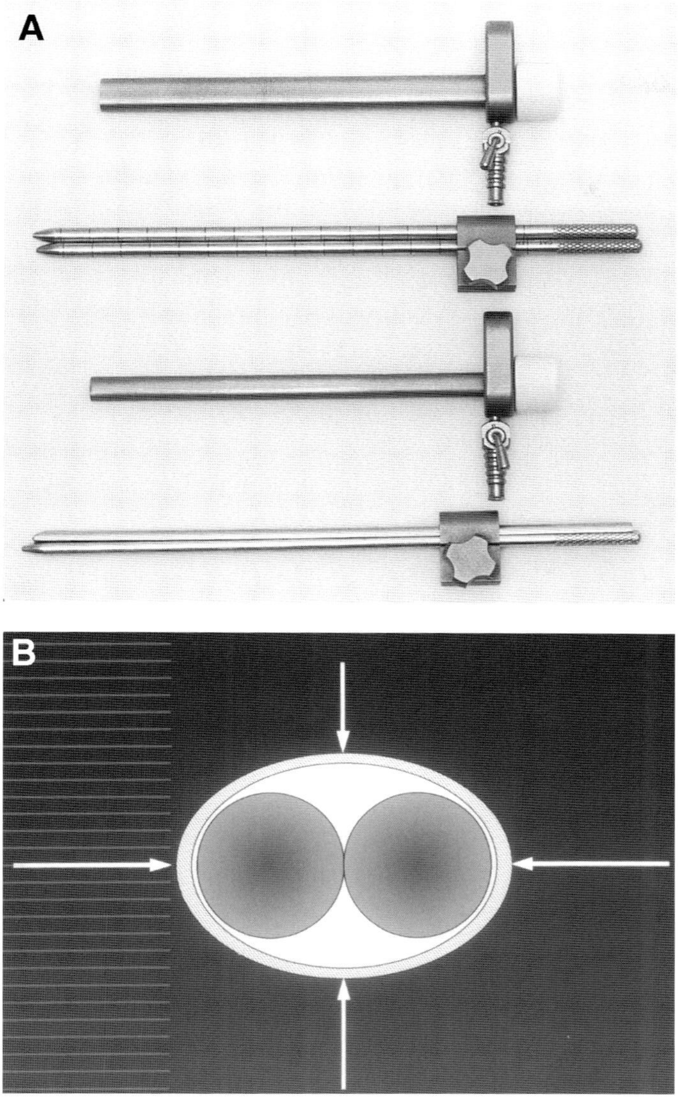

Fig. 17. **(A)** From top: 5 × 10 mm id oval cannula; two cannulated obturators are passed through the appropriate jig in preparation of insertion of a 5 × 10 mm oval cannula; and a 5 × 8 mm oval cannula, a cannulated obturator, and a half-moon cannula are passed through the lumen of the appropriate jig in preparation of insertion of a 5 × 8 mm oval cannula. **(B)** Illustration demonstrating cross section of two cannulated obturators. which permits their use together prior to insertion of an oval cannula.

A meaningful use of arthroscopes and endoscopes in the field of spinal surgery was not realized until 1988, when the anatomical and radiographic appearance of the posterolateral annulus was described for safe positioning of instruments adjacent to the spinal canal *(42,56)*. Subsequently, the arthroscopic appearance of intradiscal, periannular, and neural structures was demonstrated *(42,43)*. In the mid- and late 1980s, during our investigational phase, when our efforts were being directed toward intradiscal

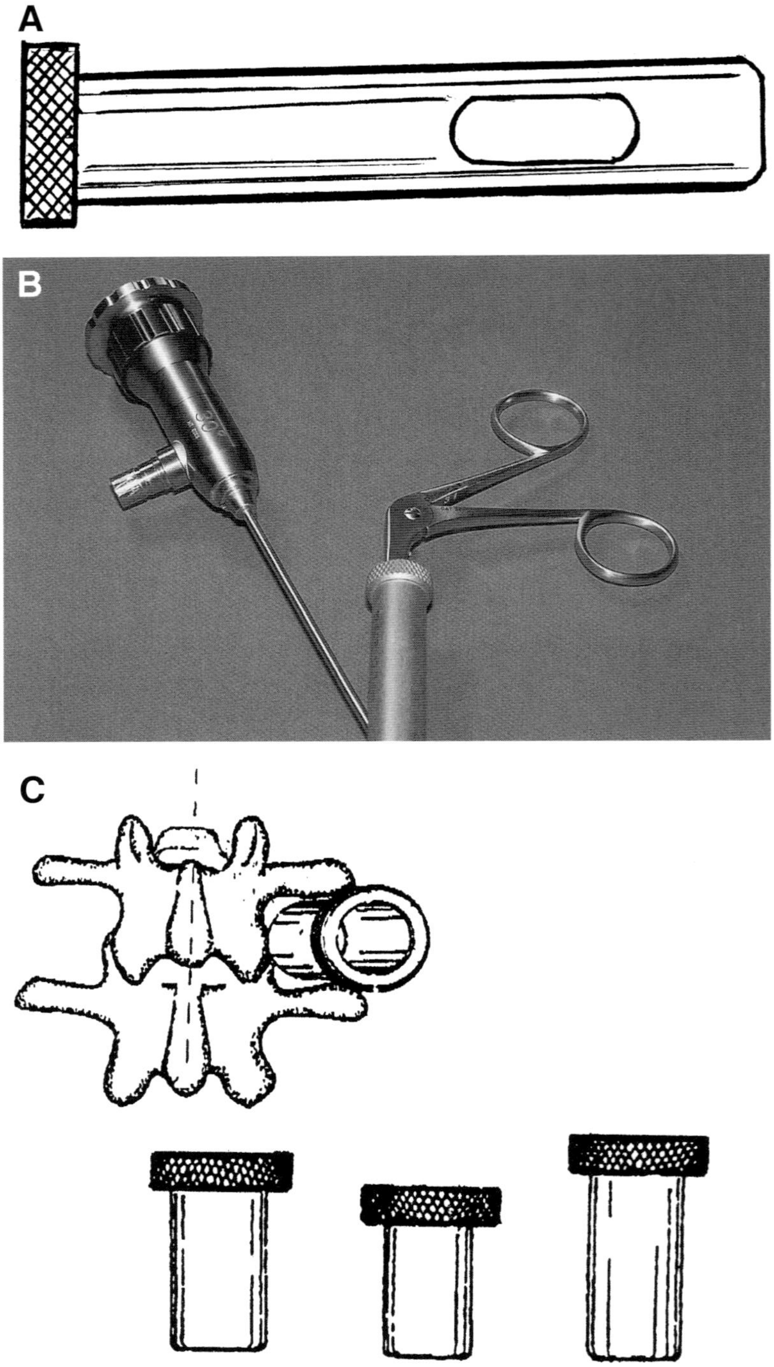

Fig. 18. **(A)** Illustration of the 10-mm-id cannula with side window used for translaminar access to the spinal canal for the removal of sequestrated disc herniation under endoscopic control; **(B)** demonstration of the use of scope through the side window and the forceps through the cannula for visualization and extraction of disc herniations from the spinal canal; **(C)** illustration of short cannulas which were used for foraminal decompression under arthroscopic control.

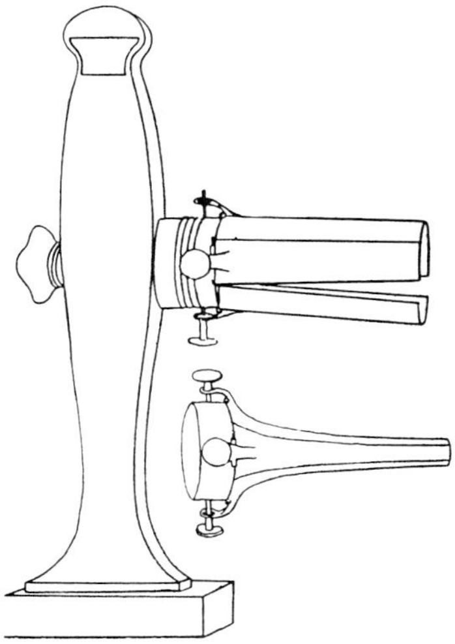

Fig. 19. Illustration of Bozzini's endoscope for visualization of internal organs.

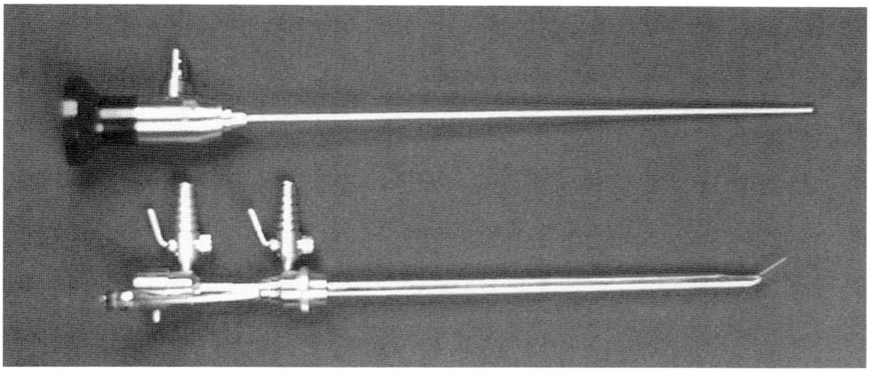

Fig. 20. Photo of our original working-channel arthroscope that permitted manipulation and angulation of inserted instruments within intervertebral disc.

access and retrieval of herniated disc fragments, with the cooperation of industry (Dyonics, Andover, MA), we developed a working channel arthroscope that provided ample space for manipulation and angulation of instruments inserted within the intervertebral disc space (Fig. 20). However, an inability to establish adequate fluid irrigation within the intravertebral disc, poor visualization, and an inability to maneuver the forceps within the disc space adequately led to discontinuation of the use of this instrument. By the mid-1990s, endoscopic examination and visualization of the contents of the spinal canal via a posterolateral, transforaminal approach became a common practice *(43,52,61,77,78)*. Our experience with the use of radiofrequency coagulators for control of epidural bleeding further facilitated access and retrieval of sequestered disc fragments from the spinal canal via a transforaminal approach *(62,64,79)*. Endoscopic laminatomy and foraminotomy has been reported *(60,66,67,80,81)*. However, the advantages of this technology in compared with conventional microscopic discectomy is currently debated.

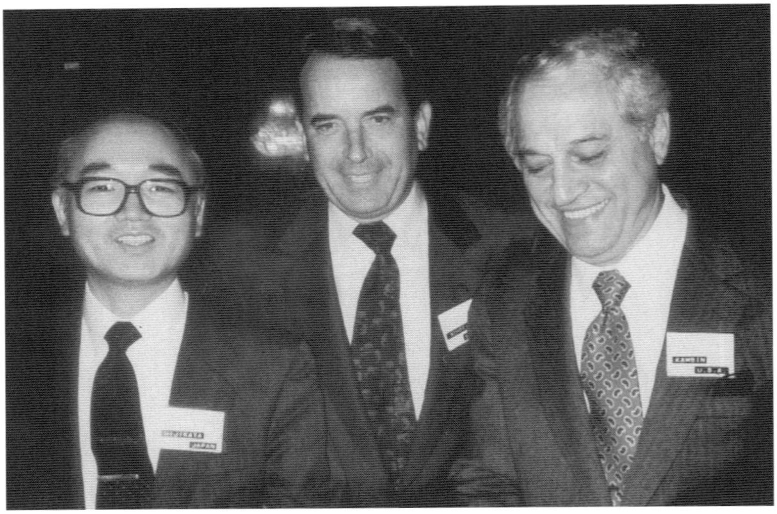

Fig. 21. Photograph taken during the First International Symposium held at the Graduate Hospital in Philadelphia in 1983. From left to right: Dr. Hijikata, Professor Adam Schreiber, Dr. Parviz Kambin.

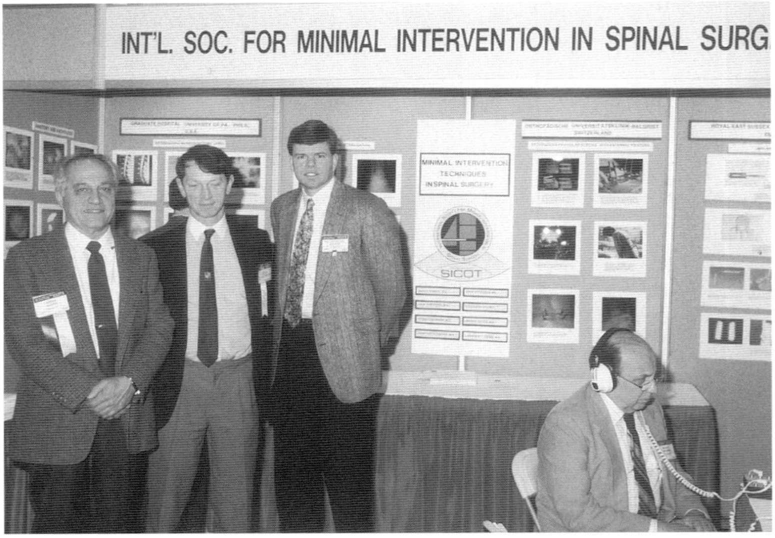

Fig. 22. Scientific exhibits at the American Academy of Orthopaedic Surgeons. From left to right: Parviz Kambin, John Sheppherd, Hal Matthew.

Although endoscopes had been widely used for laparoscopic and thoracoscopic surgery, in recent years Obenchain and other investigators have used this technology in the treatment of a variety of spinal disorders *(82–89)*.

In April 1990, the term *minimally invasive spinal surgery* was coined when a surgical approach for the treatment of a variety of spinal disorders under arthroscopic or endoscopic magnification and illumination became a reality, and the International Society

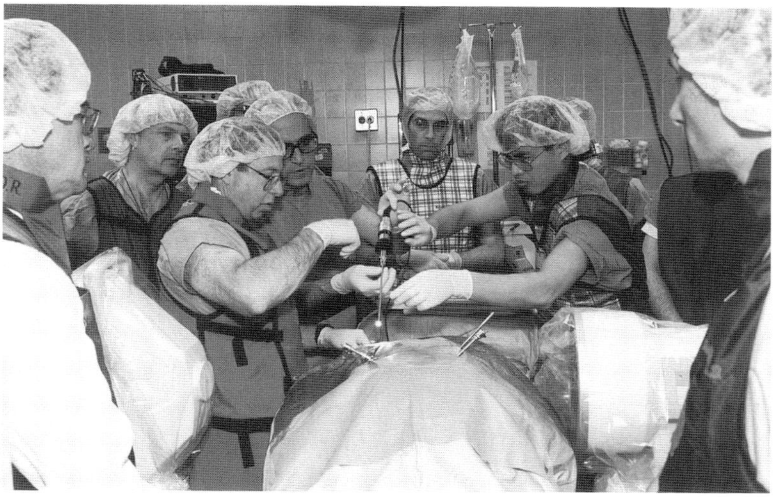

Fig. 23. Photograph from hands-on sessions held at the Graduate, Hospital and MCP Hahnemann University Hospital annually. The orthopedic and neurological surgeons had the opportunity to learn and practice the principle of arthroscopic and endoscopic surgery on cadaver specimens.

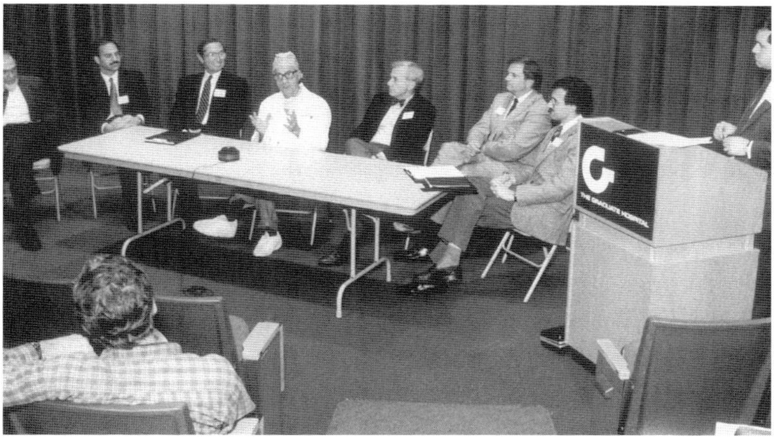

Fig. 24. Photograph of faculty during panel discussions, question-and-answer period following a closed-circuit live surgical demonstration.

for Minimal Intervention in Spinal Surgery was established. The society has held annual symposiums and workshops in both the United States and Europe, where the faculty and surgeons interested in the field of minimally invasive spinal surgery had the opportunity to communicate and interact. (Figs. 21–24).

ACKNOWLEDGMENT

I would like to extend my appreciation to Dr. Oscar Sugar, Emeritus Professor of Surgery, University of Illinois for his contribution and assistance in translating the articles by Alajouanine and Crouzon et al.

REFERENCES

1. Hippocrates in Garrison's History of neurology; Charles C Thomas, Springfield, IL, 1969, 7–8.
2. Aristotle In medicine: an illustrated history, Harry N. Abrams, New York, 1978, p. 219.
3. Erasistratos Medicine: an illustrated history, Harry N. Abrams, New York, 1978, pp. 310–312.
4. Avicenna in Medicine an illustrated history, Harry N. Abrams New York, 1978, p. 313.
5. Avicenna in The illustrated history of surgery, A B Nordbok, Gothenburg, Sweden, 1988, p. 73.
6. Avicenna in Medicine an illustrated history, Harry N. Abrams, New York 1978, p. 310.
7. Cotunio D. De Ischiade Nervosa Cammentarius. Simoncos Brothers, Naples, 1764.
8 Putti V. The Lady Jones lecture: pathogenesis of sciatic pain. Lancet 1927;2:53.
9. Valleix. Quoted from Reynolds F and Katz S: Herniated lumbar intervertebral disc, American Academy of Orthopaedic Surgeons Symposium on the Spine, CV Mosby, St. Louis, 1969.
10. Lasegue CH. Considerations sur la sciatique. Arch Gen Med 1864;2:558.
11. Brissard. Quoted from Reynolds F and Katz S: Herniated lumbar intervertebral disc, American Academy of Orthopaedic Surgeons Symposium on the Spine Mosby CV, St. Louis, 1969;84–96.
12. Virchow R. Untersuchungen uber die Entwickelung des Schadelgrundes, G Reimer, Berlin, 1857.
13. von Luschka H. Die Gelenke des menschlichen Korpers, 1858; IV G Reimer, Berlin, 1858.
14. Kocher T. Die Verletzungen der wirbelsaule. zugleich als beitrag zur phsyiologic des menschlichen ruckenmarks. Mitt Grenzgeb Med Chir 1896;1:415.
15. Schmorl G. Die pathologische anatomic der wirbelsaule. Verch Deutsch Orthop Gest 1926;21:3.
16. Goldthwait JE. The lumbosacral articulation: an explanation of many cases of alumbago, sciatica and paraplegia. Boston Med Surg J 1911;164:365.
17. Elsberg CA. Experiences in spinal surgery: observations upon 60 laminectomies for spinal disease. Surg Gynecol Obstet 1913;16:117.
18. Elsberg CA. Extradural spinal tumors, primary, secondary, metastasis. Surg Gynecol Obstet 1928;46:1.
19. Stookey B. Compression of the spinal cord due to ventral extradural cervical chondromas. Arch Neurol Psychiatry 1928;20:275.
20. Bucy PC. Chondroma of intervertebral disc. JAMA 1930;94:1552.
21. Alajouanine TH. From the presidential address by Professor Jean Cauchoix before Annual Meeting of the International Society for the Study of the Lumbar Spine, San Francisco, June 1978.
22. Alajouanine TH, Petit-Dutaillis, D. Le nodule fibrocartilageneux de la face face posterieure des disques inter-vertebraux, II. Etude clinique et therapeutique d'une variete nouvelle de compression radiculo-medullaire extra-durale. Presse Med 1930;38:1749–1751.
23. Crouzon O, Petit-Dutaillis D, Christophe J. Sur un cas de compression de la queue de cheval, d'origine traumatique, par un nodule fibro-cartilagineux du disque intervertebral: operation. Gurison Rev Neurol (session of 7 May 1931); l(5):612–617 (this is chronologically vol. 55).
24. Dandy WE. Loose cartilage from the intervertebral disk simulating tumor of the spinal cord. Arch Surg 1929;29:660.
25. Mixter WJ, Barr JS. Rupture of the intervertebral disc with involvement of the spinal canal. N Eng J Med 1934;211:210.
26. Yasargil MG. Die klinischen erfahrungen mit der mikrotechnik. Schweiz Arch Neuropsychiatry 1972;111:493–504.
27. Yasargil MG. Small approach to herniated disc. Adv Neurosurg 1997;4:81.
28. Williams RW. Microsurgical lumbar discectomy: report to American Association of Neurology and Surgery, 1975. Neurosurg 1979;4(2):140.

29. Hult L. Retroperitoneal disc fenestration in low back pain and sciatica. Acta Orthop Scand 1956;20:342–348.
30. Virgin WJ. Experimental investigation into the physical properties of the intervertebral disc. J Bone Joint Surg 1951;33B:60.
31. Brown T, Hansen RJ, Yorra AJ. Some mechanical tests on the lumbosacral spine with particular reference to the intervertebral disc: a preliminary report. J Bone Joint Surg 1957;39A:1135.
32. Nachemson A. Lumbar intradiscal pressure. Acta Orthop Scand (Suppl) 1960;43:104.
33. Nachemson A. In vivo discometry in lumbar discs with irregular myelogram. Acta Orthop Scand 1965;36:418.
34. Kambin P, Brager M. Percutaneous posterolateral discectomy: anatomy and mechanism. Clin Orthop 1987;223:145–154.
35. Kambin P: History of disc surgery, in Minimal Intervention in Spinal Surgery. (Kambin ed), Urban & Schwarzenberg, Baltimore, 1991, pp. 3–8.
36. Sakamoto T, Yamakawa H, Tajima T, Sawaumi A. A study of percutaneous lumbar nucleotomy and lumbar intradiscal pressure. March 1989 International Symposium on Percutaneous Nucleotomy, Bruxelles, 1989.
37. Hampton D, Laros G, MacCarron R, Franks D: Healing potential of annulus fibrosis. Spine 1989;14(4):398–401.
38. Smith L, Garvin PJ, Gesler RM, Jennings RB. Enzyme dissolution of the nucleus pulposus. Nature 1963;198:1311,1312.
39. Thomas L. Reversible collapse of rabbit ears after intravenous papain. J Exp Med 1956;104:245.
40. Kambin P, Gellman H. Percutaneous lateral discectomy of the lumbar spine: a preliminary report. Clin Orthop 1983:174:127–132.
41. Kambin P, Sampson S. Posterolateral percutaneous suction—excision of herniated lumbar intervertebral discs: report of interim results. Clin Orthop 1986;207:37.
42. Kambin P. Arthroscopic microdiscectomy, in Minimal Intervention in Spinal Surgery (Kambin pr ed.), Urban & Schwarzenberg, Baltimore, 1991, pp. 67–1100.
43. Kambin P. Arthroscopic microdiscectomy. Arthroscopy 1992;8:287–295.
44. Hijikata S. Percutaneous diskectomy: a new treatment method for lumbar disk herniation. J Toden Hosp 1975;5:5–13.
45. Schreiber A, Suezawa Y, Leu H. Does percutaneous nucleotomy with discoscopy replace conventional discotomy? Clin Orthop 1989;238:35–42.
46. Blum RS, Swartz A, Morris J. Percutaneous nucleotomy. May 1981;presented at the International Society of Lumbar Spine: Paris, France.
47. Hoppenfield S. Percutaneous removal of herniated lumbar disc through the tube technique. May 1983; Presented at the American Association of Bone and Joint Surgeons, Sea Island, Georgia.
48. Friedman WA. Percutaneous discectomy: an alternative to chemonucleolysis. J Neurosurg 1983;13:542.
49. Onik G, Helms C, Ginsburg L, et al. Percutaneous lumbar discectomy using new aspiration probe. AJR 1985;144:1137–1140.
50. Ascher PW, Holzer P. Laser denaturation of the nucleus pulposus of herniated intervertebral discs, in Arthroscopic Microdiscectomy Mininal Intervention in Spinal Surgery (Kambin pr, ed.), Urban & Schwarzenberg, Baltimore, 1991, pp. 137–140.
51. Kambin P. Endoscopic laser discectomy. Jan 1990;FDA, IDE G890238–S1.
52. Kambin P. Arthroscopic microdiscectomy: lumbar and thoracic spine in Spine Care (White All, ed.), CV Mosby, St. Louis, 1995, pp. 1002–1016.
53. Craig, FS. Vertebral-body biopsy. J Bone Joint Surg 1956;38-A:93–102.
54. Ottolenghi, CE. Vertebral body biopsy, aspiration biopsy. J Bone Joint Surg 1955;37–A.
55. Valls J, Ottolenghi CE, Schajowicz F. Aspiration biopsy in diagnosis of lesions of vertebral bodies. JAMA 1948;136:376.

56. Kambin P. Percutaneous lumbar discectomy: current practice. Surg Rounds Orthop 1988; 31–35.
57. Kambin P, McCullen G, Parke W, et al. Minimally invasive arthroscopic spinal surgery. Instruct Course Lect 1997;46:143–161.
58. Mirkovik SR, Schwartz DG. Anatomic considerations in posterolateral procedures. Spine 1995;20:1965–1971.
59. Kambin P. Unilateral biportal percutaneous surgical procedures and instrumentation. US patent 1991;5,395,317.
60. Kambin P. Arthroscopic foraminal surgical procedures performed through a working channel scope. Patent application 08/207831,1994.
61. Kambin P. Diagnostic and therapeutic spinal arthroscopy. Neurosurg Clin N Am 1996;(1): 65–76.
62. Kambin P. Arthroscopic microdiscectomy and lumbar intervertebral fusion, in The Adult Spine: Principles and Practice (Frymoyer J W, Ducker T, Hadler N, et al. eds.), New York, 1996, pp. 2037–2047.
63. Kambin P. Arthroscopic techniques for spinal surgery, in Operative Arthroscopy (McGinty JB, Casperi RB, Jackson RW, Poehling GG, eds.), Lippincott-Raven, Philadelphia, 1996, pp. 1215–1225.
64. Kambin P, Gennarelli T, Hermantin F. Minimally invasive techniques in spinal surgery: current practice. Neurosurg Focus 1998;4(2):l–l0.
65. Shepperd JAN. Percutaneous and minimal intervention spinal fusion. in Arthroscopic Microdiscectomy Minimal Intervention in Spinal Surgery (Kambin p, ed), Urban & Schwarzenberg, Baltimore, 1991, pp. 127–129.
66. Kambin P. Principles and experiences with monoportal arthroscopic microdiscectomy. Video presentation of endoscopic laminatomy and foraminatomy. Bulgrist Orthopaedic Hospital, University of Zurich School of Medicine, Zurich, Switzerland, December 2, 1993.
67. Foley KT, Smith MM. Microendoscopic discectomy. Techniques Neurosurg 1997;3(4): 301–307.
68. Bozzini PD. Lichleiteroder beschreibank einer einfachen vorrichtung und inhern anwendsung surerlechtung innerer hohlen und zwischenraume des lebenden animalischen korpers.Weimer, 1807.
69. Jacobaeus HC. Possibility of the use of the cystoscope for investigations of serious cavities. Munch Med Wochenschrift 1910;57:2090–2092.
70. Burman MS. Myeloscopy or the direct visualization of the spinal canal and its contents. J Bone Joint Surg 1931;13:695–696.
71. Pool JL. Direct visualization of dorsal nerve roots of the cauda equina by means of the myeloscope. Arch Neurol Psychol 1938;39:1308–1312.
72. Pool JL. Myeloscopy: diagnostic inspection of the cauda equina by means of the endoscope. Bull Neurol Inst NY 1938;7:178–189.
73. Ooi Y, Morisaki N. Intrathecal lumbar endoscope [1st report in Japanese]. Clin Orthop Surg 1969;4:295.
74. Ooi Y, Satoh Y, Mita F, Schaffer JL. Myeloscopy and endoscopic nucleotomy, in Spine Care (White AH, Schofferman J, eds.), CV Mosby, St. Louis, 1995, pp. 1009–1073,
75. Hausmann B, Forst R. Nucleoscope: instrumentation for endoscopy of the intervertebral disc space. Arch Orthop Trauma Surg 1983;102:37–59.
76. Kambin P, Zhou L. History and current status of percutaneous arthroscopic disc surgery. Spine 1996;21(24).
77. Kambin P, O'Brien E, Zhou L, Schaffer JL. Arthroscopic microdiscectomy and selective fragmentectomy. CORR 1998;(347):150–167.
78. Mathews HH, Kyles M , Lang BH, Fiore SM, Gordon CL. Spinal endoscopy: indications, approaches and applications. Orthop Trans 1995;19:219.

79. Kambin P, Casey K, O'Brien E, et al. Transforaminal arthroscopic decompression of lateral recess stenosis. J Neurosurg 1996;84:462–467.
80. Destandau J. A special device for endoscopic surgery of the lumbar spine. Neurol Res 1999;21:39–42.
81. Roh SW, Kim D, Cardoso A, Fessler RG. Endoscopic foraminotomy using Spine Med System in cadaveric specimens. Spine 2000;25(2):260–264.
82. Mathews HH, Evans MT, Molligan HJ, Long BH. Laparoscopic diskectomy with anterior lumbar interbody fusion: a preliminary review. Spine 1995;20:1797–1802.
83. Connolly PJ, Yuan HA, Kolata RJ, Clem MF. Endoscopic approach to the lumbar spine using the insufflation technique. in Atlas of Endoscopic Spine Surgery (Regan, McAffee, Mack, eds.), Quality Medical Publishing, St. Louis, 1995.
84. Horowitz MB, Moossy JJ, Julian T, Ferson PF, Huneke K. Thoracic discectomy using video assisted thoracoscopy. Spine 1994;19:1082–1086.
85. Mack MJ, Regan JJ, Bobechko WP, Acuff TE. Application of thoracoscopy for disease of the spine. Ann Thorac Surg 1993;56:736–738.
86. Obenchain TG. Laparoscopic lumbar diskectomy. a case report. J Laparoendosc Surg 1991;1:145–149.
87. Obenchain TG, Cloyd D, Slavin M. Outpatient laparoscopic lumbar discectomy. Description of technique and review of first twenty-one cases. Surg Tech Int 1993;2:415–418.
88. Regan JJ. Technique and approach for laparoscopic discectomy and fusion, Atlas of Endoscopic Spine Surgery (Regan, Mcaffee, Mack, eds). Quality Medical Publishing st. Louis, pp. 130–135.
89. Regan JJ, Mack M J, Picetti GDI, A technical report on video-assisted thoracoscopy in thoracic spinal surgery: preliminary description. Spine 1995;20: 831–837.

2
Arthroscopic and Endoscopic Anatomy of the Lumbar Spine

Parviz Kambin, MD

INTRODUCTION

The success of arthroscopic and endoscopic spinal surgery hinges by and large on clear visualization and identification of various anatomical structures. During intracanalicular surgery, venous bleeding may obstruct the surgeon's visual field. This must be controlled with topical anticoagulants, radiofrequency probes, cold irrigation fluid, and a simple increase in its inflow.

THORACOLUMBAR FASCIA

The thoracolumbar fascia appears as a heavy band of interwoven, whitish fibers that lacks a blood supply (Fig. 1).

PARASPINAL MUSCLES

The sacrospinalis, quadratus lumbrorum, and psoas major muscles appear as reddish bundles that are readily visualized under arthroscopic magnification and illumination (Fig. 2). The muscle fibers are moderately vascular. At the end of arthroscopic spine surgery, it is not unusual to see extravasation of blood through the small incision used for insertion of instruments. This bleeding can be controlled by applying compression to the skin and the paraspinal muscles.

TRIANGULAR WORKING ZONE

The triangular working zone is a safe zone on the posterolateral surface of the annulus adjacent to the spinal canal. It is suitable for safe lodging of instruments during posterolateral access to the intervertebral disc and the spinal canal (Fig. 3) (*see* Chapters 3 and 4). The annular surface in the triangular working zone is bordered anteriorly by the exiting root, inferiorly by the proximal plate of the inferior lumbar segment, medially by the dural sac and the traversing root, and posteriorly by the articular processes of the adjacent segment *(1,2)*. The annular surface in the triangular working zone is covered with loosely woven globules of adipose tissue (Fig. 4A,B). It should be noted that the fatty tissue is relatively stationary and does not

From: *Arthroscopic and Endoscopic Spinal Surgery: Text and Atlas: Second Edition*
Edited by: P. Kambin © Humana Press Inc., Totowa, NJ

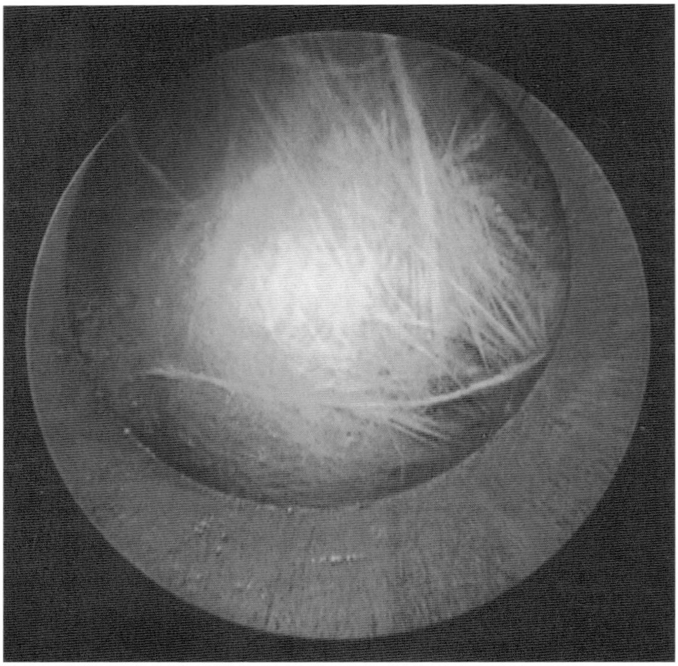

Fig. 1. Arthroscopic view showing the thoracolumbar fascia as an avascular heavy band of interwoven fibers.

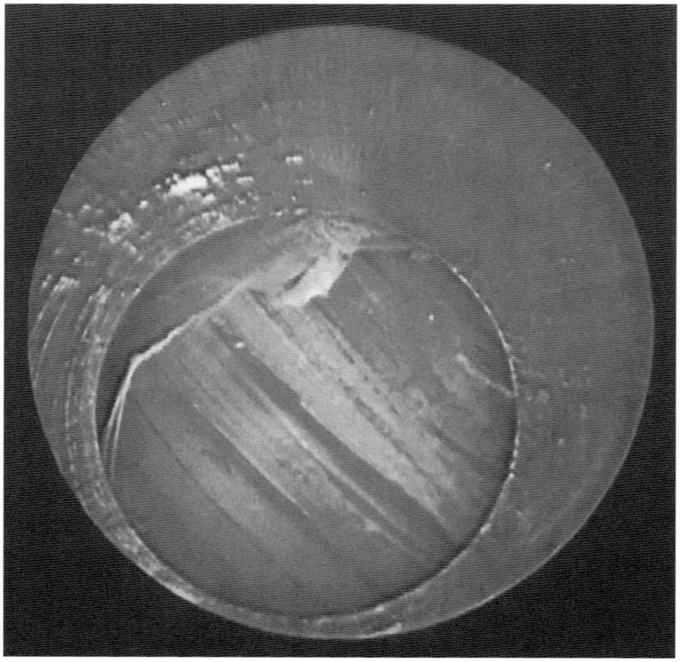

Fig. 2. The paravertebral muscles of the lumbar spine are seen as a moderately vascular muscle bundle.

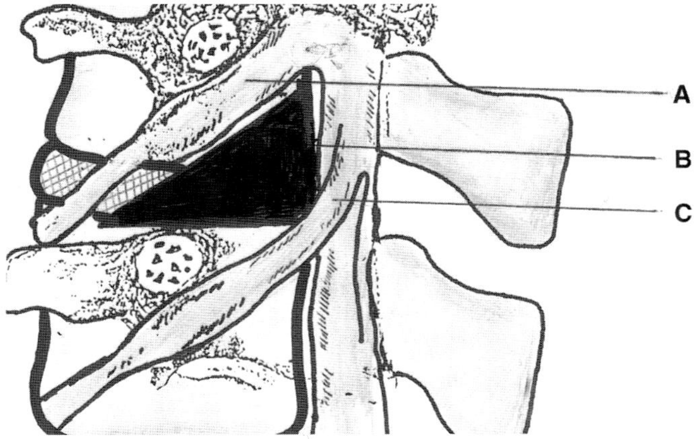

Fig. 3. Illustration of triangular working zone: A, exiting root that forms anterior boundary of triangular working zone; B, triangular working zone; C, traversing root.

move in and out of the cannula as the patient breathes. Small-caliber veins that may have to be coagulated may be observed on the surface of the triangular working zone (Fig. 5A,B). Coarse fibrous bands of the annulus are observed after removal of the adipose tissue (Fig. 6A,B). At times, a thin layer of fibers of the psoas muscle are observed on the dorsolateral surface of the annulus in the triangular working zone (Fig. 7).

NERVE ROOTS AND ROOT GANGLIA

Both exiting and traversing roots that form the lateral and medial boundaries of the triangular working zone are in the path of dorsolaterally inserted instruments and may be subject to insult during intradiscal or extraannular approaches to the lumbar spine. At the onset of arthroscopic disc surgery, the final and proper positioning of the instruments is best determined by accurate placement and documentation of the tip of the inserted instruments (18-gage needle or guide wire) on the annular surface in the triangular working zone. The fibers of the posterior longitudinal ligament extend laterally into the triangular working zone and extraforaminal region *(4–8)* (Fig. 8). These fibers are innervated by branches of sinu-vertebral nerve and are highly sensitive to palpation by the inserted instruments. The superficial layer of the annulus and the expansion of the posterior longitudinal ligament must be adequately anesthetized during the operative procedure and annular fenestration. The exiting root is well protected in the triangular working zone, where it lays under the pedicle in the pedicular notch and is accompanied by the radicular artery, radicular vein, and branches of the sinu-vertebral nerve. The posterior sensory nerve fibers and the anterior motor fibers usually join one another prior to their departure from the dural sac. However, at times they part individually from the dura. The posterior sensory root is larger than the anterior motor root, and it continues into the fusiform root ganglia and then joins the anterior motor root. Usually the L4 and L5 dorsal root ganglia are intraforaminal and must be protected during foraminal access to the intervertebral disc or the spinal canal. The S1 root ganglion is likely to be intraspinal.

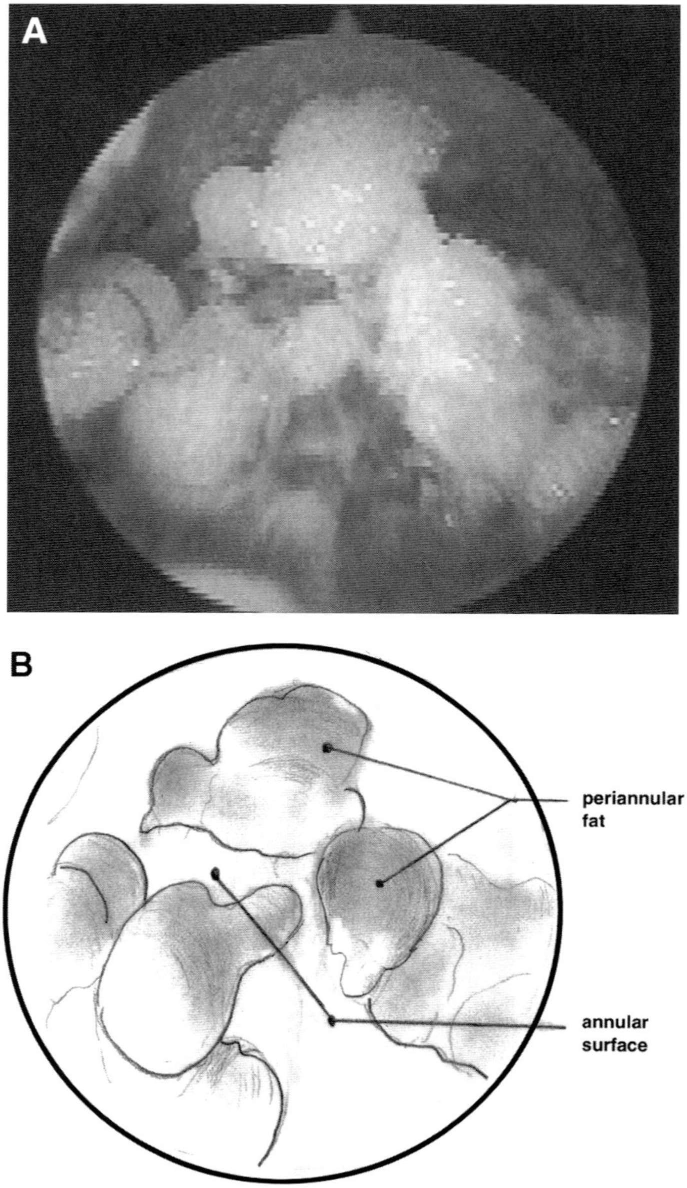

Fig. 4. (A,B) Arthroscopic view of annular surface in triangular working zone. Note the loose/woven adipose tissue on the surface of annulus.

The mobility of the traversing and exiting roots at the lower lumbar region allows the operative surgeon to retract these structures during both arthroscopic and open spinal surgery. However, limited mobility of the nerve roots in the upper lumbar spine and at the thoracolumbar junction, combined with the bulk of the cauda equina and conus medullaris in the subarachnoid space, demands protection of neural tissue by accurate positioning of the instruments, clear visualization, and careful handling of the resecting instruments.

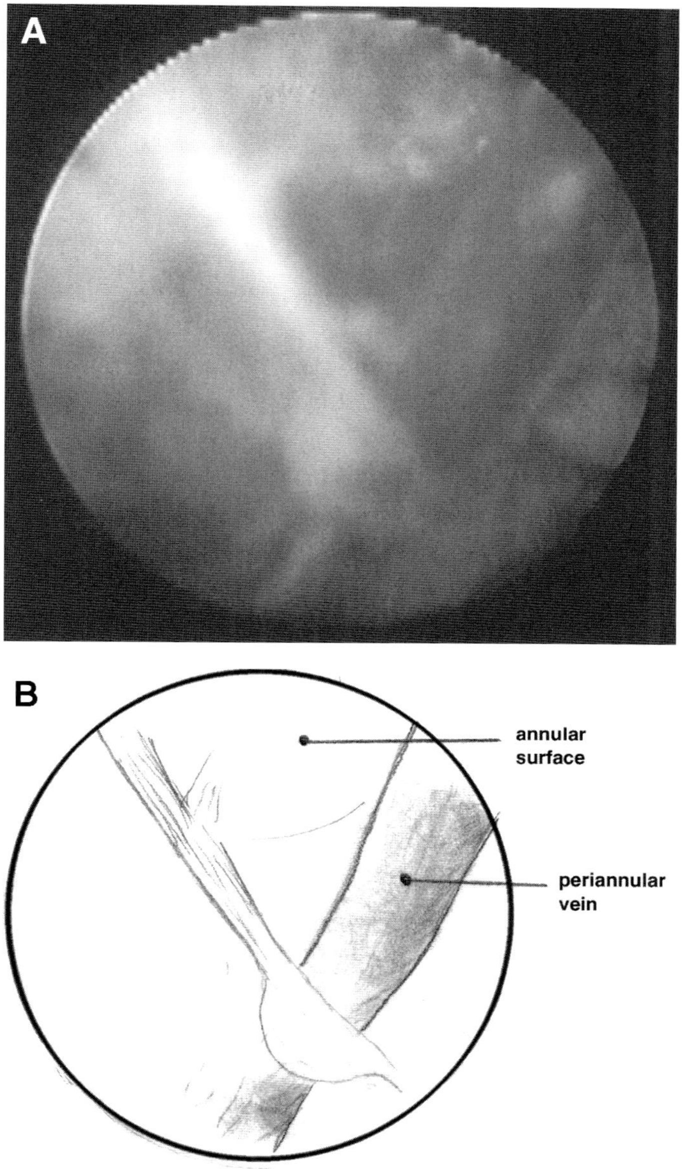

Fig. 5. Interoperative photo demonstrating presence of superficial veins on surface of annulus.

In a series of T1 imaging studies of the thoracolumbar junction, the end of the conus was identified at the L1 level in 50% of individuals but at the L2 segment in 20% of patients. Therefore, great care must be exercised while performing arthroscopic or endoscopic surgery adjacent to these two segments. The nerve roots appear as pale yellow, multifiber structures under arthroscopic illumination and magnification. Fine vessels are present on the surfaces of the nerve root and root ganglia (Fig. 9A–D). The inflamed nerve roots are highly sensitive to palpation and compression. The traversing root may be

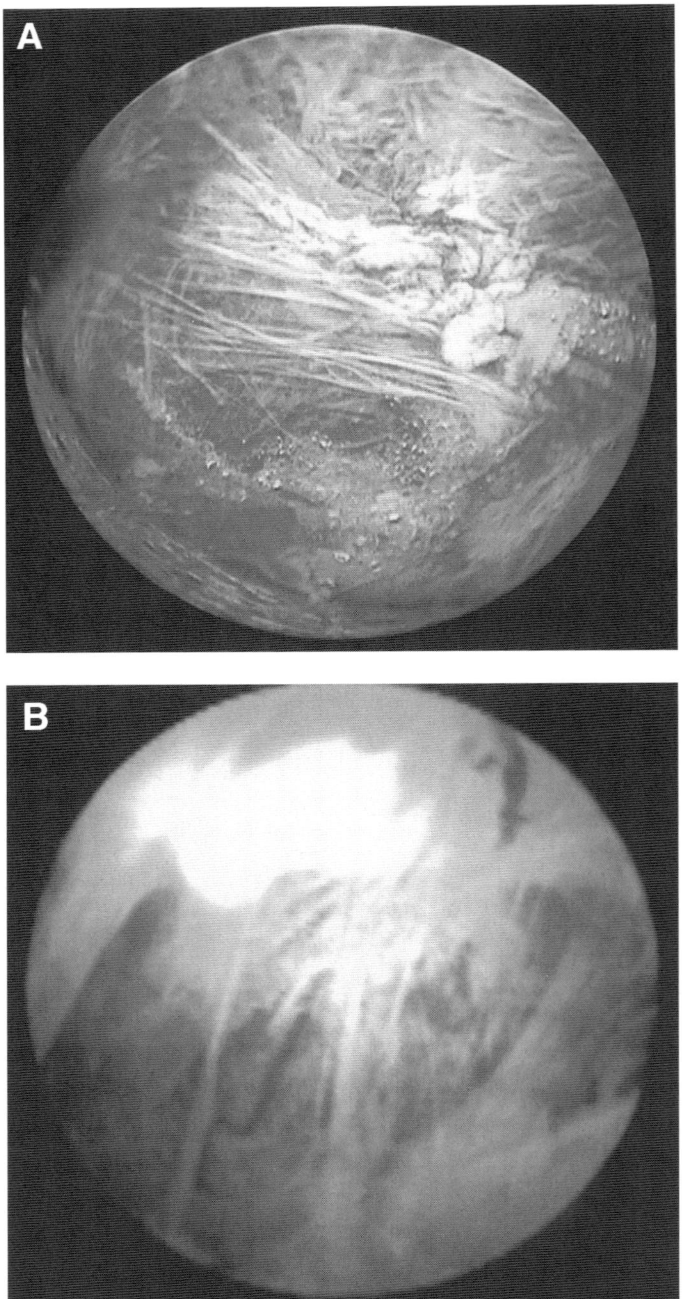

Fig. 6. Interoperative photos showing **(A)** annular surface following removal of adipose tissue and **(B)** magnified view of avascular fibers of annulus following extraction of superficial adipose tissue.

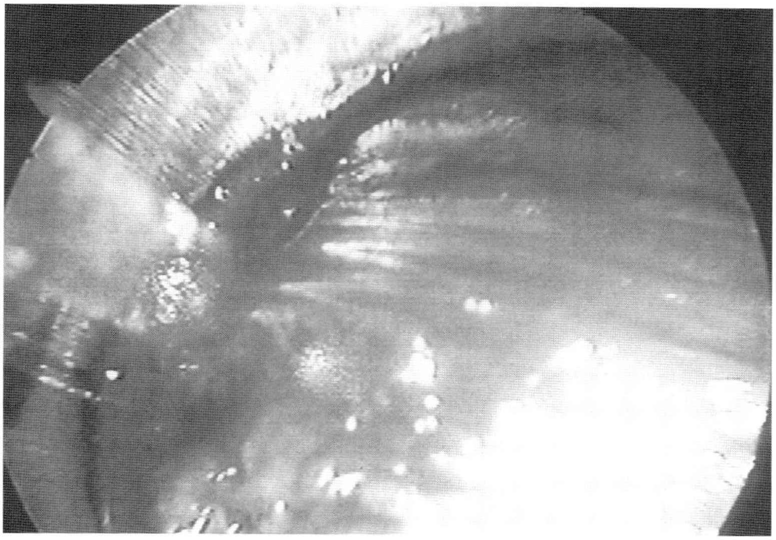

Fig. 7. A thin layer of psoas muscle that covers the triangular working zone is observed and is being removed with the aid of laser light.

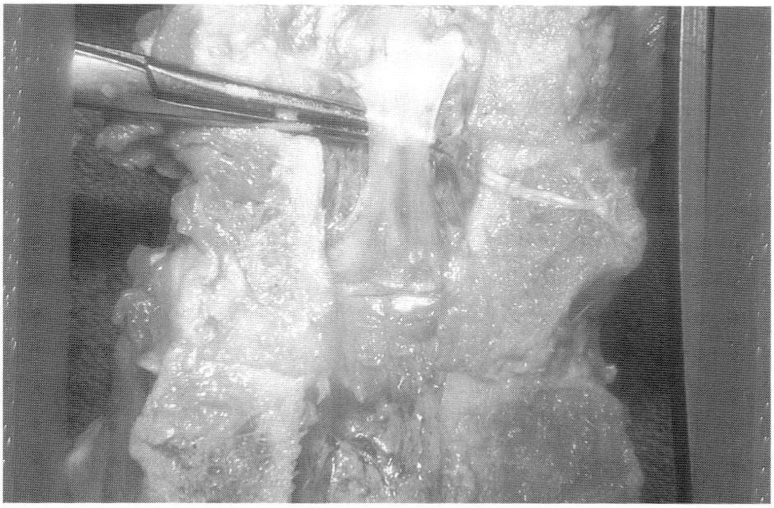

Fig. 8. Cadaveric dissection showing fibers of posterior longitudinal ligamentum, which extends to dorsolateral aspect of annulus, foraminal, and extraforaminal region.

observed adjacent to the dural sac in the medial pedicular line region and is usually surrounded by epidural veins and adipose tissue.

VASCULAR STRUCTURES

Vascular structures of epidural and neural tissue play an important role in the pathophysiology of pain that is commonly observed in individuals with symptomatic disc herniation, spinal stenosis, and failed back surgery syndrome. It has been shown that

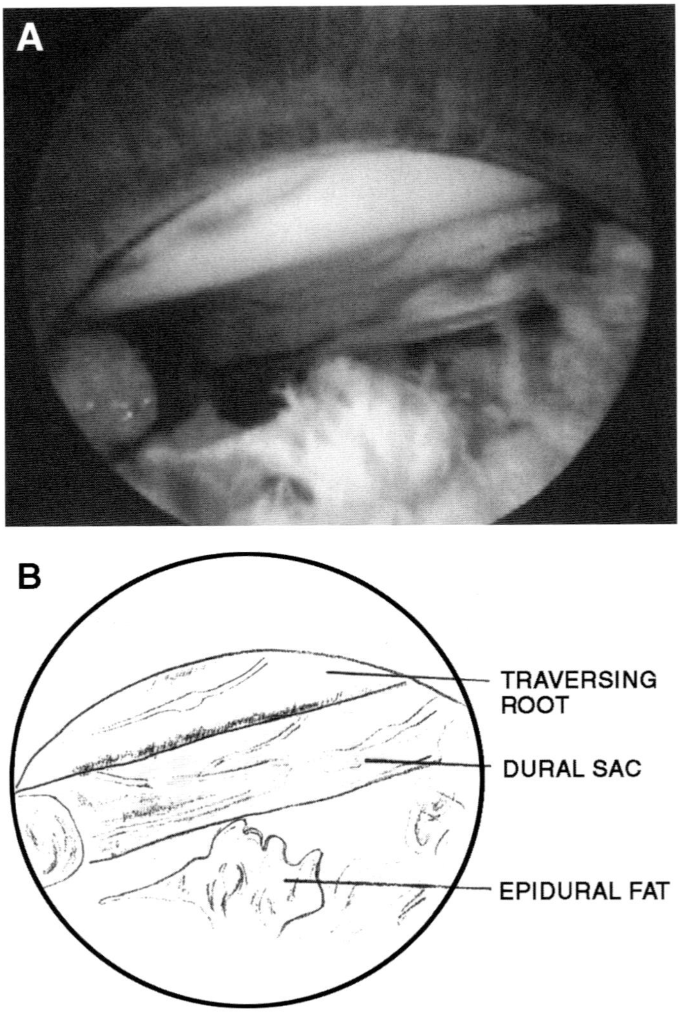

Fig. 9. Endoscopic view of content of (**A,B**) spinal canal and (**C,D**) herniated lumbar disc. (Reprinted from ref. *12*, with permission [A].)

interference with the normal blood flow of delicate neural and epidural venous systems (Fig. 10) may cause venous stasis edema of the nerve root, neural fibrosis, and chronic pain *(4,8)*. This phenomenon is usually observed in patients presenting with symptomatic disc herniation and spinal stenosis. Segmental arteries, branches from the aorta and the internal iliac artery, provide blood supply to the neural, osseous, and muscular structures of the spinal column. Branches from the lumbar arteries depart from the segmental arteries and enter the intervertebral foramen (radicular artery) with the exiting root to supply the medullary arteries of the spinal cord and the nerve roots.

Segmental arteries distal to L4 originate from the hypogastric arteries that are branches of the internal iliac arteries *(10)* (Fig. 11). When the posterolateral approach is used for either discectomy or anterior column stabilization and the instruments are directed and properly positioned in the triangular working zone, these segmental arteries are not sub-

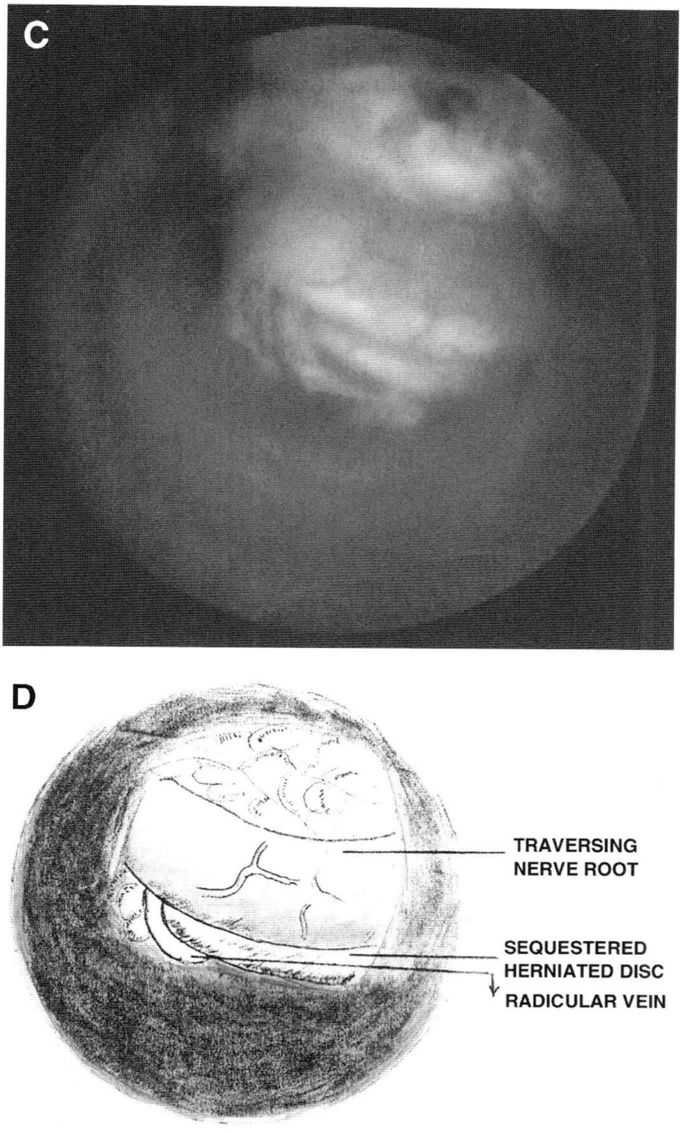

Fig. 9. *(Continued)*

ject to insult and injury. However, when the instruments are inserted too far anteriorly (vertically), they may penetrate the iliac artery or vein, causing rapid blood loss requiring immediate emergency exploration and repair of the injured vessels. By contrast, during laparoscopic or open retroperitoneal or transabdominal spinal surgery, the hypogastric and infraaortic arteries as well as sympathetic ganglia are in the path of the inserted instruments and must be protected.

When the instruments are properly lodged in the triangular working zone, the radicular arteries remain protected under the pedicular notch. However, during decompression

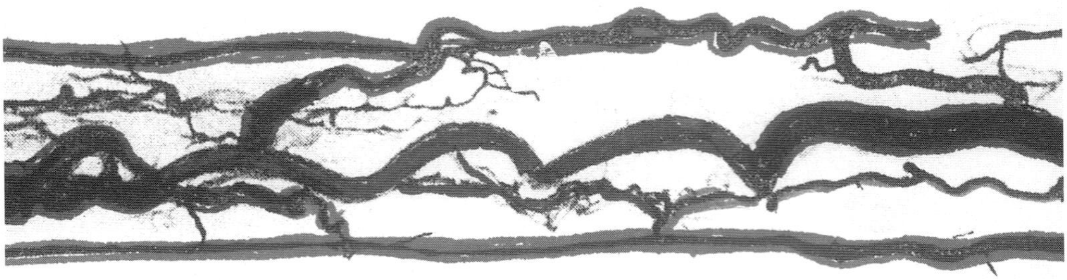

Fig. 10. Photograph demonstrating arteries and venous system of nerve root and A.V. anastomosis (courtesy of Wesley Parke).

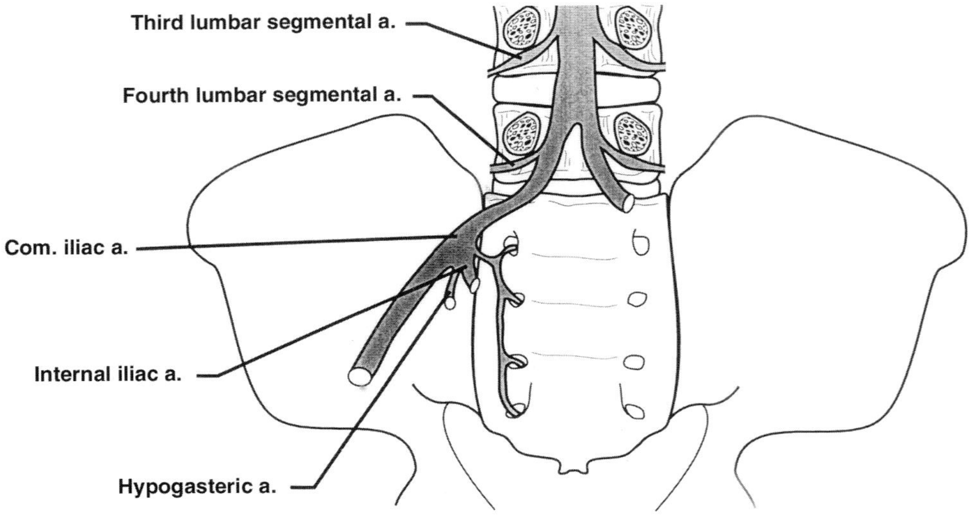

Fig. 11. Illustration showing origin of segmental arteries of lumbar spine.

of the lateral recess in the treatment of lateral recess stenosis, particularly when a back-firing laser light is being used, great care must be exercised to protect the vascular structures and their accompanying exiting root in the pedicular notch. Only a small portion of the exiting root that is situated between the lateral pedicular line and the superior border of the transverse process is subject to insult during the posterolateral approach for the removal of extraforaminal herniations *(7)*. However, positioning the instruments medial to the lateral pedicular line at the onset of operative procedures will help avoid any complications (see Chapter 4).

EPIDURAL ADIPOSE TISSUE

Epidural adipose tissue is usually seen as rather large globules of fat that move in and out of the cannula when a patient inhales and exhales. This adipose tissue is surrounded by the epidural venous system, which must be controlled when transforaminal intracanalicular access is employed for the removal of a sequestered disc.

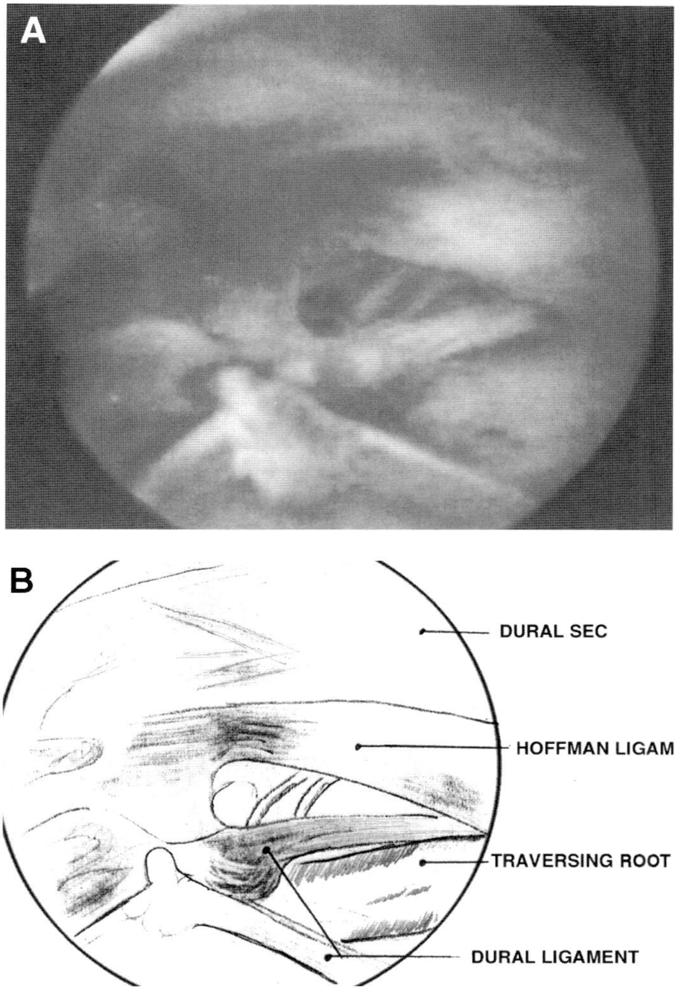

Fig. 12. (A,B) Ligamentous structures of ventral dura and nerve root.

DURAL SAC

The dural sac is seen as grayish tissue surrounded by epidural veins that readily bleed (Fig. 9A,B).

INTRACANALICULAR LIGAMENTS

In a virgin spine, fine and mobile vascular and ligamentous structures on the floor of the spinal canal may be seen under endoscopic magnification (Fig. 12A,B). Hoffman's ligament, which extends from the ventral and lateral dura to the posterior longitudinal ligament, and the dural ligament, which extends from the dura and traversing root to the posterior longitudinal ligament and periosteum, may be identified following adequate hemostasis.

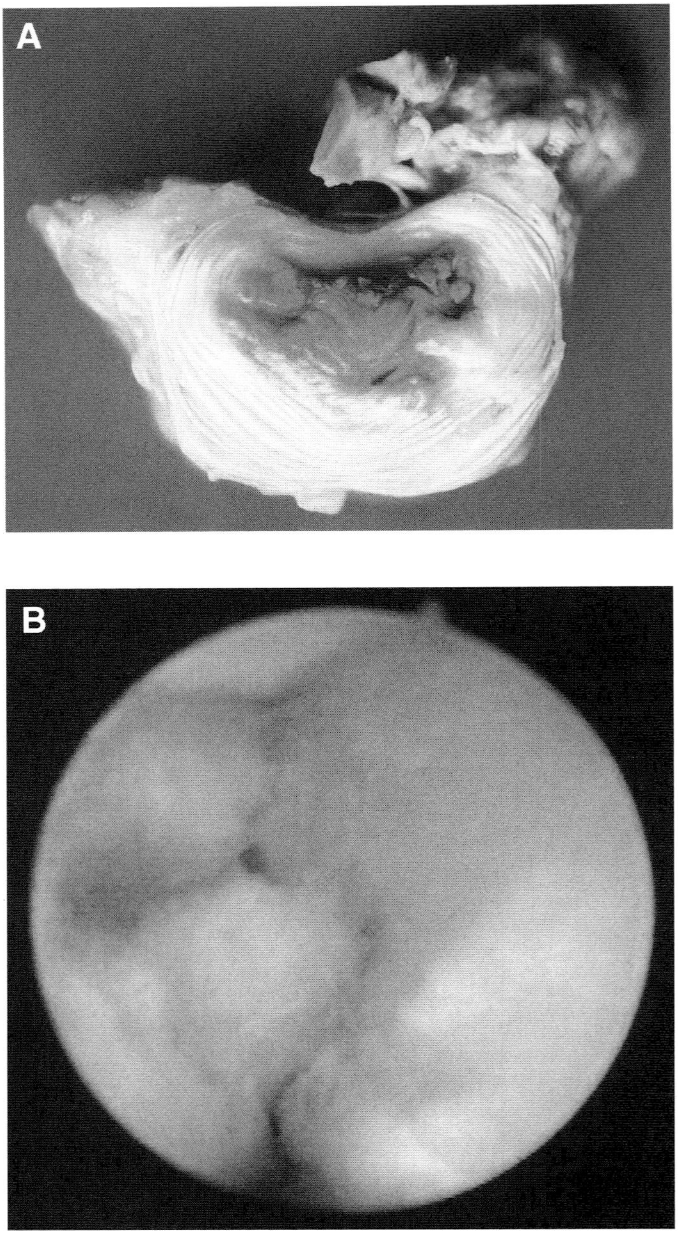

Fig. 13. **(A)** Gross anatomy of annulus fibrosus and NP in young cadaver specimen. The nucleus has been injected with methylene blue. Note, however, the thickness of the annulus fibrosus anteriorly and posterolaterally. **(B)** Cotton-ball appearance of nucleus in adolescence (arthroscopic view).

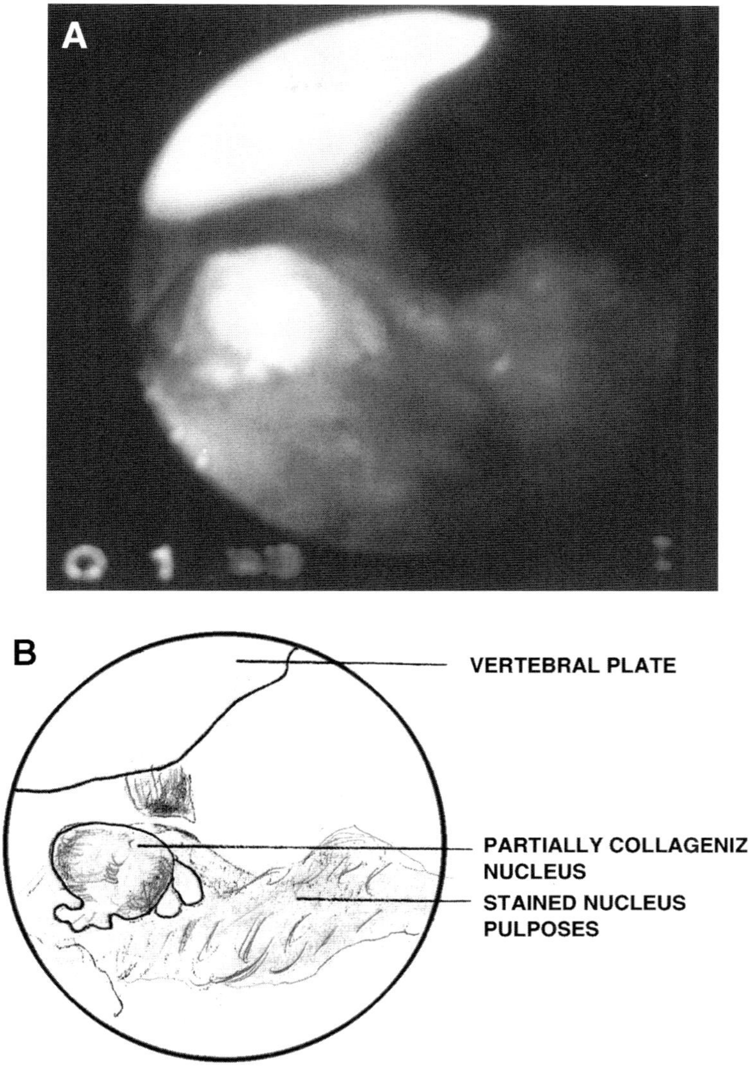

Fig. 14. (A,B) Arthroscopic view of NP in a 45-yr-old male following interdiscal injection of diluted indigo carmine. Note the unstained partially collagenized nucleus mixed with stained soft nuclear tissue.

NUCLEUS PULPOSUS

In adolescence the nucleus pulposus (NP) is well contained within the annular ring (Fig. 13A). It has a whitish, cotton-ball appearance (Fig. 13B). The nucleus breaks off and separates easily. It is not liquid and does not flow. Nuclear tissue absorbs a considerable amount of fluid and has a tendency to swell. By contrast, the nucleus will become dehydrated and partially collagenized in the fifth and sixth decades of life. A mixture of collagenized tissue and whitish soft nucleus may be observed within the intervertebral disc in this older group of patients (Fig. 14A,B). In addition, multiple collagenized free fragments floating within the disc space may also be seen (Fig. 15A,B).

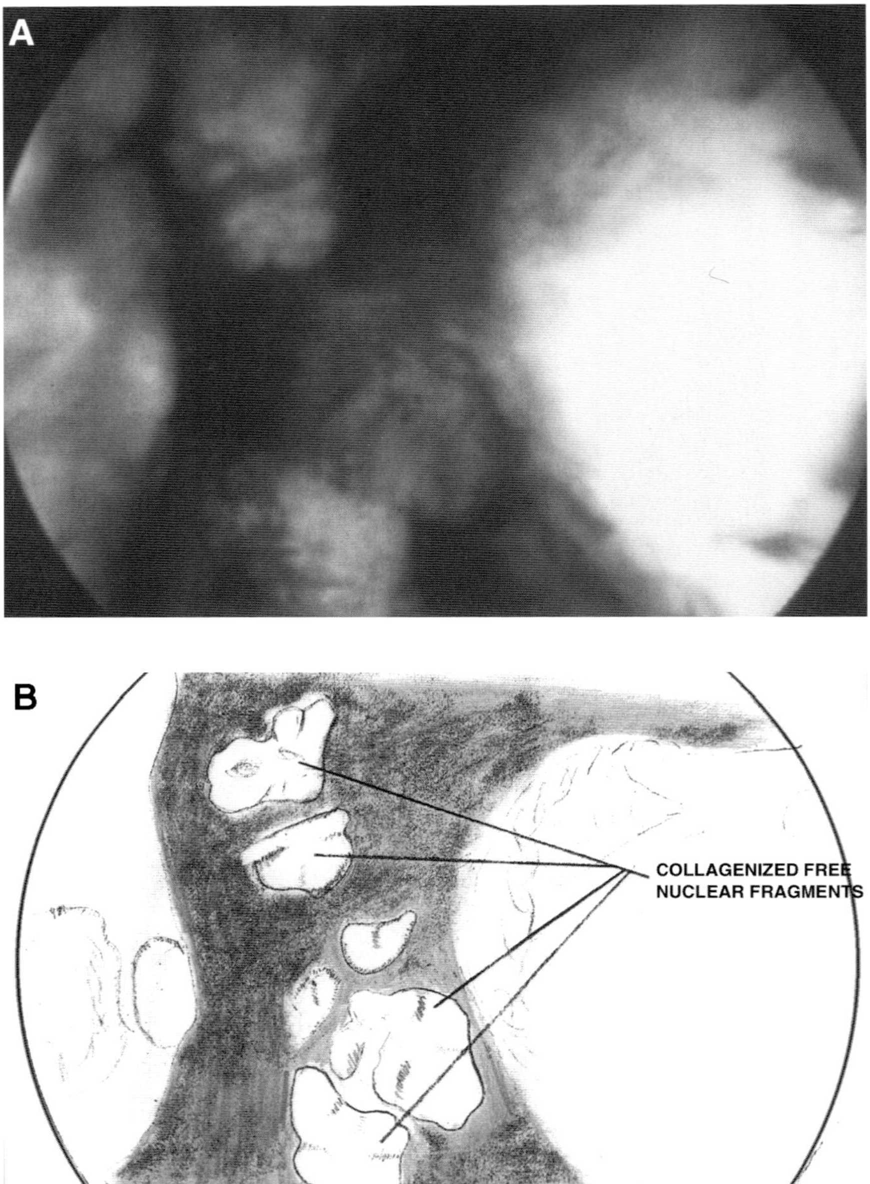

Fig. 15. **(A,B)** Interoperative arthroscopic view of intervertebral disc. Note multiple collagenized free fragments floating within a degenerated intervertebral disc (intradiscal sequestration).

ANNULUS FIBROSUS

In elderly patients, the nucleus becomes dehydrated and collagenized and begins to migrate posteriorly through the torn fibers of the annulus (Fig. 16). From a clinician's point of view, the dorsolateral migration of the nuclear tissue will present three distinct

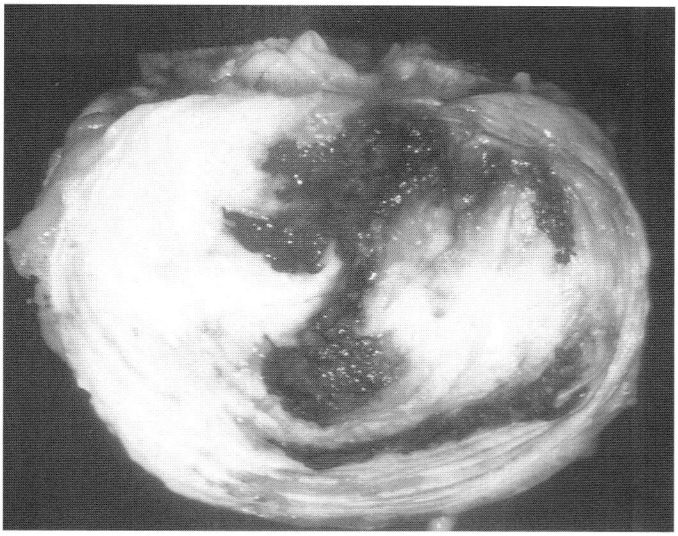

Fig. 16. Fresh cadaveric specimen of a degenerated disc following injection of methylene blue. Note the disorganization of the nuclear tissue, annular tear, and migration of the nucleus into the periphery.

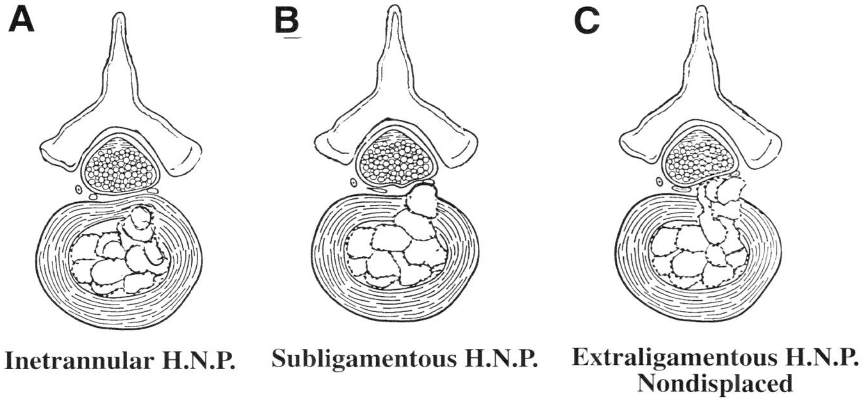

Fig. 17. Schematic drawing demonstrating **(A)** interannular, **(B)** subligamentous, and **(C)** extraligamentous, herniation of nucleus pulposus (H.N.P.).

anatomical and imaging presentations. A partial tear of the annular fibers may cause an intraannular herniation with imaging evidence of a small and gradually developed bulge or protrusion of the annulus (Fig. 17A) *(11)*. By contrast, a subligamentous migration of the collagenized nuclear tissue is associated with a sudden change in the external geometry of the annulus, with an imaging appearance of a distinct herniation having smooth borders (Fig. 17B). When the integrity of the posterior longitudinal ligamentum has been altered, the collagenized nuclear fragments are dislodged into the spinal canal. Imaging studies will reveal a large extradural sequestered fragment with irregular and uneven borders (Fig. 17C).

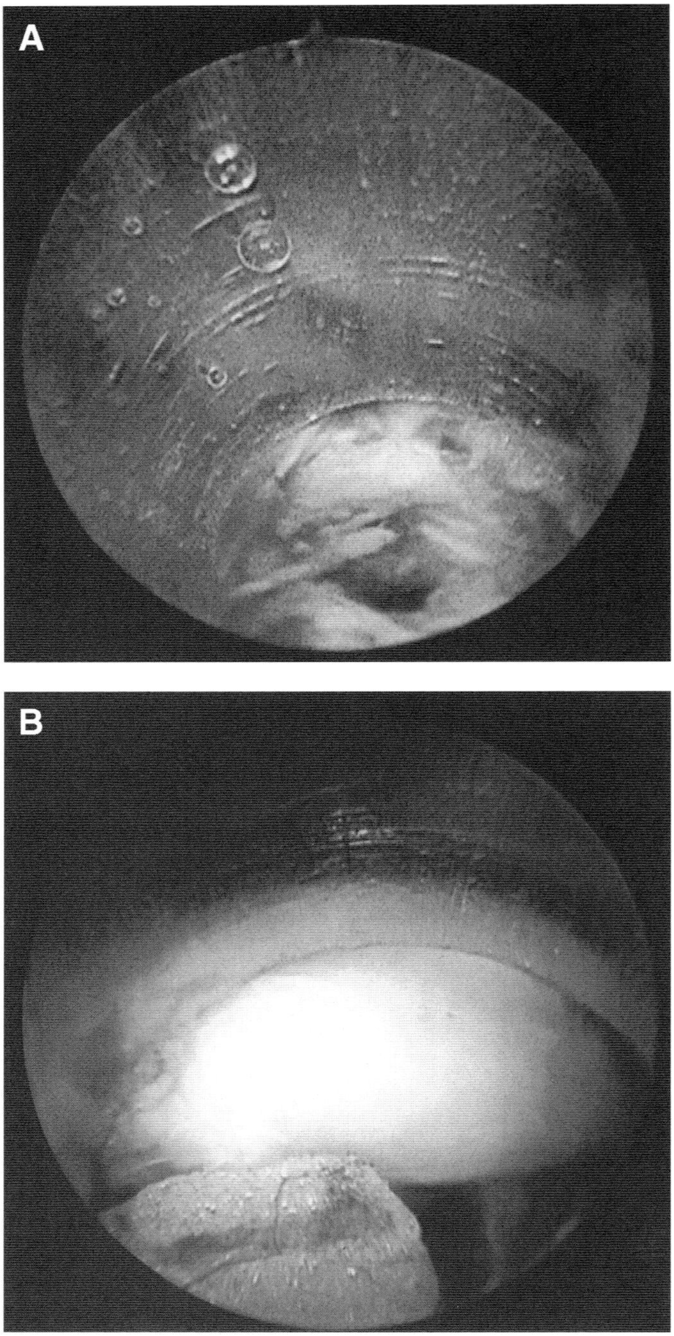

Fig. 18. **(A)** Endoscopic view of capsular ligamentum flavum complex; **(B,C)** magnified view of capsular ligamentum flavum complex, which appears as an avascular structure.

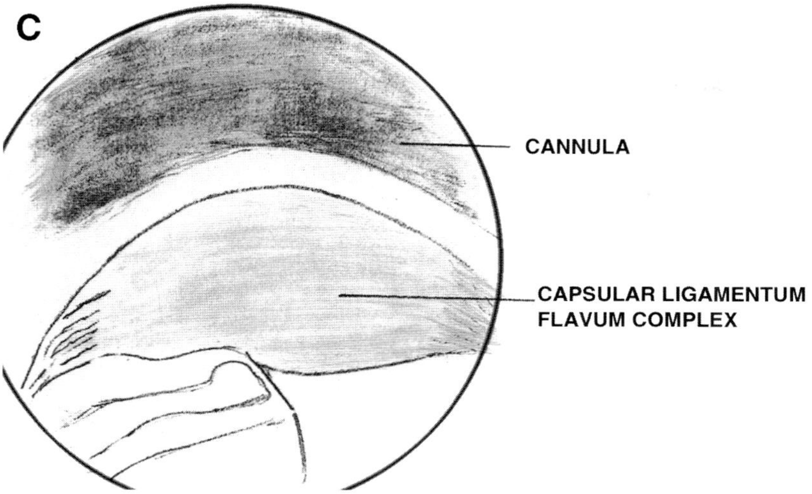

Fig. 18. *(Continued)*

Arthroscopic differentiation between the torn annulus and nucleus may be difficult. Intraoperative injection of diluted indigo carmine has a tendency to stain the nucleus and the torn fibers of annular tissue while sparing intact annular fibers. Schreiber and Leu originally introduced this technique for intraoperative tissue differentiation *(12)*.

CAPSULAR, LIGAMENTOUS FLAVUM COMPLEX

During foraminal or transforaminal intracanalicular surgery *(3,4,9)*, the capsule of the facet joints combined with a thickened inflamed ligamentous flavum may interfere with free passage of instruments for surgical removal, or vaporization of the content of the spinal canal.

In our experience, removal of the fibers of the posterior longitudinal ligamentum invariably is adequate and will provide ample access to the ventral surface of the dural sac and traversing root *(13)* (*see* Chapter 4). In contrast to the traversing root, the capsule and the ligamentum flavum complex are observed as an avascular tissue (Fig. 18A–C).

POSTERIOR LONGITUDINAL LIGAMENTUM

The ventral surface of the posterior longitudinal ligamentum may be observed when subligamentous access to a contained disc herniation has been attempted. Visualization of the ventral surface of the posterior longitudinal ligamentum signifies that adequate decompression of the nerve root and dural sac has been accomplished. Following extraction of the torn fibers of the annulus, partial nucleotomy, and creation of a small cavity ventral to the posterior longitudinal ligamentum, a 30 or 70° arthroscope may be used for visualization of the above structures. In contrast to the annulus, the fibers of the posterior longitudinal ligamentum run perpendicular to the vertebral plates and are seen as avascular structures (Fig. 19A–C).

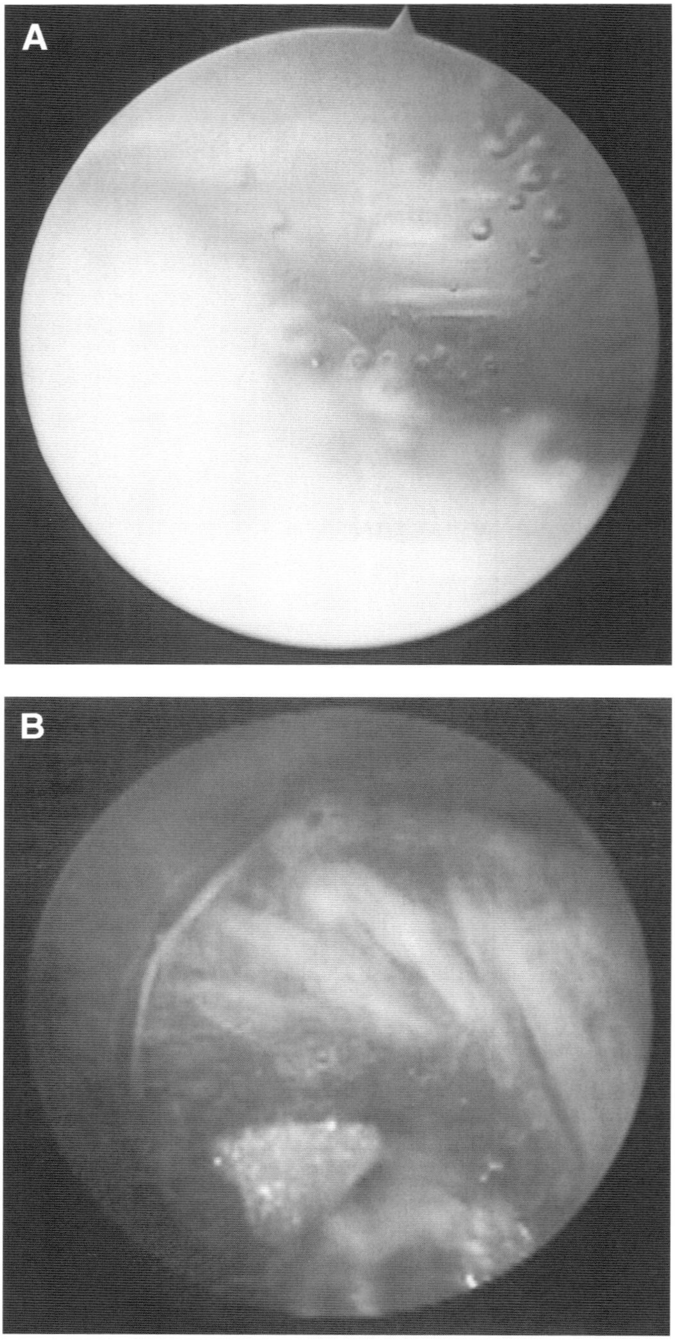

Fig. 19. **(A)** Intraoperative photo demonstrating ventral surface of posterior longitudinal ligamentum following evacuation of a contained disc herniation; **(B,C)** magnified view of ventral surface of posterior longitudinal ligamentum (PLL) shown in Fig. 17A.

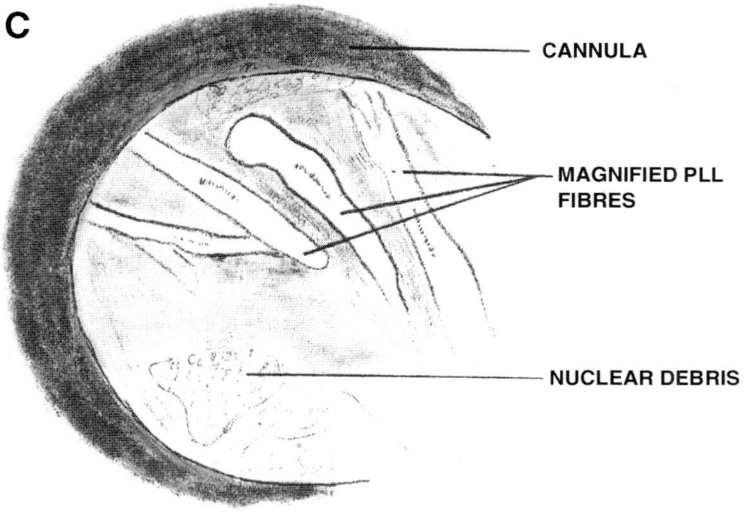

Fig. 19. *(Continued)*

REFERENCES

1. Kambin P. Percutaneous lumbar discectomy: current practice. Surg Rounds Orthop 1988;31–35.
2. Kambin P. Arthroscopic Microdiscectomy: Minimal Intervention in Spinal Surgery R (Kambin P, ed.), Urban & Schwarzenberg, Baltimore, 1991, pp. 67–100.
3. Kambin P. Gross and arthroscopic anatomy of the lumbar spine, in Operative Arthroscopy (McGinty JB, Casperi RB, Jackson RW, Poehling GG, eds.), Lippincott-Raven, Philadelphia, 1996, pp. 1207–1214.
4. Kambin P, McCullen G, Parke W et al. Minimally invasive arthroscopic spinal surgery. Instruct Course Lect 1997;46:143–161.
5. Kambin P. Arthroscopic microdiscectomy lumbar and thoracic spine, in Spine Care, vol. 2 (White A, Schoffeman JA, eds.), Mosby, St. Louis, 2002. pp. 1002–1016.
6. Mirkovik SR, Schwartz DG. Anatomic considerations in posterolateral procedures. Spine 1995;20:1965–1971.
7. Kambin P, Brager M. Percutaneous posterolateral discectomy: anatomy and mechanism. Clin Orthop 1987;223:145–154.
8. Park WW. Anatomy of spinal nerve and it's surrounding structures. Semin Orthop 1991;6(2):65.
9. Mathews HH, Kyles MK, Lang BH, Fiore SM, Gordon CL. Spinal endoscopy: indications, approaches and applications. Orthop Trans 1995;19:219.
10. Park WW, Whalen JL, VanDemark RE, Kambin P. The infra-aortic arteries of the spine: their variability and clinical significance. Spine 1994;19(1):1–5.
11. Schaffer JL, Kambin P. Minimally invasive spine surgery. Textbook of Rheumatology Update 1994;9:2–12.
12. Schreiber A, Leu HJ. Biportal percutaneous lumbar nucleotomy, in Spinal Surgery (Kambin P, ed.), Urban & Schwarzenberg Baltimore, 1991, pp. 67–100.
13. Hermantin FU, Peters T, Quartaro L, Kambin P. A prospective, randomized study comparing the results of open disectomy with those of video-assisted arthroscopic microdisectomy. J Bone Joint Surg Am 1999;81:958–965.

3

Instruments and Surgical Approaches for Minimally Invasive Spinal Surgery Via Posterolateral Access

Parviz Kambin, MD

INSTRUMENTS

A variety of instruments have been marketed by at least five industries. All of them share the already published principles *(1–4)*:

1. Precise positioning of needle or guide pin under fluoroscopic control in the triangular working zone.
2. Use of a blunt-ended cannulated obturator or soft-tissue dilator over the previously positioned guide pin. The blunt end of the obturator will have a tendency to bypass the traversing or exiting root as it descends toward the triangular working zone.
3. Final positioning of a working cannula that is passed over the previously positioned soft-tissue dilator.

The instruments include the following:

1. An 18-gage needle, 15 cm (6 in.) in length (Fig. 1).
2. A blunt-end cannulated obturator with a 4.9-mm outer diameter (od).
3. Cannulas: A number of cannulas are available and have been used by various surgeons for arthroscopic spinal surgery. The round universal cannula has a 6.4-mm od that provides an inner diameter (id) working area of 5 mm. Recently, a round, bevel-ended cannula has been introduced and utilized by some surgeons (T. Yeung, personal communication).

   Two sizes of oval cannulas are available (Fig. 1): a cannula with a 6.4 × 10 mm od that provides a 5 × 8 mm id working area; and a larger oval cannula, primarily used for arthroscopic anterior column stabilization, that provides a 10 × 5 mm id working area *(4,5)* (available from Stryker, Howmedica, Osteonics, Allendale, NJ).

   I and others have used a series of telescoping oval cannulas (Fig. 2) in order to maximize access to the intervertebral disc for the introduction of bone grafts. These cannulas were designed to fit within the dimensions of the triangular working zone. Because the height of the triangular working zone is somewhat limited by the height of the intervertebral disc, oval cannulas will not exert undue traction to the neural structures when it lies within the triangular working zone. A 10- and a 12- mm oval cannular jig permits parallel insertion of both a cannulated obturator and a half- or full-moon auxiliary obturator in preparation of insertion of 10- or 12-mm cannulas (Fig. 3A,B).
4. Triphens: Two sizes of triphens are available that can be used for annular fenestration or cutting and removing osteophytes. Both triphens fit within the lumen of the 5-mm cannula, which was previously described (Fig. 4). Three working scopes are available in 0, 8, and

From: *Arthroscopic and Endoscopic Spinal Surgery: Text and Atlas: Second Edition*
Edited by: P. Kambin © Humana Press Inc., Totowa, NJ

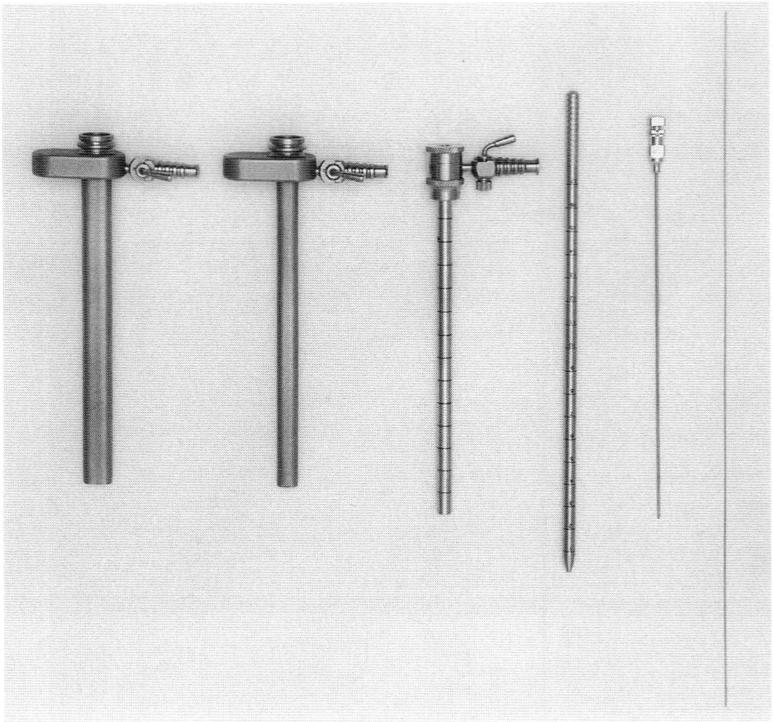

Fig. 1. Instruments for spinal surgery. Shown are from left to right a 5 × 10 mm id oval cannula, a 5 × 8 mm id oval cannula, a 5 × 5 mm id cannula, a cannulated obturator, an 18-gage needle, and guide wire.

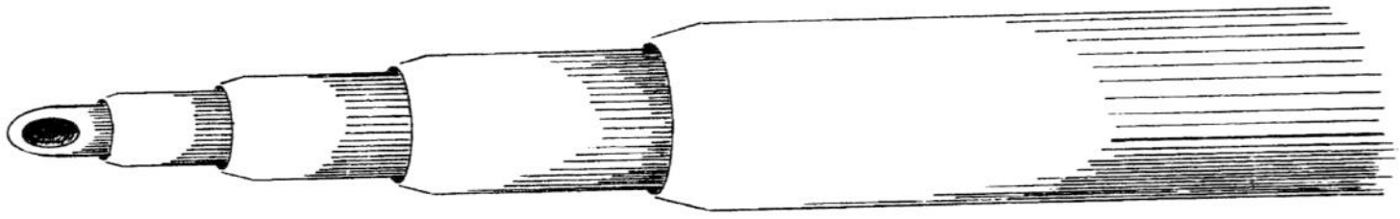

Fig. 2. Schematic drawing of a series of telescopic cannulas.

20° models. The working channel of these instruments accommodates small-caliber forceps, knives, curettes, a radiofrequency coagulator, and palpating instruments (Fig. 5).

5. Arthroscopes: A variety of 0, 30, and 70° arthroscopes are available for intradiscal and periannular surgery. These scopes may be used with the appropriate irrigation sheaths in conjunction with round or oval-shaped cannulas (Fig. 6).
6. Straight-upbiting and flexible-tipped forceps (Fig. 7).
7. Articulating suction forceps.
8. Deflecting tube that permits 40° dorsal angulation of the flexible-tipped forceps when it is fully inserted into the deflecting tube.
9. Variety of powered trimmer blades (disc shavers).
10. Monopolar or bipolar radiofrequency coagulator.
11. Video equipment that is available in most operating room settings.

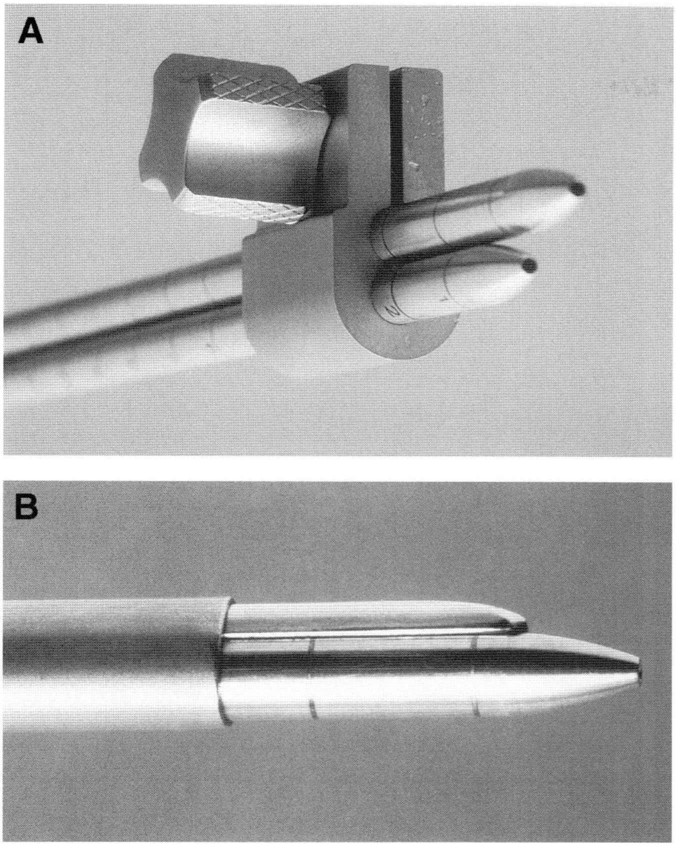

Fig. 3. (A) Jig for insertion of two cannulated obturators in preparation of insertion of 5 × 10 mm oval cannula. **(B)** A cannulated obturator and a half-moon obturator are inserted into the intervertebral disc in preparation of insertion of a 5 × 8 mm id oval cannula.

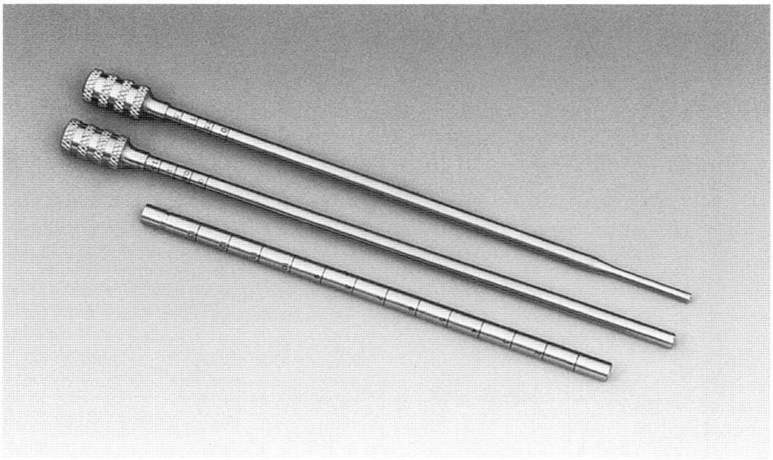

Fig. 4. Shown are from top to bottom a 3-mm triphen, a 5-mm triphen, and a universal 5-mm-id cannula.

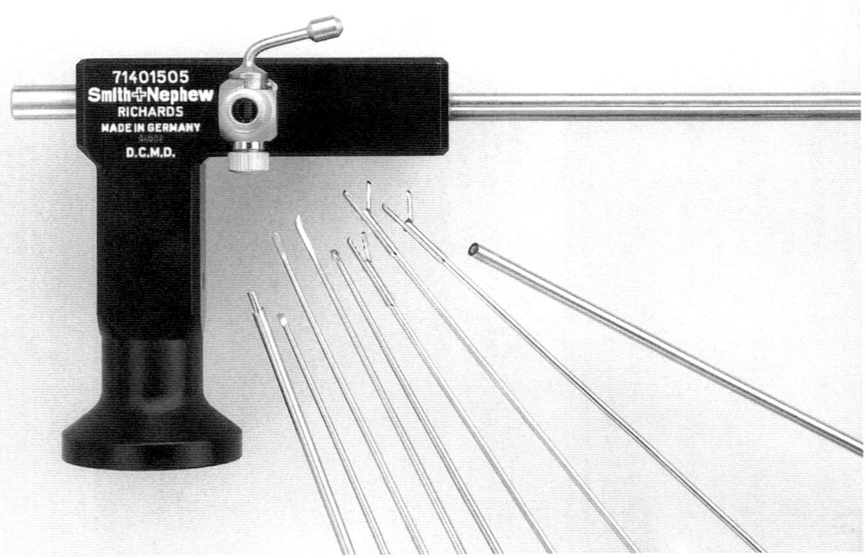

Fig. 5. Working-channel scope with a variety of instruments that can be used in conjunction with working scope.

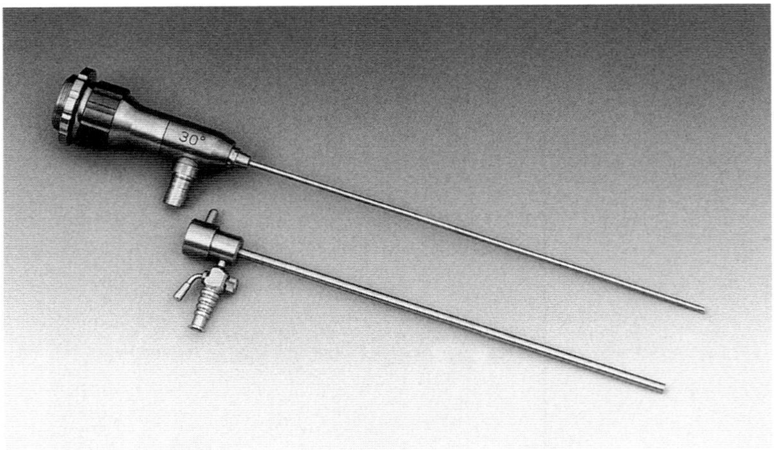

Fig. 6. Three video discoscopes are available: 0, 30, and 70°. The scopes are inserted into the scope sheath, which is used for inflow of saline solution. The scope and the scope sheath assembly fit within the lumen of the 5-mm-id cannula, as well as of the oval cannulas.

SURGICAL APPROACHES

A variety of approaches have been used to access the intervertebral discs and vertebral bodies in the lumbar region. Selection of the surgical approach is largely dictated by the site of the pathology and the experience of the operating surgeon with the particular approach.

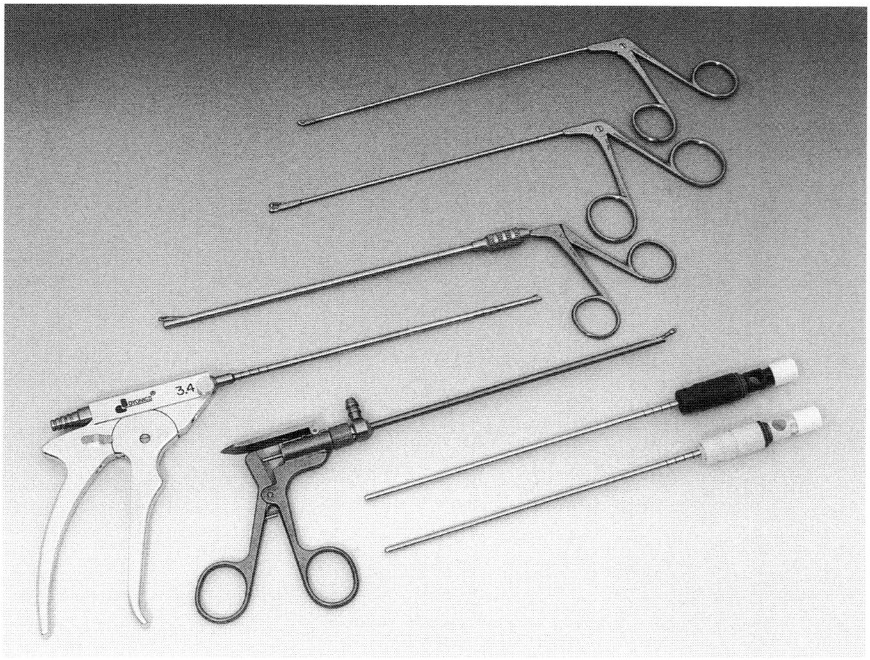

Fig. 7. Additional instruments used for arthroscopic and endoscopic spinal surgery. From top to bottom, upbiting forceps, straight punch forceps, deflecting tube and flexible-tip forceps, punch forceps, deflecting suction forceps, and a variety of trimmer blades (disco shavers).

Uniportal Approach

A 5 × 5 mm or 5 × 8 mm id cannula is commonly used for uniportal access to the herniated disc fragments in the lumbar region *(1,2,5)* (Fig. 8A,B). A larger-diameter cannula may also be telescoped over the 5 × 5 mm id cannula to provide wider access to the intervertebral disc. A working channel scope is usually used with a 5-mm-id cannula. However, a 5 × 8 mm id cannula provides additional advantages by simultaneously accommodating a 0 or 30° arthroscope, larger forceps, and resecting instruments *(3–5)* (Fig. 9A,B).

The uniportal approach is commonly utilized for retrieval of paramedial, small central, foraminal, and extraforaminal herniations (see Chapter 4). Uniportal use of a 5 mm id cannula also provides adequate access for a transforaminal approach to the spinal canal (*see* Chapter 4).

Bilateral Biportal Approach

In the bilateral biportal technique, two cannulas are inserted contralaterally from the right and left sides of the intervertebral disc (Fig. 10A,B). A small cavity is created posteriorly adjacent to the spinal canal by resection of nuclear tissue and torn fibers of the annulus and the posterior longitudinal ligament. Communication between the right and left portals is essential to establish free inflow of saline into one portal and outflow from the opposite portal. A radiofrequency probe has been most helpful in vaporizing nuclear tissue and establishing communication between the two portals *(2,3,5)*. Adequate

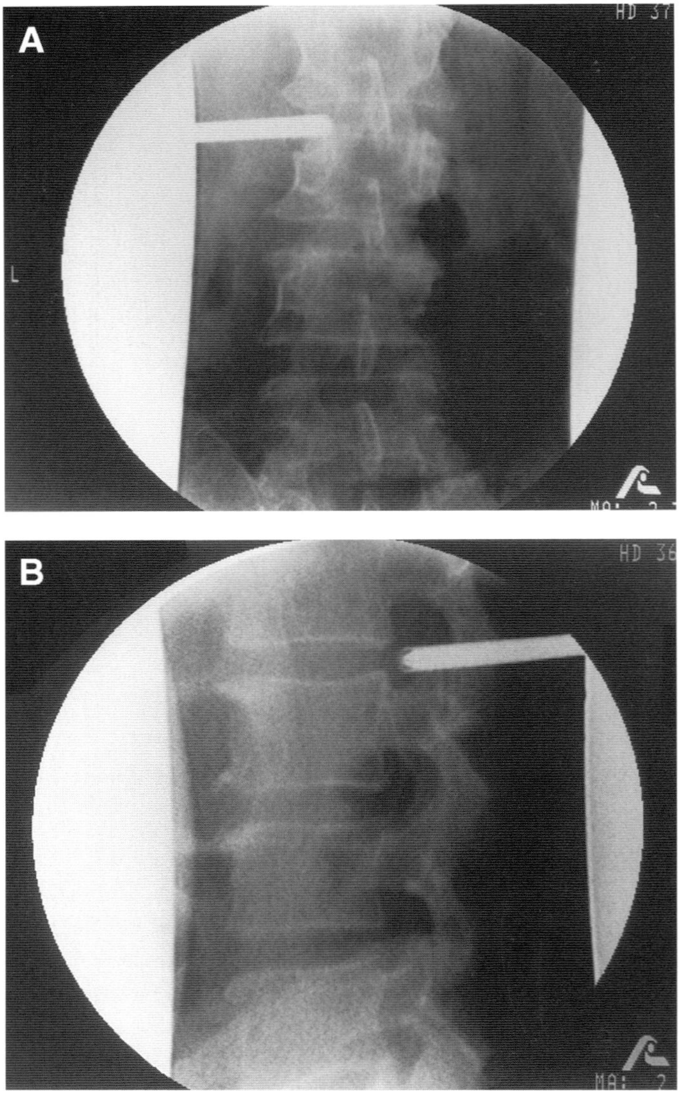

Fig. 8. **(A)** Properly positioned cannula at medial pedicular line for access to content of spinal canal at L2-L3 level; **(B)** lateral interoperative fluoroscopic view of position of tip of cannula adjacent to posterior boundary of L2-L3.

visualization is accomplished by insertion of a 70 or 90° arthroscope from one portal and introduction of articulating or upbiting forceps from the opposite portal. The bilateral biportal approach is suitable for removal of large central herniations and sequestered nonmigrated disc fragments. Following retrieval of a sequestered disc fragment, the ventral surface of the dura is usually visualized with the arthroscope that is inserted into the intervertebral disc. Retrieval of a sequestered fragment from the spinal canal is usually

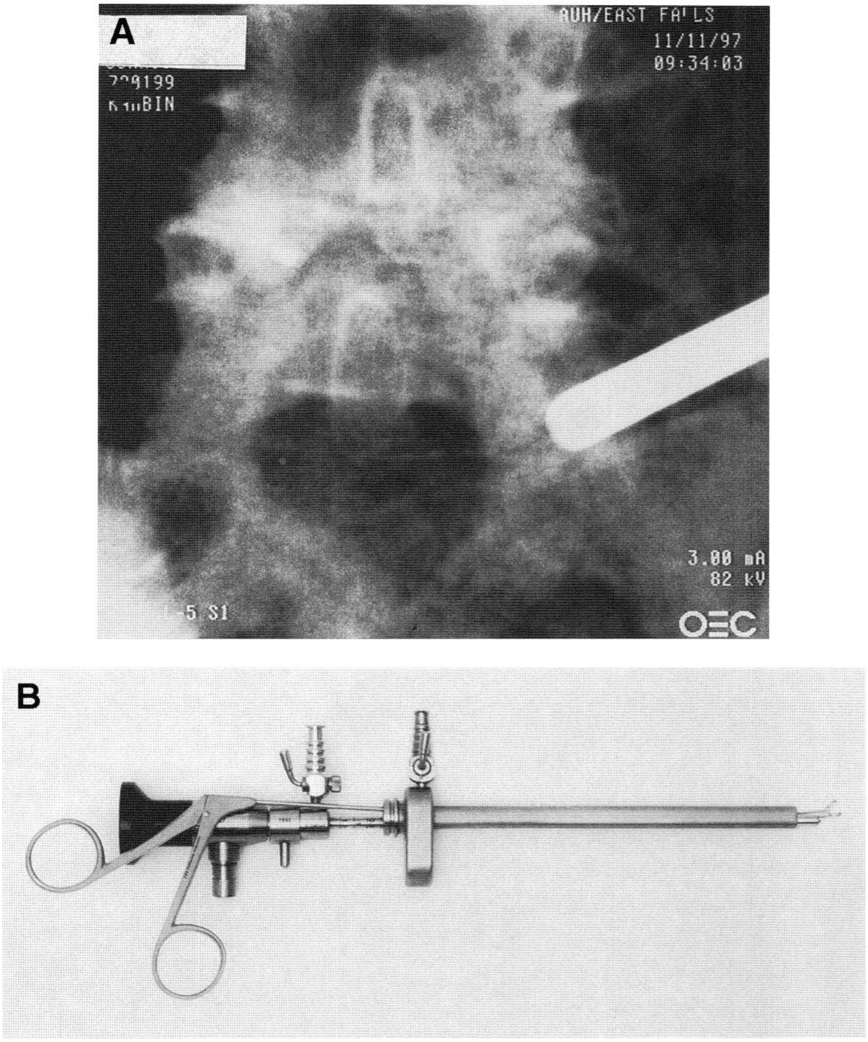

Fig. 9. **(A)** Interoperative fluoroscopic examination showing position of 5 × 8 mm id oval cannula at L5-S1 in anteroposterior projection. **(B)** Flexible-tip forceps and 30° arthroscopes are used in conjunction with a 5 × 8 mm id oval cannula for visualization and removal of larger disc fragments.

followed by a discharge of venous blood into the disc cavity. This blood has a tendency to coagulate when the instruments are removed.

In addition, bilateral biportal access is necessary for anterior column stabilization when a minimally invasive posterolateral approach is employed (*see* Chapter 5).

Unilateral Biportal Approach

In the unilateral biportal approach, two parallel or converging cannulas are positioned in the triangular working zone with the aid of specially designed jigs. The two parallel

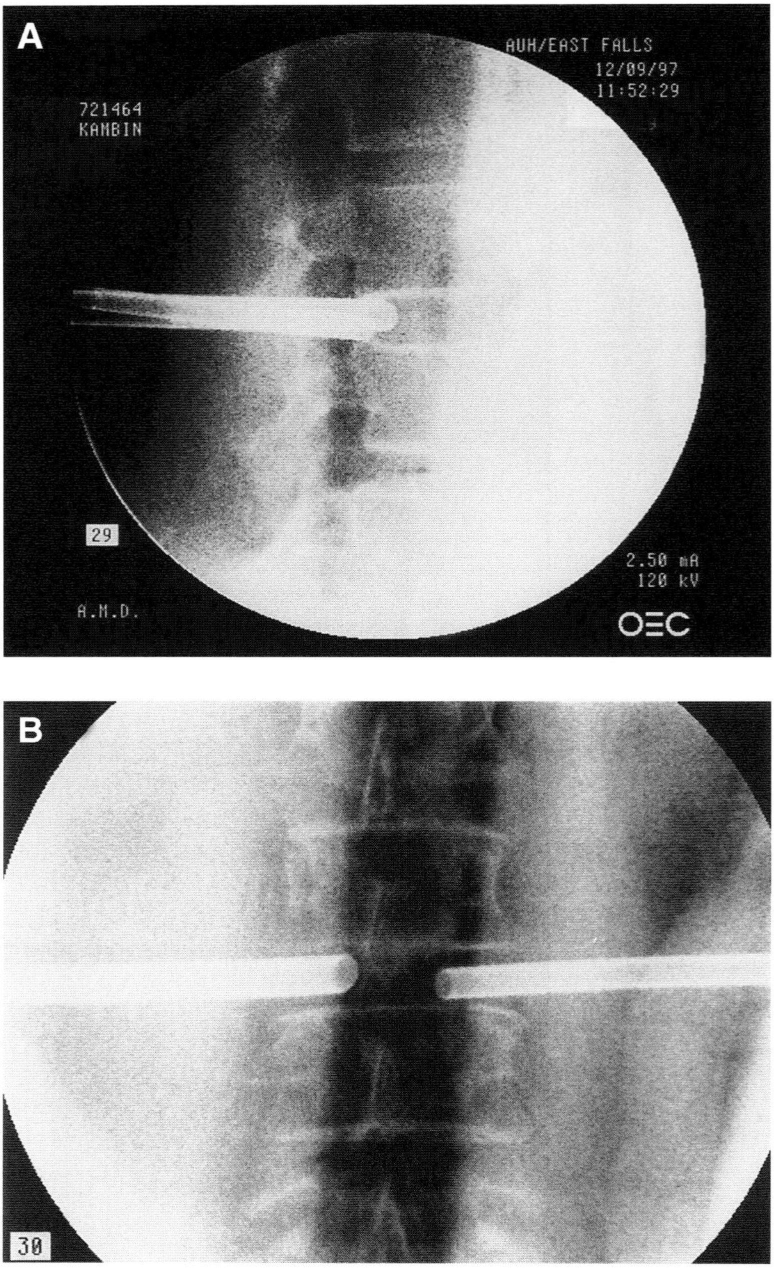

Fig. 10. **(A)** Interoperative lateral fluoroscopic examination of biportal access to L3-L4 intervertebral disc. Note the posterior position of the instruments adjacent to the spinal canal. **(B)** Anteroposterior fluoroscopic examination of position of cannulas shown in (A). Note that a 5 × 8 mm id oval cannula is used on the left and a 5-mm-id cannula on the right. The cannulas are positioned for removal of a centrally located sequestrated disc herniation.

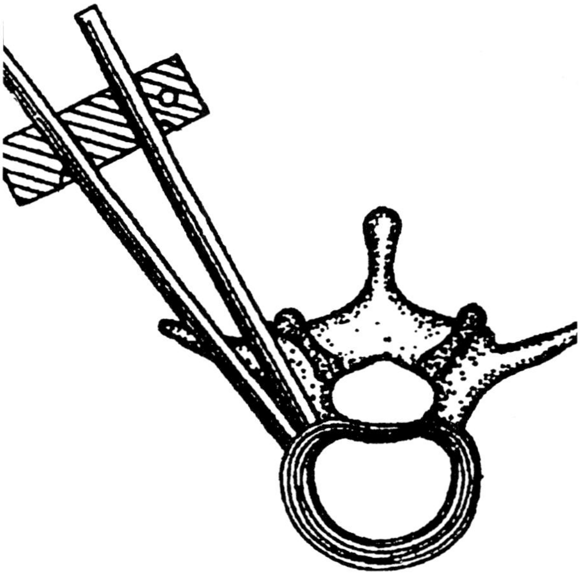

Fig. 11. Schematic drawing of unilateral biportal access to foramen utilizing specially designed jig.

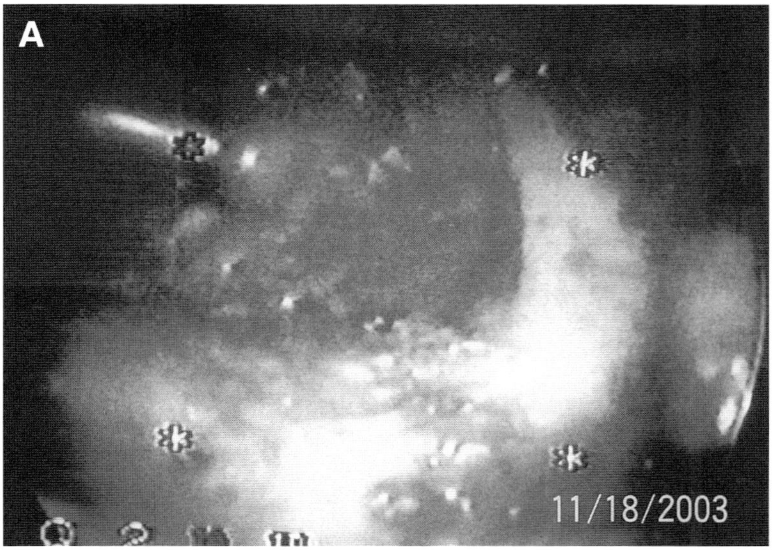

Fig. 12. (A) Intraoperative endoscopic review demonstrating how high-speed diamond burr is being used for laminatomy. **(B)** Intraoperative photograph following laminatomy and partial facetectomy. Note the dural sac at the top of the photograph and the herniated disc in the axilla of the traversing nerve root. **(C)** Schematic drawing of **(B)**.

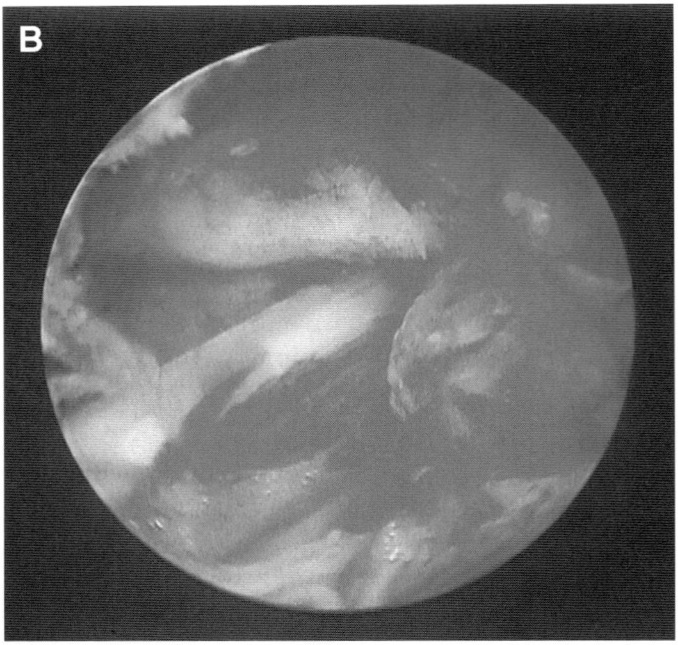

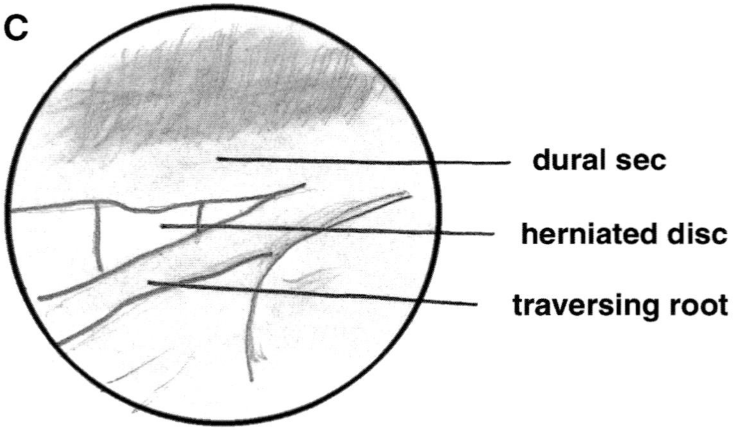

Fig. 12. *(Continued)*

obturators then may be replaced with an oval-shaped cannula that provides wider access to the intervertebral disc *(4,5)* (Figs. 1 and 3). The 5 × 8 mm id cannula (Fig. 9A,B) is suitable for intradiscal or subligamentous access to a disc herniation. It also may be used for retrieval of extraforaminal and foraminal herniations. The 5 × 10 mm id cannula (Figs. 1 and 3A) is commonly utilized in the course of arthroscopic anterior column stabilization. Two converging cannulas are useful for visualization and removal of foraminal and extraforaminal herniations (Fig. 11) *(5,6)*.

Interlaminar Access

Endoscopic interlaminar access to the content of the spinal canal and the lateral recess follows the principle of already established open operative procedures (*see* Fig. 18 in Chapter 1). Although originally my colleagues and I used a working cannula with a side window *(3–5)* for insertion of a straight arthroscope, with the availability of 45 and 90° angled arthroscopes (Figs. 3–5) in the pursuing years, we were able to introduce the arthroscope and resecting instruments directly from the proximal opening of the cannula into the surgical field. We have used a high-speed diamond burr for laminatomy (Figs. 3–12A), and the retrieval of disc fragments has been similar to that of known techniques used during open procedures.

REFERENCES

1. Kambin P, Gellman H. Percutaneous lateral discectomy of the lumbar spine: a preliminary report. Clin Orthop 1983;174:127–132.
2. Kambin P. Arthroscopic microdiscectomy. Arthroscopy 1992;8:287–295.
3. Kambin P. Arthroscopic techniques for spinal surgery, in Operative Arthroscopy (McGinty JB, Casperi RB, Jackson RW, Poehling GG, eds.), Lippincott-Raven, Philadelphia, 1996, pp. 1215–1225.
4. Kambin P, Gennarelli T, Hermantin F. Minimally invasive techniques in spinal surgery: current practice. Neurosurg Focus 1998;4(2):1–10.
5. Kambin P. Arthroscopic microdiscectomy, in The Adult Spine: Principles and Practice, 2nd ed. (Frymoyer JW, Ducker T, Hadler N, et al. eds.), Raven, New York, 1996, pp. 2023–2036.
6. Kambin P. Unilateral biportal percutaneous surgical procedures and instrumentation. US patent 5,395,317, October 1991.

4
Herniated Lumbar Disc and Lumbar Radiculopathy

Parviz Kambin, MD

DIAGNOSIS OF LUMBAR DISC HERNIATIONS: INCLUSION AND EXCLUSION CRITERIA

The satisfactory outcome of arthroscopically and endoscopically assisted management of herniated lumbar discs hinges on accurate diagnosis of the symptom-producing site. Although the mean age of onset of symptoms of disc herniation is around 35 yr, disc herniations are occasionally observed in populations older than 60 or younger than 20 yr of age. In younger children, combined slippage of the intervertebral disc and the vertebral plates may be responsible for the presenting symptomatology.

A careful assessment of the patient's complaints followed by a thorough physical examination is the essential and most reliable initial step in arriving at an accurate diagnosis. A simple questionnaire that includes a pain analog scale will provide a wealth of information to the operating surgeon. When the distribution of pain extends to a level below the knee or involves the calf or lateral aspect of the leg, the surgeon's attention is directed toward L5 or S1 root involvement. By contrast, disc herniation in the middle or upper lumbar spine is associated with anterior thigh or groin pain. Similarly, expression of numbness or "pins and needles" sensations involving the fifth toe or calf area suggests S1 root compression most likely at the L5-S1 level. However, when similar complaints are expressed on the dorsum of the great toe and lateral aspect of the leg, attention should be drawn to L5 nerve root involvement.

The presence of midline localized tenderness at the index level, sciatic tilt, and tenderness over the sciatic notch are objective confirmative findings. A thorough neurological examination to assess reflex and sensory and motor abnormalities is essential. Absence of the achilles reflex suggests an S1 root compression. Unilateral absence of the tibialis posterior reflex should draw attention to L5 root involvement. The patellar reflex may be absent when the L3 or L4 nerve roots are compressed.

Positive tension signs (Fig. 1A), which include a positive straight-leg-raising, Lazarevic test (Fig. 1A) *(1)*; positive Lasegue sign (Fig. 1B,C) *(2,3)*; or positive bow sling sign *(4)*, comprise one of the four essential criteria to consider in surgical management. A positive contralateral straight-leg-raising test suggests a midline or paramedial herniation. A positive reverse Lasegue sign or femoral stretching test indicates pressure on the L3 or L4 nerve roots.

From: *Arthroscopic and Endoscopic Spinal Surgery: Text and Atlas: Second Edition*
Edited by: P. Kambin © Humana Press Inc., Totowa, NJ

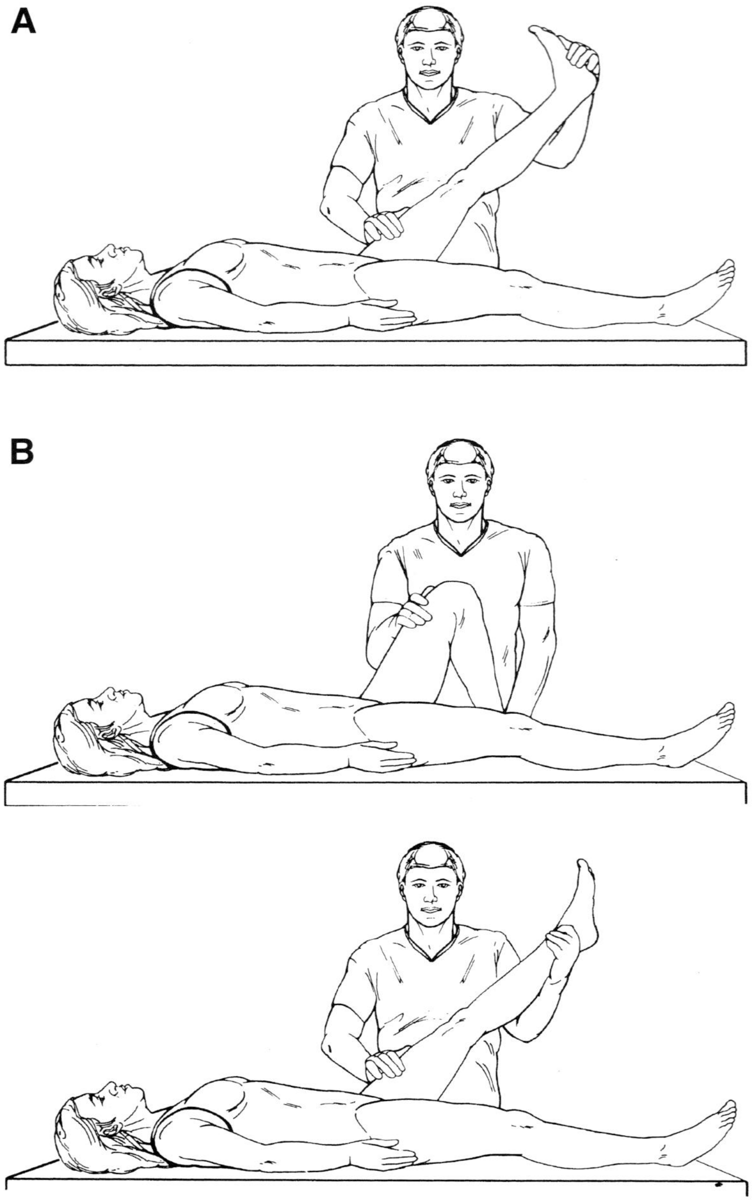

Fig. 1. **(A)** Straight-leg-raising test described by Lazarevic. While the leg is being raised and the knee is kept in full extension, the ankle is dorsoflexed. The patient's radicular pain is reproduced. **(B)** The Lasègue test consist of two phases. The hip and the knee on the symptomatic side are first flexed. If the patient has hip disorder, the pain is reproduced. In phase two of the test, the leg is raised while the hip and knee of the affected side are kept in full extension. **(C)** Bow-sling sign described by Cram. In the sitting position, the leg is raised while the knee is kept in flexion. Then the knee is gradually brought into full extension while the examiner's hand applies pressure to the sciatic trunk in the popliteal region.

C

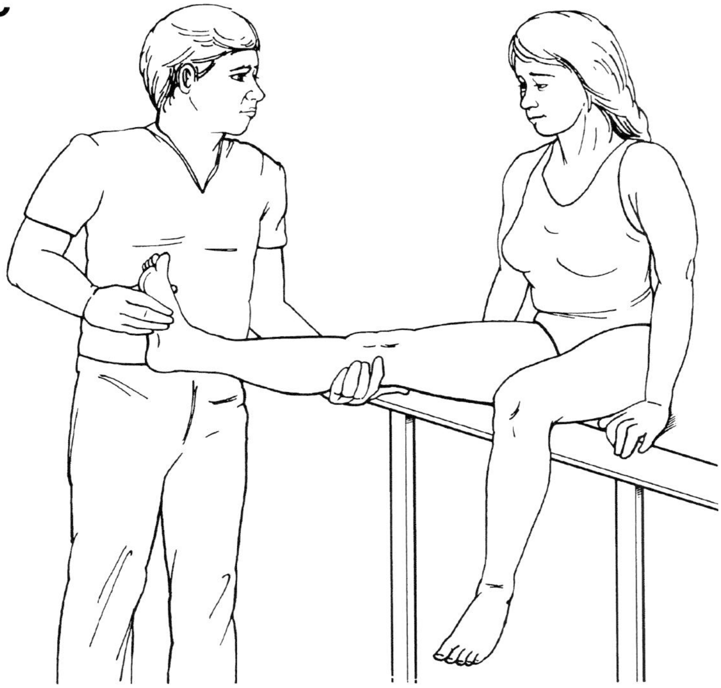

Fig. 1. *(Continued)*

Nerve root tension may be tested with the patient standing erect while the examiner evaluates the presence or absence of points of tenderness, muscle rigidity, and range of motion of the lumbar spine. In the standing position, the patient is instructed to lean forward and slightly bend laterally toward the symptomatic side while holding the knees in full extension. When a paramedial herniation is present, forward flexion with a slight lateral bending may reproduce the radicular symptoms (Fig. 2) *(5,6)*.

Individuals with a lateral disc herniation usually complain of unilateral leg pain that may be associated with positive tension signs and with sensory and motor deficits. By contrast, patients with a central or slightly paramedial disc herniation may have bilateral symptoms or alternating symptomatology affecting one lower extremity or another from time to time. The latter group of patients is more likely to have positive ipsilateral or contralateral straight-leg-raising tests.

Compression of the exiting root in the foraminal canal may be related to a contained interannular disc protrusion. This type of herniation invariably extends to the lateral boundary of the spinal canal, thus causing ipsilateral compression on both the traversing and exiting roots (Fig. 3). A sequestered foraminal herniation may migrate away from the intervertebral disc, caudal or cephalad to the pedicular region.

At times a sequestered intracanalicular disc herniation migrates laterally into the foraminal canal and causes compression on the exiting root at the index level. Foraminal herniations usually have an acute onset with intense radicular symptoms. However, low-back pain may be absent or minimal.

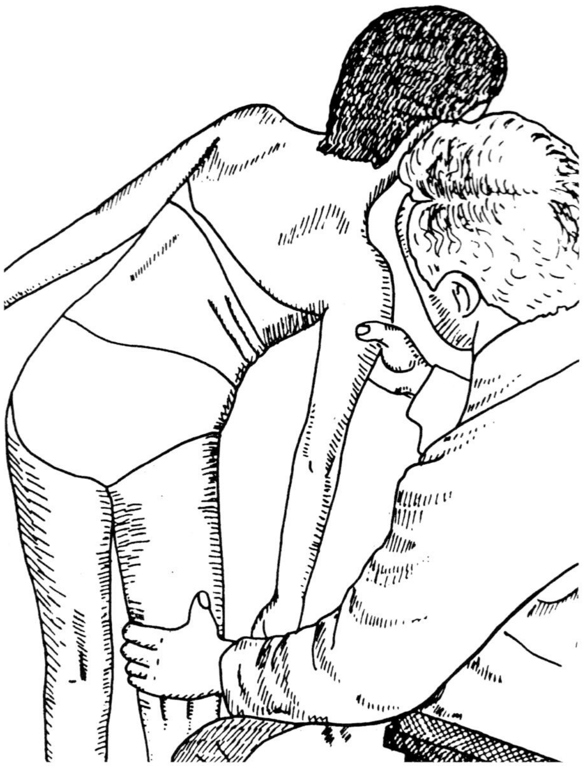

Fig. 2. As described by Kambin: in the standing position, the patient is instructed to lean forward and slightly bend toward the symptomatic leg while the examiner maintains the patient's knee in full extension. (Reprinted from ref. *43*, with permission.)

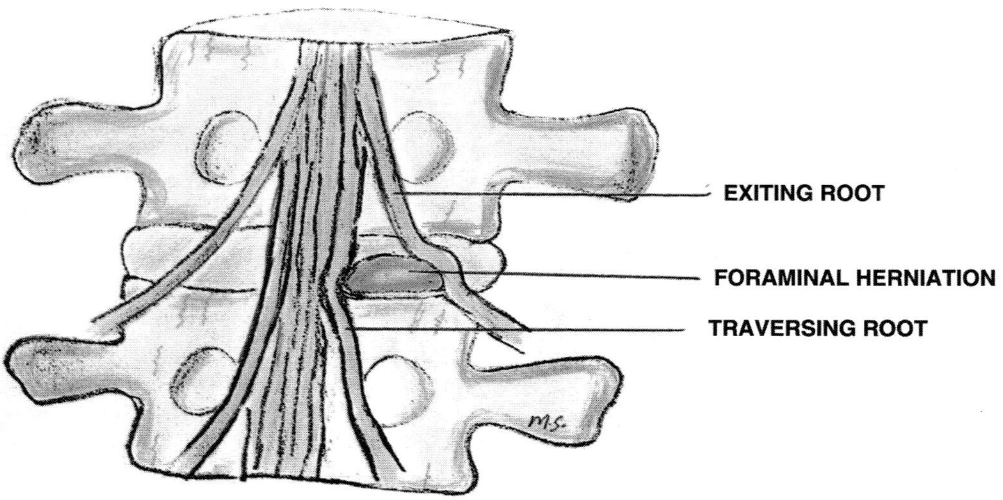

Fig. 3. Schematic drawing demonstrating how a foraminal herniation can cause compression on both exiting and traversing roots.

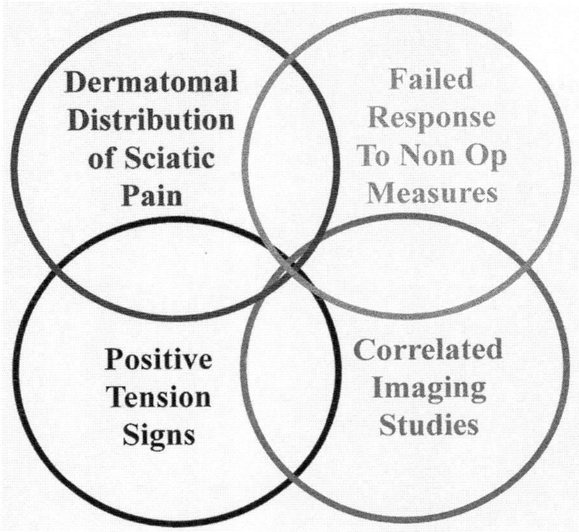

Fig. 4. The four prerequisites for surgical intervention in treatment of herniated lumbar discs.

When the nerve root ganglion has been compressed in addition to the above, patients present signs and symptoms of sympathetic nerve involvement, such as severe skin hypersensitivity to touch or a sense of coldness or excess heat in the involved limb.

As with foraminal herniations, compression and tension on the exiting root in the extraforaminal region is usually associated with intense radicular symptomatology with minimal or no low-back pain.

The history and physical examination should also include a thorough medical and psychological evaluation combined with a work history and history of drug use or dependency. Management of individuals with a history of long-term use of narcotic-based medication is best accomplished by obtaining a preoperative psychological and pain management consultation.

In summary, the inclusion criteria for arthroscopic and endoscopic management of herniated lumbar discs to treat nerve root compression are similar to the accepted criteria for open laminotomy and discectomy. They include failure to respond to a well-designed and executed nonoperative management, correlative dermatomal distribution of pain in the lower extremity, positive tension signs, and positive correlative imaging studies (Fig. 4).

At this state of the art, patients who present with signs and symptoms of cauda equina syndrome should be excluded from arthroscopically and endoscopically assisted microdiscectomy.

Transforaminal access to a large central herniation or sequestered disc at L5-S1 may be difficult in individuals with high iliac crests. However, these herniations may be accessed laterally through a circular fenestration that is made through the iliac crest. Instruments are passed through this fenestration into the intervertebral disc. Individuals with signs and symptoms of lateral recess stenosis may also successfully be treated with arthroscopic techniques. With the availability of bipolar radiofrequency probes and effective topical coagulators, adequate epidural hemostasis can be obtained and sequestered disc herniations can be extracted via endoscopically assisted posterolateral transforaminal access to the spinal canal.

ADVANTAGES OF ARTHROSCOPIC AND ENDOSCOPIC DISC SURGERY

Improvement of Visualization

The availability of small-caliber, rigid-rod endoscopes; three-dimensional cameras; and developing image modification technology has provided operating surgeons with a superior means of visualization and tissue differentiation than the naked eye and microscope. The "aquarium effect" of the technology provides clearer and larger images of anatomical structures.

Although the microscope permits visualization of the dorsolateral aspect of the contents of the spinal canal, spinal endoscopy via a posterolateral approach makes it possible to visualize the medial, lateral, and ventral surfaces of the nerve root and the dural sac without undue manipulation and retraction of neural tissue.

Lowered Incidence of Reherniation

Recurrent herniation following open laminotomy and discectomy is not uncommon. Atken and Bradford *(7)* reported an incidence of reherniation up to 24%. Balderston et al. *(8)* reported recurrent herniation of 12% in two groups of patients who underwent open discectomy with simple fragment extraction or fragment removal and curettage of the disc space. They reported similar outcomes in both groups. Recurrent disc herniations at the site of previous surgery may be diagnosed with enhanced magnetic resonance imaging (MRI) studies. However, many of these herniations are asymptomatic and do not require surgical management. During open translaminar discectomy, annular fenestration is performed at the apex of the herniation. Therefore, the containing ability of the annular ring is further weakened. This invites expulsion of nuclear tissue into the epidural space, particularly when the spine is exposed to flexion and rotational forces during the patient's work and activities. The posterolateral annulus appears to be a more desirable area for annulotomy. The natural axial width and intact fibers of the posterolateral annulus (Fig. 13A in Chapter 2) combined with its inherent contractibility may minimize the incidence of reherniation through the surgically induced annular fenestration. The anatomical position of the facet joints also inhibits undue transmission of external forces to the posterolateral boundary of the annulus fibrosis, therefore limiting expulsion of nuclear tissue through the posterolateral annular defect.

In an animal model, Hampton et al. *(9)* reported on the healing potential of a surgically induced defect in the annular fibers of 10 dogs. The dogs were sacrificed within 3–12 wk postoperatively. Dissection of the surgical site demonstrated that the defect was filled with a solid plug of fibrous structures. Postoperative imaging studies by my colleagues and I on patients who had undergone percutaneous posterolateral discectomy confirmed these findings. Markolf and Morris *(10)* reported a decrease in compressive stiffness and an increase in creep and the relaxation rate of the intervertebral disc in cadaveric specimens that were exposed to annular fenestration and then followed by exposure of the spinal unit to compressive forces. In younger specimens, extrusion of nuclear tissue had a tendency to seal off the annular defect and to restore normal function of the spinal unit.

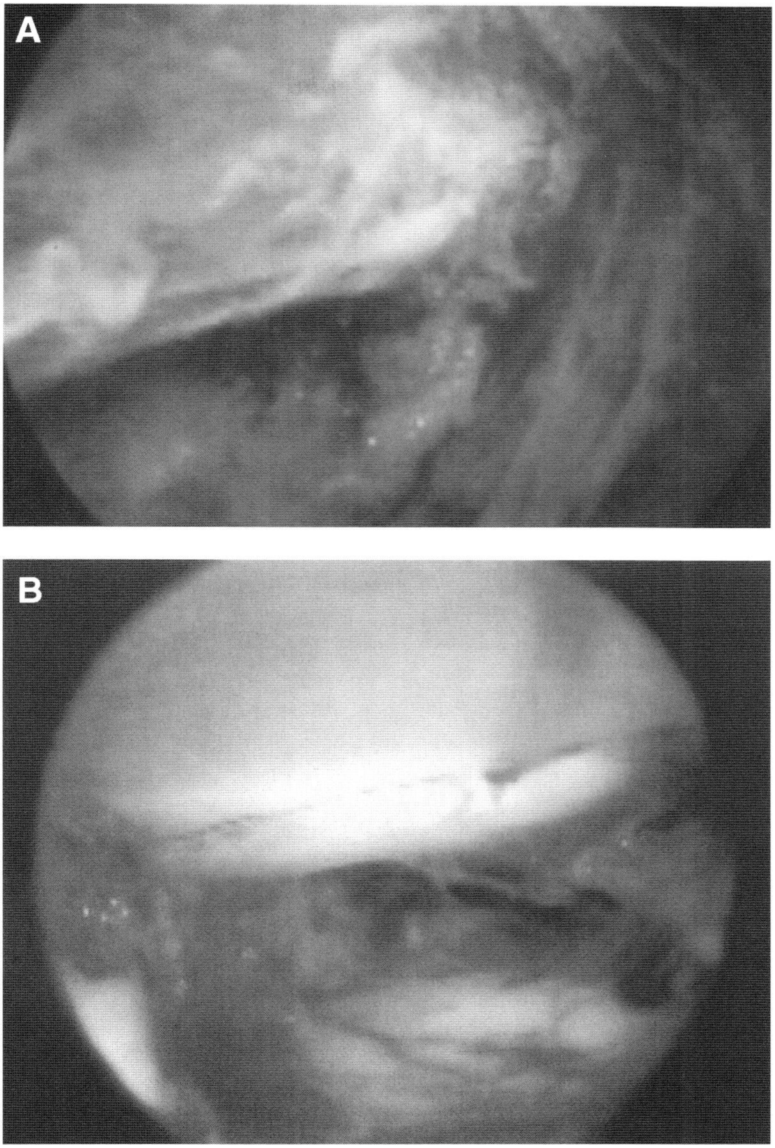

Fig. 5. **(A)** Interoperative endoscopic view of patient who had laminotomy and discectomy 2 yr earlier. Note the massive epidural and perineural scar formation. **(B)** Endoscopic view of virgin spine showing clear visualization of traversing root and epidural space.

Reduction in Incidence of Nerve Root Tethering and Formation of Epidural Scar Tissue

Although perineural and epidural scar tissue may not be pain-producing structures, tethering of the nerve root and dural sac has a tendency to inhibit smooth mobility and gliding of these structures in flexion and extension (Fig. 5A,B; *see also* Figs 9 and 12 in Chapter 2). Nerve root tethering may be responsible for recurrence of sciatic pain when the patient has resumed normal physical activities following the surgical procedure *(11)*. Epidural application of a fat graft, Gelfoam, and other artificial materials has proven to be unsatisfactory in the prevention of epidural and perineural fibrosis after open spine surgery. I have emphasized avoiding manipulation of the content of the spinal canal and suggested subligamentous access to contained and nonmigrated extraligamentous herniations *(12)*.

Protection of Epidural Venous System and Minimization of Nerve Root Trauma

The delicate venous system of nerve roots may be further traumatized by undue intraoperative manipulation and retraction. Haaland et al. *(13)*, Park *(14,15)*, and other investigators *(16)* have emphasized the importance of patency of neural venous systems in the prevention of venous stasis, which is invariably followed by neural edema, ischemia, and the development of pain (Fig. 6A) in a clinical setting. The presence of neural edema has been objectively demonstrated with postoperative MRI studies following an exercise program (Fig. 6B).

Maintenance of Integrity of Paraspinal Muscles

During arthroscopic or endoscopic spinal surgery, the paraspinal muscles, namely the erector spinalis, sacrospinalis, quadratus lumbrorum, and psoas major, are not severed, stripped, or retracted. A small soft-tissue dilator with a 4.9-mm outer diameter (od) has a tendency to separate the muscle fibers and descend toward the annulus at the index level. This reduces the postoperative morbidity and eliminates potential denervation and muscle injury *(17–20)*. The derangement of the muscle fibers and massive scar formation may be readily observed in postoperative MRI studies of patients who have been exposed to traditional open spinal surgery (Fig. 7).

Maintenance of Spinal Stability

When posterolateral arthroscopically or endoscopically assisted disc extraction is attempted, the facet joints and bony structures are not disturbed. Therefore, the incidence of postoperative instability, spondylolisthesis, and rapid collapse and narrowing of the disc spaces is reduced *(21)*.

Facilitation of Postoperative Imaging Studies

When a subligamentous approach for removal of a disc herniation is utilized, the contents of the spinal canal are not manipulated nor disturbed. The absence of epidural and perineural fibrosis (Fig. 8A–D) facilitates accurate postoperative imaging evaluation of the contents of the spinal canal if it becomes necessary *(22)*. My clinical observation has been that even when transforaminal access for retrieval of sequestered fragments under fluid medium was attempted, the incidence of postoperative scar formation appeared to be less prevalent than with open laminotomy and discectomy.

Facilitation of Accurate Intraoperative Documentation

The entire operative procedure may be documented for future reference or teaching purposes via either intraoperative photography or videotape.

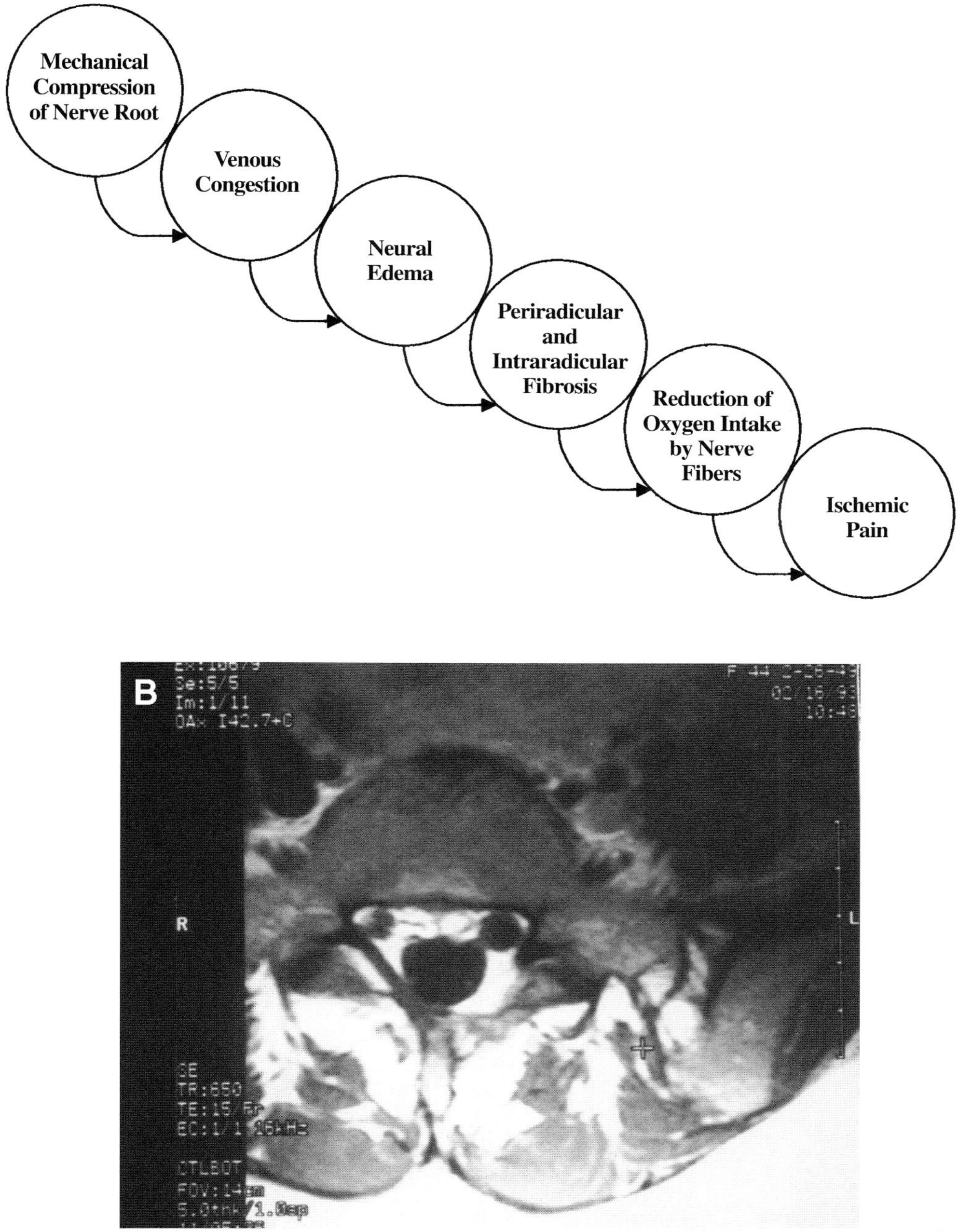

Fig. 6. **(A)** Schematic drawing demonstrating how venous obstruction of nerve root and neural edema can become symptom producing. **(B)** Postlaminotomy MRI study of surgical site following exercise program associated with recurrence of symptoms and MRI evidence of ipsilateral neural edema.

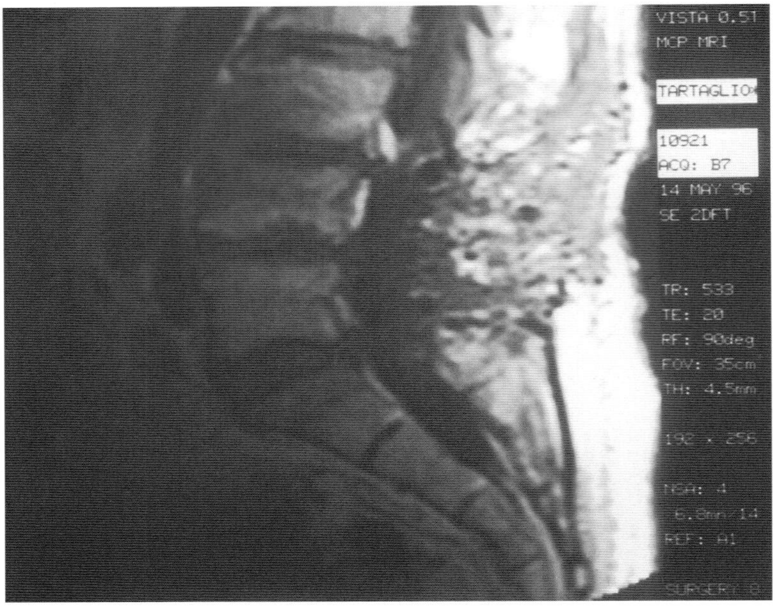

Fig. 7. Post open surgery MRI study of lumbar spine demonstrating disruption and derangement of muscular tissue.

Cost-Effectiveness

The use of regional anesthetics during arthroscopic and endoscopic spinal surgery combined with minimal postoperative morbidity has eliminated the need for hospitalization and lengthy postoperative rehabilitation. Currently, most minimally invasive operative procedures are being performed in short-procedure units on an ambulatory basis. This has contributed to the cost-effectiveness of minimally invasive spinal surgery.

ABCs OF OPERATIVE TECHNIQUES

Arthroscopic or endoscopic spinal surgery via a posterolateral approach is performed through the triangular working zone located on the posterolateral annulus *(5,23,24)*. Considering that the intervertebral disc is an amphiarthrosis when the surgery is being performed via an intradiscal approach, the term *arthroscopic surgery* is applicable. Some investigators have used the term *endoscopic spinal surgery* to describe the posterolateral approach to the contents of the spinal canal. However, note that the spinal canal is not a cavity, so the term *extra-articular* or *periannular arthroscopic discectomy* may be more appropriate.

Choice of Operating Room Table

The operating room table for arthroscopic spinal surgery must be radiolucent and relatively narrow so that the C-arm can be rotated from the anteroposterior (AP) to the lateral projection with minimal risk of contaminating the surgical field.

A pacemaker extension may be attached to the available operating room table and used for minimally invasive spinal surgery. A disadvantage of this arrangement is the

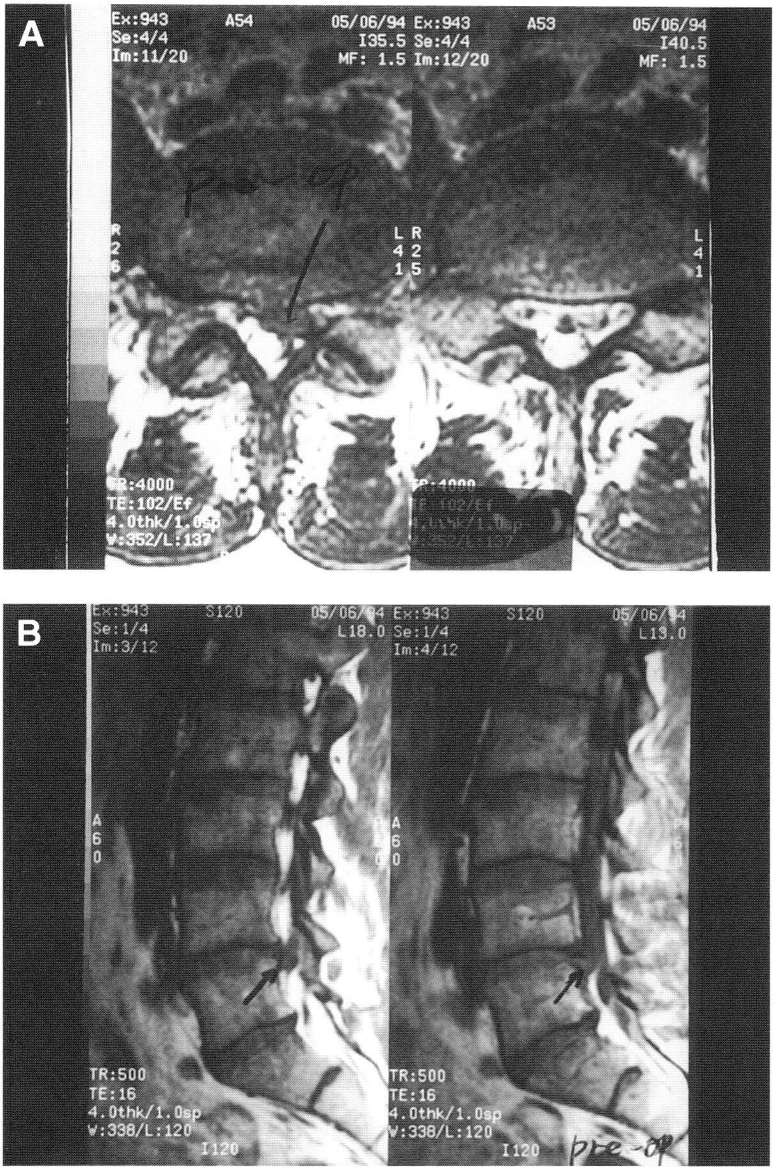

Fig. 8. **(A)** Preoperative axial MRI demonstrating sequestrated disc herniation at L4-L5; **(B)** sagittal MRI findings shown in (A); **(C)** postoperative axial MRI study shown in (A) demonstrating annular defect at site of disc herniation and evidence of fibrovascular invasion at site of extracted disc fragment; **(D)** sagittal view of findings shown in (C).

potential of inadvertently tilting the pacemaker extension and the table, particularly when an overweight patient is positioned for the surgery. In addition, the anesthesiologist may have difficulty reaching and monitoring the patient's status from the top of the table.

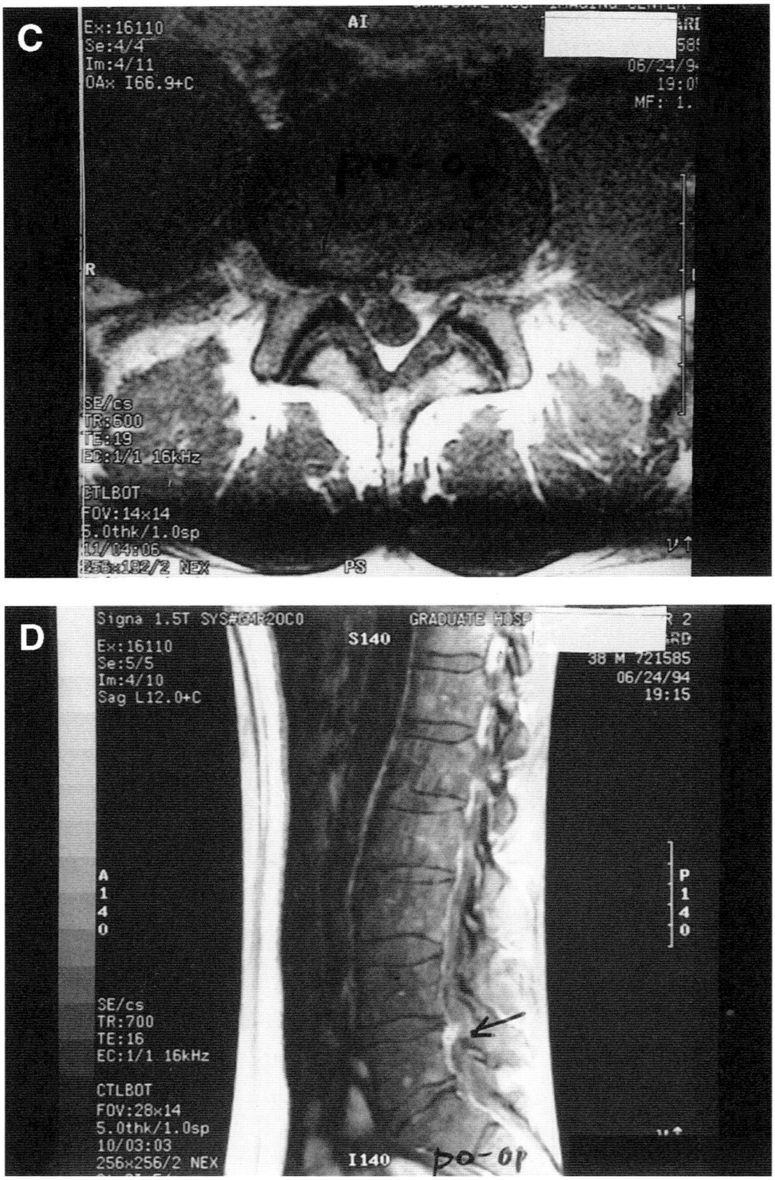

Fig. 8. *(Continued)*

Fracture tables have been used for minimally invasive spinal surgery. The extension of these tables used for positioning of the lower extremities is narrow and suitable for positioning the radiofrequency frame and the patient. This provides ample space for rotation of the C-arm intraoperatively. The AMSCO 3080 table appears to be the table of choice for arthroscopic spinal surgery. It is available in most operating rooms. This table has a long extension that is designed for positioning the lower extremities during surgery. During arthroscopic spinal surgery, we rotate the table and position the radiolucent frame and the patient's trunk and head on the distal end of the table. This allows free rotation of the C-arm around the patient. To further facilitate intraoperative movement of the C-arm, it is advisable to remove the foam mats from the top of the table and place the frame directly on the table.

Radiolucent Frame

Most arthroscopic spinal procedures are performed when the patient is in a prone position. This positioning becomes more critical when biportal access to the intervertebral disc is utilized. The available bolsters (US Medical, Paoli, PA) are comfortable and well padded. They provide ample room for the rib cage and adequate support for the patient's iliac crest and anterior superior iliac spine, thereby allowing reversal of lumbar lordosis (Fig. 9A), slight flexion of the hip joints, and widening of the dimensions of the foramen, so that the inserted instruments can be passed into the foramen and triangular working zone.

Prior to positioning of the patient, the bolsters of the frame should be adjusted to the size of the patient. The proximal ends of the bolster should be placed far enough apart to provide space for the patient's rib cage. In addition, the distal ends of the bolsters should be brought together so that they provide adequate support under the patient's iliac crest (Fig. 9B).

C-Arm

Although a number of C-arms are available in the marketplace, a C-arm with a wide arch is most desirable for arthroscopic and endoscopic spinal surgery. This permits unrestricted rotation of the C-arm for both AP and lateral exposure. Whether the C-arm should be positioned next to the operating surgeon or on the opposite side of the table is not important. I prefer positioning the C-arm on the symptomatic side of the patient while the operating surgeon stands on the opposite side (Fig. 10). If the patient presented with right sciatica, the C-arm is positioned on the right side and the instruments are inserted from the right posterolateral access. This permits a favorable radiographic visualization and a better approach to the compressed and inflamed nerve root at the index level. It is advisable to adjust the height of the operating room table and the C-arm at the onset of the procedure to make certain that the C-arm can be moved from the lateral to AP position without obstruction and potential contamination.

The C-arm should be covered with a sterile sheet or plastic and secured with a Kling bandage by wrapping it around the C-arm. The C-arm should always rotate under the table, rather than on top of the operating table.

To have a reproducible AP and lateral image, the C-arm must be rotated 90° for lateral X-ray exposure. One should make certain that the sterile sheet or plastic does not prevent the full 90° rotation of the C-arm.

Positioning of Patient

Prone positioning of the patient on an adjustable radiolucent frame is most desirable for arthroscopic or endoscopic spinal surgery. In this position, any inadvertent movement of the patient during the surgery can be readily corrected by repositioning the patient, thus allowing repeated reproducible interoperative imaging studies *(5,24–26)*.

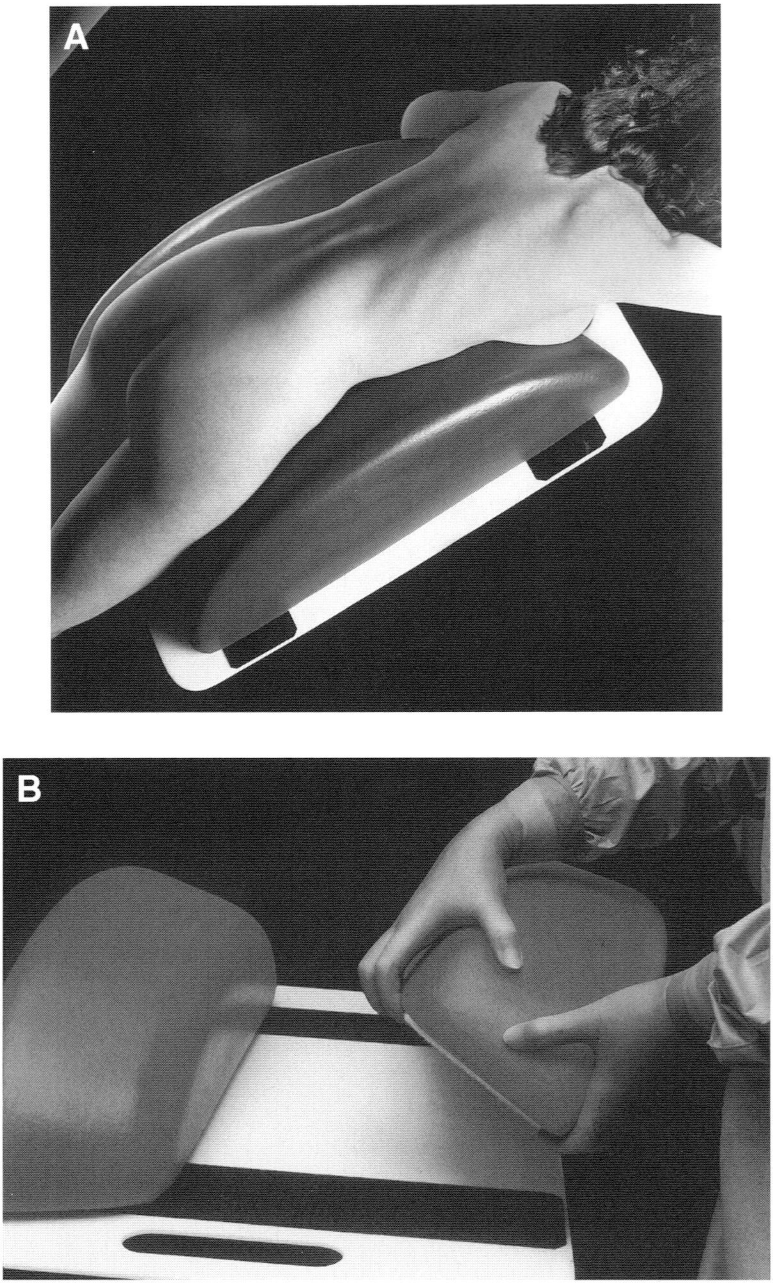

Fig. 9. **(A)** Proper positioning of patient on radiolucent frame. Note the flattening of the lumbar lordosis. **(B)** Adjustment of bolsters to provide support under anterior, superior iliac spine of patient and room for expansion of chest wall. (Frame produced by USA Medical, a division of Universal Services Associates, Inc., Broomall, PA 19008.)

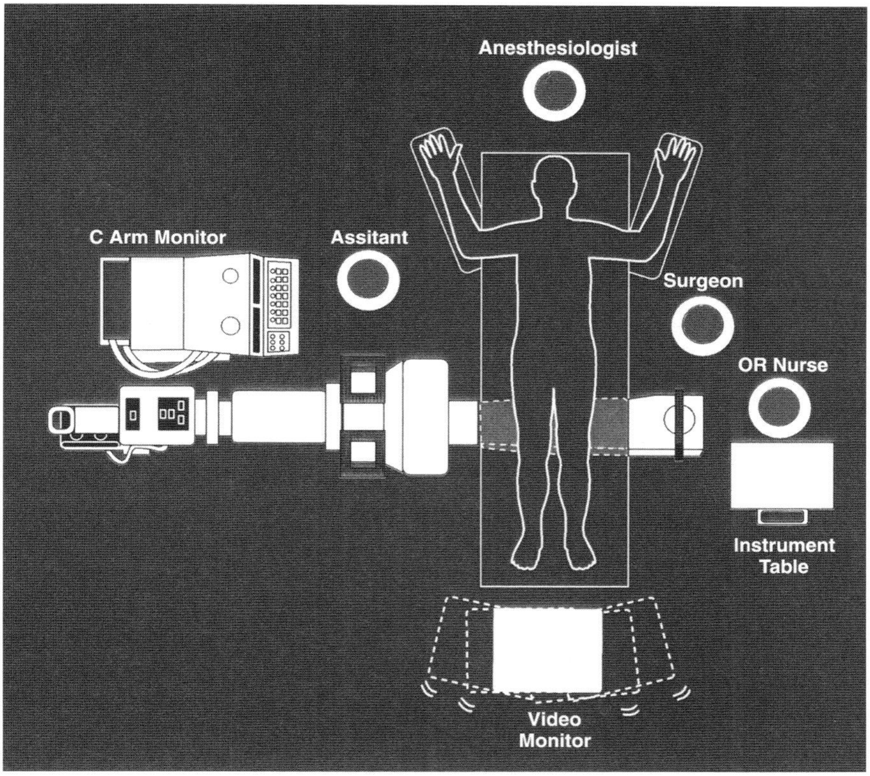

Fig. 10. Drawing demonstrating position of patient and operating room setup for minimally invasive spinal surgery.

In addition, prone positioning of the patient is essential for bilateral biportal access to the intervertebral discs.

It is essential that adequate padding be placed under the kneecaps while the patient is lying in the prone position. If straps are placed on the dorsum of the thighs to secure the patient on the operating room table, adequate padding should be provided to make certain that the peroneal nerve is well protected. Lateral positioning of the patient may be attempted when uniportal access to the L5-S1 intervertebral disc is being attempted. Maintaining the symptomatic side of the patient up and wedging the table will widen the disc space at the index level. This positioning allows the iliac crest to move away from the skin entry site (Fig. 11). In a clinical setting, the lateral positioning of the patient may be practical in younger and more flexible patients. When lateral positioning is used for arthroscopic disc surgery, the patient must be secured on the operating room table with bolsters and adhesive tape. This prevents inadvertent movement and rotation of the trunk during surgery.

Anesthesia

A majority of arthroscopic and endoscopic discectomies can be performed under local anesthesia with the assistance of an anesthesiologist using conscious sedation.

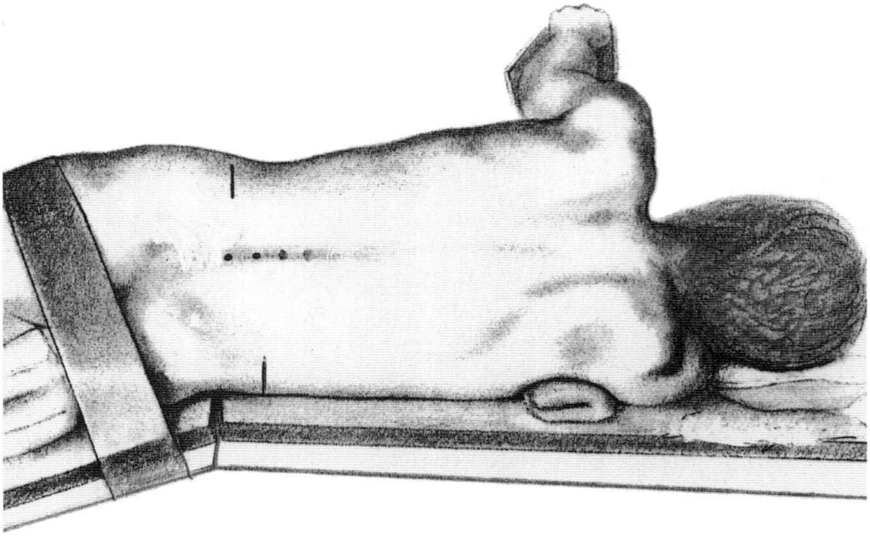

Fig. 11. Lateral positioning of patient on operating room table for access to L5-S1 intervertebral disc.

However, general anesthesia may be employed when ample experience with the operative technique and visual differentiation of the anatomical structures are gained. At the onset of the operative procedure, a 20-gage needle is used and skin, subcutaneous tissue, and muscle layers are infiltrated with 1% Xylocaine® solution. This is then followed by insertion of an 18-gage needle 6 in. in length. The needle is directed toward the foramen at the index level. Injection of a mixture of 1 cc of fentanyl (Elkins Sinn, Cherry Hill, NJ) with 3 cc of saline solution into the foramen as soon as the correct position of the tip of the needle in the triangular working is established may minimize interoperative pain and reduce the incidence of postoperative development of dysesthesia, which has been reported in the literature *(12–27)*. Considering that the expansion of the posterior longitudinal ligamentum in the foramen and the extraforaminal region is highly innervated, prior to annulotomy the annular fibers should be anesthetized with Xylocaine solution via a long 18-gage needle inserted through the previously positioned cannula.

Prophylactic Antibiotic Therapy

In our practice, we have used 1000 mg of Ancef™ (cefazolin sodium) intravenously preoperatively in most of our patients. This is usually administered in the waiting area before the patient is transferred to the operating room. Two additional doses of Ancef are administered at 8 and 16 h postoperatively. Because most of the discectomies are performed on an ambulatory basis, patients are instructed to take two additional 1000-mg doses of Keflex™ (cephalexin hydrochloride) orally every 8 h after their discharge. When a patient presents with a history of sensitivity to cefazolin, this antibiotic is replaced with 500 mg of vancomycin injected preoperatively.

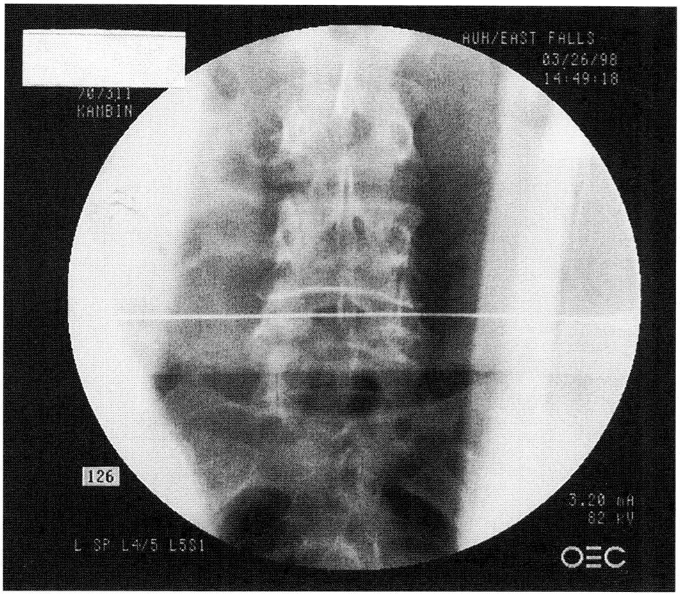

Fig. 12. Interoperative fluoroscopic examination of surgical site. A needle is placed on the skin at the L4-L5 level. An Ap X-ray shows proper positioning of the needle. The skin is marked accordingly prior to surgery.

In addition, we use a dilute solution of gentamicin (Elkin's Sinn) (80 mg in 1000 cc of normal saline) for final irrigation of the surgical site prior to withdrawal of the instruments and final closure.

Identification of Surgical Site

The surgical site must first be identified with an AP and a lateral X-ray study. While the patient is positioned prone, a long needle or a Steinman pin is placed on the top of the skin over the disc space at the index level. The C-arm is then moved into place for AP radiographic exposure. The C-arm may be slightly tilted cephalad to direct the X-ray beams into the intervertebral disc at the surgical site. By moving the needle or Steinman pin cephalad or caudally, the surgical level is identified and the skin is marked accordingly by drawing a transverse line (Fig. 12). One should make certain that the patient is not tilted to the side and is symmetrically positioned on the frame and the table. The spinal processes should be seen in straight alignment on the midline (Fig. 13).

In addition, some surgeons prefer to place an opaque instrument at the patient's side. They take an X-ray to determine the direction of the intervertebral disc in the lateral projection. This helps to direct the needle toward the index level (Fig. 14).

Insertion of Needle

Proper positioning of the tip of the needle in the triangular working zone may be time-consuming. However, it is essential for successful evacuation of herniated disc fragments and the final outcome of minimally invasive spinal surgery.

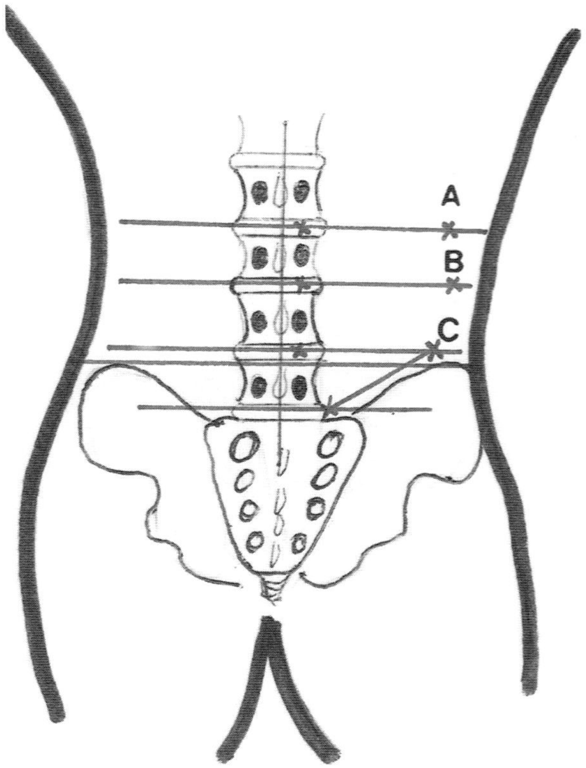

Fig. 13. Schematic drawing demonstrating that patient is symmetrically positioned on table. The spinal processes are well aligned on the midline. A–C represent the skin entry site. The site of annular lodging of the instruments is shown at the midpedicular line.

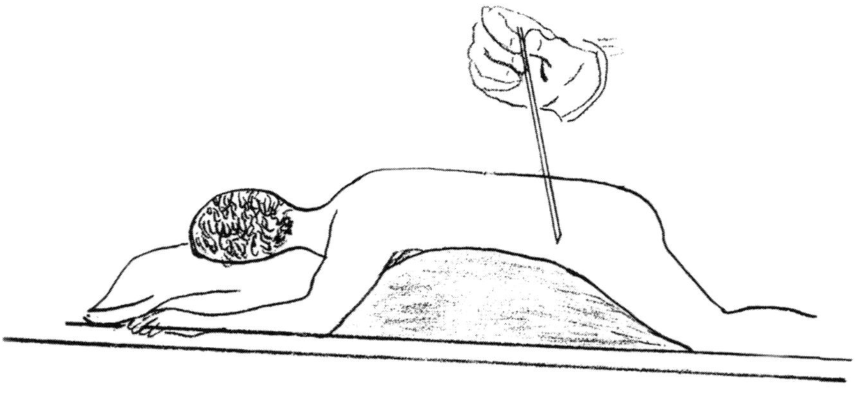

Fig. 14. Schematic drawing showing proper direction of inserted needle in lateral projection. The needle is held on the side of the patient and the lateral X-ray is exposed.

Table 1
Selection of Skin Entry Site

11–12 cm from midline	7–9 cm from midline	2–5 cm from midline
• Arthroscopic subligamentous discectomy	• Discography	• Arthroscopic facet arthrodesis
• Transforaminal endoscopic discectomy (confirm skin entry site via preoperative prone CT)	• Chemonucleolysis	• Interlaminar microlaminatomy and discectomy
• Arthroscopic foraminal decompression	• Vertebral body biopsy (Ottolenghi-Craig)	• Arthroscopic foraminotomy and partial facetectomy
• Diagnostic endoscopy (confirm skin entry point with preoperative CT study of surgical site)	• Arthroscopic anterior column stabilization	• Minimally invasive posterolateral interbody fusion and instrumentation

Proper needle placement encompasses two essential steps: (1) selection of the skin entry site; and (2) proper positioning of the needle in the triangular working zone, the site of annular fenestration (Table 1).

Skin Entry Site

Various techniques have been used for selection of the skin entry point. The size and weight of the patient certainly influence the choice. In addition, the operative technique and location of herniation affect selection of the skin window (Table 1). When transforaminal access to the contents of the spinal canal is contemplated, it is desirable to position the skin entry site more laterally. By contrast, when the evacuation of an extraforaminal herniation is desired, a skin entry point 8 to 9 cm from the midline may be adequate. At times, degenerative and hypertrophic changes in the facet joints prevent proper positioning of the needle in the triangular working zone, and it is therefore necessary to use a skin entry site more laterally to bypass the facet joints. However, far lateral positioning of the skin window or vertical insertion of the needle may direct the tip of the needle into the peritoneal cavity and cause contamination and complications. With the patient in the prone position, a needle may be held at the patient's side, and the tip of the needle placed at the center of the intervertebral disc at the index level under lateral fluoroscopic control. The distance from the center of the disc to the skin level then is selected to represent the required distance between the skin entry site and the midline *(28)*. This technique exposes the patient and the operating surgeon to additional radiation. Although this technique may be used for central nucleotomy, note that during arthroscopic or endoscopic fragmentectomy the instruments are positioned posteriorly adjacent to the spinal canal and not in the center of the intervertebral disc. Therefore, the accuracy of such measurements has been questioned. Generally, in the lumbar spine, a skin entry site of about 10–12 cm from the midline is appropriate for insertion of the needle. If the needle cannot be properly positioned on the annulus, then the needle may be withdrawn, a more lateral entry site selected, and the needle reinserted.

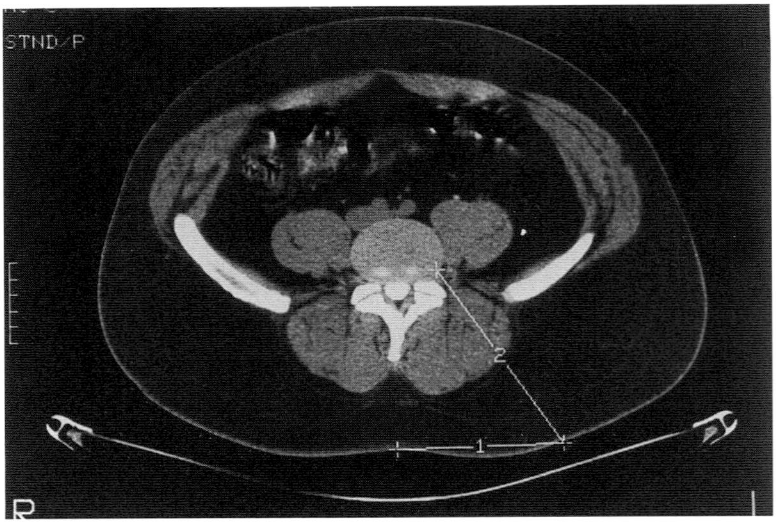

Fig. 15. Preoperative prone CT scan study of surgical site demonstrating desired distance of skin entry point from midline.

The most reliable method for selecting the skin entry site is a preoperative computed tomography (CT) study of the surgical site with the patient in a prone position (Fig. 15) *(5,24,29)*. This study should always be performed when arthroscopic or endoscopic surgery in the thoracic spine or at the thoracolumbar junction and transforaminal access to the spinal canal are planned.

While inserting the needle and directing it toward the triangular working zone, it is safer to position the C-arm for the lateral exposure. To prevent deviation of the beveled tip of the 18-gage needle and to palpate tissue resistance, the needle should be advanced with a slow rotary movement. Advancement of the needle should be stopped when its tip has reached the superficial layer of the annulus. The needle should not penetrate the annular fibers, and there is no reason to insert the needle into the center of the disc at this stage of the operative procedure.

It is difficult to ascertain the required angle for insertion of the needle. The size of the patient, the skin entry site, and the desired site for the annular window dictate the angle of insertion. Conducting a preoperative CT study in the prone position is the only way to predetermine the required angle of insertion.

It is always safer to insert the needle in a more horizontal plane. This allows palpation of the facet joints with the tip of the needle. Then the needle may be partially withdrawn and reinserted in a more vertical direction, thus bypassing the facet joint and entering the triangular working zone.

When transforaminal access to the spinal canal for retrieval of a sequestered disc herniation is attempted and the needle is positioned medial to the midpedicular line, the stylet of the needle should be removed as the tip of the needle is advanced toward the annular surface. If the spinal fluid begins to drip out, the needle should be withdrawn and repositioned.

The operating surgeon should pay close attention to the length of the needle that is inserted into the paraspinal muscles. Standard needles used for arthroscopic or endoscopic surgery are 6 in. (15 cm) long. If the skin entry point is 11 cm from the midline, at approx 11 cm of penetration the tip of the needle should reach the posterior annulus in the triangular working zone and annular resistance should be palpated. If the target is not reached after 11 cm of penetration, AP and lateral X-rays should be taken to confirm that the tip of the needle is equidistant from the target at the midpedicular line. Note that redirecting the needle while it is embedded in the deep muscle layers is difficult. To reposition the tip of the needle, the needle should be pulled back into subcutaneous tissue and then redirected and properly positioned.

Selection of Site of Annular Lodging of Instruments

Proper selection of the site where instruments are to be lodged on the annulus during intracanalicular, foraminal, and extraforaminal surgeries is essential at the onset of the operative procedure. To avoid inadvertent insertion of the tip of the needle and the subsequent instruments into the spinal canal and penetration of the dural sac and the neural structures, a safe point of resistance adjacent to the spinal canal has been identified and its radiographic landmarks have been described *(5,15,23,24,30)* (*see* Fig. 3 in Chapter 2).

When attempting subligamentous access to a disc herniation, midpedicular positioning of the tip of the needle as observed in the AP C-arm images (Fig. 16A–C) is desired (Table 2). However, for evacuation of an extraforaminal herniation, adequate access to the herniation, site is achieved by positioning the instruments on the lateral pedicular line, as is observed in the AP X-ray projection.

Intraoperative Radiographic Landmarks

Proper positioning of the needle in the triangular working zone must be monitored intraoperatively, by both AP and lateral fluoroscopic examinations. Although in the lateral projection the position of the tip of the needle may appear to be satisfactory, the AP projection may demonstrate an improper and potentially dangerous site for annulotomy and introduction of instruments (Fig. 17A).

If the needle is inserted too vertically in the AP fluoroscopic examination, the tip of the needle may appear to be satisfactory. However, the LA projection shows the unacceptable vertical insertion (Figs. 17B and 18A–D). By contrast, if the needle is inserted flat or close to the horizontal line in the lateral X-ray projection, the tip of the needle will be observed posterior to the vertebral bodies, and the AP projection will falsely show that the needle has been inserted into the intervertebral disc or the spinal cannal.

When the needle is properly positioned in the lateral X-ray projection, the tip of the needle is aligned with the posterior vertebral bodies (Fig. 16C). In the AP projection, the tip of the needle is observed in alignment with the midpedicular or lateral pedicular line (Fig. 16B).

Positioning of Cannulated Obturator and 5 × 5 mm Inner Diameter Access Cannula

Prior to introduction of a blunt-end cannulated obturator (soft-tissue dilator), the stylet of an 18-gage needle is replaced with a fine guide wire and the needle is then withdrawn. The cannulated obturator is positioned over the guide wire with the operating hand used to advance the obturator toward the triangular working zone with a slow rotary

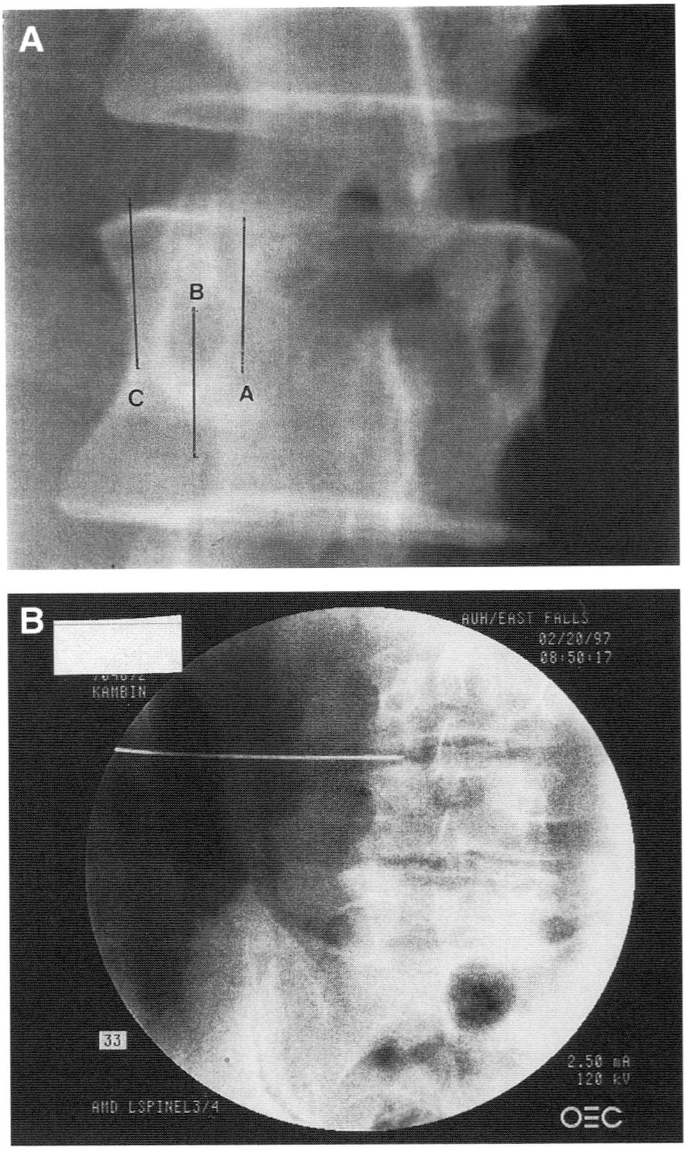

Fig. 16. **(A)** AP X-ray of lumbar segment for selection of position of instruments in triangular working zone: A, medial pedicular line; B, midpedicular line; C, lateral pedicular line. **(B)** Proper positioning of needle on midpedicular line at L3-L4. **(C)** Lateral positioning of needle shown in (B), which is in alignment with posterior boundary of adjacent vertebrae.

movement (Fig. 19) while the other hand maintains the proper direction of the inserted obturator. If the needle has been positioned at the midpedicular line or slightly medial to it, the guide wire should be withdrawn about 1 cm prior to its full insertion (Fig. 20D). This maneuver permits the blunt end of the obturator to bypass the traversing root and move it away from the surgical site (Fig. 20C). While holding the obturator firmly against the annular surface, a 5 × 5 mm inner diameter (id) universal cannula is placed over the obturator and directed toward the annular surface in the triangular working

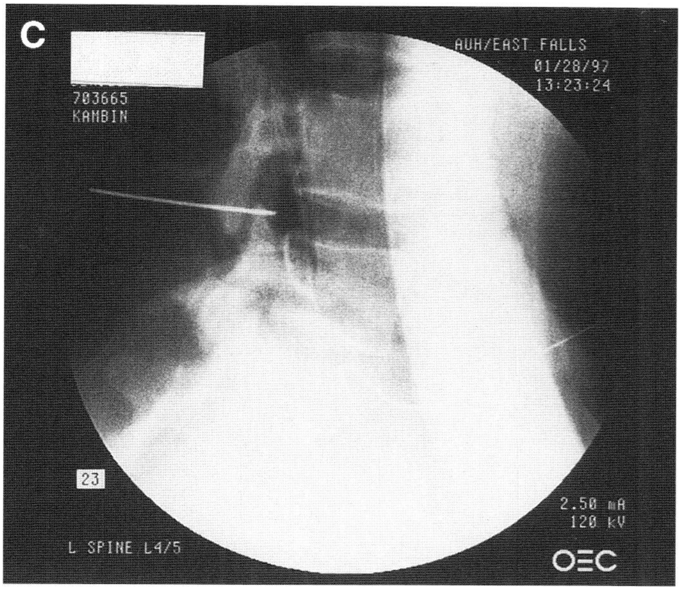

Fig. 16. *(Continued)*

Table 2
Selection of Annular Window Position

Medial pedicular line in AP projection	Midpedicular line in AP projection	Lateral pedicular line in AP projection
Use C-arm and document annular lodging site in AP projection		
• Endoscopic inspection of spinal canal's contents	• Subligamentous arthroscopic microdiscectomy	• Removal of extraforaminal herniation
• Removal of sequestered disc fragment	• Removal of foraminal herination	• Arthroscopic anterior column stabilization • Discography • Chemonucleolysis

zone. It is advisable to confirm and document the correct position of the cannula with an AP and a lateral fluoroscopic examination (Fig. 20E,F).

Arthroscopic and Endoscopic Examination of Triangular Working Zone

To establish adequate inflow and outflow of saline solution and clear visualization of intracanalicular and extra-annular structures, a suction irrigation valve is first attached to the proximal end of a universal cannula (Fig. 21). Practitioners have also used cannulas with a permanently attached suction irrigation valve to achieve the same goal. A 0° arthroscope or a working channel scope may be used for inspection of these structures. If the cannula is not held firmly against the posterolateral annulus in the triangular working zone, venous bleeding may obstruct visualization of these structures.

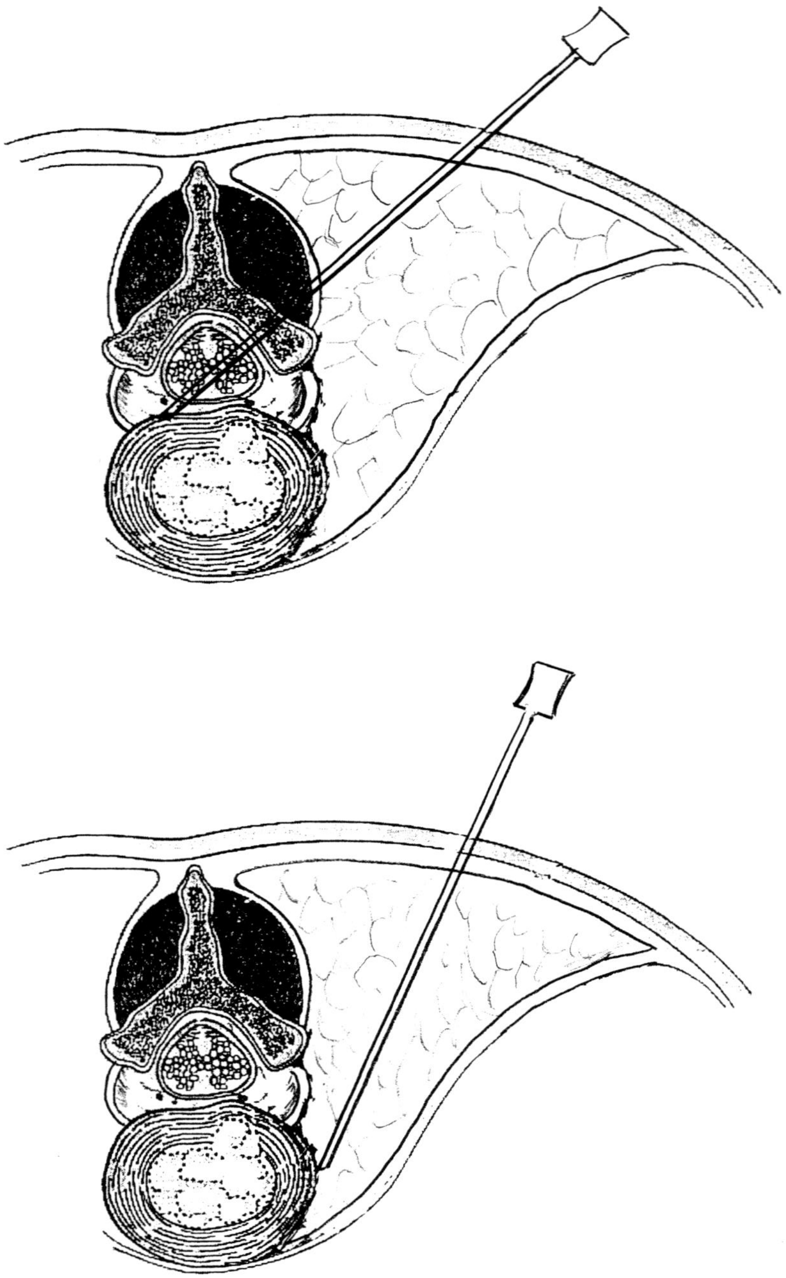

Fig. 17. (A) Schematic drawing of axial view of improper positioning of needle. This signifies the importance of having both AP and lateral intraoperative images in order to confirm the proper positioning of the needle. A lateral X-ray study will show a satisfactory positioning of the needle. However, an AP fluoroscopy will demonstrate that needle has not been properly positioned. **(B)** Schematic drawing of axial positioning of a needle. In the AP fluoroscopic examination, the tip of the needle may appear to be in a satisfactory position. However, in the lateral fluoroscopic images, improper positioning of needle is identified.

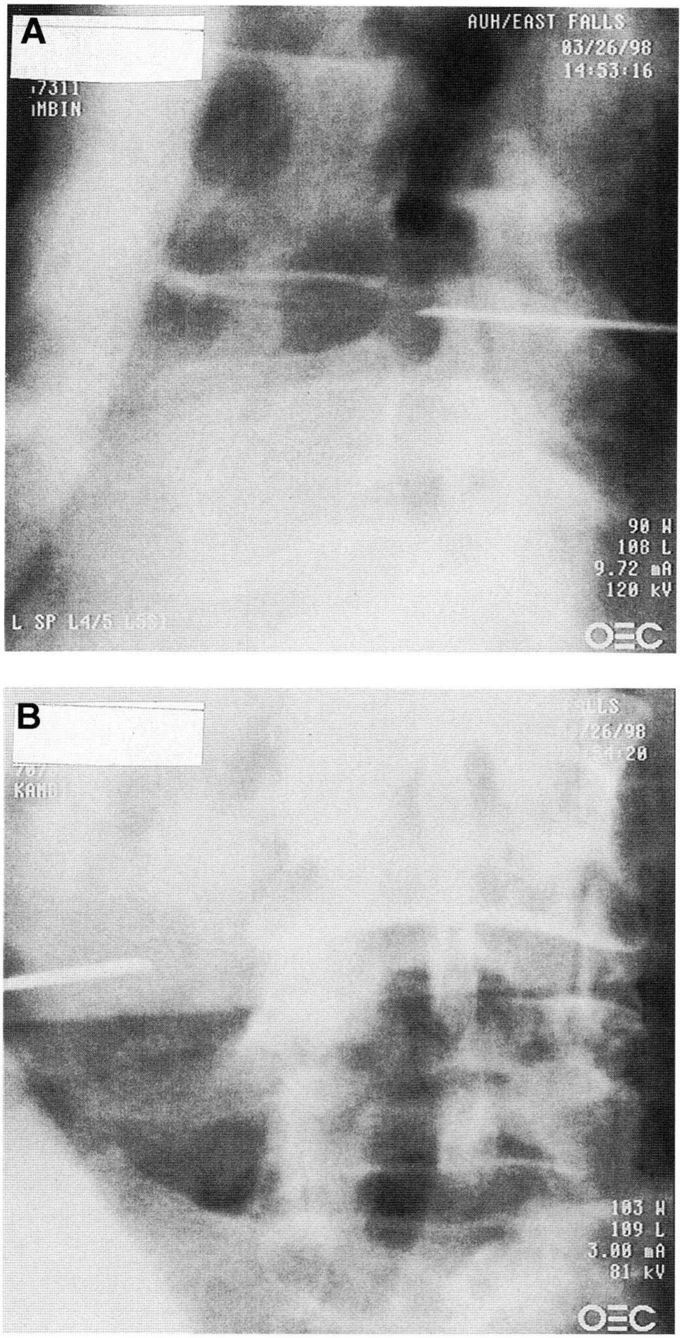

Fig. 18. **(A)** Improper vertical position of needle. In the lateral projection, the position of the needle appears to be satisfactory. **(B)** AP fluoroscopic examination shown in (A). The tip of the needle remains away from the intervertebral disc. **(C)** Improper horizontal insertion of needle. In the AP projection, it appears that the needle has reached the midpedicular line. **(D)** Lateral fluoroscopic examination shown in (C) demonstrating that needle is far away from L4-L5 intervertebral disc.

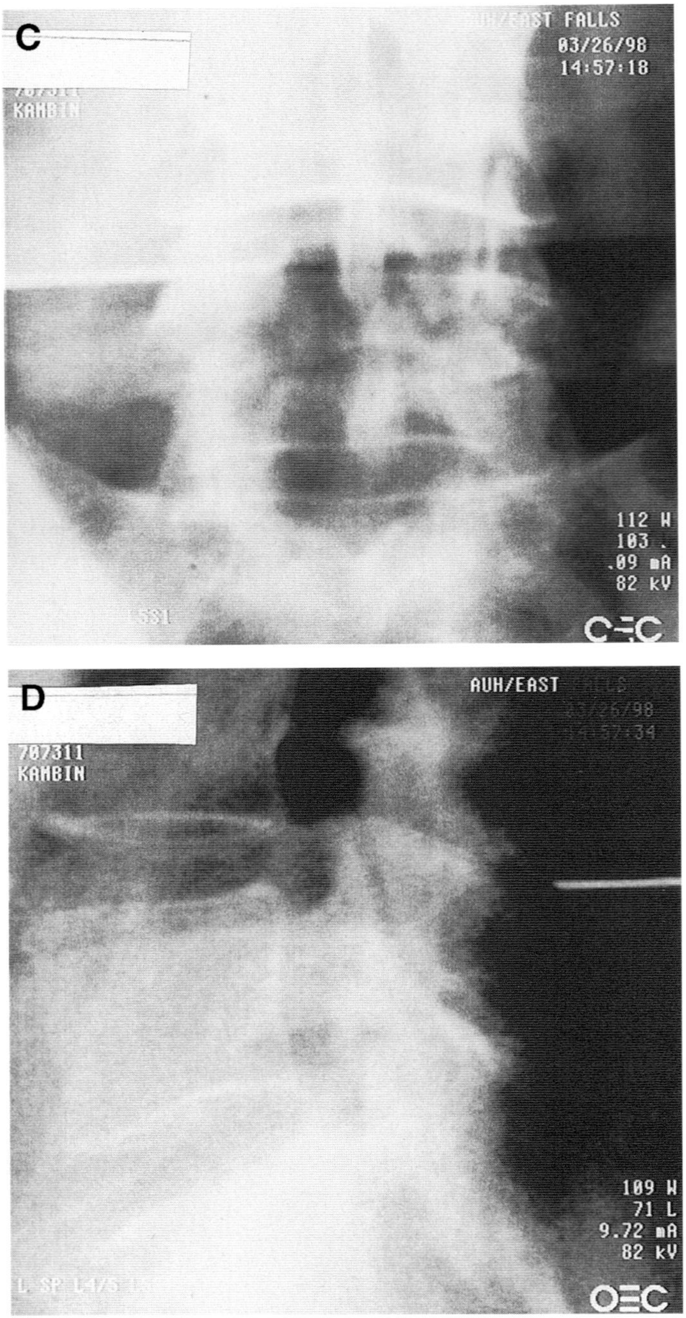

Fig. 18. *(Continued)*

Loosely woven adipose tissue that covers the surface of the posterolateral annulus is usually observed in the triangular working zone (*see* Fig. 4A,B in Chapter 2). This adipose tissue may be wiped out with a cottonoid or removed with a radiofrequency (Fig. 22) probe for clear visualization of the annulotomy site (*see* Fig. 6A,B in

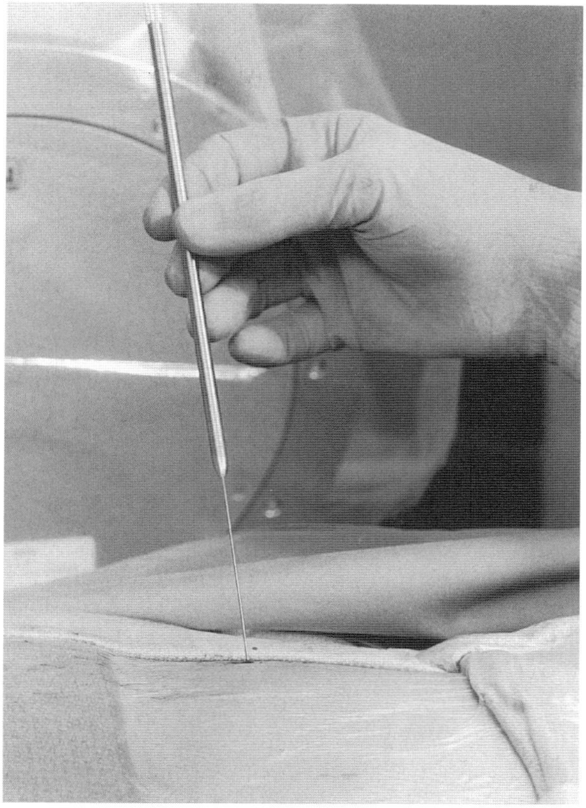

Fig. 19. Interoperative photograph showing advancement of cannulated obturator over guide wire with slow rotatory movement to prevent deviation of obturator and bending of guide wire.

Chapter 2). The exiting roots accompanying radicular arteries and veins are located under the pedicular notch and are not seen on the surface of the posterolateral annulus. If the cannula has been positioned medial to the midpedicular line, epidural adipose tissue, epidural veins, the traversing root, and the dural sac will be observed (Fig. 5B; *see also* Fig. 9A,B in Chapter 2). Note that globs of epidural adipose tissue are usually larger than periannular fat, and they have a tendency to move into the cannula when the patient inhales. If the cannula is positioned in the midpedicular region, a slight tilt of the medial end of the cannula dorsally will permit inspection of the contents of the spinal canal. However, prior to introduction of the trephine or resecting instrument, the medial end of the cannula should be turned away and brought into a more vertical position to prevent injury to the neural structures.

Annulotomy

Most annulotomies are performed in the triangular working zone *(12,30,31)*. Subligamentous approach provides access to paramedial and medial herniations (Fig. 23). If access to the spinal canal is desired, lateral fibers of the posterior longitudinal ligament must be removed to expose the ventral surface of the traversing root and the dural sac (Fig. 23A,B).

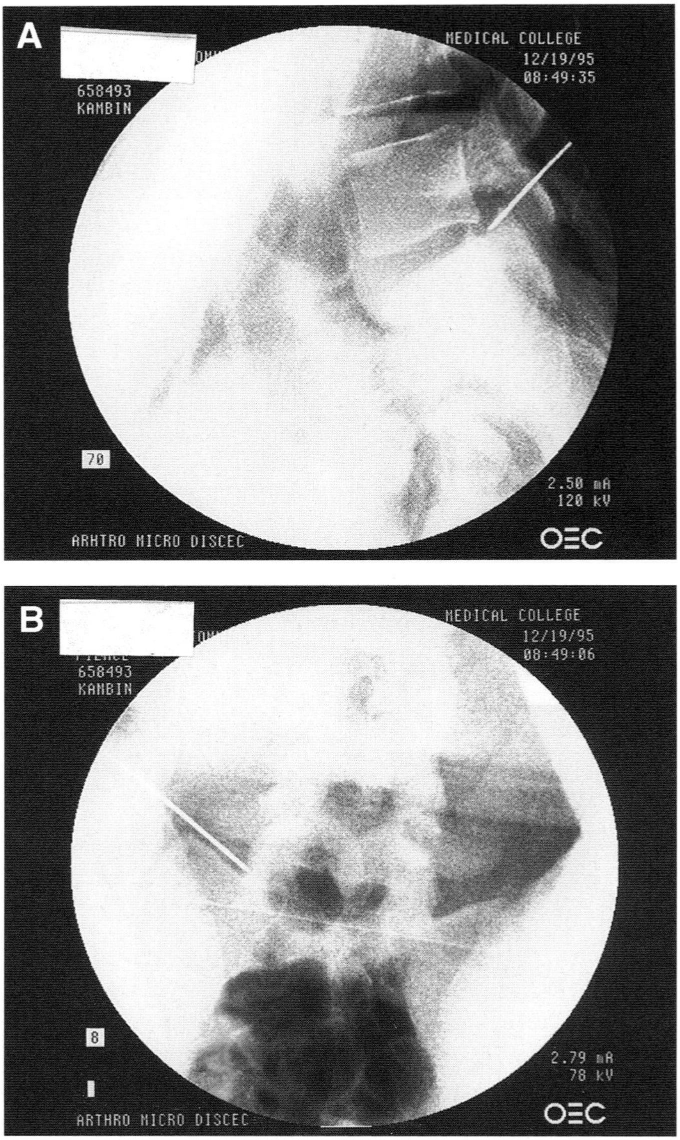

Fig. 20. **(A)** Proper positioning of needle at L5-S1 in lateral fluoroscopic examination; **(B)** proper positioning of needle at L5-S1 shown in **(A)**. **(C)** Demonstrates that obturator has reached intervertebral disc and guide wire has been removed; **(D)** Demonstrates that cannulated obturator is approaching L5-S1 intervertebral disc and signifies withdrawal of guide wire. **(E)** final and proper position of cannula at L5-S1; **(F)** final position of instrument in AP fluoroscopic examination.

Annulotomy may be performed with a trephine or under direct visualization by using a working scope. The superficial layers of the annulus should be anesthetized with topical anesthetic and then with a local injection of lidocaine (Xylocaine) solution. The four corners of the annular fibers inside the cannula are perforated with an 18-gage needle. This is a useful test to ensure that the cannula is not seated on the vertebral plates and is well centered on the disc space.

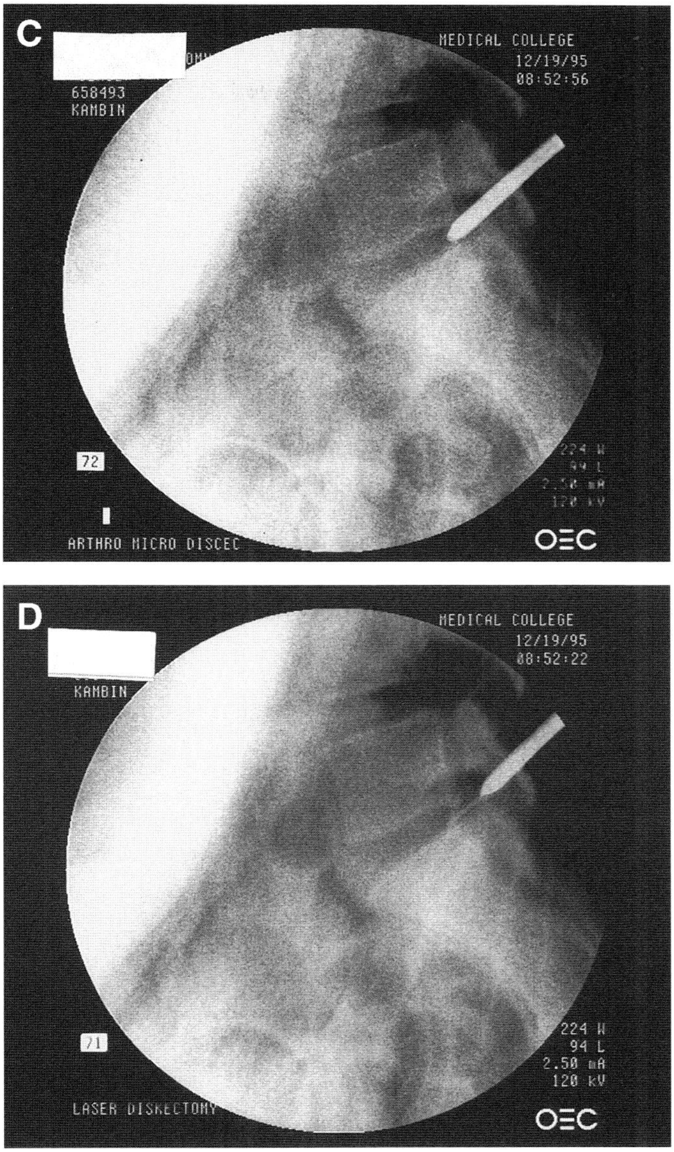

Fig. 20. *(Continued)*

Positioning of Oval Cannulas

The proper positioning of the 5 × 8 or 5 × 10 mm id oval cannulas is accomplished via the following steps *(26,30,32,33):*

1. Reinsert the blunt cannulated obturator into the lumen of a 5 × 5 mm id universal cannula, and insert the distal end of the obturator into the intervertebral disc.
2. Withdraw the 5 × 5 mm universal cannula.
3. Position a 10- or 12-mm od jig template over the proximal end of the inserted cannulated obturator. This jig is provided with an oval-shaped bore that accommodates both

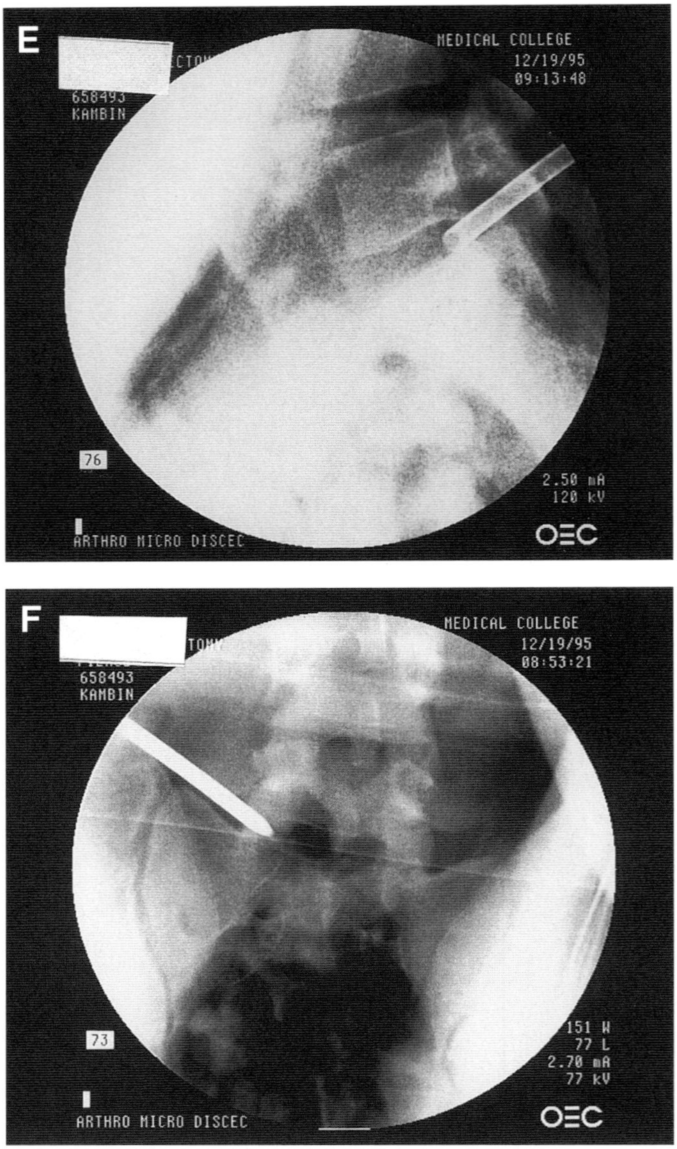

Fig. 20. *(Continued)*

the cannulator obturator and a half- or full-moon auxiliary obturator (*see* Fig. 3A,B in Chapter 3).

4. Insert a half-moon auxiliary obturator through the bore of the jig template, and direct it toward the intervertebral disc at the index level.
5. Remove the jig template and insert an appropriate-size oval cannula by sliding it over the previously positioned cannulated obturator and half- or full-moon auxiliary obturators. Then gently tap the oval cannula into position and engage in the superficial layer of the annular fibrosis (Fig. 24A,B).

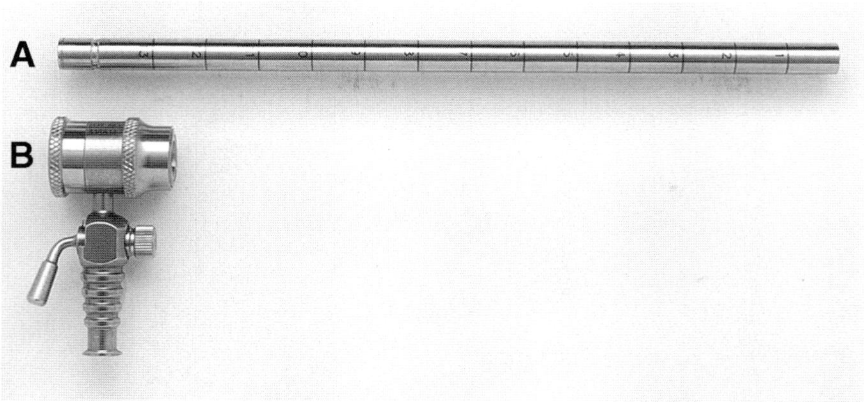

Fig. 21. (**A**) A 5 × 5 mm id universal cannula; (**B**) a removable suction irrigation valve.

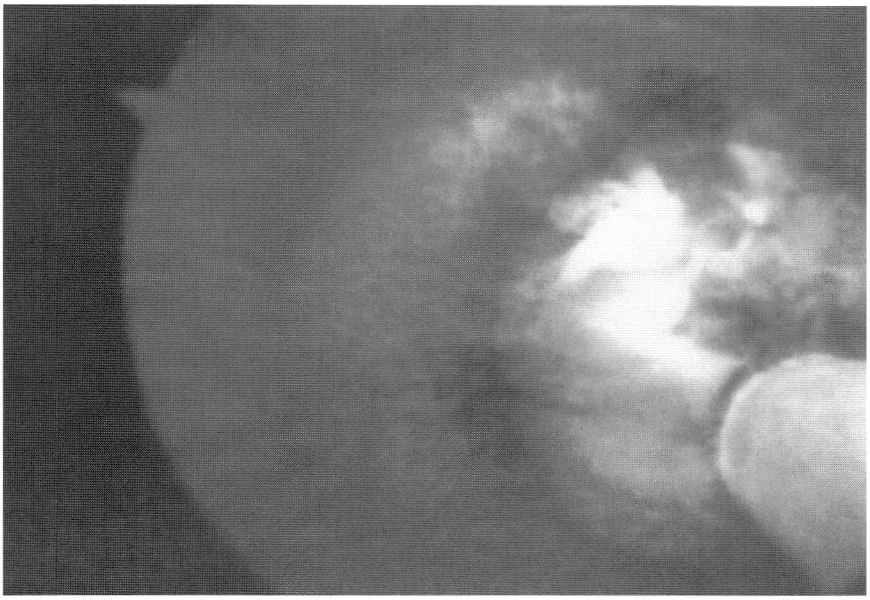

Fig. 22. Interoperative photograph demonstrating how radiofrequency probe is used for periannular hemostatsis and removal of adipose tissue in triangular working zone.

Retrieval of Herniated Disc Fragments

When subligamentous access to the herniation site is being used *(6,12,22)*, the access cannula is first engaged into the superficial annular fibers and the position of the access cannula is maintained with one hand throughout the surgical procedure. A straight and an upbiting forceps are used to grasp and remove the herniated disc material that may be dislodged posterolaterally adjacent to the tip of the inserted cannula. The inserted trephine and forceps will have a tendency to sweep ventral to the posterior longitudinal ligamentum, traversing root and lateral dura, thus facilitating evacuation of the herniated fragments.

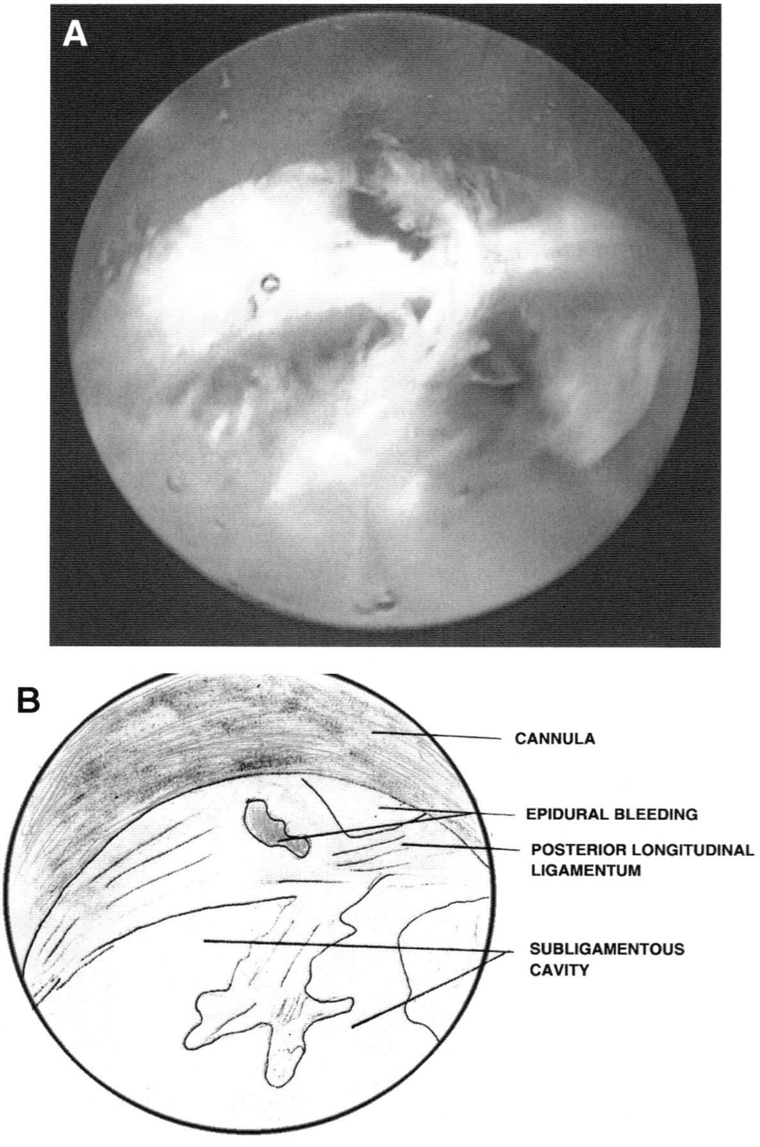

Fig. 23. **(A,B)** Intraoperative arthroscopic view demonstrating subligamentous access to disc herniation.

The oval cannula permits insertion of a 0 of 30° scope and resecting instruments for visualization of the surgical site during retrieval of the herniated disc fragments (Fig. 25; *see also* Fig. 9A,B in Chapter 3).

Fluid Management

Because most arthroscopic spinal surgeries are currently performed with the use of fluid media, proper intraoperative fluid management makes it possible for the operating surgeon to better differentiate between anatomical and pathological structures. Most of the

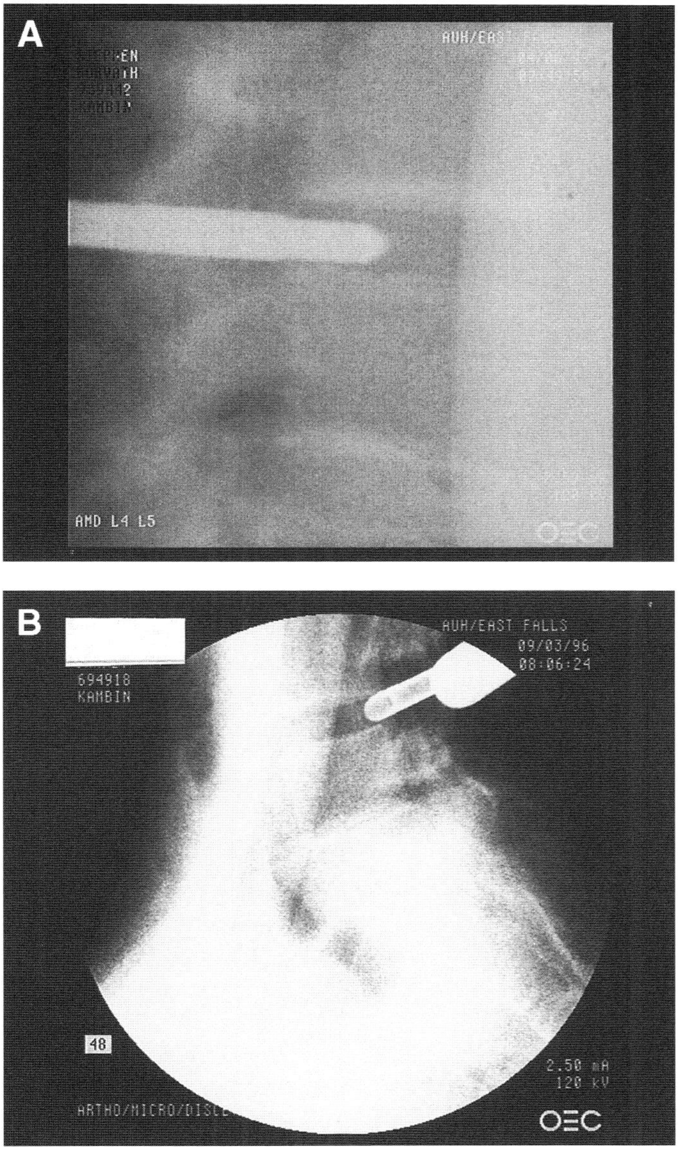

Fig. 24. **(A)** Lateral fluoroscopic examination demonstrating that cannulated obturator and auxiliary obturator are inserted into intervertebral disc and oval cannula has reached surface of annulus; **(B)** lateral fluoroscopic examination shown in (A) demonstrating withdrawal of obturators and anchorage of oval cannula in superficial layer of posterolateral annulus.

arthroscopes and endoscopes used for minimally invasive spine surgery, including the working-channel scope, are provided with at least two channels for the inflow and outflow of saline solution. However, fluid management may have to be adapted to the surgical access selected and the technique utilized in the management of a given patient. Most surgeons who have employed our original technique of uniportal intradiscal access to posteriorly lodged disc fragments have experienced extreme difficulty in establishing the inflow

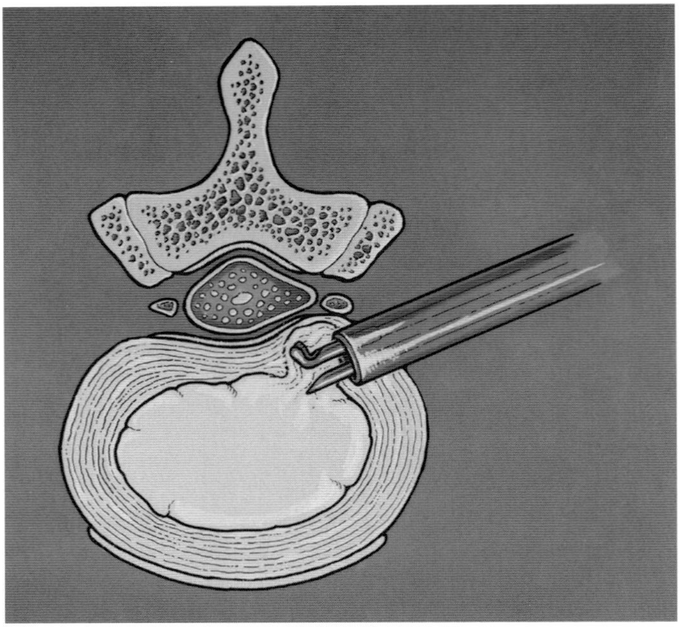

Fig. 25. Schematic drawing demonstrating how scope and upbiting forceps are used in conjunction with oval cannula for visualization and extraction of herniated disc fragments.

and outflow of saline solution. Nuclear debris invariably blocks the outflow channel of the arthroscope and the free flow of saline solution in the cavity that is created in the intervertebral disc. To obtain a quick view of the surgical site, we previously advocated the use of a 50-cc syringe for a bulk delivery of saline solution into the disc cavity *(24,34)*. However, this technique has been abandoned and is no longer used.

Currently, most of the arthroscopic procedures that were previously performed via an intradiscal access are now performed by using a subligamentous *(12,22)* approach, a transforaminal approach *(29,31,35,36)*, or bilateral biportal access *(22)*.

In our experience, allowing free gravitation of outflow saline solution has been most effective and has reduced the incidence of intraoperative bleeding and formation of air bubbles in the surgical field. During both subligamentous and transforaminal intracanalicular access, a large volume of saline solution may be introduced into the surgical field and allowed to gravitate out from the end of the cannula and collect in a sterile plastic bag that is attached to the surgical drapes. The volume of inflow saline solution may be increased by elevating the inflow bag or applying a pressure cuff around the inflow bag. The gravitation of outflow solution may be used in conjunction with a 5×5 mm id. Universal cannula or an oval 5×8 mm id cannula.

When bilateral biportal access to the intervertebral disc is employed (*see* Fig. 10A,B in Chapter 3), inflow of saline solution is connected to the inflow valve of the arthroscope. This tends to remove nuclear debris and blood away from the arthroscope, thus permitting visualization of the surgical site. The saline solution is then retrieved through the cannula that was introduced into the intervertebral disc from the opposite portal.

During transforaminal access to the contents of the spinal canal *(29,31,35–36)*, epidural bleeding invariably obstructs clear visualization of the anatomical and pathological structures. The following steps have proven useful in controlling epidural bleeding:

1. If the bleeding site is visible and can be located, use a radiofrequency probe or bipolar electrocoagulator to control the bleeding points.
2. Close the outflow valve of saline solution and increase the volume and pressure through the inflow valve.
3. Use cold saline solution for irrigation.
4. Introduce a small cottonoid saturated with topical anticoagulants into the surgical site by holding it with the tip of a forceps.
5. Some surgeons have reported adequate epidural hemostasis with injection of diluted epinephrine solution (1:500,000) into the surgical site. After injecting the solution, use a clear saline solution for further irrigation and completion of the operative procedure.
6. Use hypotensive anesthesia.

Retrieval of Foraminal and Extraforaminal Herniations

With the introduction and availability of MRI and CT scans, orthopedic and neurological surgeons have been able to establish an early definitive diagnosis of disc herniations in the lateral zone and render appropriate surgical management when deemed necessary.

The hidden zone, which was well described by MacNab, now is readily diagnosed by high-resolution CT and MRI evaluations. The lateral zone has been divided into three sections: subarticular, foraminal, and extraforaminal regions *(38)* (Fig. 26A). Wiltse described the paraspinal sacrospinalis splitting approach for the removal of far-out extraforaminal disc herniations *(39)*.

The midline approach has also been used to access the lateral zone. Both of these approaches, in particular the midline approach, require extensive soft-tissue dissection, partial facetectomy, and bone removal, which may become complicated by segmental instability. Therefore, the midline approach should be reserved for management of patients with severe lateral recess stenosis and facet hypertrophy. In our experience, arthroscopic microdiscectomy is the procedure of choice for the management of the majority of foraminal and extraforaminal disc herniations.

In contrast to intracanalicular disc herniations, foraminal and extraforaminal herniations are associated with signs and symptoms of compression and tension on the exiting root. Therefore, a patient with a disc herniation at L4-L5 most likely will exhibit signs and symptoms of L4 root involvement, whereas a patient with intracanalicular paramedial disc herniation at the same level will present objective and subjective evidence of L5 root involvement (Fig. 26B). A sequestered disc fragment in the lateral zone may migrate distally and cause pressure on the traversing root and the dural sac.

A patient with an acute ruptured disc in the foraminal or extraforaminal region (Fig. 27A) will present all signs and symptoms of disc herniations, including positive tension signs, with or without neurological deficit. By contrast, an individual with a contained bulging and protruding disc associated with small marginal posterolateral osteophytes may present signs and symptoms of lateral stenosis, having radicular pain but lacking positive tension signs.

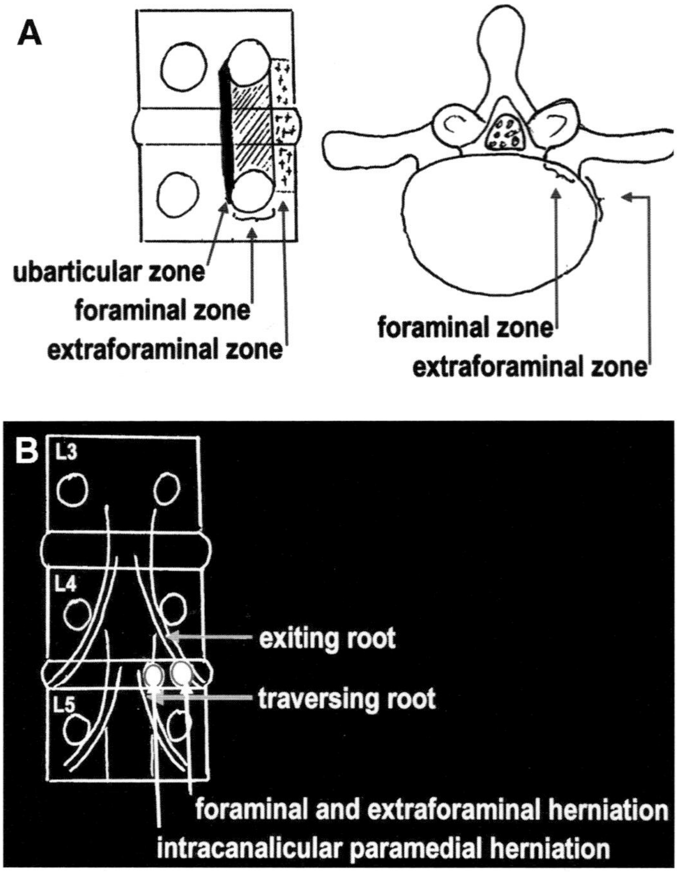

Fig. 26. **(A)** Schematic drawing showing subarticular foraminal and extraforaminal zone in AP and axial projection; **(B)** schematic drawing demonstrating that a paramedial herniation at L4-L5 produces compression at L5 root whereas a foraminal and an extraforaminal herniation at same level can produce compression of L4 root.

The positioning of the patient, draping of the C-arm, and locating of the surgical site are similar to those described previously (*see* Chapters 3 and 4). The skin entry site is usually about 9 or 10 cm from the midline. For removal of an extraforaminal herniation, the tip of an 18-gage needle is positioned over the lateral pedicular line, as is observed in the AP radiographic evaluation. However, one should be aware of the fact that in the lateral X-ray images the tip of the needle may not appear to be aligned with the posterior boundary of the adjacent vertebral bodies, because the bulk of the herniation prevents alignment of the tip of the needle with the posterior vertebral line.

Following initial annular fenestration and subligamentous evacuation of the disc material (Fig. 27B,C), the cannulated obturator is reinserted into the lumen of the cannula and the cannula and obturator assembly are gradually moved laterally into a more vertical position. This maneuver permits further access and evacuation of the remainder of disc fragments. In addition, the cannula has a tendency to move laterally and protect the

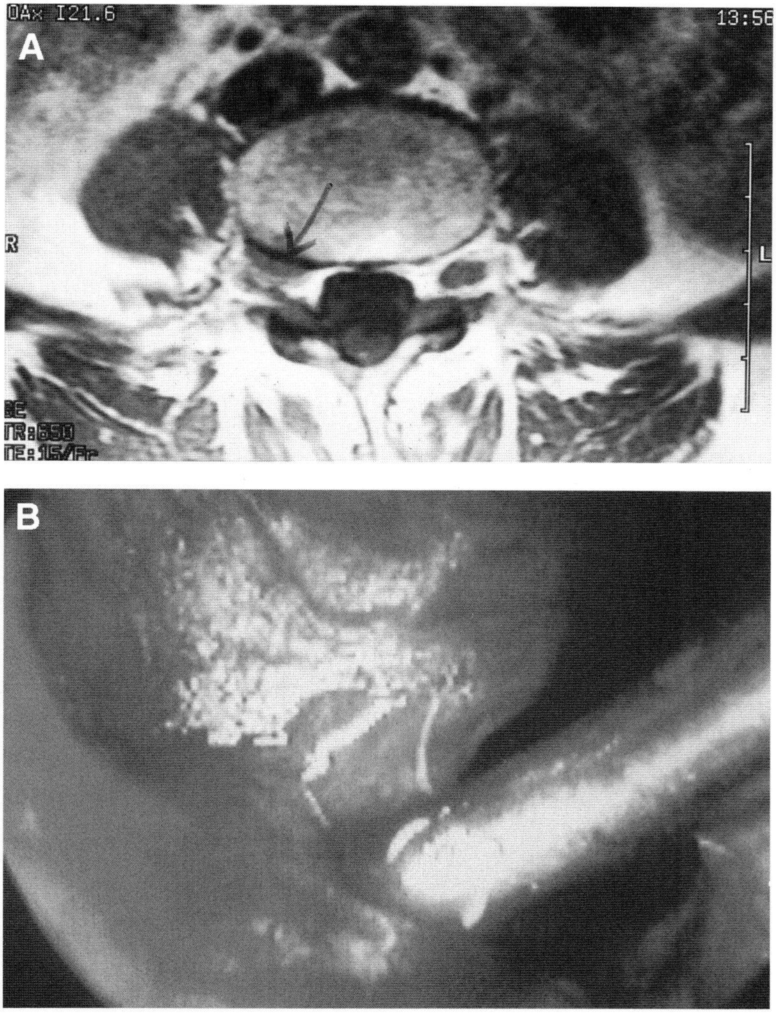

Fig. 27. **(A)** Preoperative axial MRI study of foraminal and extraforaminal herniation at L3-L4. **(B)** Interoperative arthroscopic view of herniation site. Note that the probe is being used to isolate the herniation from the surrounding tissue. (Reprinted from ref. *43*, with permission.) **(C)** Interoperative arthroscopic view demonstrating that herniation has been evacuated and subligamentous region is being probed in search of additional disc fragments.

exiting root during the evacuation stage. If marginal posterolateral osteophytes are deemed to be responsible for the development of lateral recess stenosis, a trephine or powered instruments may be used for annulectomy and evacuation of the osteophytes *(27,40)*. In our hands, the oval cannula with an id of 5 × 8 mm has been particularly helpful for access and retrieval of extraforaminal herniations. At times a sequestrated herniated disc migrates to the foraminal and subpedicular region of the proximal segment (Fig. 28A). The retrieval of herniated fragments requires positioning of the 5 mm id cannula in the subpedicular region for extraction of sequestrated disc fragments (Fig. 28B–F).

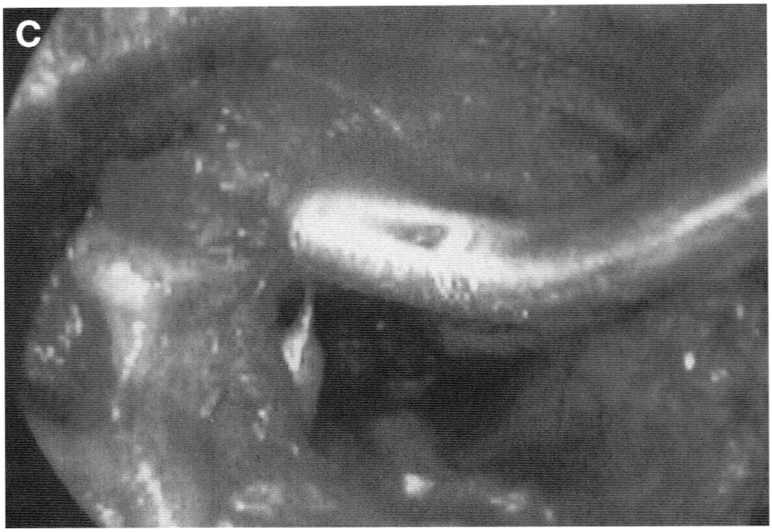

Fig. 27. *(Continued)*

Retrieval of Paramedial or Central Disc Herniations

Subligamentous access to disc herniations requires that the skin entry site be more lateral (*[12,22]*; Table 1). The needle and instruments are positioned at the midpedicular line. Following inspection of the annulotomy site, the medial end of the cannula is tilted toward the patient's dorsum, and the contents of the spinal canal are inspected (Fig. 29A–C). The medial end of the cannula is then tilted ventrally so that the open end of the cannula is not in the spinal canal (Fig. 30). Annular fenestration is performed with a working channel scope in accordance with the principles that were described previously. The cannulated obturator is reinserted into the lumen of the cannula and is driven into the intervertebral disc. This maneuver makes it possible to advance the cannula over the obturator and to engage it with the superficial layer of the annulus fibrosus. A cavity is then created ventral to the posterior longitudinal ligament by partial nucleotomy and evacuation of the torn fibers of the posterior annulus (Fig. 31A,B). The intradiscal tail of nonmigrated sequestered fragments or a subligamentous herniation is then identified under direct visualization and removed.

The subligamentous approach is particularly desirable for evacuation of a contained disc herniation, thus making it unnecessary to enter the spinal canal.

Retrieval of Sequestered Disc Herniation

Transforaminal access *(22,29,31,36)* requires that the skin entry site be more lateral and that the needle be positioned slightly medial to the midpedicular line (Fig. 32A,B) (Tables 1 and 2). It is advisable to confirm the skin entry site via a prone preoperative CT study. The principle of the surgical approach is similar to that described for subligamentous access. Following the creation of a cavity under the posterior longitudinal ligament, lateral fibers of the posterior longitudinal ligament adjacent to the tip of the inserted cannula are also removed with a forceps or a radiofrequency probe (Fig. 33A–C).

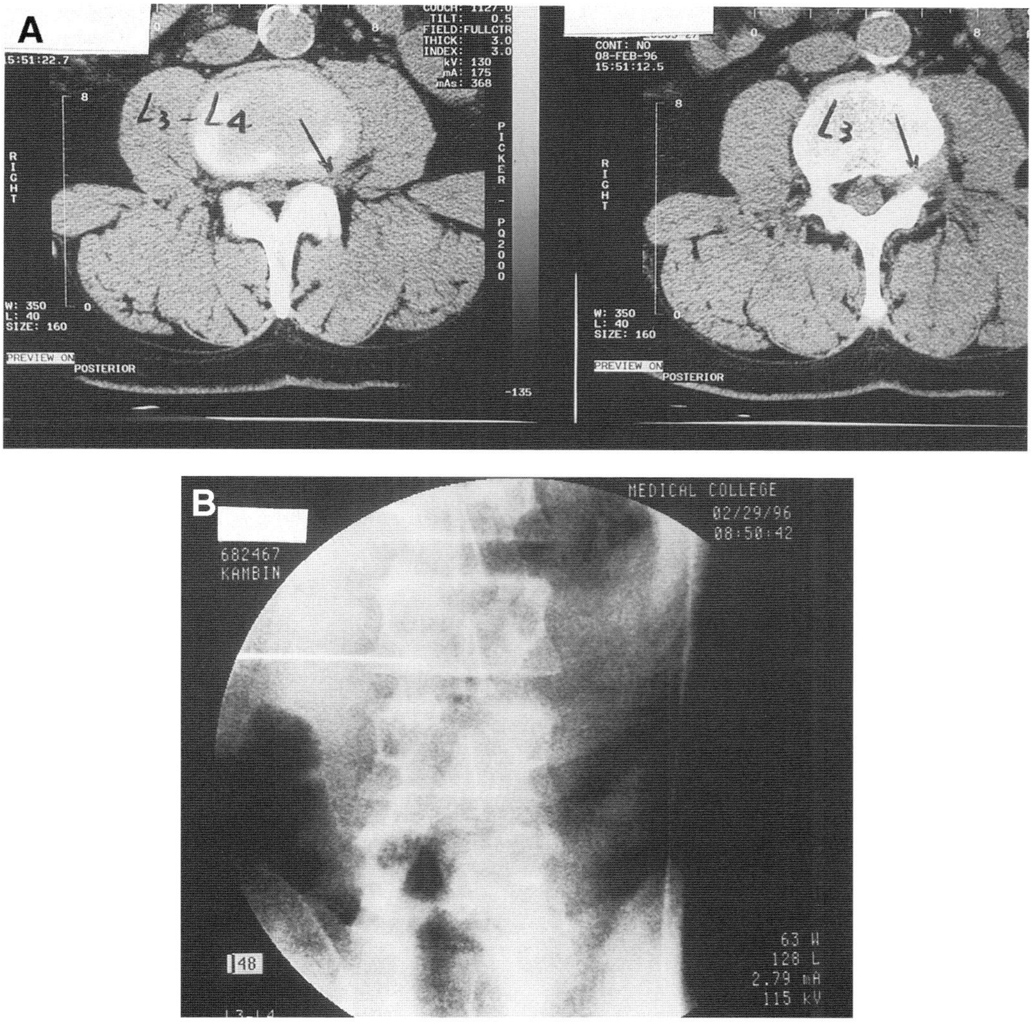

Fig. 28. **(A)** Axial view of migrated sequestrated disc herniation. Note that at disc level (left) the herniation is not seen. However, at the subpedicular region (right), a large free fragment is demonstrated. **(B)** Proper positioning of needle in subpedicular region in AP projection. **(C)** Lateral view of needle positioning illustrated in (B). **(D)** Positioning of cannula in subpedicular region. **(E)** Interoperative photograph demonstrating retrieval of sequestrated disc fragments with straight forceps. **(F)** Interoperative photograph showing partial removal of sequestrated fragments and exposure of nerve root ganglia.

Epidural bleeding and adipose tissue may obstruct clear visualization of intracanalicular structures. Epidural bleeding may be controlled by temporarily increasing the pressure of the saline solution through the inflow valve and closing the outflow valve. The use of cold saline solution has also been useful in controlling epidural bleeding. We have used cottonoids saturated with topical anticoagulants and radiofrequency probes to stop bleeding. Excess epidural adipose tissue may also be evacuated with the aid of forceps and easily with the use of a radiofrequency probe. Some surgeons

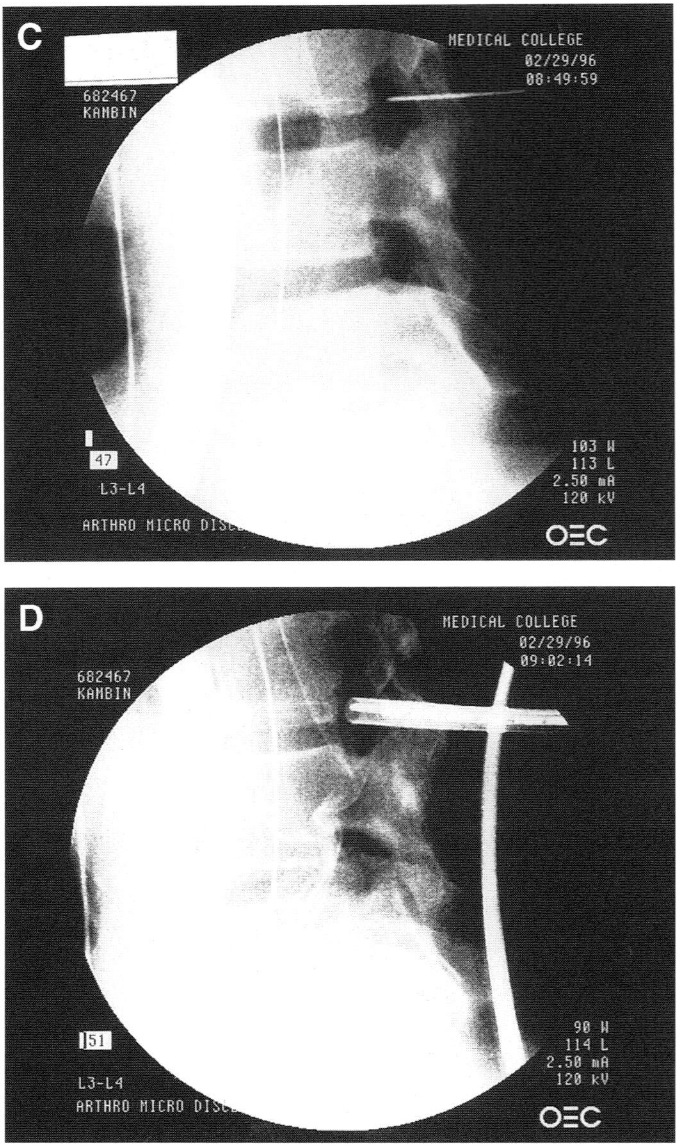

Fig. 28. *(Continued)*

have used a cold dilute epinephrine solution (1 mg/1000 cc of saline solution) for control of multiple, minute epidural bleeders.

Once epidural bleeding has been controlled and excess epidural adipose tissue removed, a working channel scope is introduced into the lumen of the cannula and the disc fragments are visualized and evacuated. The cannula may be tilted cephalad or caudad for further access to the migrated disc fragments within the spinal canal.

Bilateral biportal intradiscal (Fig. 34A–D) access may be used for evacuation of a nonmigrated sequestered disc herniation. This approach is most effective for retrieval of central herniations. It prevents undue intraoperative manipulation of the neural

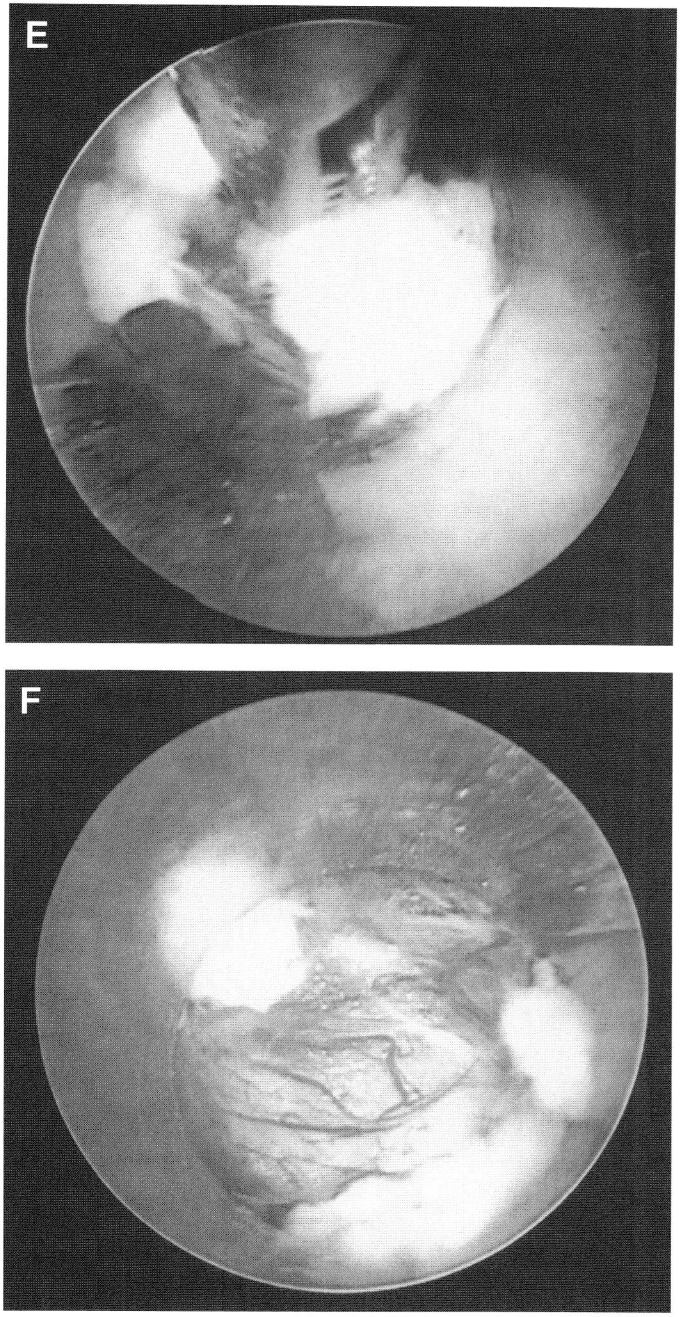

Fig. 28. *(Continued)*

structures. A cavity is created ventral to the posterior longitudinal ligamentum. Communication between the right and left portal is developed via resection of the nucleus with forceps or with the aid of a radiofrequency probe. Inflow and outflow of saline solution is established between the two portals. The intradiscal segment of the sequestrated

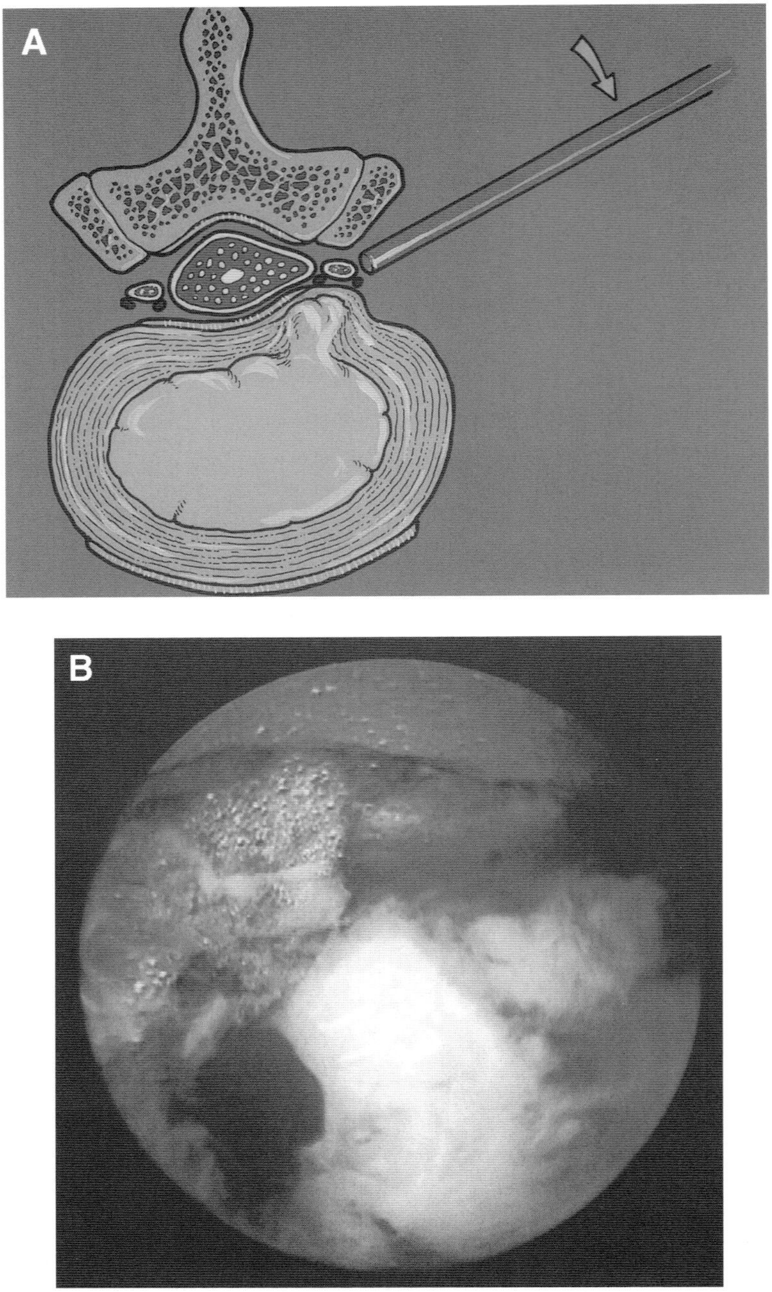

Fig. 29. **(A)** Schematic drawing demonstrating how medial end of cannula is tilted toward dorsum of patient by pushing lateral end of cannula ventrally, therefore allowing visualization of contents of spinal canal; **(B,C)** interoperative photograph demonstrating visualization of contents of spinal canal following dorsal tilt of medial end of cannula.

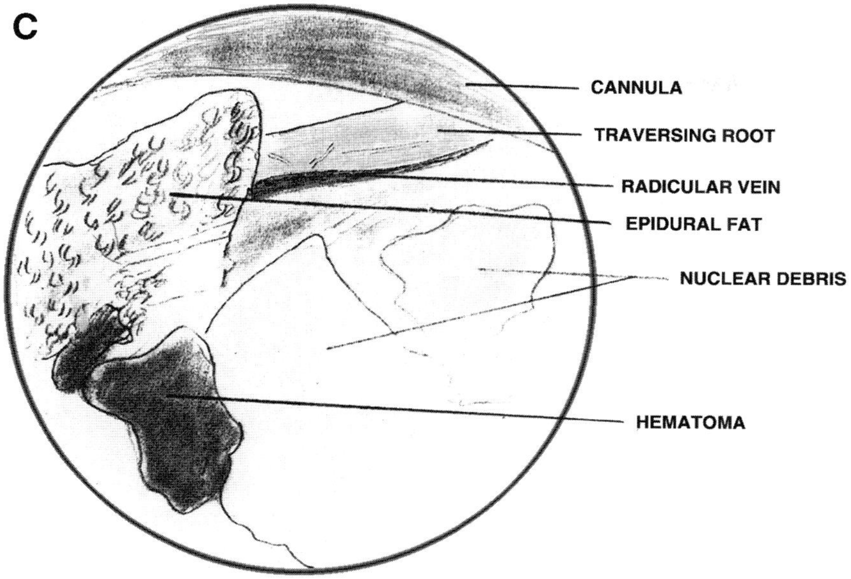

Fig. 29. *(Continued)*

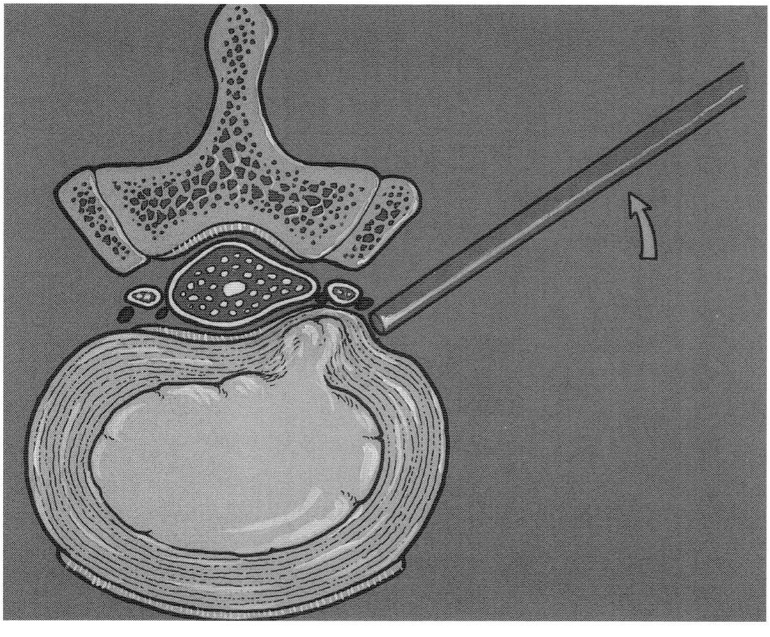

Fig. 30. Schematic drawing showing ventral tilt of medial end of cannula in preparation of annulotomy.

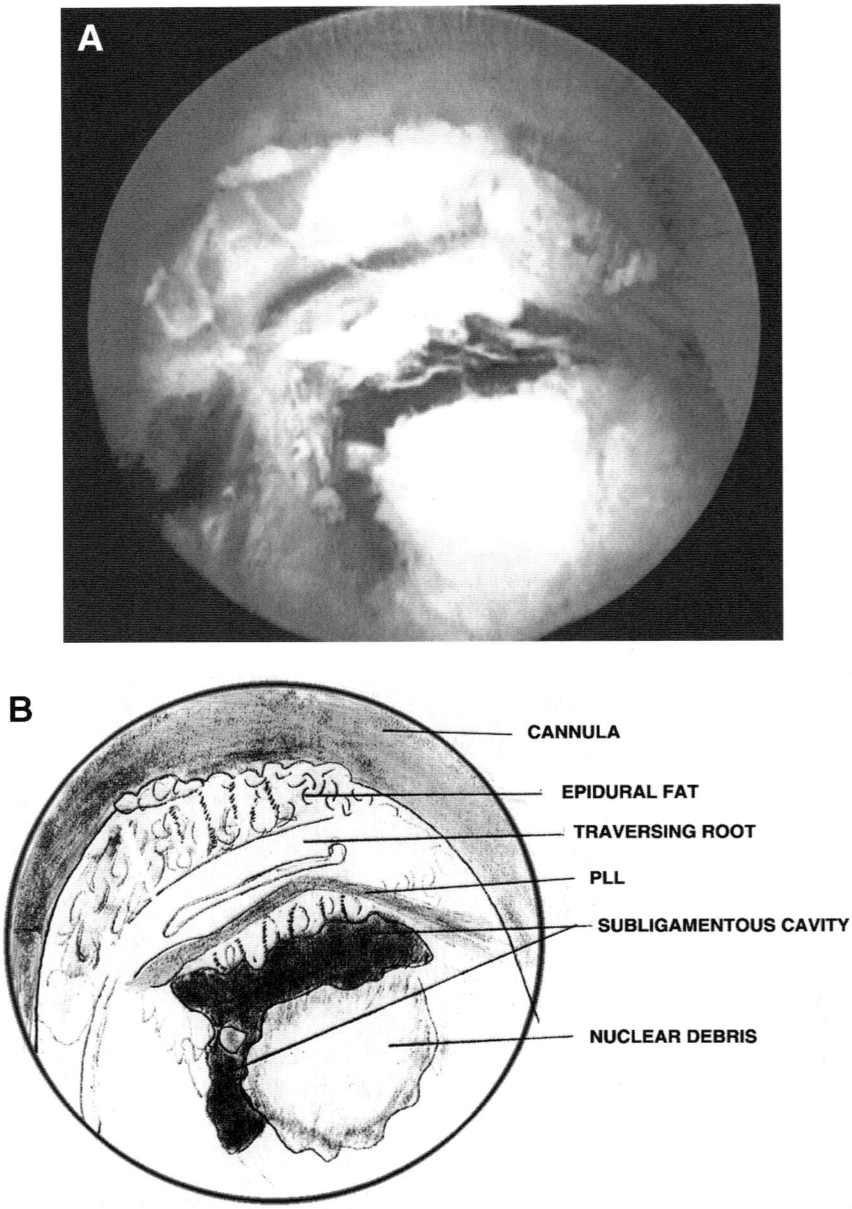

Fig. 31. **(A)** Interoperative photograph demonstrating subligamentous annulotomy. The traversing root is seen at the top of photo above. PLL, posterior longitudinal ligamentum.

disc herniation is then identified and grasped with forceps and removed (Fig. 35A–C). Although this technique is more time-consuming than the uniportal approach, it spares the neural and vascular structures from undue manipulation and potential injury (Fig. 36; *see also* Fig. 10 in Chapter 2). At the completion of the operative procedure, the ventral dura and torn fibers of the posterior longitudinal ligamentum are observed via a

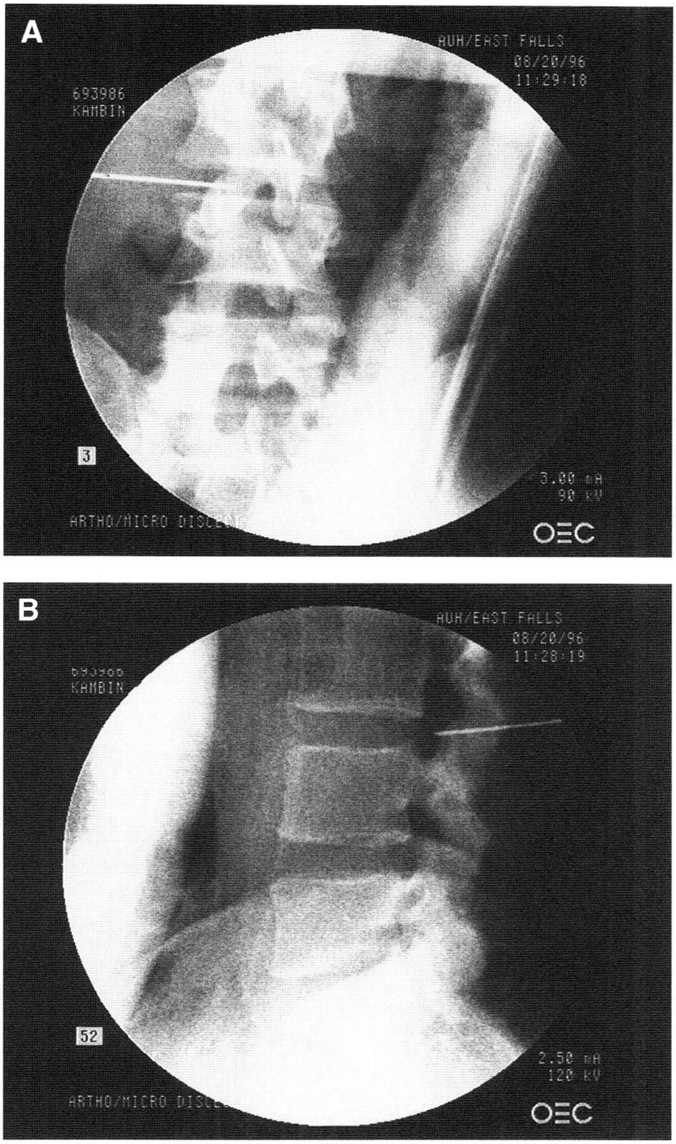

Fig. 32. (A) AP fluoroscopic examination demonstrating proper positioning of needle on medial pedicular line for intracanalicular access; **(B)** lateral positioning of needle as shown in (A); **(C)** proper positioning of cannula for intracanalicular surgery.

30 or 70° arthroscope (Fig. 37A–C). To ensure adequate decompression of the traversing nerve root, the spinal canal may be examined prior to withdrawal of instruments (Fig. 38A,B).

A larger-diameter cannula may be positioned at the interlaminar space under fluoroscopic control from a distance of 2 cm from the midline for mini-laminatomy and retrieval of sequestered disc fragments under endoscopic visualization. In the past, we have used

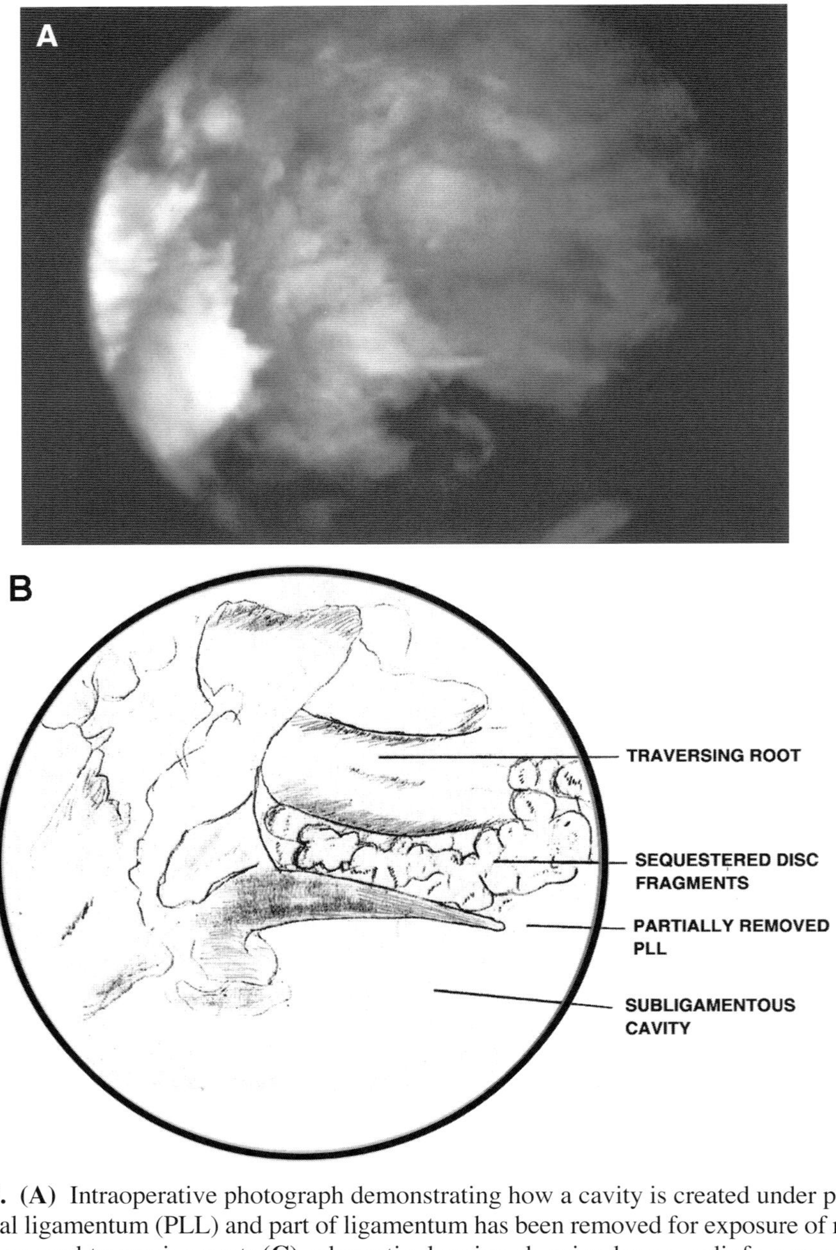

Fig. 33. **(A)** Intraoperative photograph demonstrating how a cavity is created under posterior longitudinal ligamentum (PLL) and part of ligamentum has been removed for exposure of massive herniation around traversing root; **(C)** schematic drawing showing how a radiofrequency probe is used for vaporization of PLL and torn fibers of annulus and exposure of herniated fragments and nerve root, under endoscopic visualization.

cannulas with side windows for introduction of straight endoscopes (Fig. 18A,B in Chapter 1). This allowed the insertion of a variety of instruments through the proximal opening of the cannula *(6,26,37)*. With the later availability of angled endoscopes, we were able to insert both endoscopes and instruments through the proximal opening of a larger-diameter cannula *(40)*.

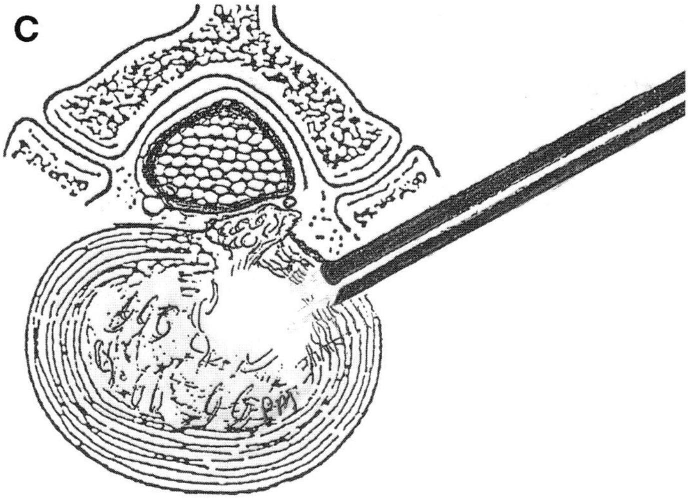

Fig. 33. *(Continued)*

Retrieval of Thoracic or Thoracolumbar Herniation

Considering the limited muscle mass in the thoracolumbar area, thorough preoperative planning becomes an essential part of retrieving a thoracic or thoracolumbar herniation.

The skin entry site should be determined and selected by using a prone CT study of the index level before surgery (Fig. 15) *(5,29)*. Accurate placement of the skin entry site will prevent inadvertent violation of the thoracic or abdominal cavity by the inserted instruments. Because many extradural defects in the thoracic region do not represent a soft disc herniation, a preoperative CT scan study of the surgical site is helpful in differentiating between soft herniations and osteophytes. Owing to anatomical limitations, which are imposed by the rib cage and the limited muscle mass, it is invariably difficult to place the skin entry site far enough laterally and to use a subligamentous approach to the herniation site. Bilateral biportal access to the intervertebral disc may be necessary for visualization and decompression of the ventral surface of the dural sac and the nerve roots. Great care should be exercised not to use trimmer blades or vibrating instruments adjacent to the spinal cord during an intradiscal approach to the thoracic or thoracolumbar region.

Retrieval of Recurrent Disc Herniations

Recent technological advances in the field of minimally invasive spinal surgery have opened a window of opportunity to access, isolate, and retrieve recurrent herniated disc fragments. Neurolysis of tethered nerve root under endoscopic control is the essential first step (Fig. 39). The surgical approach for retrieval of recurrent disc herniations is similar to that previously described for subligamentous access to the intervertebral disc. A small cavity is first created under the posterior longitudinal ligament by removing part of the nucleus and torn annular tissue. This is then followed by partial resection of

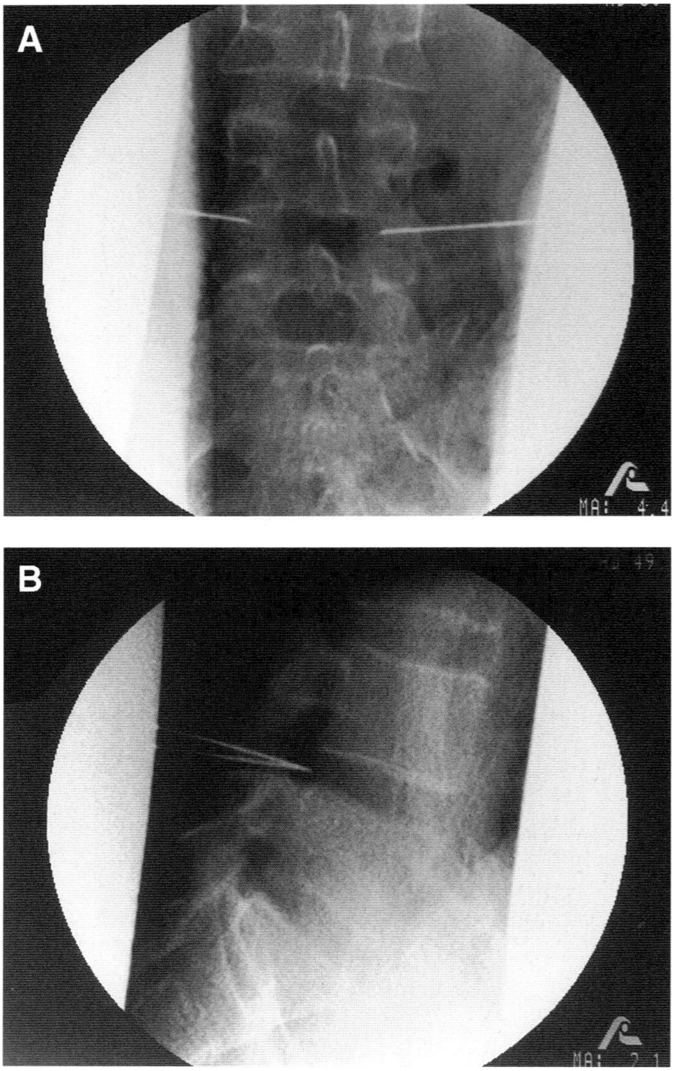

Fig. 34. **(A)** Proper positioning of two needles in AP projection for bilateral biportal access to a large nonmigrated central disc herniation. **(B)** Proper positioning of needles shown in (A) in lateral radiographic examination. **(C)** Insertion of two cannulas from right and left side of patient. This accommodates ipsilateral insertion of forceps and introduction of the arthroscope from the opposite portal for intradiscal triangulation. **(D)** Position of inserted instruments in lateral radiographic examination.

lateral fibers of the posterior longitudinal ligament adjacent to the tip of the inserted cannula (Fig. 33A,B). This permits exposure of the ventral surface of the traversing root and the dural sac. The recurrent disc herniation then may be isolated and retrieved via a working channel scope. If it becomes necessary, a bipolar radiofrequency probe may be utilized for hemostasis and vaporization of epidural and perineural scar tissue. Prior to retrieval of the cannula at the end of the operative procedure, a steroid compound may be used to infiltrate epidural and perineural structures.

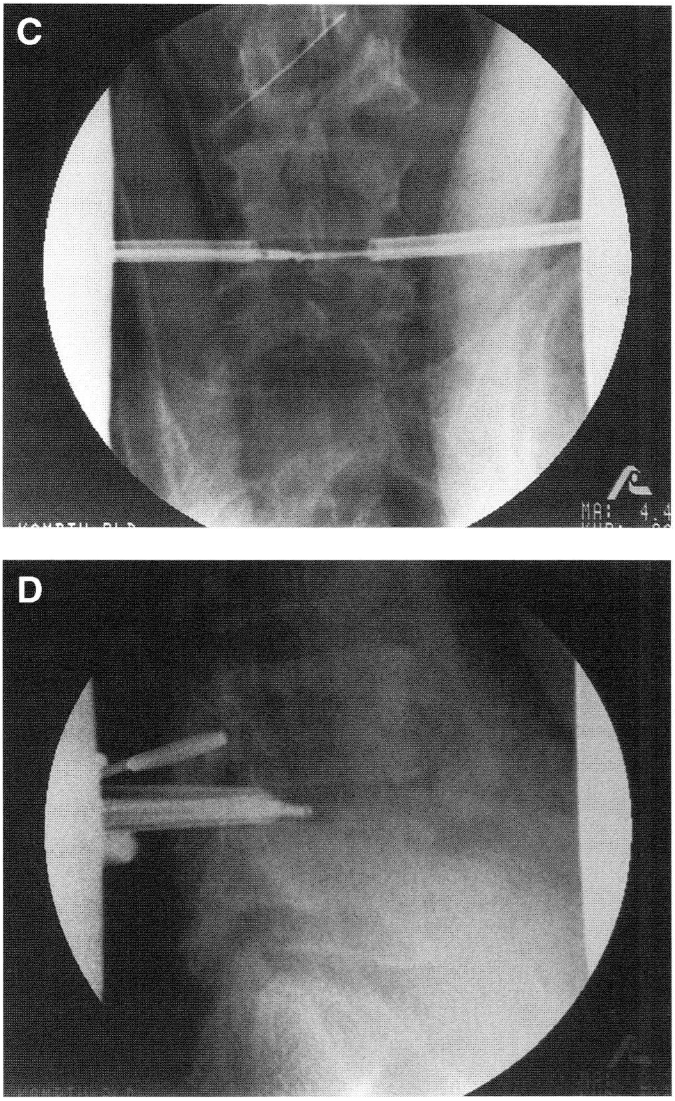

Fig. 34. *(Continued)*

HOW TO PREVENT COMPLICATIONS

Hazards Associated With Needle Insertion

A far lateral or vertical insertion of needles at the onset of a minimally invasive posterolateral approach to the intervertebral disc should be avoided. When performing surgery in the upper lumbar spine or at the thoracolumbar junction, the surgeon should request a preoperative prone CT study of the surgical site in order to determine accurately the distance of the skin entry site from the midline and the appropriate angle of needle insertion. Inadvertent vertical insertion of the needle may cause injury to the iliac arteries and veins or may penetrate the contents of the abdominal cavity.

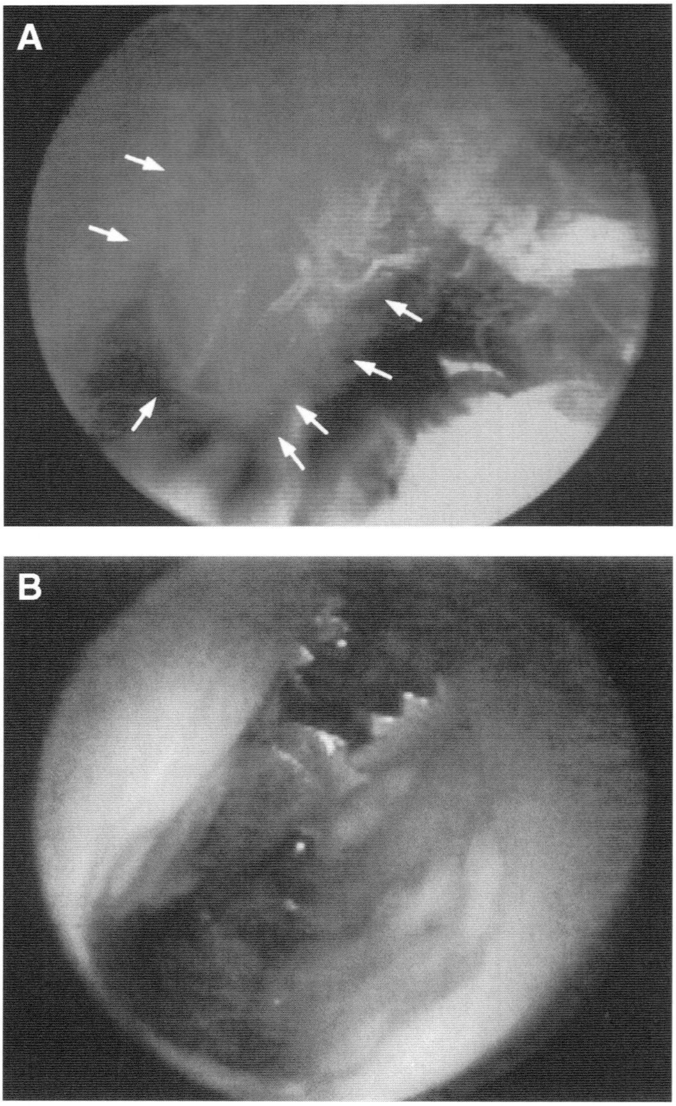

Fig. 35. **(A)** Interoperative photograph demonstrating how a cavity is created within intervertebral disc and intradiscal extension of sequestrated fragment is identified (arrows). (Reprinted from ref. *43*, with permission.) **(B)** Interoperative photograph showing use of deflecting suction forceps to access herniated disc fragments. **(C)** Intraoperative photograph demonstrating use of radiofrequency probe to develop communication between right and left portals.

Horizontal insertion of the needle at the onset of the operative procedure is always a safer practice.

Hazards Associated With Placement of Cannulated Obturator

The cannulated obturator should smoothly descend toward the triangular working zone as it advances over the previously positioned guide wire. The surgeon should maintain the direction of the insertion of the obturator with one hand while using the

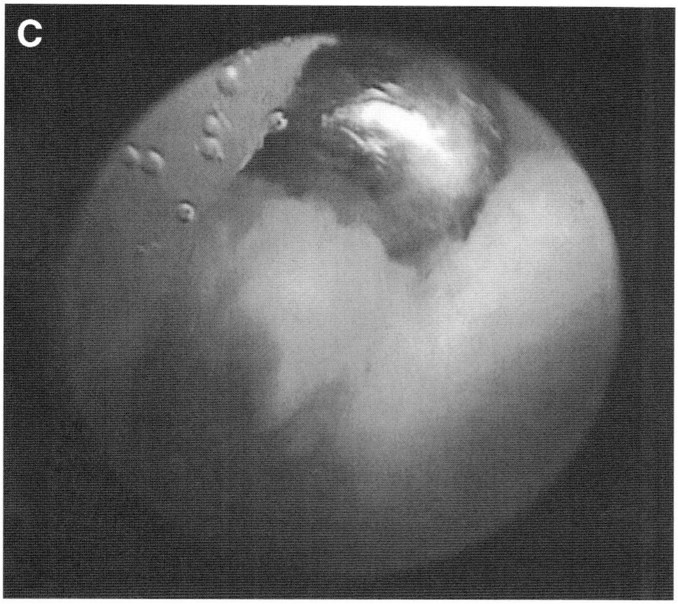

Fig. 35. *(Continued)*

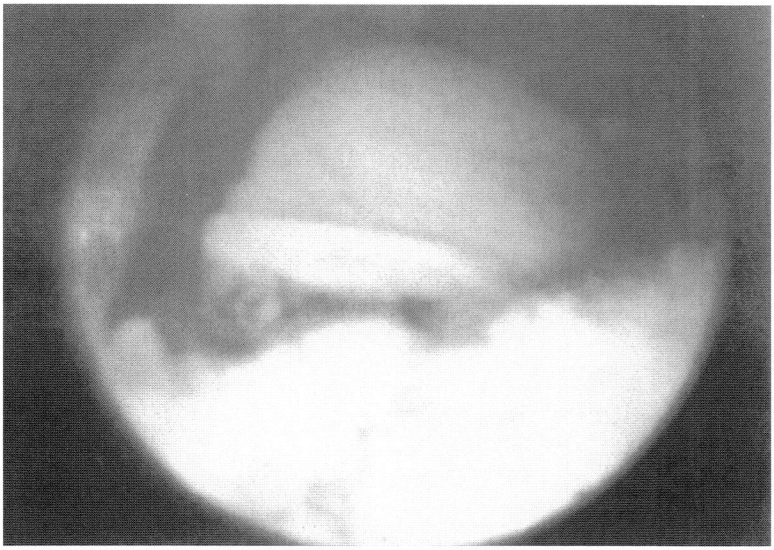

Fig. 36. Endoscopic view of undisturbed traversing root with intact accompanying fine vascular structures.

opposite hand to advance the obturator with a slow rotary movement. If the obturator is not aligned with the guide wire, forceful insertion of the obturator will tend to bend the inner end of the guide wire that is anchored into the annular fibers; misalignment also makes withdrawal of the guide wire difficult. If in doubt, intraoperative fluoroscopic examination should be conducted to confirm that the direction of the obturator and the guide wire has remained satisfactory (Fig. 19).

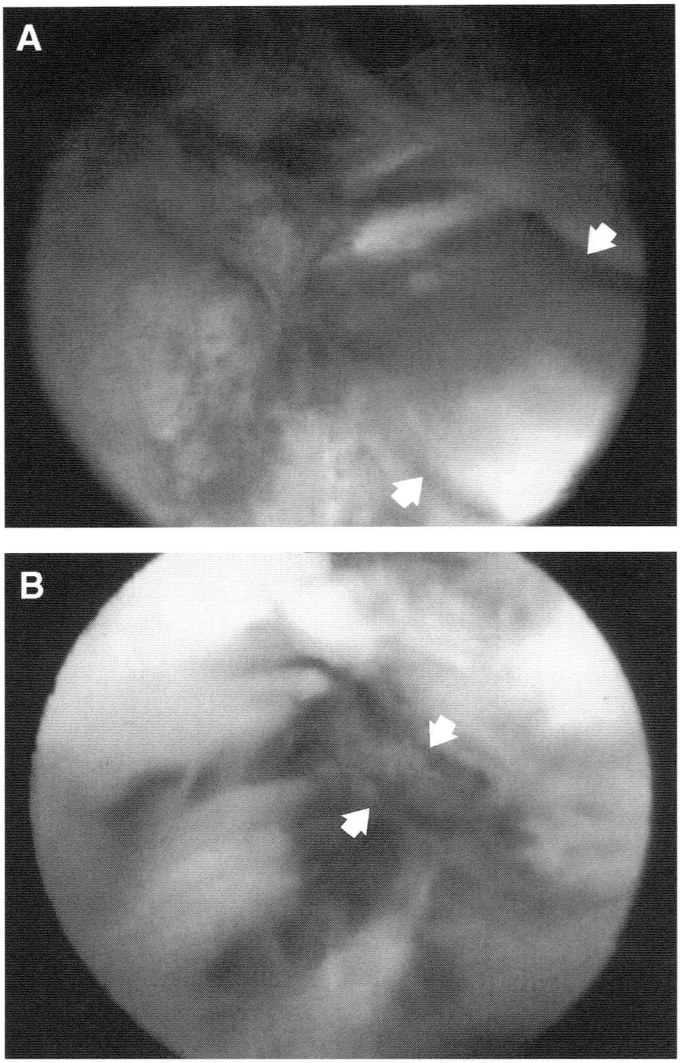

Fig. 37. (**A**) Interoperative photograph following intradiscal evacuation of large central herniation. Note the exposure of the ventral dura (arrows) and magnified view of a few fibers of the posterior longitudinal ligamentum shown at the top. (**B**) Intradiscal view of ventral dura following evacuation of sequestrated disc herniation. (**C**) Note torn fibers of the posterior longitudinal ligamenum and exposure of ventral dura (arrow) following intradiscal biportal evacuation of sequestrated disc herniation.

Hazards Associated With Migration of Cannula

The design of most instruments does not permit them to penetrate more than 2 cm beyond the distal extremity of the inserted cannula. Inadvertent intradiscal migration of the cannula will allow deep penetration of the tip of the forceps and other instruments into the intervertebral disc. This will cause complications if the instruments enter the abdominal cavity. When an intradiscal or subligamentous approach to the intervertebral

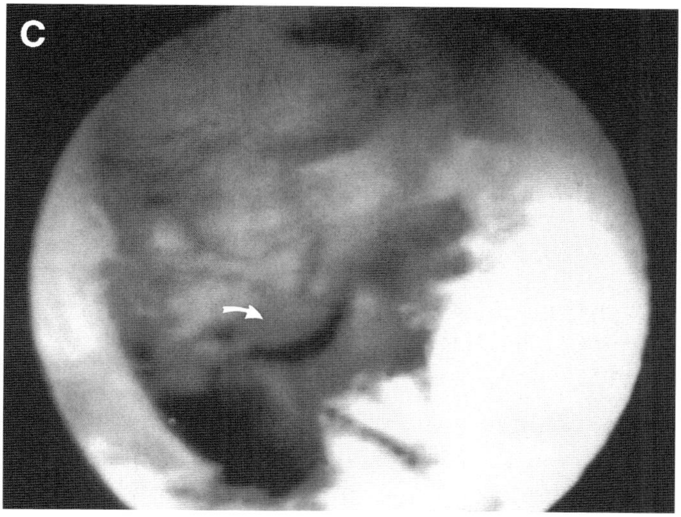

Fig. 37. *(Continued)*

disc is attempted, the distal end of the cannula should be engaged in the superficial layers of the annulus and held in this position by the operating surgeon throughout the surgical procedure.

Hazards Associated With Periannular or Intracannicular Bleeding

Periannular bleeding usually occurs when the cannula is not firmly held against the annular fibers in the triangular working zone. If excessive bleeding is encountered, the cannulated obturator should be reintroduced into the lumen of the cannula and firmly held against the annular surface. The cannula should then be advanced over the obturator and held in position. If the bleeding remains uncontrolled, AP and lateral X-rays should be taken to establish that the cannula is on the midpedicular line in the AP projection and has not been introduced into the spinal canal. Superficial veins on the surface of the annulus in the triangular working zone are invariably observed; they should be coagulated with a radiofrequency probe or by introducing a cottonoid saturated with topical anticoagulants. Epidural bleeding is common during transforaminal access to the spinal canal and should be meticulously controlled to achieve a clear view prior to insertion of grasping instruments.

Potential Hazards Associated With Use of Power-Driven Suction Nuclear Resectors

Great care must be exercised when a subligamentous approach is utilized for retrieval of herniated disc fragments. The use of suction and trimmer blades directly under the traversing root and dura is extremely dangerous and will cause serious complications. During a biportal approach to an intervertebral disc, a trimmer blade is invariably used to create a cavity and communication between the two portals. When the trimmer blade is retracted into the cannula to free nuclear debris, the open end of the trimmer blade should be turned ventrally and away from the neural structures and dural sac. Recently, we successfully used radiofrequency probes to resect nuclear tissue with no undue complications.

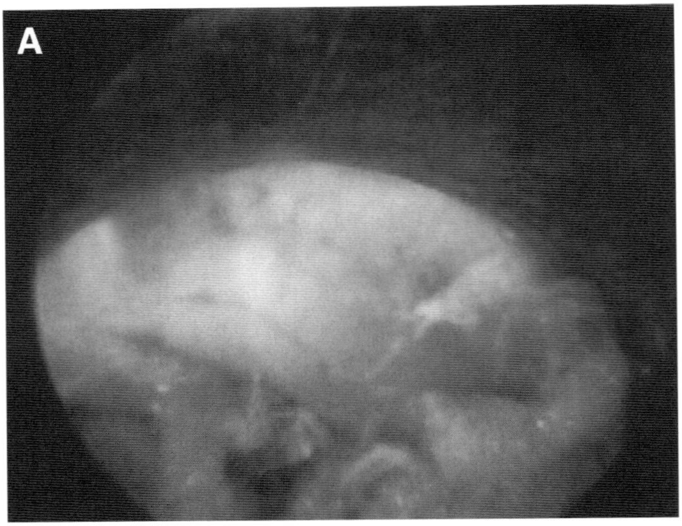

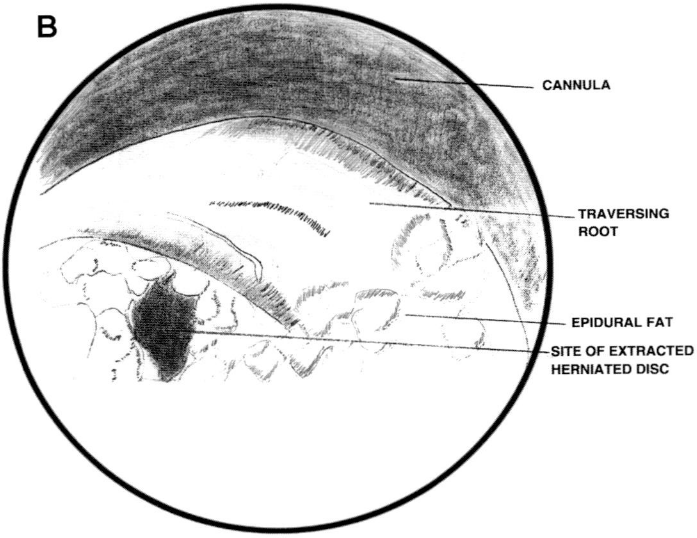

Fig. 38. (A,B) Intraoperative photograph demonstrating final examination of traversing root following intradiscal retrieval of sequestrated disc herniation. Note the site of extracted disc fragment.

Reducing Incidence of Postoperative Dysesthesia

Development of skin hypersensitivity following arthroscopic or endoscopic spine surgery via posterolateral access has been reported *(22,27)*. Symptoms usually occur 4 to 5 d following surgery and involve the preoperative symptomatic extremity. The presenting symptoms include complaints of a burning sensation, a causalgic type of pain, and an inability to wear a stocking or keep the limb under covers. Intraoperative trauma to the nerve root ganglia of the exiting or the traversing root may be responsible for the presenting symptoms. In our experience, this complication was more prevalent when transforaminal access to the spinal canal or decompression of the lateral recess stenosis was attempted *(27)*. The use of power-driven disc shavers or laser light in the foramen may also contribute to development of this complication.

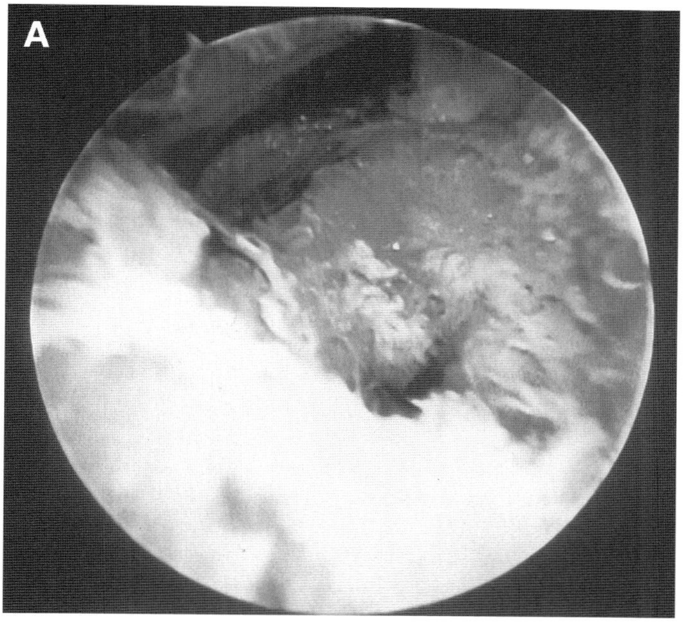

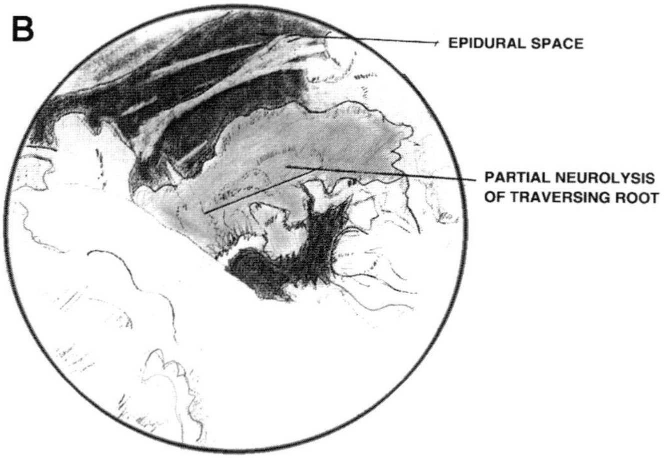

Fig. 39. (A,B) Intraoperative photograph showing neurolysis of traversing root surrounded by scar tissue and isolation of recurrent disc herniation.

Intraoperative injection of a mixture of fentanyl and normal saline solution around the nerve root ganglia at the onset of the operative procedure following proper positioning of an 18-gage needle in the triangular working zone has proven to be helpful in prevention of these complications.

Although most patients respond to oral administration of nonsteroidal or short-term steroid therapy, in our clinic we have had success with the intraforaminal steroid injection particularly in the first few days following the onset of the symptomatology. Under a sterile environment, an 18-gage needle is inserted into the foramen at the site of the previous surgery. Following radiographic confirmation of the position of the tip of the needle, a diluted mixture of a steroid compound is injected into the foramen around both the traversing and exiting nerve roots.

Preventing Postoperative Discitis and Infection

The incidence of postoperative bacterial discitis in the literature has been <0.5% *(22,41,42)*. When surgery is performed in an operating room setting and there is adherence to the principle of surgical technique including draping of the patient and C-arm, the chance of developing a postoperative infection will be greatly reduced. The use of prophylactic antibiotics is essential in the prevention of this serious complication.

REFERENCES

1. Lazarevic LK. Ischias postica Cotunni. Sypski Arch 1980;7:23.
2. Forst JJ. Contribution a l'etude clinique la sciatique. Paris, These 33:1881.
3. Lasegue EC. Consideration aure la sciatique. Arch Gen Med 1864;6:558–580.
4. Cram RH. A sign of nerve root pressure. J Bone Joint Surg 1953;35-B:192–195.
5. Kambin P. Arthroscopic microdiscectomy. Arthroscopy 1992;8:287–295.
6. Kambin P. Arthroscopic techniques for spine surgery, in Operative Arthroscopy (McGinty JB, Casperi RB, Jackson RW, Poehling GG, eds.), Lippincott-Raven, Philadelphia, 1996, pp. 1215–1225.
7. Atken AP, Bradford CH. End result of ruptured intervertebral disc in industry. Am J Surg 1947;73:365.
8. Balderston RA, Gilyard GG, Jones AM, et al. The treatment of lumbar disc herniation: simple fragment and excision versus disc space curettage. J Spinal Disord 1991;4:22–25.
9. Hampton D, Laros G, MacCarron R, Franks D. Healing potential of annulus fibrosis. Spine 1989;14(4):398–401.
10. Markolf KL, Morris JM. The structural components of the intervertebral disc: a study of their contributions to the ability of disc to withstand compressive forces. J Bone Joint Surg 1974;56-A:675–687.
11. Ross JS, Robertson JT, Frederickson RC, Petric JL, Obuchowski N, Modic MT, deTribolet N. Association between peridural scar and recurrent radicular pain after lumbar discectomy: magnetic resonance evaluation. ADCON-L European Study Group. Neurosurgery 1996;38:855–863.
12. Hermantin F, Quartararo L, Peters T, Kambin P. A prospective, randomized study comparing the results of open discectomy versus video-assisted microdiscectomy. J Bone Joint Surg 1999;81-A(7):958–965.
13. Haaland AK, Graver V, Ljunggren AE, Loeb M, Lie H, Magnaes B, Godal HC. Fibrinolytic activity as a predictor of the outcome of prolapsed intervertebral disc surgery with reference to background variables: results of a prospective cohort study. Spine 1992;17:1022–1027.
14. Park WW. The significance of venous return impairment in ischemic radiculopathy and myelopathy. Orthop Clin North Am 1991;22:213–221.
15. Park WW. Clinical anatomy of the lower lumbar spine, in Arthroscopic Microdiscectomy: Minimal Intervention in Spinal Surgery (Kambin P, ed.), Urban & Schwarzenberg, Baltimore, 1991, pp. 11–29.
16. Hoyland JA, Freeman AJ, Jayson ML. Intravertebral foramen venous obstruction: a cause of periradicular pain fibrosis. Spine 1989;14:558–568.
17. Dullerud R, Graver V, Haakonsen M, Haalaud AK, Loeb M, Magnaes B. Influence of fibrinolytic factors on scar formation after lumbar discectomy: a magnetic resonance imaging follow-up study with clinical correlation performed 7 years after surgery. Spine 1998;23:1464–1469.

18. Pountain GD, Keegan AL, Jayson ML. Impaired fibrinolytic activity in defined chronic back pain syndromes. Spine 1987;12:83–86.
19. Rantanen J, Hurme M, Falck B, Alaranta H, Nykvist F, Lehto M, Einola S,Kalimo H. The lumbar multifidus muscle five years after surgery for a lumbar intervertebral disc herniation. Spine 1993;18:568–574.
20. Weber BR, Grob D, Dvorak J, Muntener M. Posterior surgical approach to the lumbar spine and its effect on the multifidus muscle. Spine 1997;22:1765–1772.
21. Kambin P, Cohen L, Brooks ML, Schaffer JL. Development of degenerative spondylosis of the lumbar spine after partial discectomy: comparison of laminatomy, discectomy and posterolateral discectomy. Spine 1995;20:599–607.
22. Kambin P, O'Brien E, Zhou L. Arthroscopic microdiscectomy and selective fragmentectomy. Clin Orthop 1998;347:150–167.
23. Kambin P. Percutaneous lumbar discectomy: current practice. Surg Rounds Orthop 1988;31–35.
24. Kambin P. in Arthroscopic Microdiscectomy: Minimal Intervention in Spinal Surgery (Kambin P, ed.), Urban & Schwarzenberg, Baltimore, 1991, pp. 67–100.
25. Kambin P. The role of minimally invasive surgery in spinal disorders. Adv Oper Orthop 1995;3:147–171.
26. Kambin P. Arthroscopic microdiscectomy, in The Adult Spine: Principles and Practice Edition, (Frymoyer JW, Ducker T, Hadler N, et al. eds.), Raven, New York, 1996, pp. 2023–2036.
27. Kambin P, Casey K, O'Brien E, et al. Transforaminal arthroscopic decompression of lateral recess stenosis. J Neurosurg 1996;84:462–467.
28. Yeung A, Tsou PM. Posterolateral endoscopic excision for lumbar disc herniation, surgical technique: outcome and complications in 307 consecutive cases. Spine 2002;27:722–731.
29. Kambin P. Arthroscopic microdiscectomy: lumbar and thoracic in Spine Care, vol. 2 (White A, Schofferman JA, eds.), Mosby, St. Louis, 1995, pp. 1002–1016.
30. Kambin P, McCullen G, Park W, et al. Minimally invasive arthroscopic spinal surgery. Instruct Course Lect 1997;46:143–161.
31. Kambin P. Diagnostic and therapeutic spinal arthroscopy. Neurosurg Clin North Am 1996;7(1):65–76.
32. Kambin P. Unilateral biportal percutaneous surgical procedures and instrumentation. US patent 5,395,317, 1991.
33. Kambin P, Gennarelli T, Hermantin F. Minimally invasive techniques in spinal surgery: current practice. Neurosurg Focus 1998;4(2):1–10.
34. Kambin P, Sampson S. Laminectomy versus percutaneous lateral discectomy—a comparative study. Paper presented at 51st AAOS Meeting, February 1984, Atlanta, GA.
35. Kambin P, Casey K. Posterolateral arthroscopic and endoscopic microdiscectomy of lumbar spine. In Spinal Cord Surgery (Zileli M, ed.) Vol. 1 2002; pp 705–718.
36. Mathews HH, Kyles MK, Lang BH, Fiore SM, Gordon CL. Spinal endoscopy: indications, approaches and applications. Orthop Trans 1995;19:219.
37. Kambin P. Principles and experiences with monoportal arthroscopic microdiscectomy. Video presentation of endoscopic laminectomy and foraminatomy. Bulgrist Orthopaedic Hospital University of Zurich School of Medicine, Zurich, Switzerland, December 2, 1993.
38. Wiltse LL, Rothman SLG, Chafetz N. Stenosis in spondylolisthesis of the lumbar spine (Anderson GBJ, McNeill TW, eds.), Mosby Yearbook 1992, pp. 179–207.
39. Wiltse LL, Bateman JG, Hutchinson RH, et al. The paraspinal sacrospinalis-splitting approach to the lumbar spine. J Bone Joint Surg (Am) 1968;50:919–926.
40. Kambin P. Arthroscopic foraminal surgical procedures performed through a working channel scope. US patent application 08/207831 March 1994.

41. Hadjipavlou AG, Kambin P, Lander PH, Crow WN, Simmons JW. Imaging-guided minimally invasive surgery for low back pain, sciatica and spinal infection. J Intervent Radiol 1999;14:1–22.
42. Schaffer JL, Kambin P. Percutaneous posterolateral lumbar diskectomy and decompression with a 6.9 millimeter cannula: analysis of operative failures and complications. J Bone Joint Surg (Am) 1991;73:822–831.

5

Management of Discogenic Pain and Spinal Instability Using Minimally Invasive Surgical Techniques

Parviz Kambin, MD

INTRODUCTION

Although a causal relationship between lumbar disc herniation and radiculopathy has been well established by many clinical studies and scientific tests, the role of other pain generators of the lumbar spine in clinical manifestations of pain and disability is still being debated. The purpose of this chapter is to identify these pain generators and offer an alternative treatment modality for their management using minimally invasive surgical techniques.

PAIN GENERATORS AND THEIR MANAGEMENT

Degenerated and Bulging Intervertebral Discs

Fibers of the posterior longitudinal ligament, as well as superficial layers of the annulus fibrosis, are innervated by the sinovertebral nerve. The fibers of the posterior longitudinal ligamentum extend laterally to the foramena and into the extraforaminal region *(1)* (*see* Chapter 2). These fibers are extremely sensitive and cause pain when subjected to compression and tension. As early as 1948, Falconer et al. *(2)* reported reproduction of back pain and a referral type of leg pain when the intervertebral disc was compressed during surgery under local anesthesia. With the advent of minimally invasive spinal surgery, the sensitivity of the posterior longitudinal ligament and its lateral expansion has been well documented in recent literature. Kambin et al. *(3)* studied the pathophysiology of the bulging annulus that is associated with a degenerated intervertebral disc; partial tear of annular fibers; and peripheral migration of degenerated, collagenized nuclear tissue. Parke *(1)* demonstrated the role of the bulging intervertebral disc in producing tension on the fibers of the posterior longitudinal ligament and in the clinical presentation of low-back pain.

Peripheral Tear of the Annulus

Although discography has been the subject of controversy, the usefulness of computed tomography (CT) discography in identification of pain-producing peripheral

From: *Arthroscopic and Endoscopic Spinal Surgery: Text and Atlas: Second Edition*
Edited by: P. Kambin © Humana Press Inc., Totowa, NJ

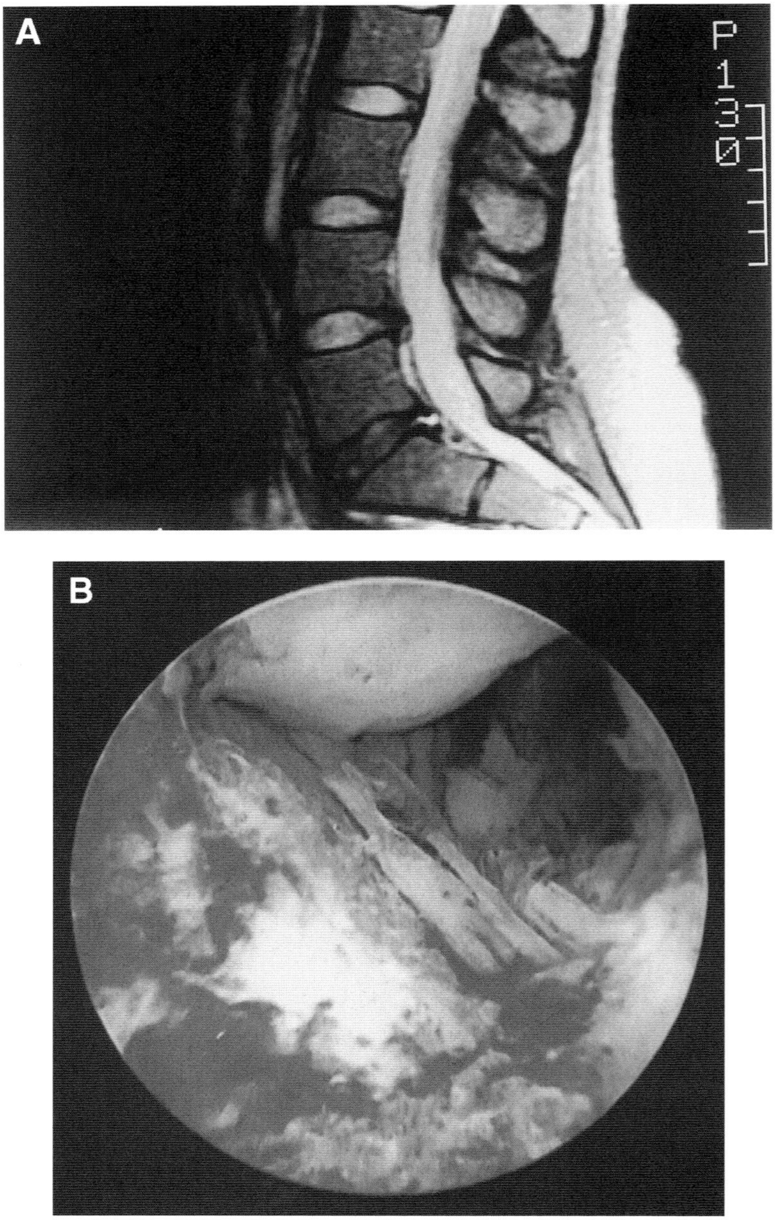

Fig. 1. (**A**) MRI study showing area of high intensity at L5-S1 level; (**B,C**) interoperative photograph demonstrating detachment of annulus from proximal vertebral plate and partial tear of annular fibers associated with ingrowth of granulation tissue that has been evacuated.

annular tears has been documented *(4–6)*. In addition, the successful relief of disabling pain following anterior column stabilization further confirms the importance of careful diagnosis of this pathological condition. Detachment of the annular rim that may be associated with ingrowth of innervated granulation tissue may be a source of disabling

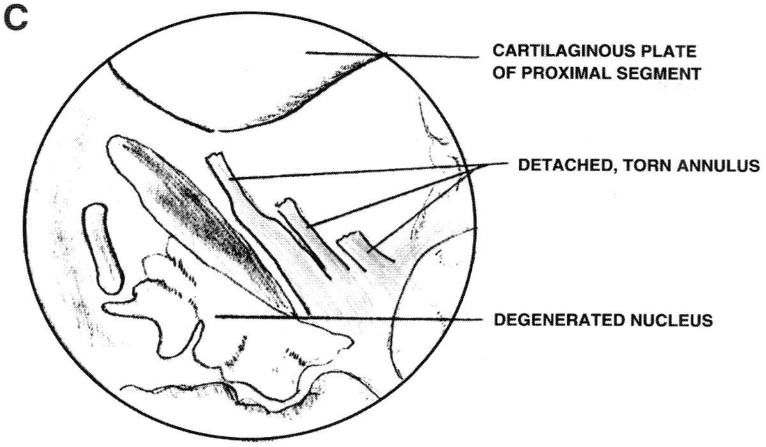

Fig. 1. *(Continued)*

low-back pain *(7)*. In magnetic resonance imaging (MRI) studies, the presence of a high-intensity zone in the posterior annulus appears to be owing to ingrowth of fibrovascular tissue into the torn annular fibers (Fig. 1A–C). At times, the high-intensity zone does not communicate with the nucleus pulposus and therefore makes the diagnosis of this condition with CT discography extremely difficult. In endoscopic diagnosis studies by my colleagues and I, we have found that the above structures are highly sensitive to palpation and compression via the instruments that are inserted through the previously positioned cannula and have been a useful diagnostic tool in our surgical armamentarium *(8)*.

Degenerative Facet Joint

Facet joints are weight-bearing synovial joints and, like joints of the extremities, are capable of producing pain. They may be treated with minimally invasive techniques. Posterolateral osteophytes arising from the vertebral plates and hypertrophic changes in the facet joints may be responsible for symptoms of lateral recess stenosis that require specific surgical management *(9)*.

Inflammatory Agents

The role of inflammatory agents in the development of pain has been extensively reviewed in the literature. It has been suggested that pain produced by discography is related to manipulation of the intervertebral disc that indirectly affects the vasoactive intestinal peptide (VIP) and substance P found in dorsal root ganglia *(6)*. A variety of neuropeptides, including calcitonin, gene-related peptide, and substance P, have been found in dorsal root ganglia. A relationship has been reported between low-frequency vibration and the amount of substance P and VIP in the dorsal root ganglia. A high level of phospholipase A2 activity has been found in lumbar disc herniation *(10)*. It has been speculated that loss of annular integrity and expulsion of nuclear material are associated with local inflammatory response in the epidural space and the nerve roots. The addition of mechanical compression on the already inflamed nerve root by the herniated disc is then associated with the onset of symptomatology and the clinical development of pain.

Diagnostic Modalities

In the absence of radiculopathy, the diagnosis and localization of a pain-producing intervertebral disc is unfortunately not a simple task. Although MRI studies invariably demonstrate the presence of annular tears, it is extremely difficult to establish that the MRI findings are responsible for the presenting symptomatology. However, MRI studies remain an excellent modality for diagnosis of the extent of hydration and degeneration of the intervertebral disc, the presence or absence of bulging or annular protrusion, and the identification of a high-intensity zone within the annular fibers (Fig. 1A,B). CT discography and provocative and anesthetic testings are reliable diagnostic modalities in identifying a pain-producing intervertebral disc. The presence of posterior and posterolateral subligamentous tears and fissures that reproduce the patient's symptomatology is a reliable guide for diagnosis of an abnormal and symptomatic intervertebral disc. The diagnostic task becomes simpler when degeneration is limited to a single spinal unit. However, in our experience, the identification of a single, symptom-producing intervertebral disc in the presence of multilevel degenerative changes has been difficult and somewhat unreliable.

Diagnostic arthroscopic probing that was described by Shepperd *(8)* may be a useful test for identifying a painful high-intensity zone that has been diagnosed with an MRI study. Under local anesthesia, a 5-mm-inner diameter (id) cannula is positioned in the triangular working zone adjacent to the spinal canal (see Chapter 4). A working scope is used, and a blunt-end probe is employed to palpate the posterior annulus and the site of the high-intensity zone. Severe pain simulating the patient's symptomatology is invariably experienced by the patient on palpation of the granulation tissue. In addition, the cessation of symptoms following local infiltration of xylocaine solution into the annular fibers further confirms the presence of annular pathology.

TREATMENT MODALITIES

Transforaminal Epidural and Perineural Steroid Therapy

The technique of transforaminal steroid therapy is an offspring of foraminal needle placement, which was developed in the early stages of percutaneous lumbar discectomy *(11–13)* (*see* Chapter 4). Invariably, owing to the presence of epidural adhesions in an already operated spine, the injected steroid in the middle or upper lumbar spine will not descend to the site of inflamed structures in the lower lumbar region. Therefore, transforaminal access allows delivery of the steroid compound directly to the epidural space, traversing and exiting the roots. In our experience, transforaminal steroid therapy has been helpful in the management of patients who are suffering from chronic radiculopathy or those who present with localized low-back pain owing to degenerated bulging intervertebral discs. The procedure is performed in a sterile environment. Needle positioning is similar to what was described under arthroscopic and endoscopic microdiscectomy in previous chapters. Under fluoroscopic control, the tip of an 18-gage needle is positioned at the midpedicular line in anteropasterior (AP) fluoroscopic examination. Then a mixture of appropriate steroid compound and anesthetics is injected into the foramen adjacent to the epidural space and the nerve roots.

Arthroscopic Annular Debridement

Subligamentous access to the intervertebral disc at the index level is first established (*see* Chapter 2). Then a posterior quadrant nucleotomy is performed, and the torn annular fibers are excised with a forceps and vaporized with a radiofrequency probe under fluid medium. Sometimes it is difficult to differentiate visually the nucleus and torn annular tissue. However, intradiscal injection of diluted indigen carmine will stain the nucleus and torn annular fibers, thus assisting the visual diagnosis of torn annular fibers. When torn annular tissue has been extracted, the fibers of the posterior longitudinal ligament that run perpendicular to the vertebral plate are identified. This indicates that adequate debridement has been accomplished (*see* Fig. 19A–C in Chapter 2).

Endoscopic Neurolysis of Nerve Roots

Recurrence of sciatic pain owing to perineural scar and tethering of the nerve roots following a successful laminatomy and discectomy is not uncommon. In our limited experience, we have had impressive success with endoscopic neurolysis and excision of epidural and perineural scar formation (*see* Fig. 39 in Chapter 4).

Reduction of Nuclear Mass and Partial Arthroscopic Decortication of Vertebral Plates

Using a uniportal approach, the nucleus is resected and the vertebral plates are partially decorticated. Pain relief following this procedure may be attributed to a reduction in intradiscal pressure; decreased tension on the posterior longitudinal ligament; and a gradual reduction in the height of the intervertebral discs, fibrous union, and autostabilization.

My limited experience with this technique has proven satisfactory in approx 65% of individuals with a single degenerated disc. None of the patients in this group had clinical or imaging evidence of lateral stenosis preoperatively. The outcome was more gratifying when free fragments of collagenized nucleus were found within the intervertebral disc and extracted (*see* Fig. 15A,B in Chapter 2).

Expandable Cages

An expandable cage may be introduced into the intervertebral disc through a cannula positioned posterolaterally. The cage is then filled with cancellous bone *(14)*.

Shepperd *(8)* experimented with a rigid metallic disc spacer that was introduced into the intervertebral disc using a posterolateral approach. However this procedure remains investigational.

Disc Prosthesis

In the last 10 yr, many investigators have attempted to design and implant a disc prosthesis that provides stability and allows physiological motion between the lumbar motion segments *(15–19)*. Long-term clinical studies dealing with this technique are not yet available. Various endoprosthetic designs have been proposed: low-friction ball-and-socket surfaces *(20)*, an artificial disc with contained fluid chambers *(21)*, a spring and hinge system *(22)*, and an artificial disc made of rubber and various elastomers. The ongoing investigation in our institution for replacement of the nucleus pulposus alone via a minimally invasive technique appears promising *(23)*. In this technique, the nucleus is replaced with a dehydrated biocompatible hydrogel polymer that is passed through a cannula and positioned in the center of the intervertebral disc by using a posterolateral approach. The hydrogel is then hydrated and allowed to expand and reach its predetermined shape and size within the confines of the annulus.

Thermal Intradiscal Therapy

Saal and Saal *(24)* recently reported on their experience with intradiscal thermal therapy on 25 patients presented with chronic discogenic low-back pain. A thermal catheter was introduced into the intervertebral disc via a posterolateral approach. The catheter's temperature was gradually raised to 90°C over a period of 13 min and was maintained for 4 min *(24)*. I have had no experience with this technology.

SEGMENTAL INSTABILITY AND ITS MANAGEMENT

The term *segmental instability* has not been well defined in the literature. However, it is commonly used as an indication for surgical fusion of a spinal unit. White and Panjabi *(9)* defined clinical instability as "loss of the ability of the spine under physiologic loads to maintain relationships between vertebrae in such a way that there is neither damage nor subsequent irritation to the spinal cord or nerve roots."

There are various kinds of segmental instabilities. Frymoyer and Selby *(25)* classified the various instabilities as axial, rotational, translational, retrolisthetic, and postsurgical.

There has been no uniform consensus among surgeons on the indications for spinal fusion. No generally accepted criteria have been developed or published on this subject. The following criteria described in the literature appear to be arbitrary and subjective: "prolapsed intervertebral disc in a young patient who wishes to return to the same type of manual work," "prolapsed intervertebral disc with disc-space narrowing," "primary central disc herniation," "disc herniation with a long-standing history of back pain," and "back pain being greater than leg pain."

Although these criteria are useful in deciding whether or not to fuse a given motion segment, they do not provide an objective assessment of the source of pain and disability, nor does they ensure that the patient will indeed benefit from the arthrodesis.

Clinically, the surgical stabilization of a motion segment is justified under the following set of circumstances:

1. When the integrity of the stabilizing structures of the motion segment has been compromised: This includes developmental instability associated with a defect in the pars interarticularis; surgically induced instability; and posttraumatic fracture or ligamentous injuries, infection, and osteomyelitis.
2. When the ability of the intervertebral disc to contain and transmit the external forces has been altered: This includes localized degenerative disc pathology as well as degenerative spondylolisthesis and retrolisthesis associated with radiographic evidence of hypermobility on lateral flexion and extension or AP side-bending films. In addition, symptom-producing adult scoliotic curves fall in this category.

In a clinical setting, generally there are three requisites for surgical stabilization of spinal units: disabling back pain, positive provocative and anesthetic testing, and abnormal dynamic studies (Fig. 2).

Fusion of the vertebrae is the oldest and still the most common and acceptable method of treating disabling low-back pain. Posterior stabilization, advocated by Albee *(26)* in 1911 and Hibbs *(27)* in 1912 for the treatment of Pott's disease, has also been

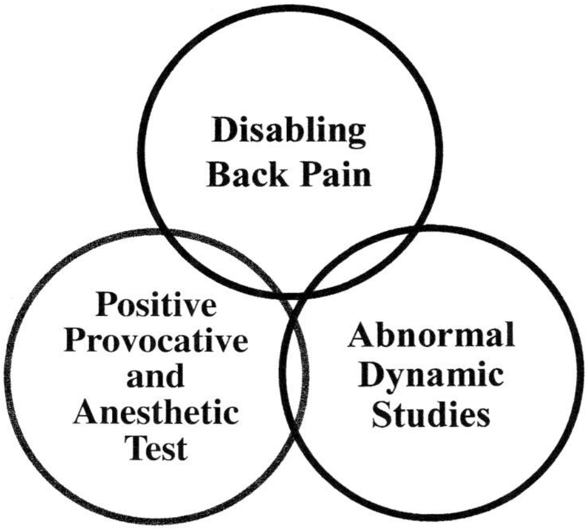

Fig. 2. The three prerequisites for surgical stabilization of the spinal unit.

used by clinicians for stabilization of painful degenerative conditions of the lumbar spine. The contributions of Watkins *(28)* and Wiltse et al. *(29)* to the concept of postero-lateral fusion also deserve recognition.

Cloward *(30)* should be credited for the description and popularization of anterior column stabilization. This remains the cornerstone of the current method for treating painful and unstable discogenic lumbar spine pain. The broad contact surface of the vertebral plates in the lumbar region, its adequate blood supply, and a natural exposure of interbody grafts to compression forces while the patient is ambulatory *(12–31)* have contributed to the high success rate and wide acceptance of anterior column stabilization when fusion of lumbar segments is deemed necessary. The addition of internal skeletal fixators by Harrington and other investigators further revolutionized the art of stabilizing spinal segments without the need to use casts or bulky braces *(32,33)*.

The following advances in the field of minimally invasive spinal surgery may be responsible for the renewed interest in arthroscopic interbody fusion:

1. Identification of radiographic and arthroscopic landmarks of the triangular working zone on the dorsolateral corner of the annulus fibrosis for safe positioning of cannulas *(11,12,34)*.
2. Development of technology for percutaneous insertion of pedicular fixators *(13,33,35)*.
3. Availability of manual and power-driven tools that may be passed through cannulas to access and decorticate the concave surfaces of the vertebral plates.
4. Availability of osteoinductive bone proteins, gene therapy, and tissue engineering to enhance osteogenesis at the fusion site.

The concept of percutaneous interbody fusion that was initiated in the mid-1980s evolved from earlier experience by my colleagues and I with percutaneous discectomy. This was followed by positioning of pedicular screws through inserted cannulas and subcutaneous (sc) placement of the plates in the early 1990s *(36)*, therefore adding a new dimension to the final outcome of the operative procedure.

Although Magerl *(33)* utilized percutaneously inserted screws and external fixators for stabilization of thoracolumbar spine fractures, we thought there was a need for more control and more accurate placement of pedicular screws. Therefore, we positioned a guide pin in the medullary canal of the pedicle under fluoroscopic control. This was

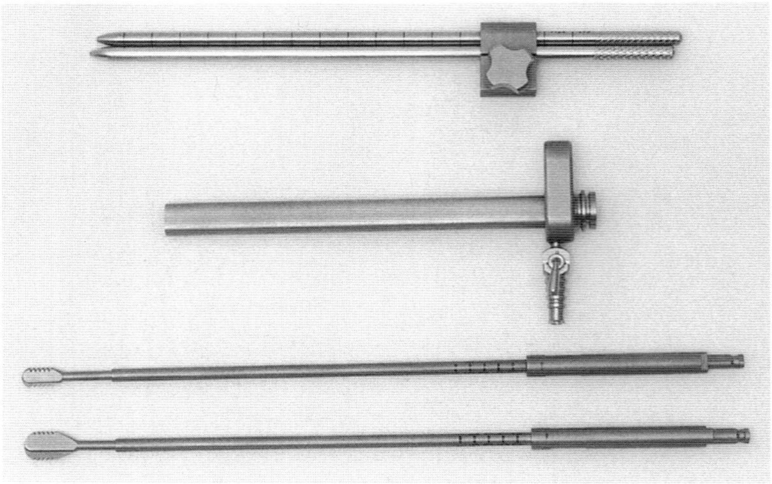

Fig. 3. Tools to facilitate successful performance of anterior column stabilization: from top to bottom, two cannulated obturators inserted into obturator jig, 5 × 10 mm id oval cannula, and two sizes of vertebral plate decorticators.

then followed by introduction of a 10-mm-id cannula adjacent to the site where the guide pin entered the pedicle. This permitted tapping of the medullary canal in the pedicle and probing of its cortices prior to final insertion of the pedicular screws. In addition, sc placement of the plates eliminated the incidence of pin tract infection and complications associated with the use of bulky external fixators.

Leu and Schreiber *(37)* have published on their experience with percutaneous lumbar fusion and the use of AO external fixators using the bull's-eye technique.

Arthroscopic Anterior Column Stabilization Augmented With Percutaneously Inserted Pedicular Bolts and sc Plates

In addition to arthroscopic microdiscectomy instruments, special tools have been developed to facilitate successful performance of anterior column stabilization. In our institution, we have discontinued the use of telescopic cannulas that allowed the insertion of a 9 × 9 mm id cannula into the intervertebral disc through which we proceeded with decortication of the vertebral plates and insertion of bone grafts *(31)*. Undue expansion of the height of the intervertebral disc was felt to be responsible for stretching of the nerve root and postoperative development of pain and dysesthesia. A 5 × 10 mm id oval cannula (Fig. 3) allows insertion of larger pituitary and cup forceps for rapid removal of nuclear tissue. In addition, this larger cannula provides passage of inserted decorticators to access the concave surfaces of the vertebral plates.

A cannulated soft-tissue dilator with a 9-mm outer diameter provides access to the pedicles without damaging the surrounding soft tissues. It also allows the proper positioning of a 10-mm-id pedicular cannula over the four pedicles adjacent to the fusion site (Fig. 4). Cannulated pedicular bolts and extension bars of various lengths (Fig. 5) permit precise positioning of the bolts within the medullary canal of the pedicles over the previously inserted guide pins.

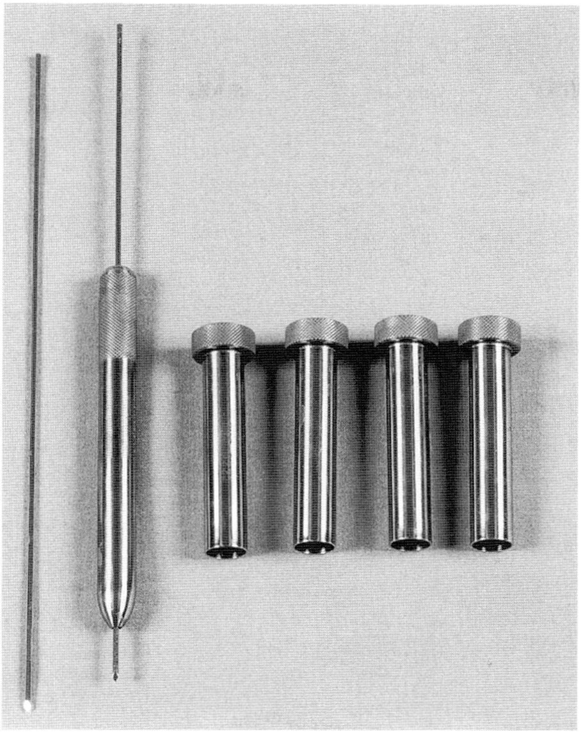

Fig. 4. Additional tools for anterior column stabilization: from left to right, Steinman pin, cannulated obturator, four 10-mm-id pedicular cannulas.

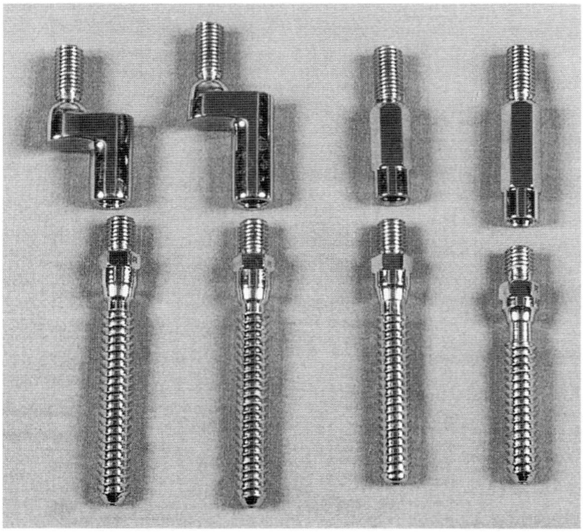

Fig. 5. Various sizes of pedicular bolts with straight and step-off extension bars.

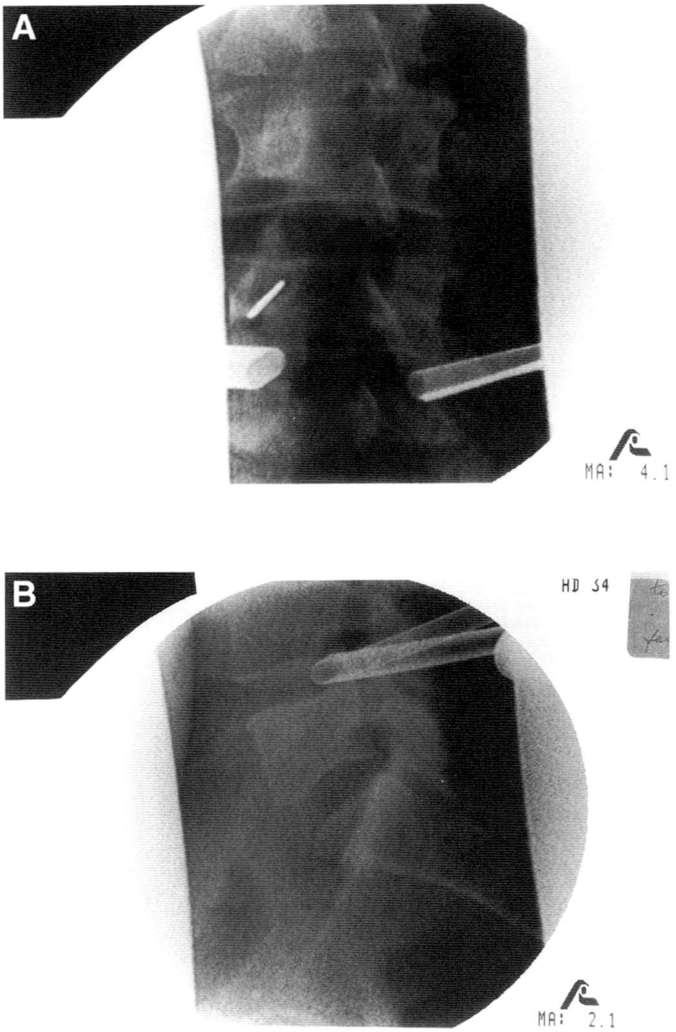

Fig. 6. **(A)** Interoperative AP view of biportal access to intervertebral disc. Note the insertion of a 5 × 10 mm id oval cannula on the left and a 5 mm id cannula on the right. A Steinman pin has been inserted into the pedicle of L4. (Printed with permission from ref. *13*.) **(B)** Lateral X-ray view of position of cannula as shown in (A).

Principles of Operative Technique

The patient is positioned prone on a radiolucent frame and table. General or spinal anesthesia is usually required. A biportal access to the intervertebral disc adjacent to the fusion site is established (*see* Chapter 3) *(7,13,31,34,37–39)* (Fig. 6A,B). The ipsilateral insertion of a 5 × 10 mm id oval cannula facilitates ample access to the intervertebral disc for extraction of the nuclear tissue, decortication, and insertion of the bone grafts (Fig. 7A–D). Meticulous nucleotomy under arthroscopic control is necessary prior to decortication of the vertebral plates. We have used both laser light and radiofrequency probes for nuclear debulking *(13–34)*. Chemopapain solution may be used for a rapid

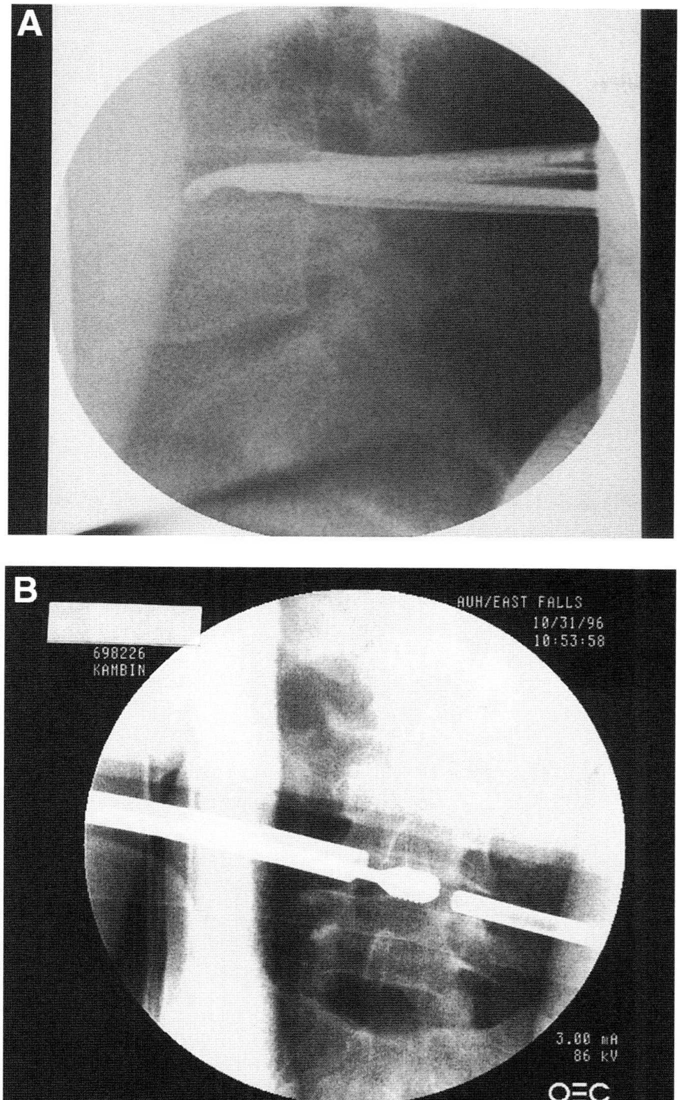

Fig. 7. **(A)** A gooseneck curette has been passed through the oval cannula for manual decortication of the vertebral plates. (Reprinted with permission from ref. *13*.) **(B)** A plate decorticator is being used for removal of the cartilaginous surface of the vertebral plates via a biportal approach. **(C)** A laser light is being utilized for removal of nuclear tissue. **(D)** Decorticated vertebral plates are shown.

and satisfactory nucleolysis. This step is then followed by ample irrigation of the intervertebral disc space. Decortication of the vertebral plates is then accomplished with appropriate decorticators and a curved curette. Bone grafts are harvested from the ilium and packed between the decorticated vertebral plates.

The use of pedicular fixation has been essential to the success of arthroscopic anterior column stabilization. To ensure accurate placement of the pedicular bolts, a

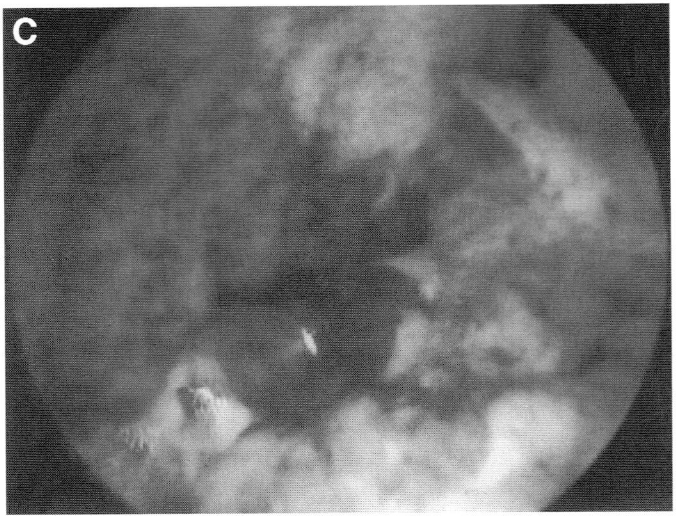

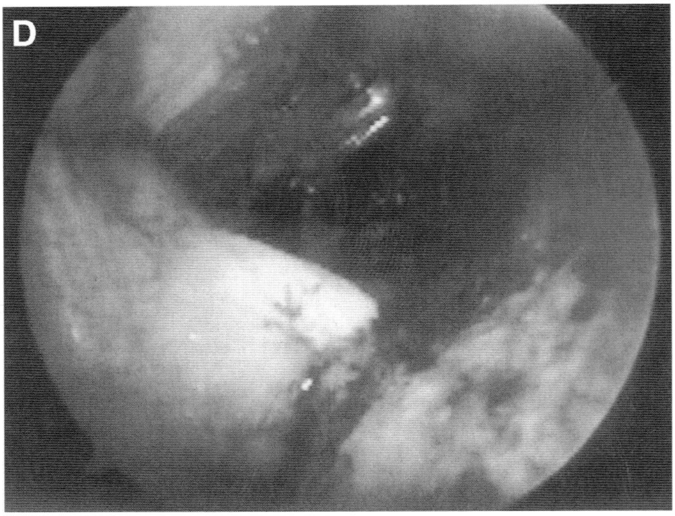

Fig. 7. *(Continued)*

Steinman pin is first inserted into the medullary canal of the pedicle of segments located above and below the fusion site. The skin entry site is determined by reviewing and measuring the preoperative axial CT study of the vertebra above and below the fusion site. Although the bull's-eye technique has been used to ensure the proper positioning of the pedicular screws *(33–37)*, we have found that positioning of the guide pin under fluoroscopic control in both the AP and lateral projections provides more information and results in better final placement of the pedicular bolts *(13–39)*.

The inherent inaccuracy of the bull's-eye technique is related to three factors:

1. The procedure requires tilting of the C-arm away from the pedicle that is being probed or, alternatively, tilting the patient and the operating table away from the C-arm that is positioned

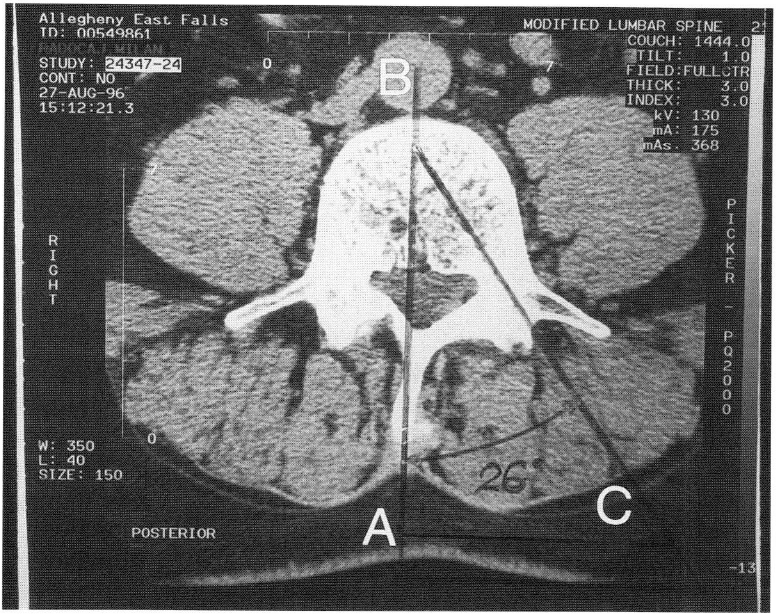

Fig. 8. Axial CT scan of segment adjacent to fusion site. Line AB passes through the spinal process and bisects the vertebra. Line BC represents the desired direction of the pedicular bolt. Line AC represents the distance from the midline and the desired site of skin incision for positioning of the pedicular cannula and insertion of the pedicular bolts. (Reprinted with permission from ref. *13.*)

for AP fluoroscopic examination. The tilt of the C-arm directly affects the direction and final position of the inserted guide pins into the pedicle. Peripheral X-ray beams may distort and alter positioning of the guide pin and, ultimately, the position of the pedicular bolt. An arbitrary 20–30° tilt of the C-arm may not ensure proper positioning of the guide pins in every individual and in various locations of the spinal column. An accurate preoperative determination of the anatomical angle of the pedicle in relation to the vertebral body of the same segment provides more specific information for insertion of the guide pins.

2. The skin entry points of the guide pins also play an important role in the final positioning of the guide pins in the pedicles. For example, excessive tilting of the X-ray tube will require that the skin entry site be placed more laterally, which might not be desirable.
3. The distance between the X-ray tube and the patient may affect the final position of the guide pins.

In our institution, prior to the surgical procedure, we perform a prone axial CT study through the pedicles of vertebrae adjacent to the fusion site. It is desirable to request an axial view that accurately reflects the exact size of the individual's vertebral bodies (Fig. 8).

A longitudinal line (AB) that bisects the vertebral bodies and extends to the center of the spinal process of the same segment is drawn on the axial CT scan film. Another line (BC) that represents the desirable position of the guide pin is drawn through the pedicle. Line AC represents the distance between the midline and the skin entry point. The angle between lines AB and BC represents the desired angle of insertion of the guide pin (or the tilt of the C-arm if the use of the bull's-eye technique is contemplated).

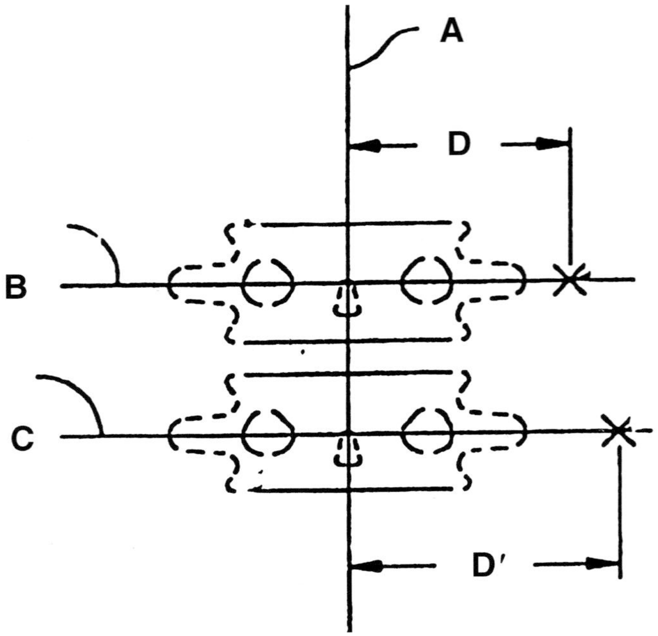

Fig. 9. Schematic drawing. Line A represents a midline drawn over the spinal processes. Lines B and C represent lines drawn through the center of the pedicles adjacent to the fusion site. Line D represents the distance from the midline and the site of the skin incision for insertion of the pedicular cannula.

At the onset of the operative procedure, while the patient is in a prone position under fluoroscopic control, a guide pin is positioned over the spinal processes of the lumbar segments. The midline of the spinal column is identified, and the skin surface is marked accordingly (Fig. 9).

Two guide pins are then placed over the pedicles of the segments that require stabilization. Accurate position of the guide wire is confirmed radiographically. A traverse line is then drawn on the skin surface perpendicular to the previous line drawn over the spinal processes. Information obtained from measurement of the axial CT scan is then transferred to the surgical site. The skin entry point (Fig. 8, lines A and C) is measured form the midline, and the guide pin is introduced manually and directed toward the pedicle with a rotary movement. AP and lateral fluoroscopic images confirm the positioning of the guide pin on the pedicle. In the AP projection the tip of the inserted guide wire should be seen in the lateral boundary of the pedicle (Fig. 10A). This step is then followed by full insertion of the guide pin into the medullary canal of the pedicle and the vertebral body of the same segment. The proper direction of the inserted guide pin should be monitored in the lateral fluoroscopic examination (Fig. 10B).

Following satisfactory positioning of the Steinman pin, a skin incision about 1 cm in length is made adjacent to the guide pin, and a blunt-end soft-tissue dilator and pedicular cannula are introduced until they reach the facet and pedicles of the vertebra (Fig. 11A). While the pedicular cannulas are firmly held against the pedicles, a cannulated pedicular tap is used and passed over the guide pin, and the medullary canal of the pedicle is tapped in preparation for final insertion of the pedicular bolts. Prior to insertion of the pedicular

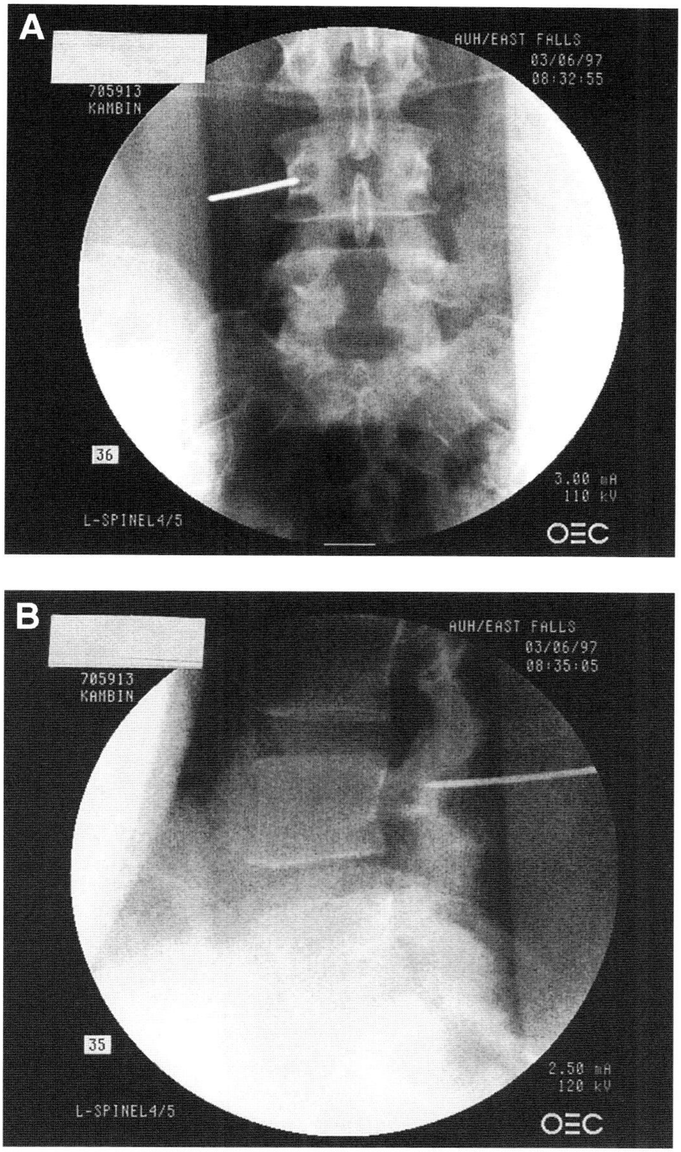

Fig. 10. **(A)** Interoperative AP fluoroscopic examination shows the proper positioning of the guide pin adjacent to the lateral boundary of the pedicle. **(B)** The lateral view of the fluoroscopic examination shown in (A) shows the appropriate direction of the guide pin in the center of the pedicle.

bolts, the medullary canal of the pedicle is examined and probed to make certain that the cortices of the pedicle have not been violated (Fig. 11B). Subcutaneous placement of the plates requires that the pedicular bolts be lengthened to reach the sc region. Extension bars (Fig. 5) of appropriate length are then selected and attached to the proximal end of the pedicular bolts. Stabilization is completed when the bolts are linked and firmly held to one another by a plate that is placed in the sc region of the lumbar spine (Fig. 12A–D).

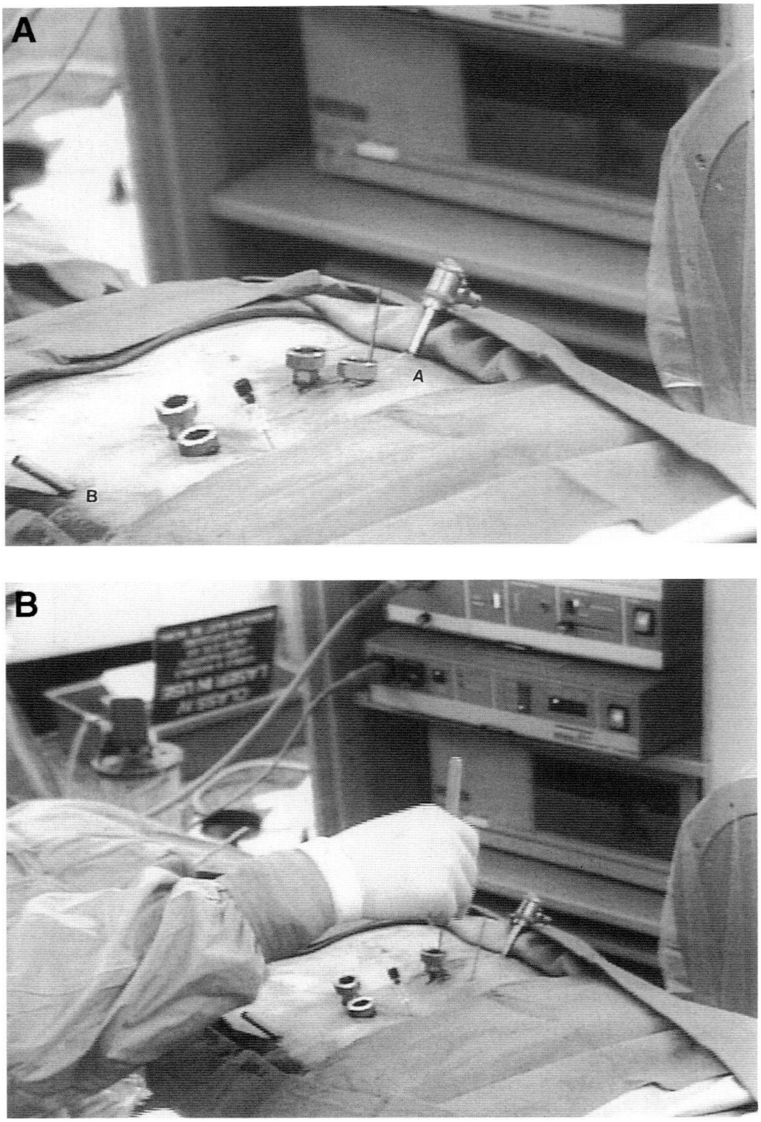

Fig. 11 (A) Interoperative photograph demonstrating that cannulas A and B have been inserted into intervertebral disc at index level and four pedicular cannulas are positioned over pedicles in preparation for insertion of pedicular bolts. The needle in the center was used for spinal anesthesia. **(B)** Interoperative photograph demonstrating how medullary canal of pedicle is being palpated to make certain that cortices of pedicle have not been disturbed.

Screw Fixation of First Sacral Segment

Percutaneous anterior column stabilization between the fifth lumbar vertebra and the sacrum has been challenging. The height of the iliac crest, particularly in male individuals, will interfere with establishing biportal access to the intervertebral disc for nucleotomy, decortication, and bone grafting. However, partial resection of the cephalad vertebral

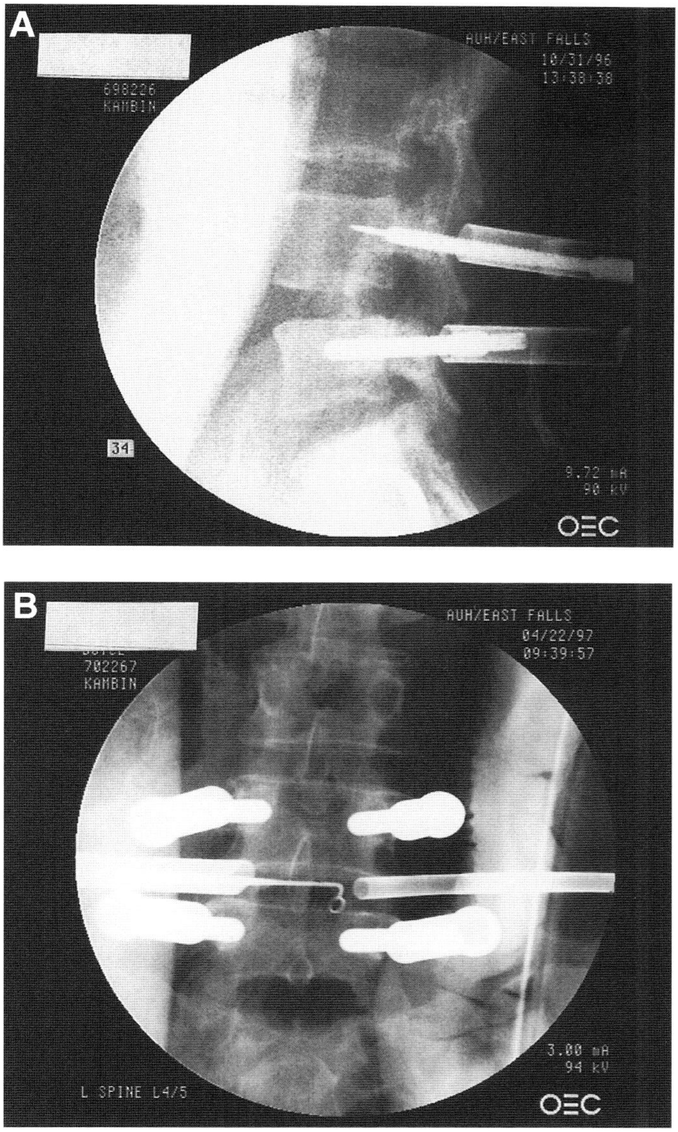

Fig. 12. **(A)** Interoperative lateral X-ray view of surgical site. Note the position of the pedicular cannulas and insertion of pedicular bolts over the previously positioned guide pins. **(B)** Interoperative AP fluoroscopy shows that four pedicular bolts are properly positioned. An angled-ring curette is used for further decortication of the vertebral plates in preparation of introduction of the bone grafts. **(C)** Postoperative X-ray study shows the proper position of the pedicular bolts and extension bars, and sc position of the plates. **(D)** Lateral fluoroscopic examination shown in (C). Note the inserted bone grafts at L4-L5 and sc position of the vertebral plates.

plates *(34)* adjacent to the fusion site through the previously positioned cannula will provide better access to the intervertebral disc at L5-S1.

Percutaneous insertion of pedicular screws to the first sacral segment also is difficult and time-consuming. Our experience with paramedial miniexposure of L5-S1 intervertebral

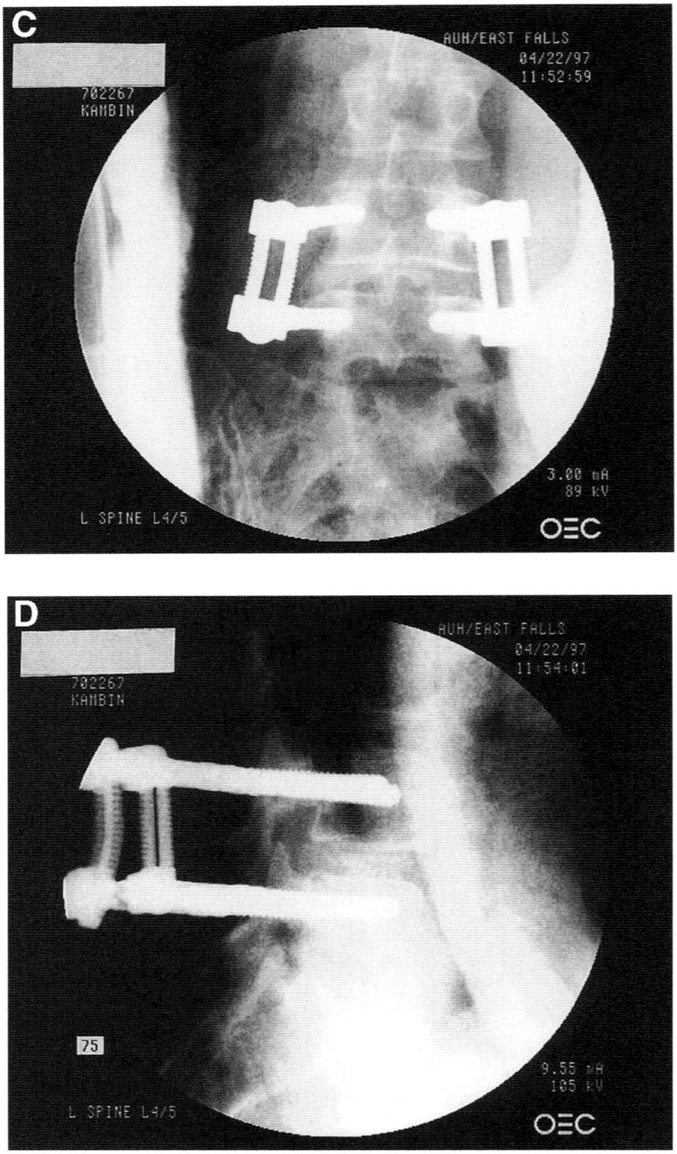

Fig. 12. *(Continued)*

disc and the facet joints for partial facetectomy and exposure of the triangular working zone has provided ample access to the intervertebral disc and articular process of the first sacral segment for insertion of the pedicular screw. Following extensive disc resection via a posterolateral approach and decortication of the vertebral plates, tricortical and cancellous bone is packed at the fusion site. Insertion of the pedicular bolt into the fifth lumbar vertebra and the sacrum is then accomplished under direct vision or via endoscopic illumination and magnification. Various approaches and techniques have been used for distal fixation of the construct to the sacrum or iliac crest. Most of the difficulties are related to inadequacy of bone quality.

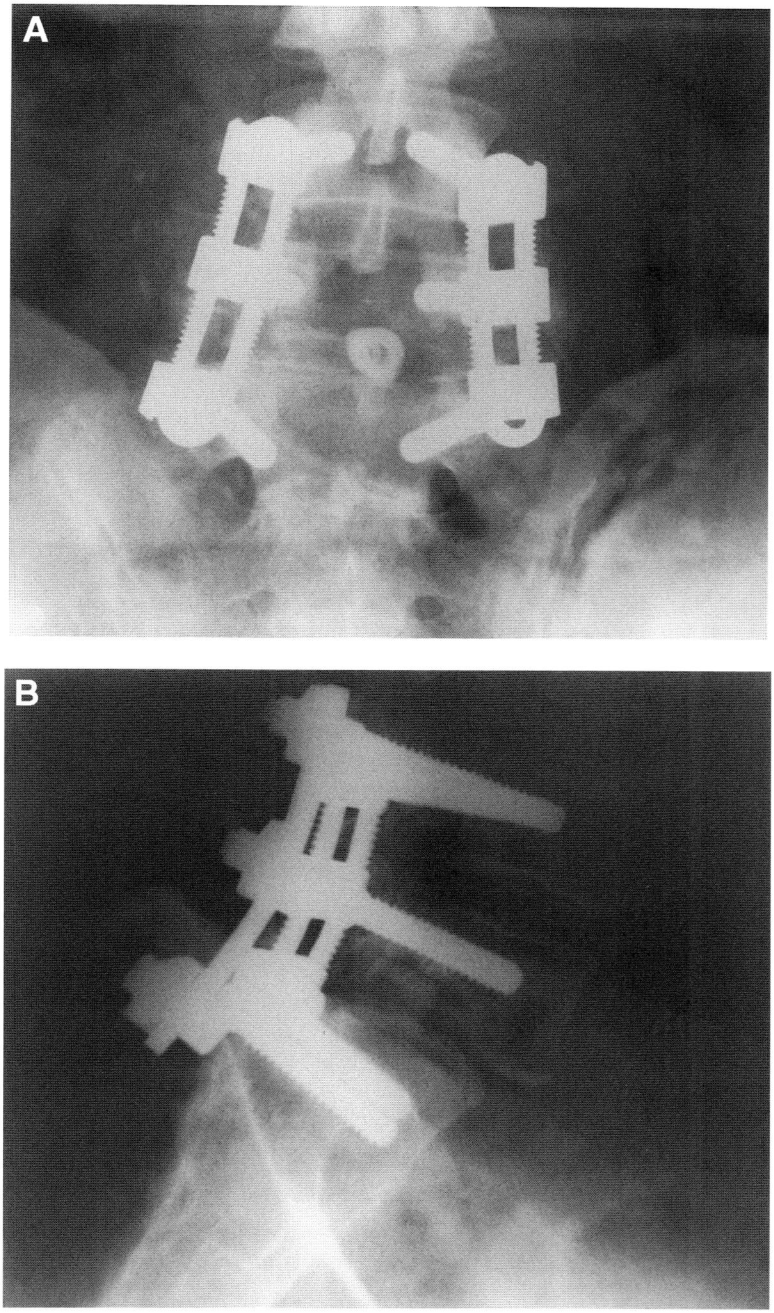

Fig. 13. **(A)** AP and **(B)** lateral postoperative X-ray study of a 45-yr-old laborer presented with Grade II spondylolisthesis of L5-S1 associated with L5 radiculopathy. The patient also had degenerative disc disease with positive CT discography and anesthetic testing at L4-L5. Percutaneous insertion of the pedicular bolts at L4-L5 with percutaneous fusion at the same level was performed. Insertion of the sacral screw and interbody fusion at L5-S1 were accomplished via a mini-incision. Note the medial and distal direction of the sacral screw. Fibular cortical bone and autogenous cancellous bone were used for fusion at L5-S1.

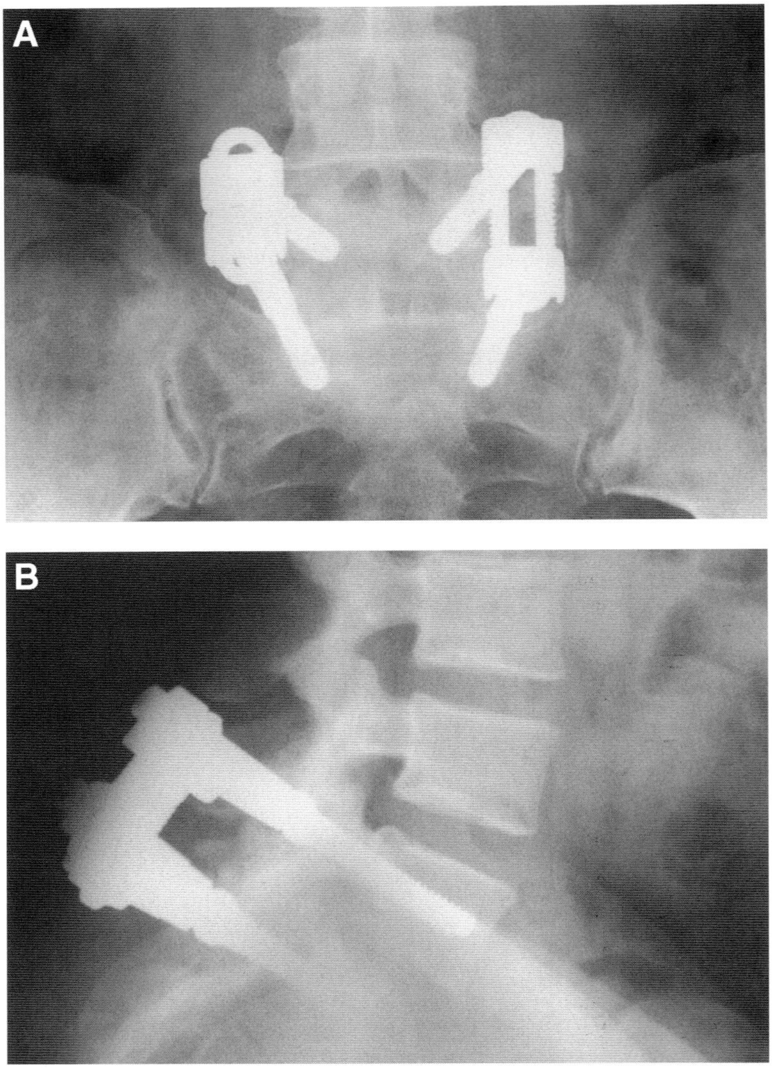

Fig. 14. **(A)** AP and **(B)** lateral postoperative X-ray study of posterolateral arthroscopic fusion at L5-S1 and sc positioning of plates.

In our clinic, we have obtained satisfactory sacral fixation by inserting the screw dorsomedially (Fig. 13A,B). The entry point is at the distal end of the articular process of the first sacral segment. A guide wire is inserted and directed anteromedially into the vertebral body of the first sacral segment. The guide wire bypasses the spinal canal and the S1 and S2 nerve root. The cortical bone of the articular process of the first sacral segment provides adequate cortical support and anchorage for the inserted screw.

The proper position of the guide wire is then evaluated via AP and lateral fluoroscopic examination. This step is followed by insertion of a cannulated pedicular tap and

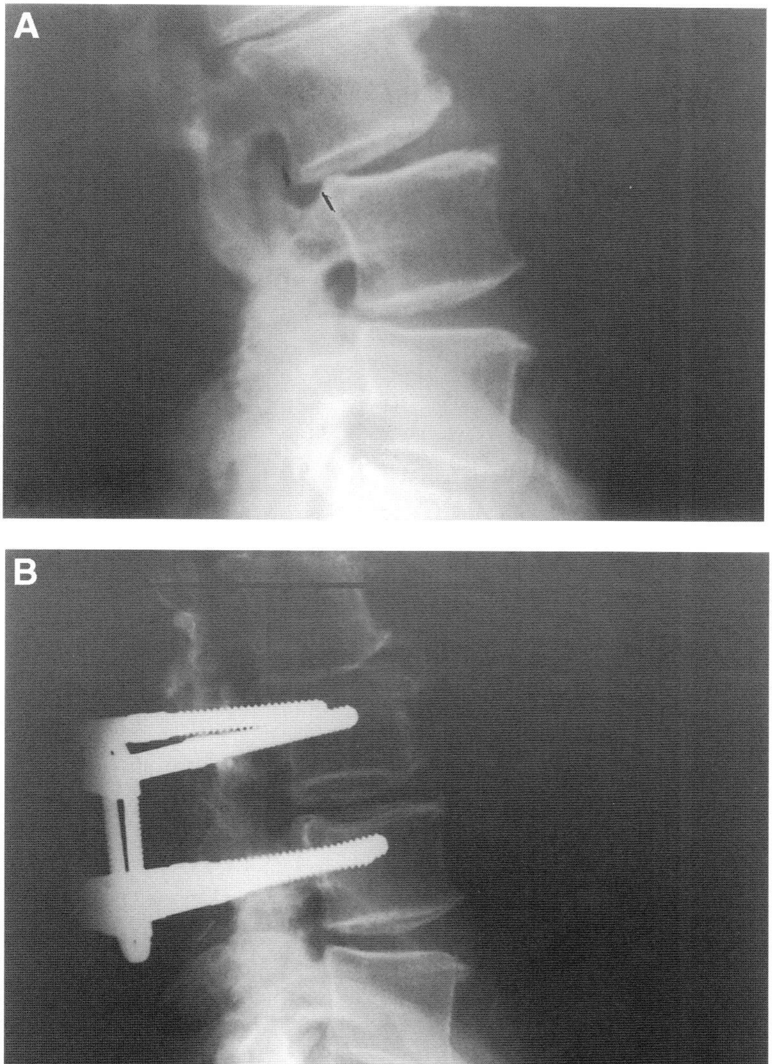

Fig. 15. (**A**) Preoperative lateral X-ray of a 40-yr-old male patient who presented with radiographic evidence of retrolisthesis at L3-L4 and intractable back and anterolateral right thigh pain. (**B**) Postoperative lateral X-ray following percutaneously inserted pedicular bolts, reduction of retrolisthesis, and sc fixation. The patient reported relief following stabilization of the above motion segment and use of a brace for 4 wk. Subsequently he underwent arthroscopic posterolateral interbody fusion with a satisfactory outcome.

of a sacral screw of appropriate length and diameter. Owing the angle of insertion of the screw into the sacrum, crowding of the proximal end of the inserted screws may occur, therefore interfering with placement of connecting plates or rods.

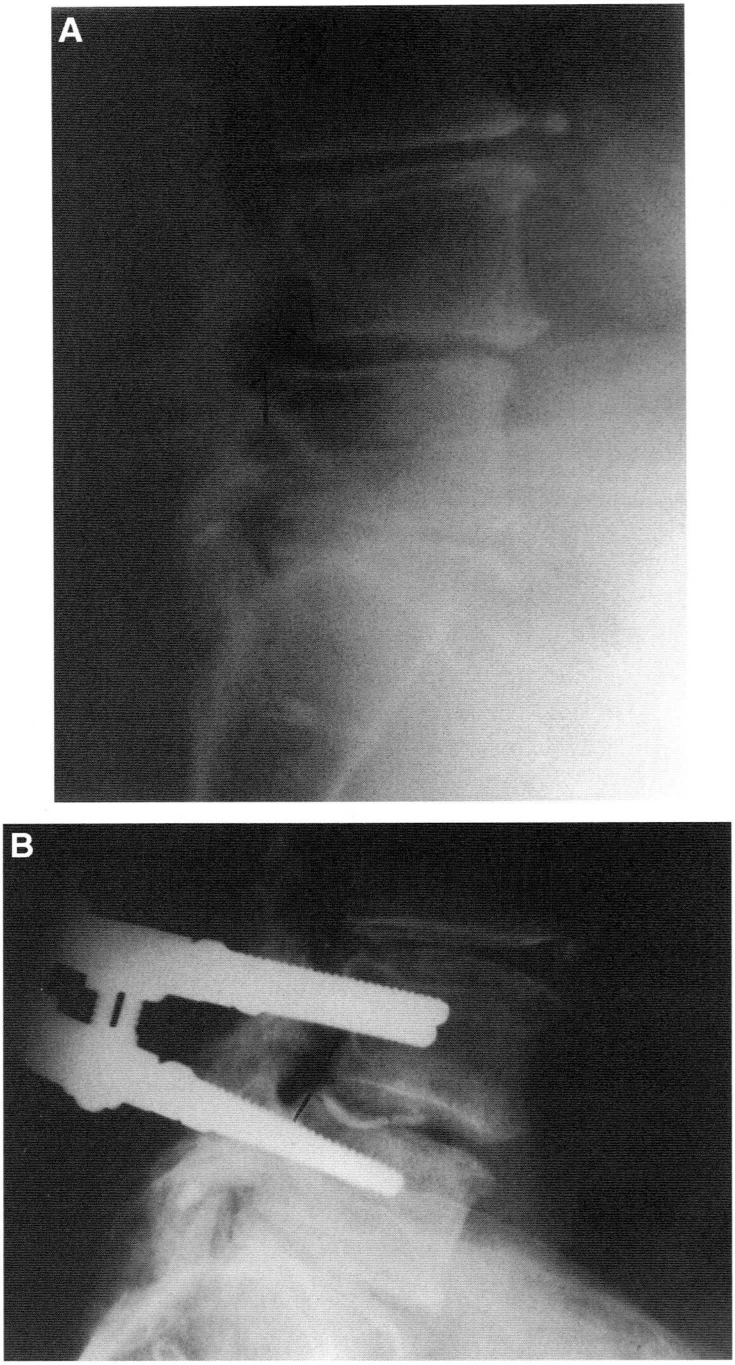

Fig. 16. **(A)** Preoperative lateral X-ray of a 54-yr-old male patient who presented with spondylolisthesis of L4-L5 and related clinical symptoms. **(B)** Postoperative lateral X-ray of same patient shown in (A) demonstrating percutaneously inserted pedicular bolts into pedicles of L4-L5 and sc placement of connecting plates. This patient had a satisfactory outcome following initial use of fixators and reduction of spondylolisthesis. He subsequently underwent percutaneous arthroscopic interbody fusion via a posterolateral approach.

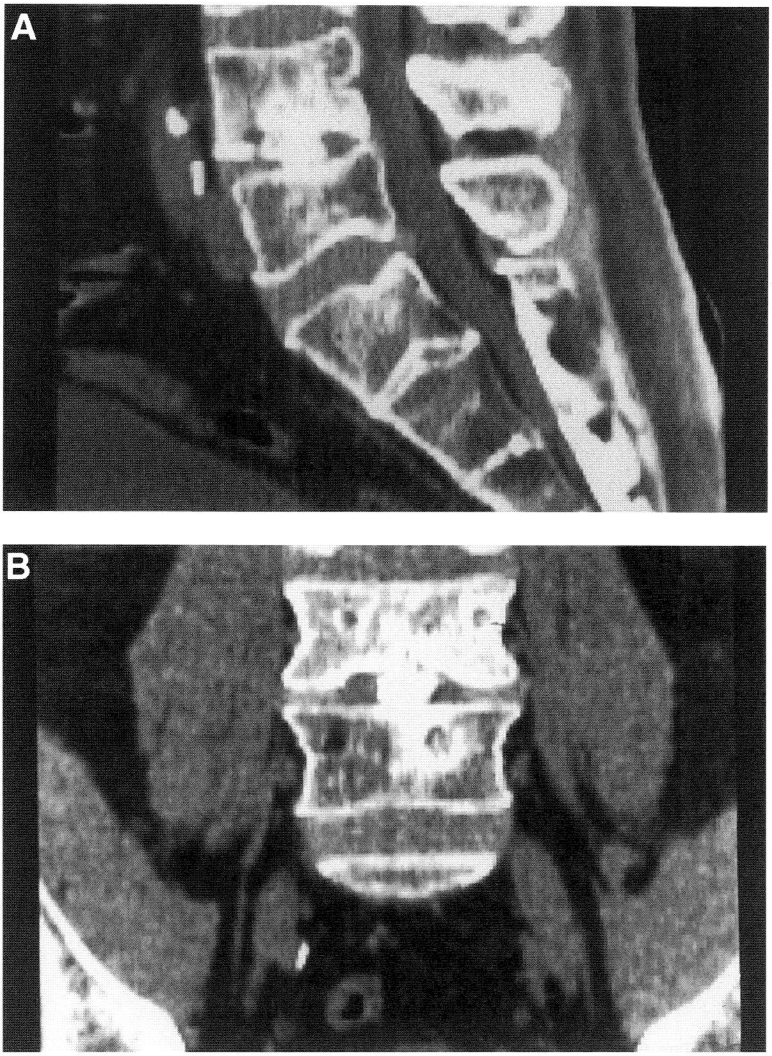

Fig. 17. (A) Postoperative CT of fusion site. Although part of the bone grafts have been absorbed, a solid fusion and extension of the bony trabeculae across the fusion site is demonstrated. (Reprinted with permission from ref. *13*.) (**B**) Reconstruction CT of fusion site shown in (A).

Attachment of an offset extension bar to the sacral screw will provide ample separation between the L5-S1 screws for insertion of the plates or rods (Fig 14A,B).

Diagnostic Stabilization of Motion Segments

Unstable lumbar segments may be stabilized percutaneously via pedicular bolts and sc plates for a period of 3 to 4 wk. If the patient's symptoms are resolved and there is evidence of objective improvement of the presenting symptomatology, arthroscopic interbody fusion is then attempted using the criteria described previously (Figs.15A,B and 16A,B).

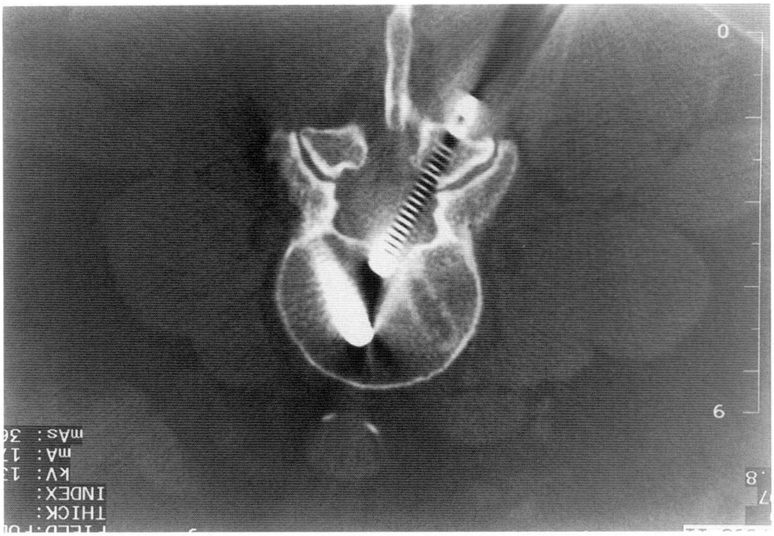

Fig. 18. Showing dislodged pedicular bolt into spinal canal. The hardware was later surgically removed.

RESULTS

In our institution, we have achieved 95% solid fusion and stabilization using the described surgical technique (Fig. 17A,B). None of our patients encountered infection or neurovascular complications. There were no instrument failures. All of the hardware was retrieved on an average of 7 mo postoperatively. In one overweight patient, a fracture of the pedicle and clinical evidence of paresthesia of the involved extremity were associated with displacement of the pedicular bolt into the spinal canal. Surgical removal of the hardware within 24 h was associated with recovery from the neurological deficit and fibrous union of the spinal unit (Fig. 18).

THORACOSCOPIC AND LAPAROSCOPIC DECOMPRESSION AND STABILIZATION

A thoracoscopic approach to thoracic and laparoscopic access to the lumbar spine has been used for stabilization of motion segments *(40)*. Although in skilled hands access to and decompression of L5-S1 segments should not present a serious difficulty, the presence of major vessels in the middle and upper lumbar spine may interfere with proper midline access, adequate decompression, fusion, or placement of spacers. A team of surgeons is usually required to perform this operative procedure. At present, this approach is being used in only a few select centers.

REFERENCES

1. Parke WW. Clinical anatomy of the lower lumbar spine, in Arthroscopic Microdiscectomy, Minimal Intervention in Spinal Surgery (Kambin P, ed.), Urban & Schwarzenberg, Baltimore, 1991, pp. 11–29.
2. Falconer MA, McGeorge M, Begg AC. Observations on the cause and mechanism of symptom-production in sciatica and low-back pain. J Neurol Neurosurg Psychiatry 1948;11,13–26.

3. Kambin P, Nixon J, Chait A, et al. Annular protrusion: pathophysiology and roentgenographic appearance. Spine 1988;13:671–675.
4. Sachs B, Vanharanta H, Spivey M, et al. Dallas discogram description: a new classification of CT/discography in low back disorders. Spine 1987;12:287–294.
5. Vanharanta H, Sachs B, Spivey M, et al. The relationship of pain provocation to lumbar disc deterioration as seen by CT/discogram. Spine 1987;12:295–298.
6. Weinstein J, Claverie W, Gibson S. The pain of discography. Spine 1988;13(12):1344–1348.
7. Kambin P. The role of minimally invasive surgery in spinal disorders. Adv Operat Orthop 1995;3:147–171.
8. Shepperd JAN. Percutaneous and minimal intervention spinal fusion, in Arthroscopic Microdiscectomy, Minimal Intervention in Spinal Surgery (Kambin P, ed.), Urban & Schwarzenberg, Baltimore, 1991, pp. 127–129.
9. White A, Panjabi MM. Clinical Biomechanics of the Spine, JB Lippincott, Philadelphia, 1978.
10. Saal, JS, Franson RC, Dobrow R, Saal JA, White AH, Goldthwaite N. High levels of inflammatory phospholipase A2 activity in lumbar disc herniations. Spine 1990;15(7): 674–678.
11. Kambin P. Percutaneous lumbar discectomy: current practice. Surg Rounds Orthop 1988;31–35.
12. Kambin P. Arthroscopic microdiscectomy. Arthroscopy 1992;8(3):287–295.
13. Kambin P, Gennarrelli T, Hermantin F. Minimally invasive techniques in spinal surgery: current practice. Neurosurgical Focus 1998;4(2):Article 8.
14. Kambin P. Expandable intervertebral cage and surgical method. US patent 5,665,122, 1997.
15. David T. Lumbar disc prosthesis, surgical technique, indications and clinical results in 22 patients with a minimum of 12 months follow up. Eur Spine J 1993;1:254–259.
16. Enker P, Stefee A, McMillin C, Keppler L, Biscup DO, Miller DO. Artificial disc replacement. Spine 1993;18:1061–1070.
17. Griffith SL, Shelokow AP, Buettner-Janz K, LeMaire JP, Zeegers WS. A multicenter retrospective study of the clinical results of the link SB Charite intervertebral disc prosthesis. Spine 1994;19:1842–1849.
18. Lemaire JP, Skalli W, Lavaste F, et al. Intervertebral disc prosthesis. Clin Orthop 1997;7:337:64–76.
19. Scott AH, Harrison OJ. Increasing age does not affect outcome after lumbar disc replacement. Int Orthop Sicot 2000;24:50–53.
20. Sali RM, Pettine KA. Intervertebral disk arthroplasty. US patent 5,258,031,2, 1993.
21. Monson GL. Synthetic intervertebral disc prosthesis. US patent 4,083,477,5, 1969.
22. Hedman TP, Kostuik JP, Fernie GR, Maki BE. An artificial spinal disc. US patent 4,759,769,12, 1988.
23. Marcolongo MS, Kambin P, Lowman A, Karduna A. Experience with minimally invasive nuclear replacement. Fourteenth International Symposium on Arthroscopic and Endoscopic Spinal Surgery May 5–6, 2000, The Graduate Hospital, Philadelphia.
24. Saal JS, Saal, JA. Management of chronic discogenic low back pain with thermal intradiscal catheter. Spine 2000;25(3):382–388.
25. Frymoyer JW, Selby DK. Segmental instability rationale for treatment. Spine 1985;10:280–286.
26. Albee FH. Transplantation of a portion of the tibia into the spine for Pott's Disease: a preliminary report. JAMA 1911;57:885–888.
27. Hibbs RA. An operation for Pott's disease on the spine. JAMA 1912;59:422–436.
28. Watkins MB. Posterolateral fusion of the lumbar and lumbosacral spine. J Bone Joint Surg Am 1953;34:1014–1018.
29. Wiltse LL, Bateman JG, Hutchinson RH, et al. The paraspinal sacrospinalis-splitting approach to the lumbar spine. J Bone Joint Surg Am 1968;50: 919–926.
30. Cloward RB. The treatment of a ruptured lumbar disc by vertebral fusion: indications, operative technique, after care. J Neursurg 1953;10:154–168.

31. Kambin P. Posterolateral lumbar interbody fusion, in Arthroscopic Microdiscectomy, Minimal Intervention in Spinal Surgery (Kambin P, ed.), Urban & Schwarzenberg, Baltimore, 1991, pp. 117–121.
32. Harrington PR, Tullos HS. Reduction of severe spondylolisthesis in children. South Med J 1969;62:1–7.
33. Magerl FP. Stabilization of the lower thoracic and lumbar spine with external skeletal fixation. Clin Orthop 1984;189:125–141.
34. Kambin P. Arthroscopic lumbar intervertebral fusion, in The Adult Spine: Principles and Practice (Frymoyer JW, Ducker T, Hadler N, et al. eds.), Raven, New York, 1996, pp. 2037–2047.
35. Kambin P. Percutaneous fixation of the vertebrae. US patent 5,242,443, 1930.
36. Kambin P. Arthroscopic lumbar fusion with pedicular bolts and subcutaneous plates. ISMISS Scientific Exhibit, Feb 20–25, 1992, AAOS Meeting, Washington, DC.
37. Leu HJ, Schreiber A. Percutaneous fusion of the lumbar spine: a promising technique. Spine State Arts Rev 1992;6:593–604.
38. Kambin P. Arthroscopic lumbar interbody fusion, in Spine Care (White AH, Schofferman JA, eds.), Mosby, St. Louis, 1995, pp. 1055–1066.
39. Kambin P. Method for percutaneous arthroscopic disc removal bone biopsy and fixation of vertebrae. US patent 6,175,758,3, 2001.
40. Regan JJ, Yuan H, McCullenG. Thoroscopic and endoscopic access to the spine. Instructional Course Lectures. AAOS 1997;46:127–141.

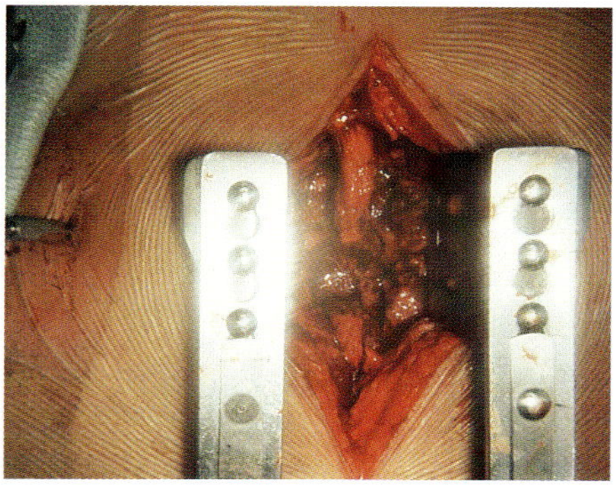

Color Plate 1, Ch. 1, Fig. 7

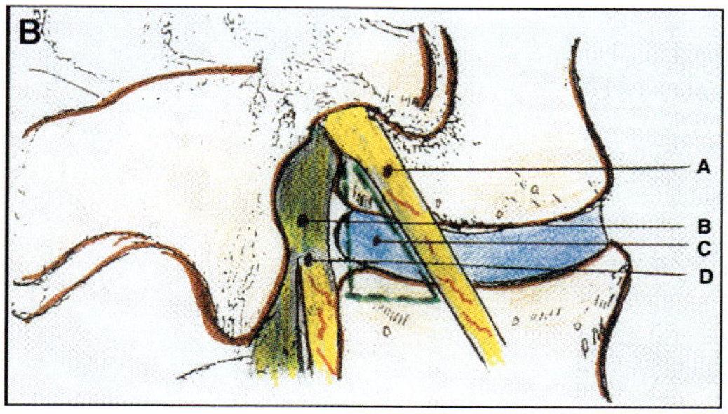

Color Plate 2, Ch 1, Fig. 16B

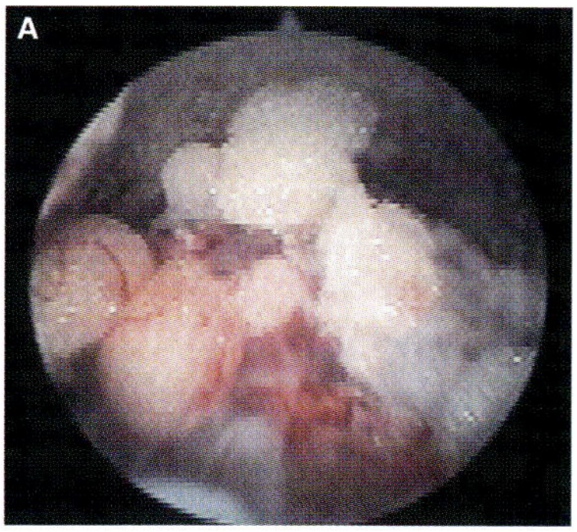

Color Plate 3, Ch. 2, Fig. 4A

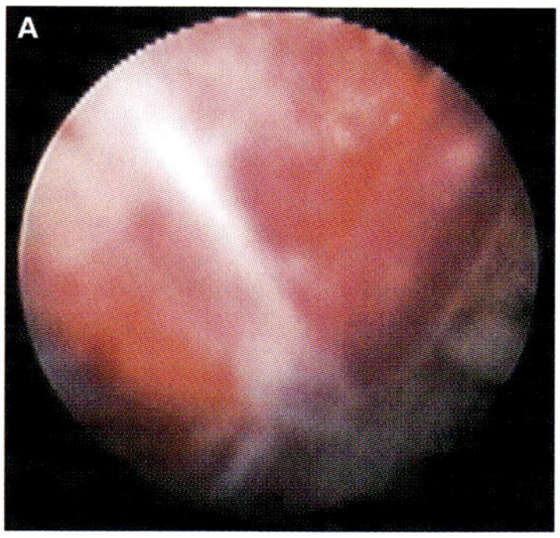

Color Plate 4, Ch. 2, Fig. 5A

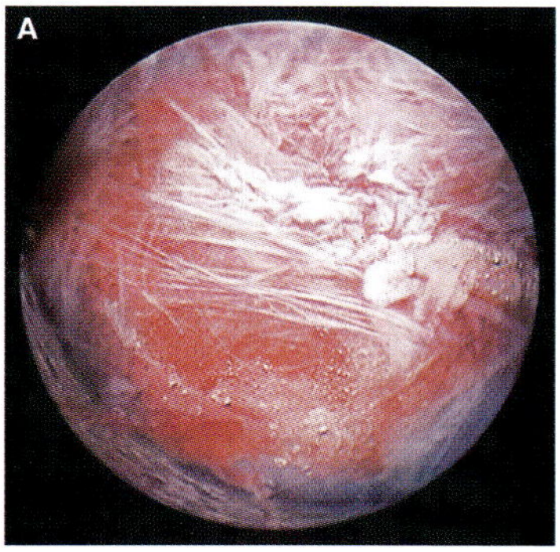

Color Plate 4, Ch. 2, Fig. 6A

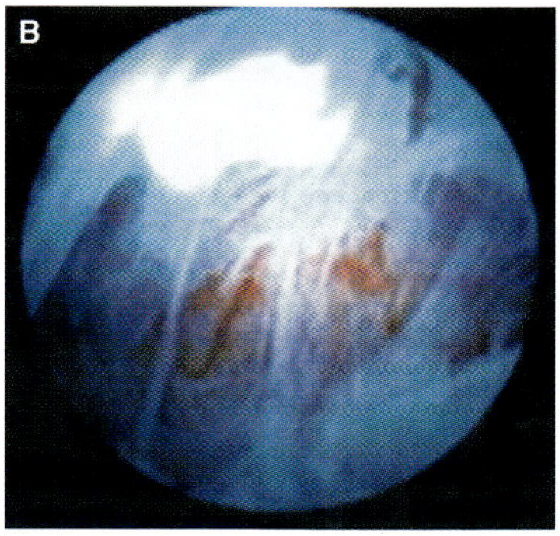

Color Plate 5, Ch. 2, Fig. 6B

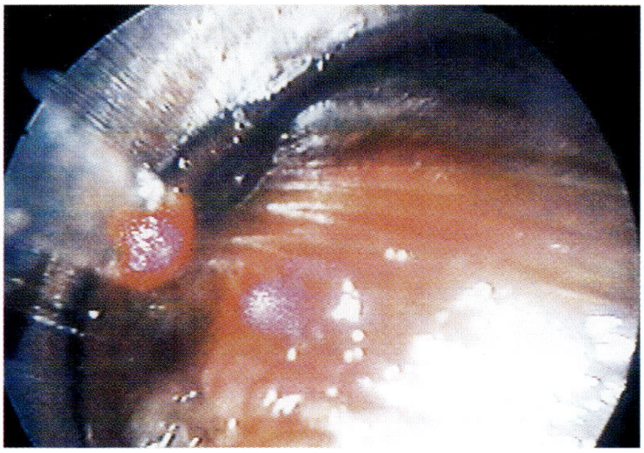

Color Plate 6, Ch. 2, Fig. 7

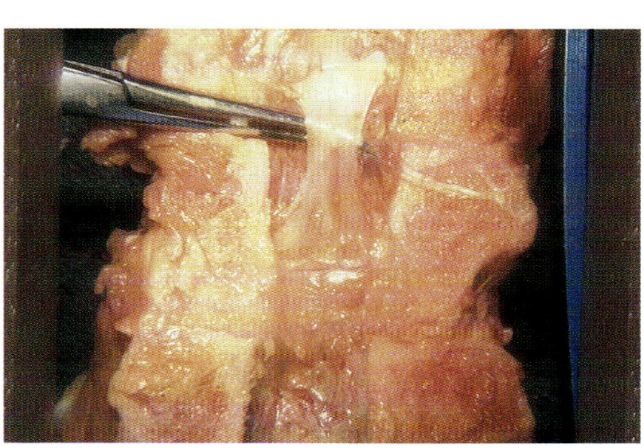

Color Plate 7, Ch. 2, Fig. 8

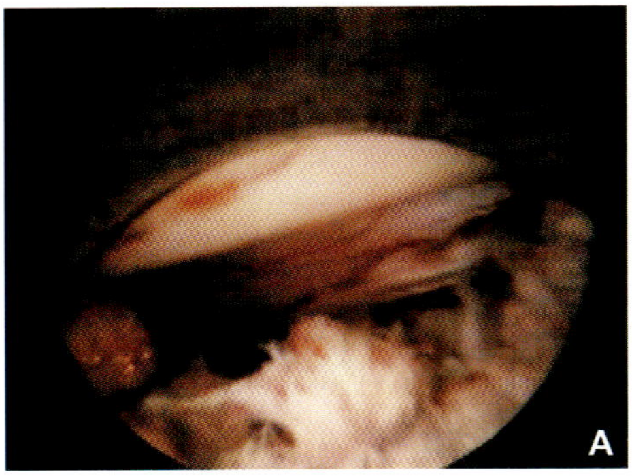

Color Plate 8, Ch. 2, Fig. 9A

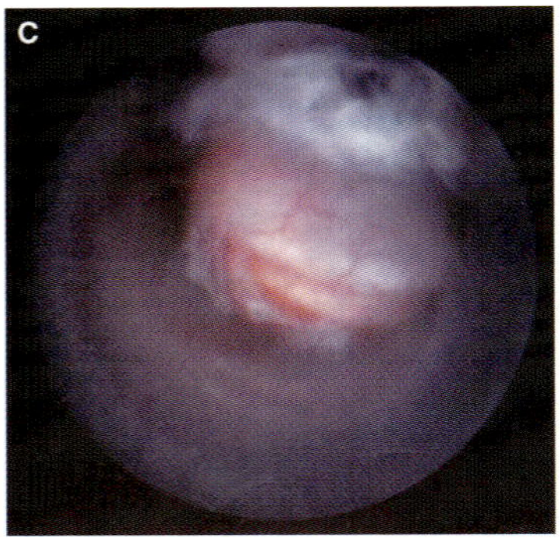

Color Plate 9, Ch. 2, Fig. 9C

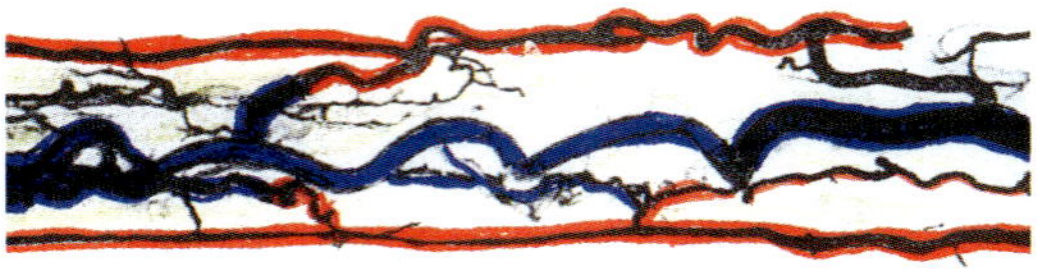

Color Plate 10, Ch. 2, Fig. 10

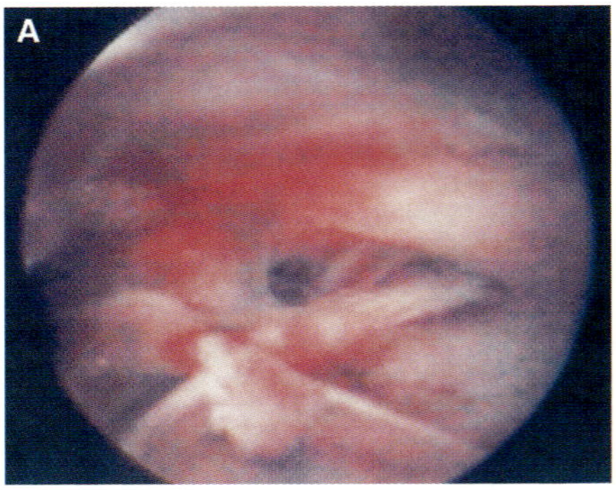

Color Plate 11, Ch. 2, Fig. 12A

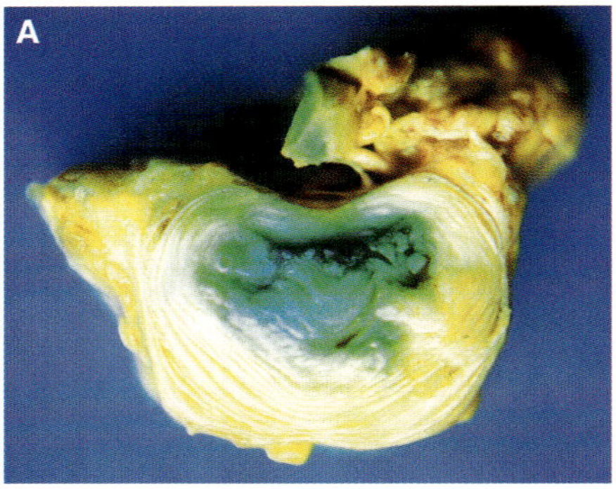

Color Plate 12, Ch. 2, Fig. 13A

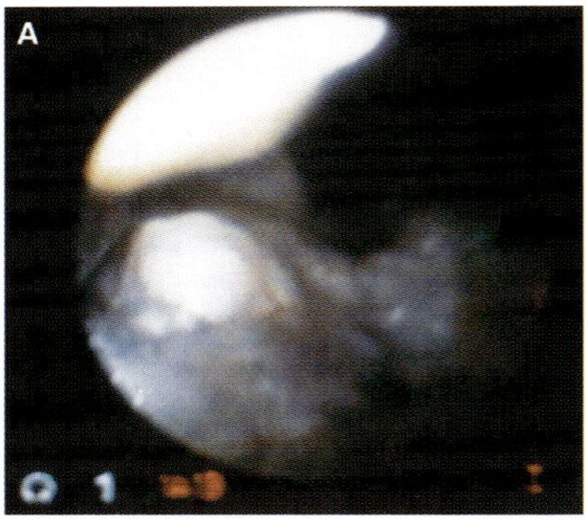

Color Plate 13, Ch. 2, Fig. 14A

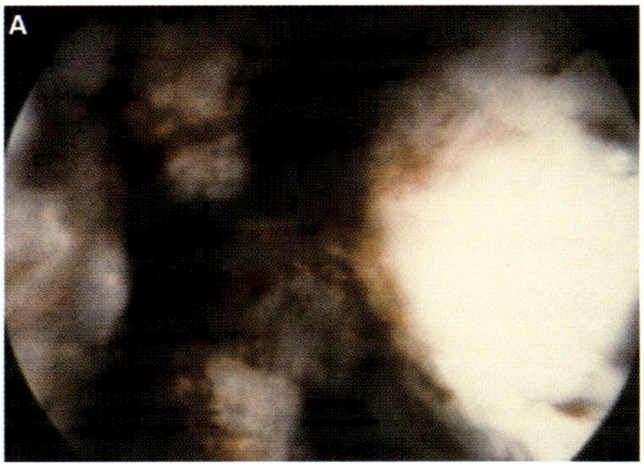

Color Plate 14, Ch. 2, Fig. 15A

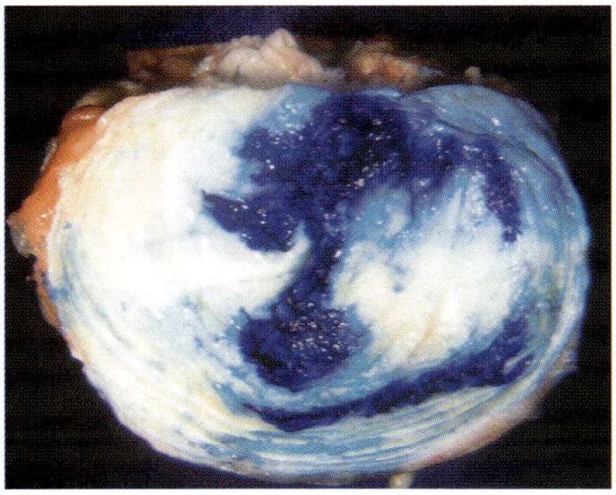

Color Plate 15, Ch. 2, Fig. 16

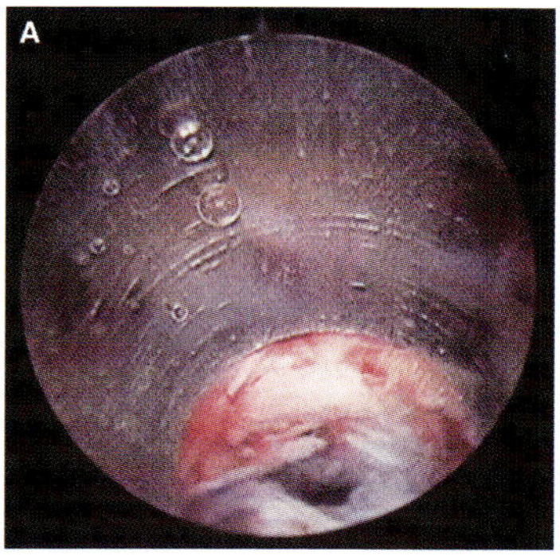

Color Plate 16, Ch. 2, Fig. 18A

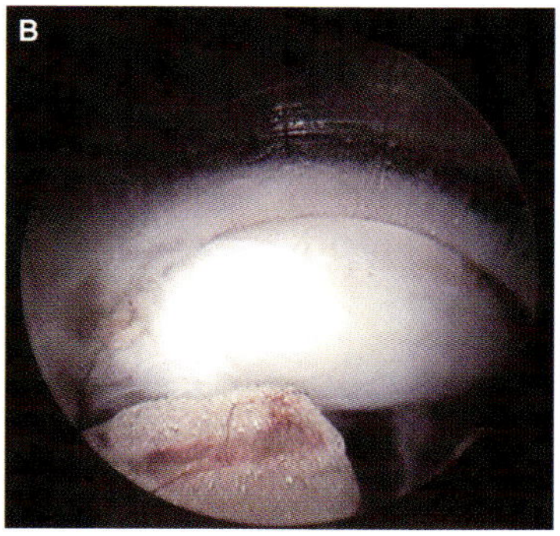

Color Plate 17, Ch. 2, Fig. 18B

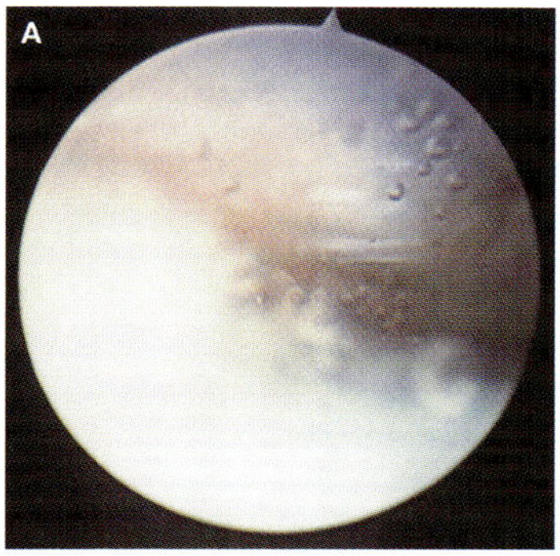

Color Plate 18, Ch. 2, Fig. 19A

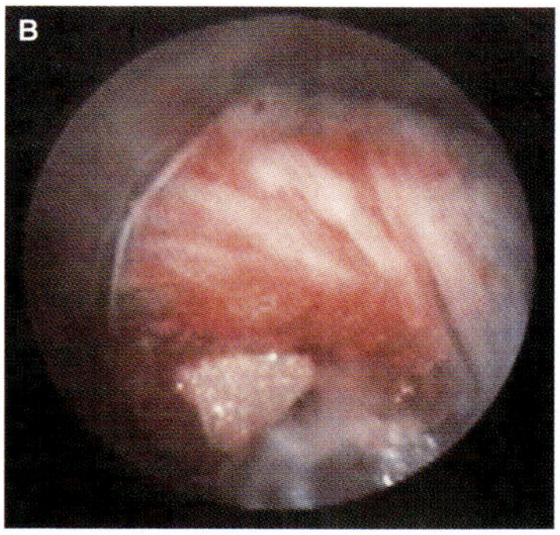

Color Plate 19, Ch. 2, Fig. 19B

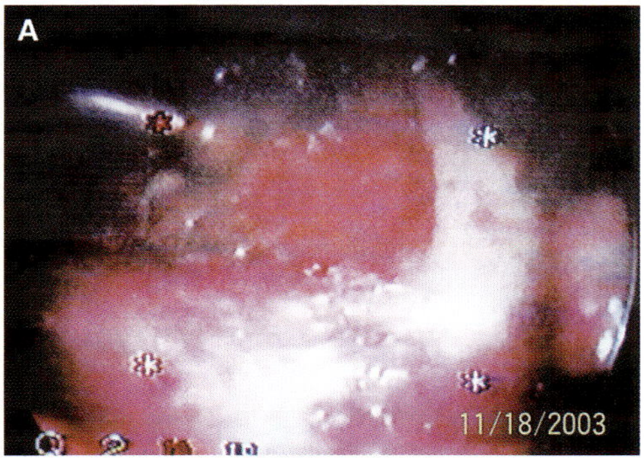

Color Plate 20, Ch. 3, Fig. 12A

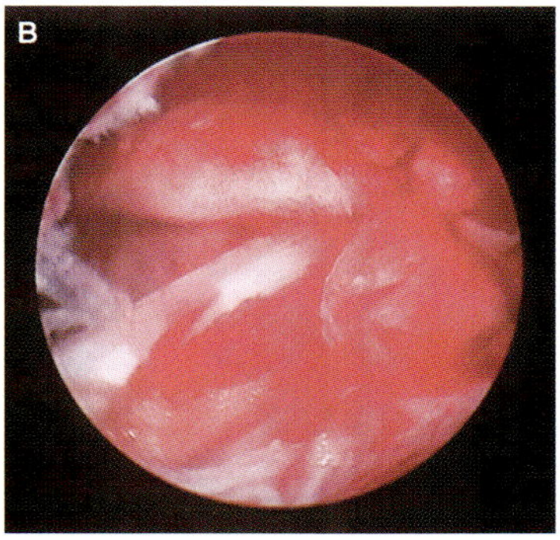

Color Plate 21, Ch. 3, Fig. 12B

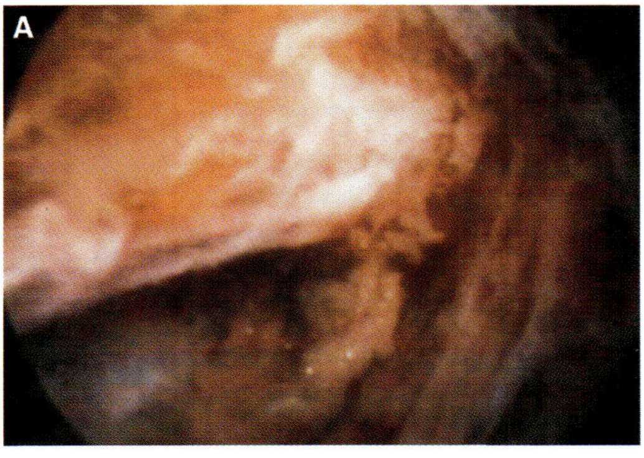

Color Plate 22, Ch. 4, Fig. 5A

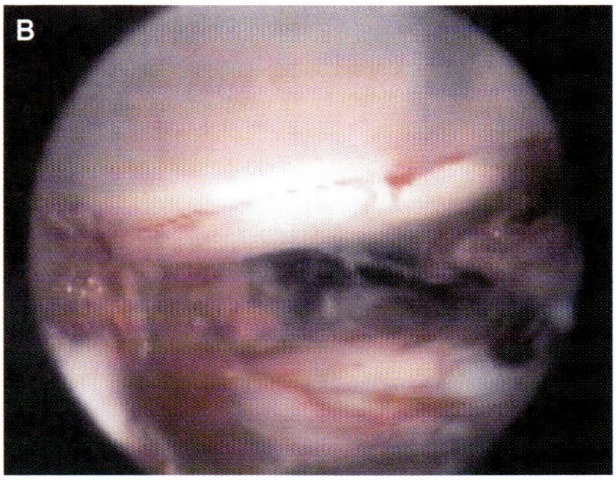

Color Plate 23, Ch. 4, Fig. 5B

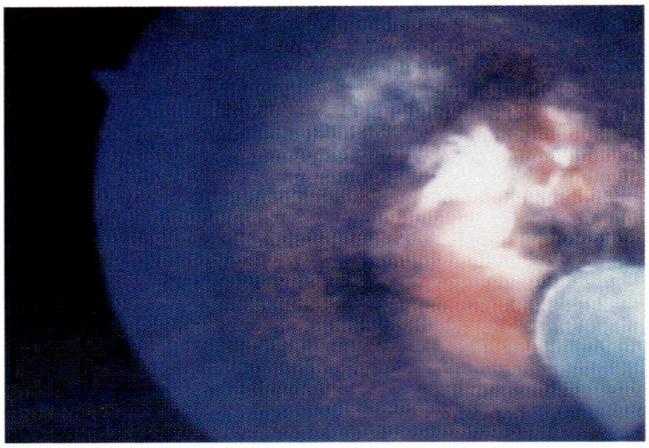

Color Plate 24, Ch. 4, Fig. 22

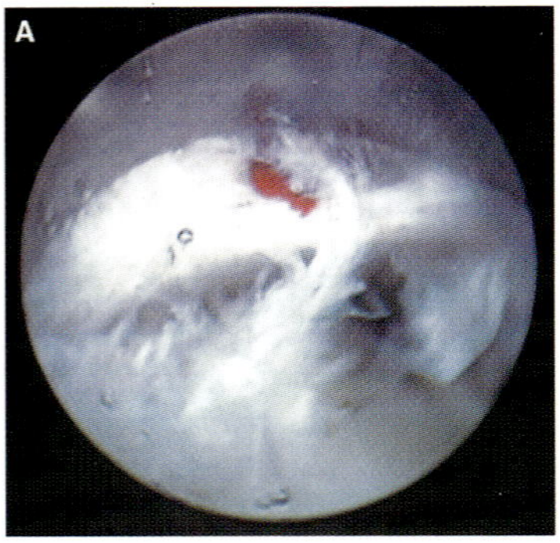

Color Plate 25, Ch. 4, Fig. 23A

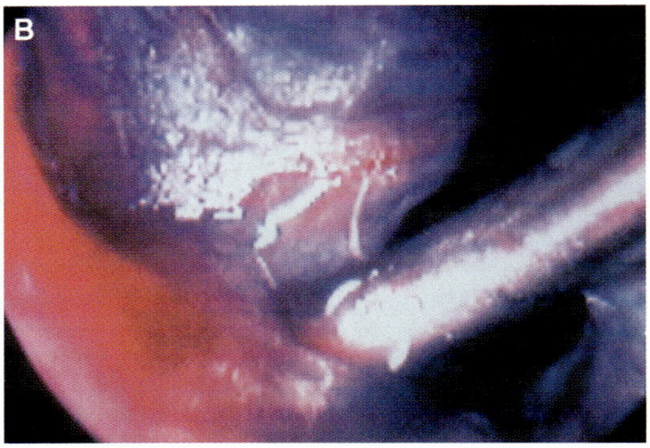

Color Plate 26, Ch. 4, Fig. 27B

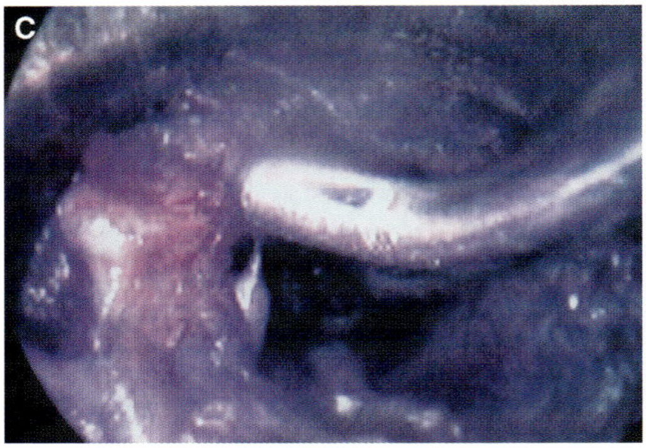

Color Plate 27, Ch. 4, Fig. 27C

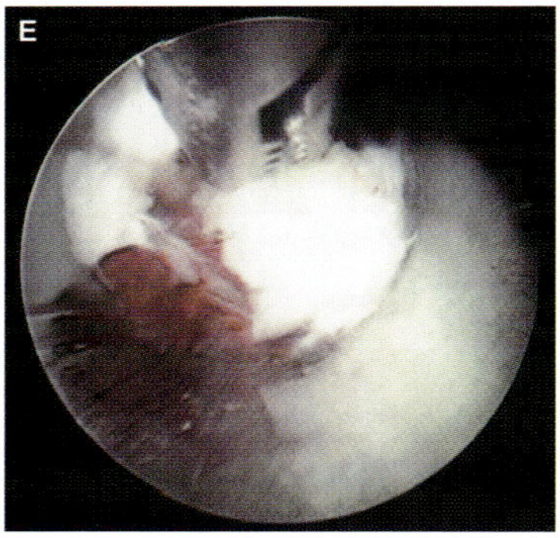

Color Plate 28, Ch. 4, Fig. 28E

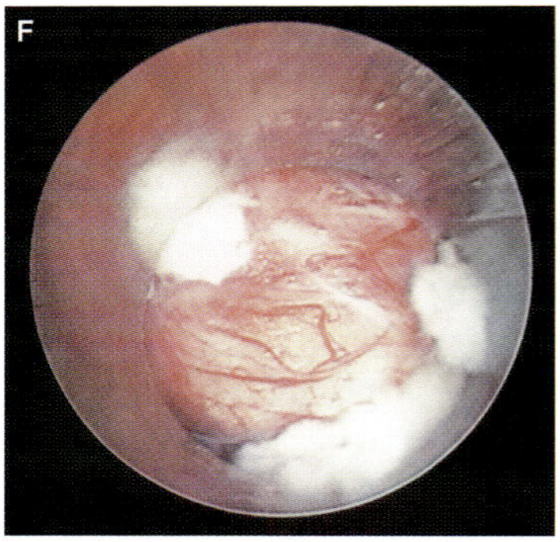

Color Plate 29, Ch. 4, Fig. 28F

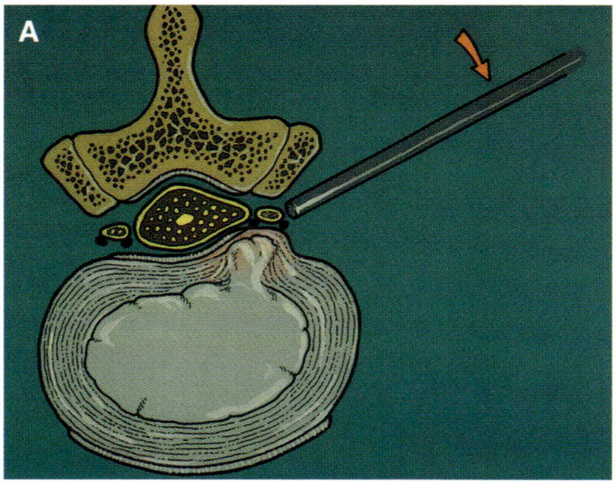

Color Plate 30, Ch. 4, Fig. 29A

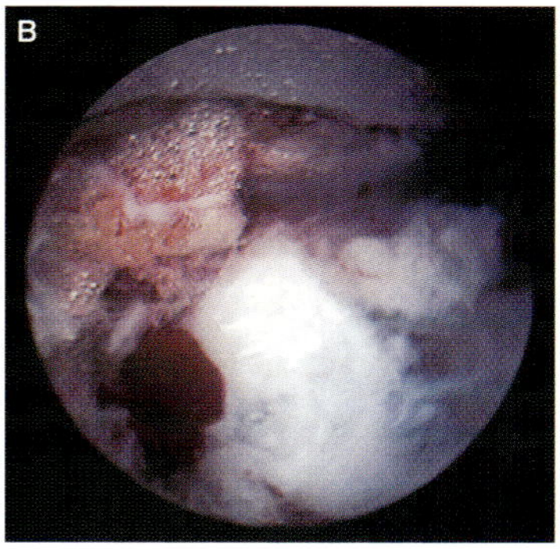

Color Plate 31, Ch. 4, Fig. 29B

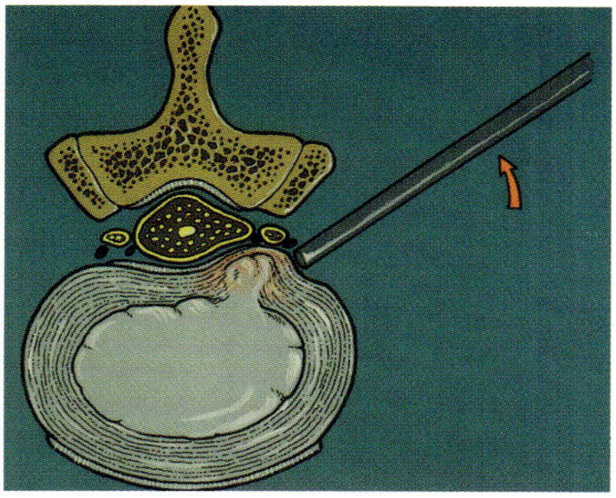

Color Plate 32, Ch. 4, Fig. 30

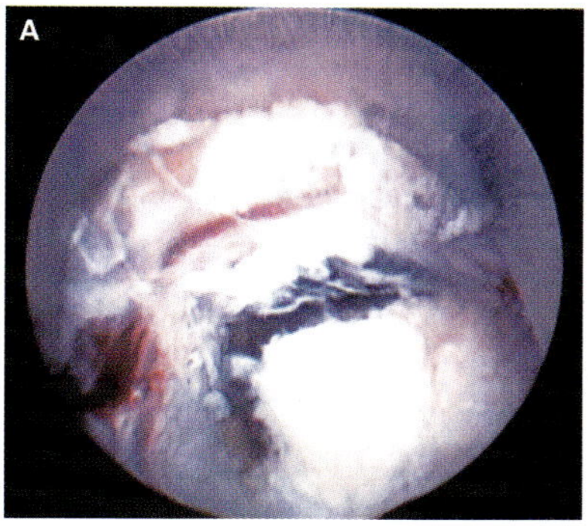

Color Plate 33, Ch. 4, Fig. 31A

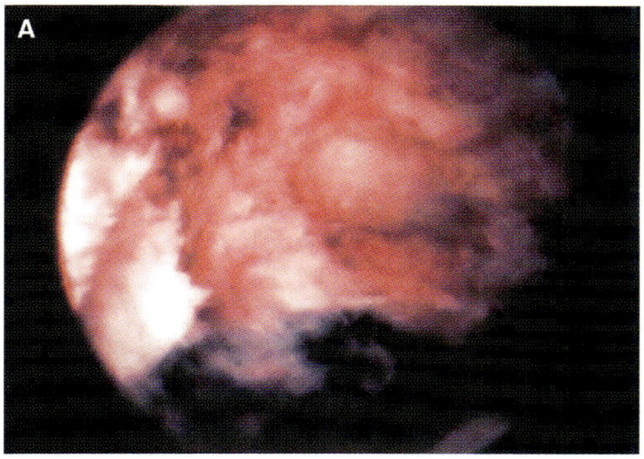

Color Plate 34, Ch. 4, Fig. 33A

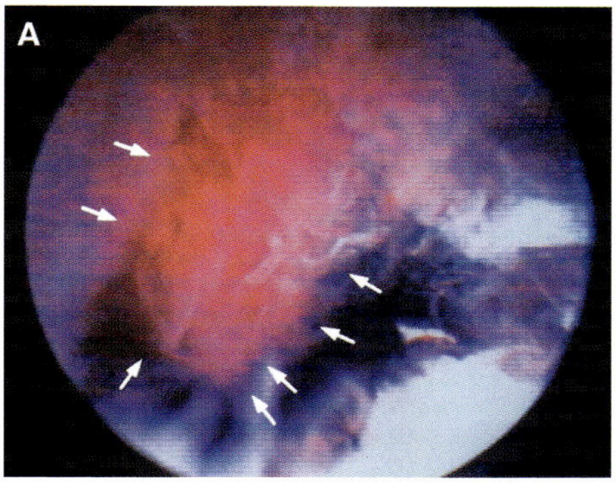

Color Plate 35, Ch. 4, Fig. 35A

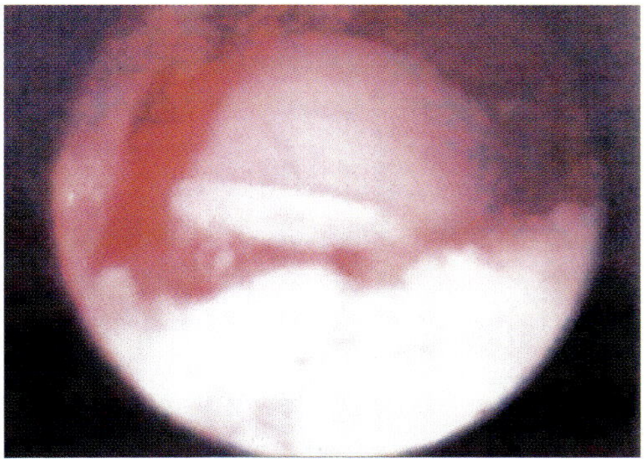

Color Plate 36, Ch. 4, Fig. 36

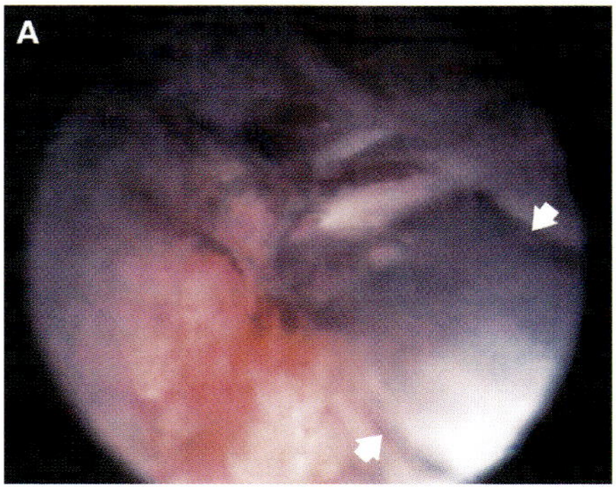

Color Plate 37, Ch. 4, Fig. 37a

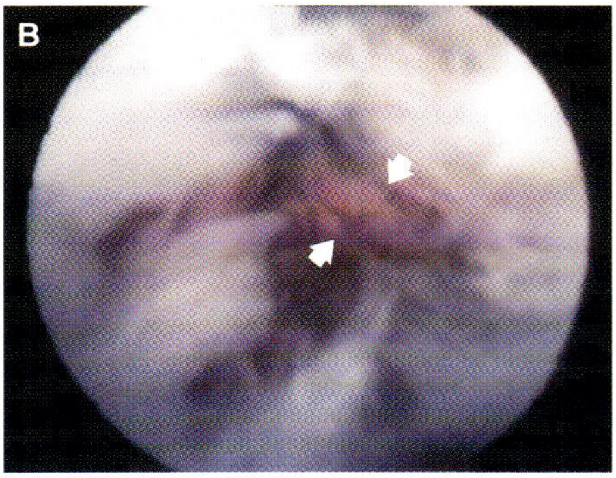

Color Plate 38, Ch. 4, Fig. 37B

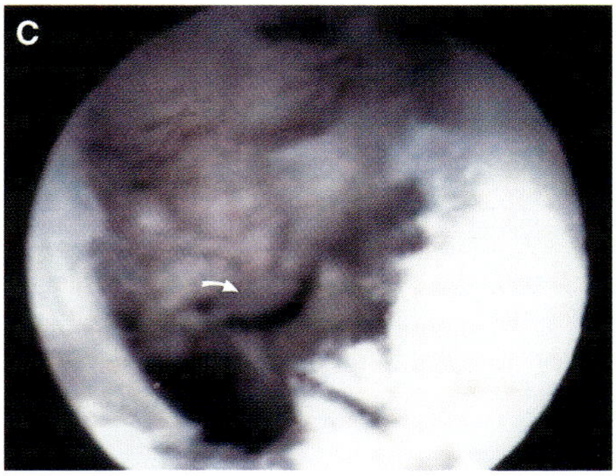

Color Plate 39, Ch. 4, Fig. 37C

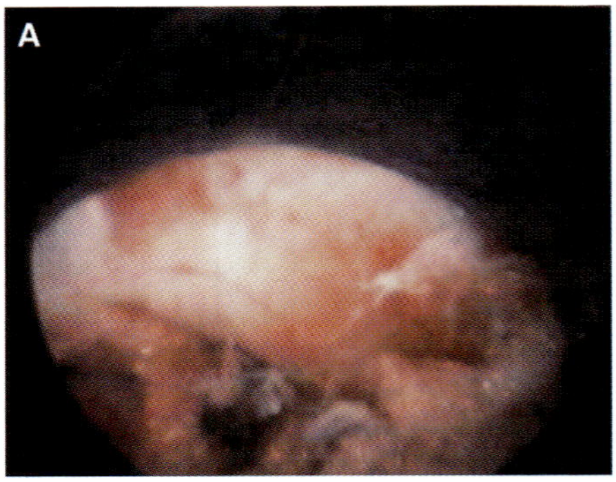

Color Plate 40, Ch. 4, Fig. 38A

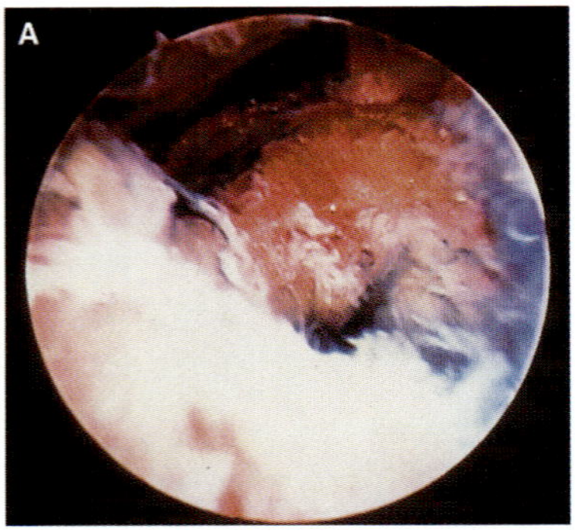

Color Plate 41, Ch. 4, Fig. 39A

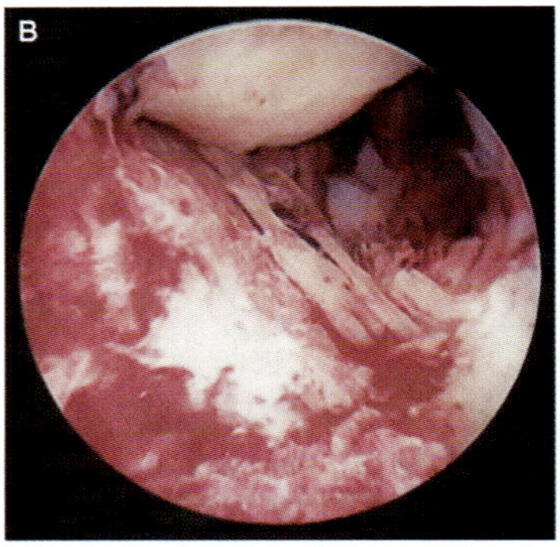

Color Plate 42, Ch. 5, Fig. 1B

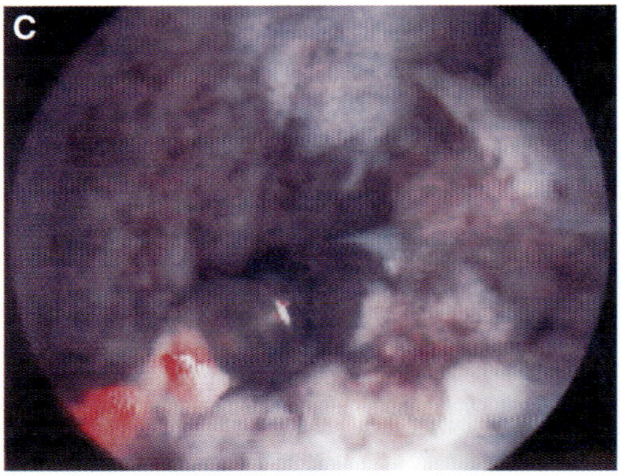

Color Plate 43, Ch. 5, Fig. 7C

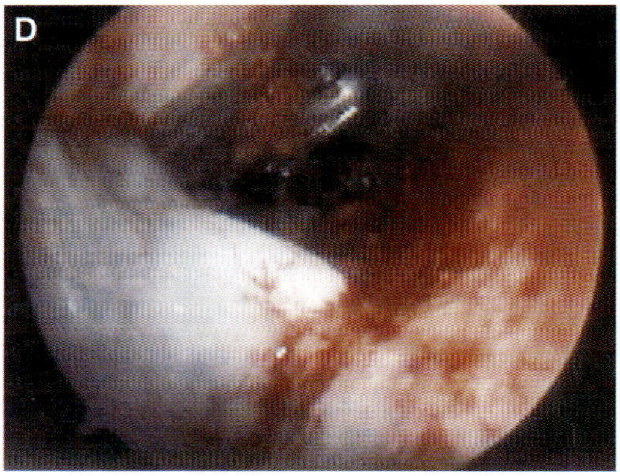

Color Plate 44, Ch. 5, Fig. 7D

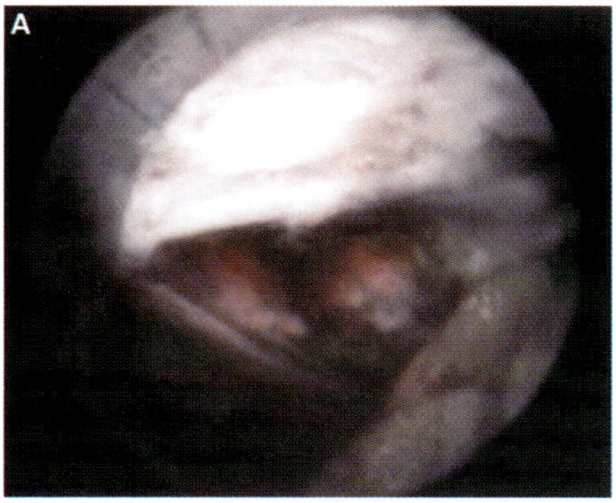

Color Plate 45, Ch. 6, Fig. 3A

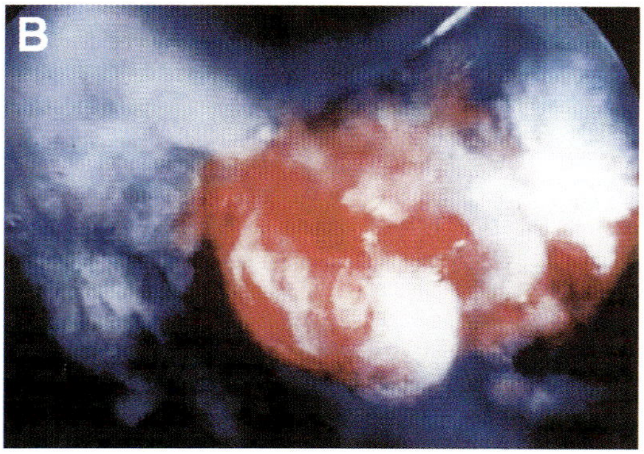

Color Plate 46, Ch. 9, Fig. 7B

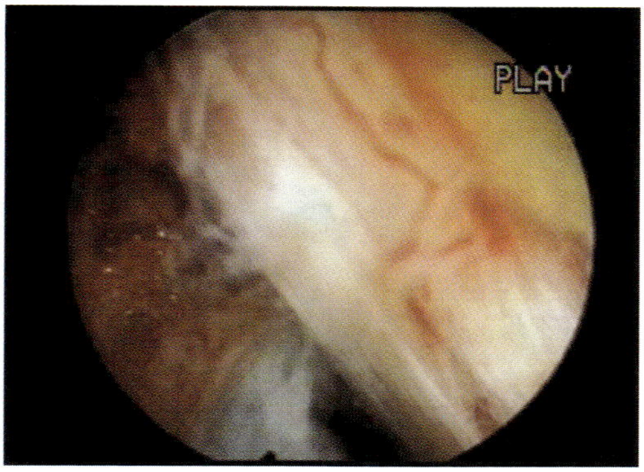

Color Plate 47, Ch. 9, Fig. 8

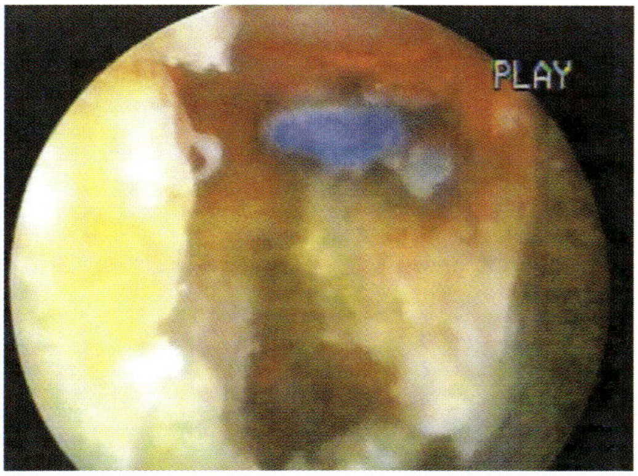

Color Plate 48, Ch. 9, Fig. 12

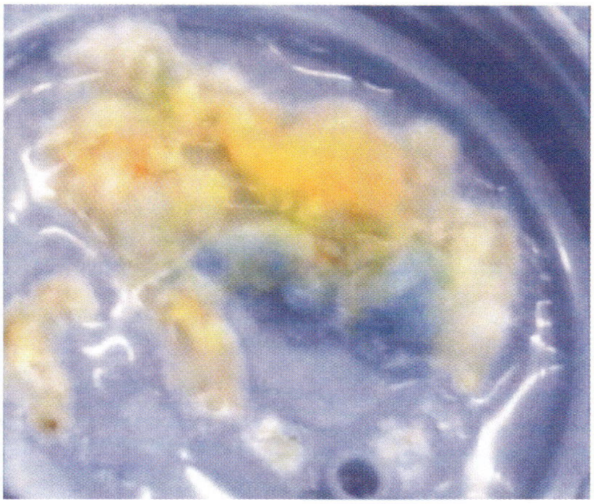

Color Plate 49, Ch. 9, Fig. 13

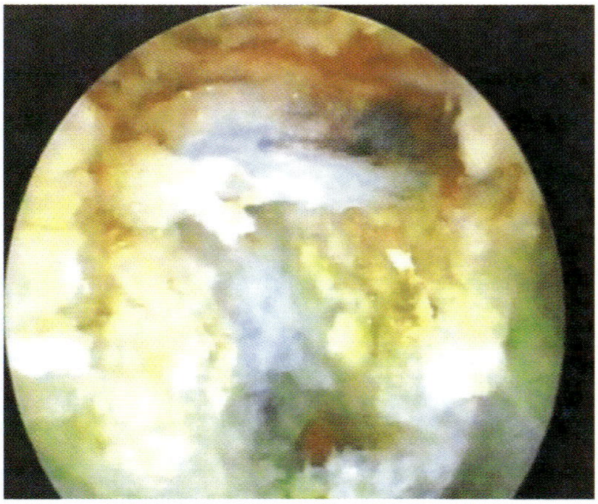

Color Plate 50, Ch. 9, Fig. 13

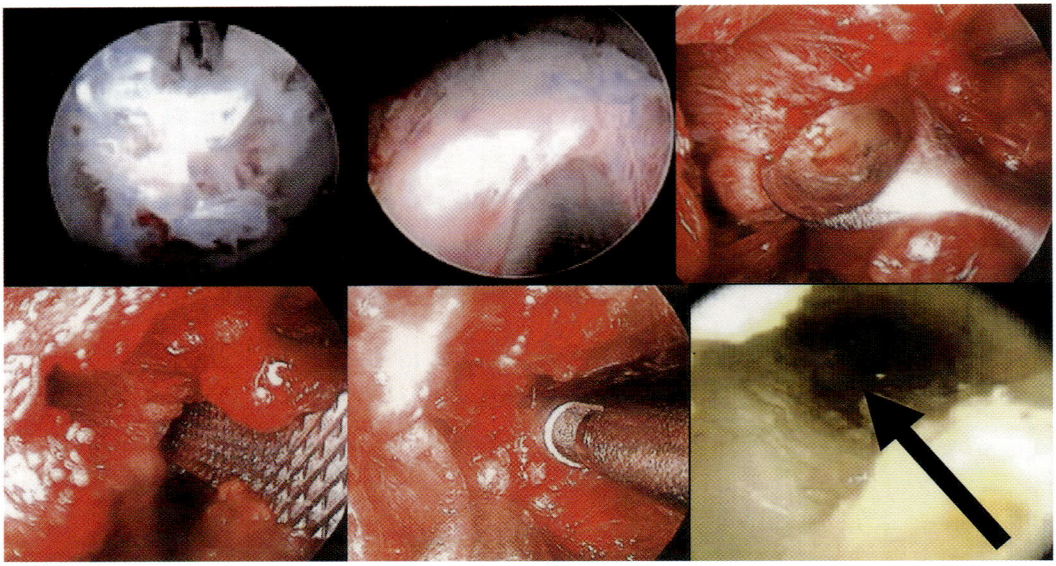

Color Plate 51, Ch. 13, Fig. 5

6

Lateral Recess Stenosis of Lumbar Spine Foraminoplasty

Parviz Kambin, MD

INTRODUCTION

In 1900, Sachs and Fraenkel *(1)* described the diagnosis and treatment of lateral recess stenosis as an entity. Epstein et al. *(2)* further clarified it as a distinct clinical entity. The availability of computed tomography (CT) and magnetic resonance imaging in recent years has facilitated visualization of the content of the lateral recess and diagnosis of this pathological condition (Fig. 1).

The nerve root canal begins from the nerve root sheath and terminates when the exiting root emerges from the foramina. The superior facet, capsular ligamentous complex (Fig. 18 in Chapter 2) forms the posterior boundary or roof of the lateral recess. Expansion of the posterior longitudinal ligamentum to the foramen, the intervertebral disc, and the posterior surface of the adjacent vertebral bodies forms the ventral or anterior surface of the foramen. The exiting root occupies the pedicular notch superiorly.

Degenerative changes in the facet joints associated with synovial hypertrophy, thickened and fibrotic facet capsules, and ligamentum flavum complex (Fig. 2) contribute to the narrowing and stenosis of the lateral recess. In addition, marginal osteophytes arising from the vertebral bodies, combined with posterior bulging and protrusion of the intervertebral disc, cause further restriction, thus adding tension and compression on the exiting nerve root and its vascular structures. It has been shown that interference with the venous return of the nerve root causes chronic edema of the root, which may become associated with intra- and perineural fibrosis *(3–5)*. The pathophysiology of the bulging annulus or protrusion has also been described *(6–8)*.

With the advancement of aging, dehydration and collagenization of the nucleus pulposus, combined with tear and disorganization of the annular fibers, plays an important role in the development of abnormal protrusion of the intervertebral disc (Fig. 17A in Chapter 2).

CLINICAL PRESENTATION

Patients with spinal stenosis are usually seen in the physician's office with signs and symptoms of neurogenic claudication and, at times, complaining of numbness or a feeling of pins and needles in the lower extremities *(9,10)*.

From: *Arthroscopic and Endoscopic Spinal Surgery: Text and Atlas: Second Edition*
Edited by: P. Kambin © Humana Press Inc., Totowa, NJ

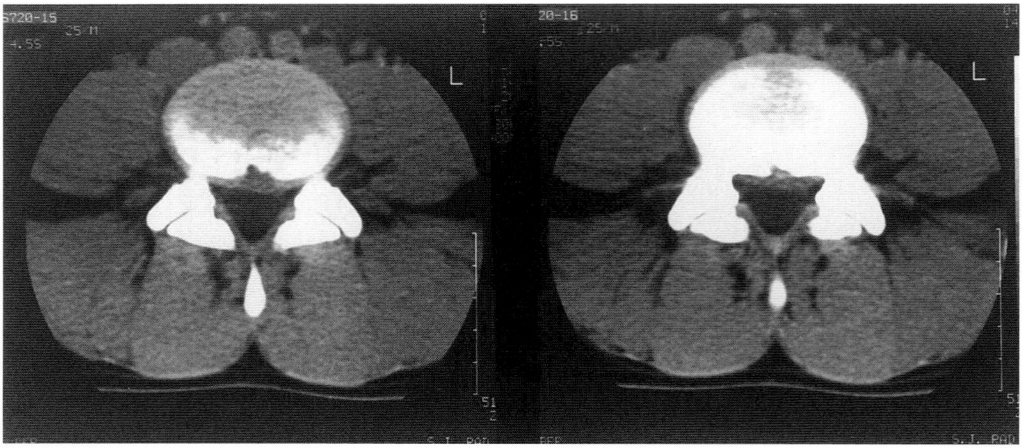

Fig. 1. Preoperative axial CT scan study of a 60-yr-old male presented with signs and symptoms of bilateral lateral recess stenosis. Note degenerative changes of the facet joints, narrowing of the foramen, bulging of the annulus.

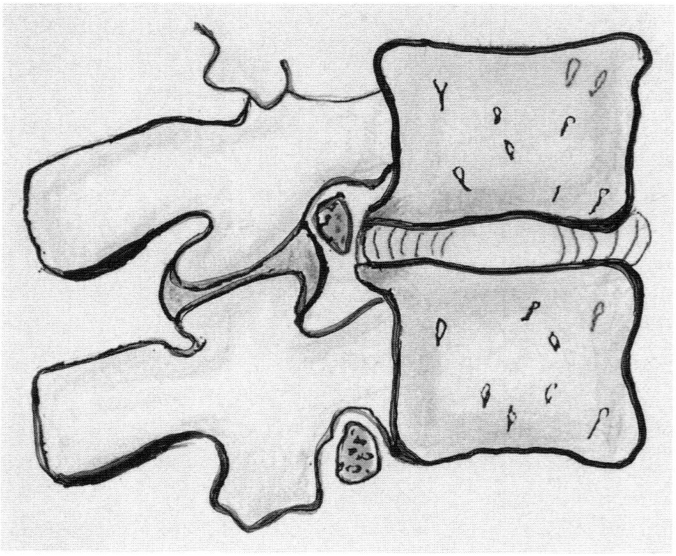

Fig. 2. Schematic drawing demonstrating how posterior marginal osteophytes from vertebral bodies combined with inflamed and hypertrophic facet capsules contribute to stenosis of nerve root canal.

The symptoms are diminished when the patient sits or reclines. This is in contrast to vascular claudication, for which the symptoms subside when the patient stops walking. Individuals with lateral recess stenosis have a tendency to bend forward while walking. Extension of the lumbar spine invariably is associated with pain. Neurological examination usually is not revealing; no reflex abnormality, sensory deficit, or positive tension signs are found.

SURGICAL MANAGEMENT

The evolution of minimally invasive spinal surgery and the availability of microbipolar electrocoagulators, radiofrequency probes, and flexible-tip microinstruments have permitted access to both the ventral and posterior boundaries of the neural canal. Reshaping of the dimensions of the lateral recess via resection of the compressive elements under arthroscopic illumination and magnification has become a standard operative procedure among minimally invasive spine surgeons.

As early as 1988, my colleagues and I used mechanical tools successfully for removal of posterior osteophytes and resection of fibrotic and bulging annulus for the treatment of lateral recess stenosis *(11,12)*. Subsequently, we were able to utilize a radiofrequency probe for vaporization of the inflamed facet capsules and the ligamentum flavum that were contributing to the clinical manifestation of lateral recess stenosis. In recent years, laser lights via a flexible-tip working scope have been used for ambulatory treatment of spinal stenosis *(13,14)*.

Arthroscopic access to the lateral recess requires further lateralization of the skin entry site. This allows insertion of the cannula in the foramen and provides access to the compressive elements on both the ventral and dorsum of the nerve root foramen. When in doubt, particularly when surgery is being attempted in the upper lumbar spine, it is advisable to secure a preoperative prone CT scan study from the surgical site. This will ensure safety of the content of the abdominal cavity and its vital structures.

The needle is positioned at the midpedicular line as observed in the anteroposterior fluoroscopic examination. This step is followed by introduction of the cannulated obturator and positioning of the working cannula (*see* Chapter 3). Under arthroscopic control, mechanical tools may be used for removal of annular protrusion and marginal osteophytes that are arising from the vertebral plates adjacent to the intervertebral disc (Fig. 3). We have used a prebent radiofrequency probe for vaporization of the articular capsule and inflamed synovial tissue.

RESULTS

The outcome of a prospective study of 40 consecutive patients who underwent arthroscopic foraminal decompression of the lateral recess stenosis was published in 1996 *(11)*. The reported outcome of patients who underwent arthroscopic decompression of lateral recess has been compatible or better than the reported result following extensive open operative procedures *(15,16)*.

DEVELOPMENT OF DYSESTHESIA

Approximately 4 to 5 d following the surgical procedure, patients began to experience a burning sensation or hypersensitivity of skin to touch affecting the involved extremity *(17)*. At times, patients are unable to use covers on their legs after this type of surgery. This subjective complaint of hypersensitivity usually is not associated with objective neurological deficit. Reflex abnormality, weakness, atrophy, or sensory deficit is not usually found. The dermatomal distribution of the dysesthesia at times is not clear. However, it may follow the pattern of sensory nerve supply of a given nerve root at the site of the surgical procedure. The etiology of this disturbing complication is attributed to manipulation, excess heat, or trauma to the nerve root ganglia.

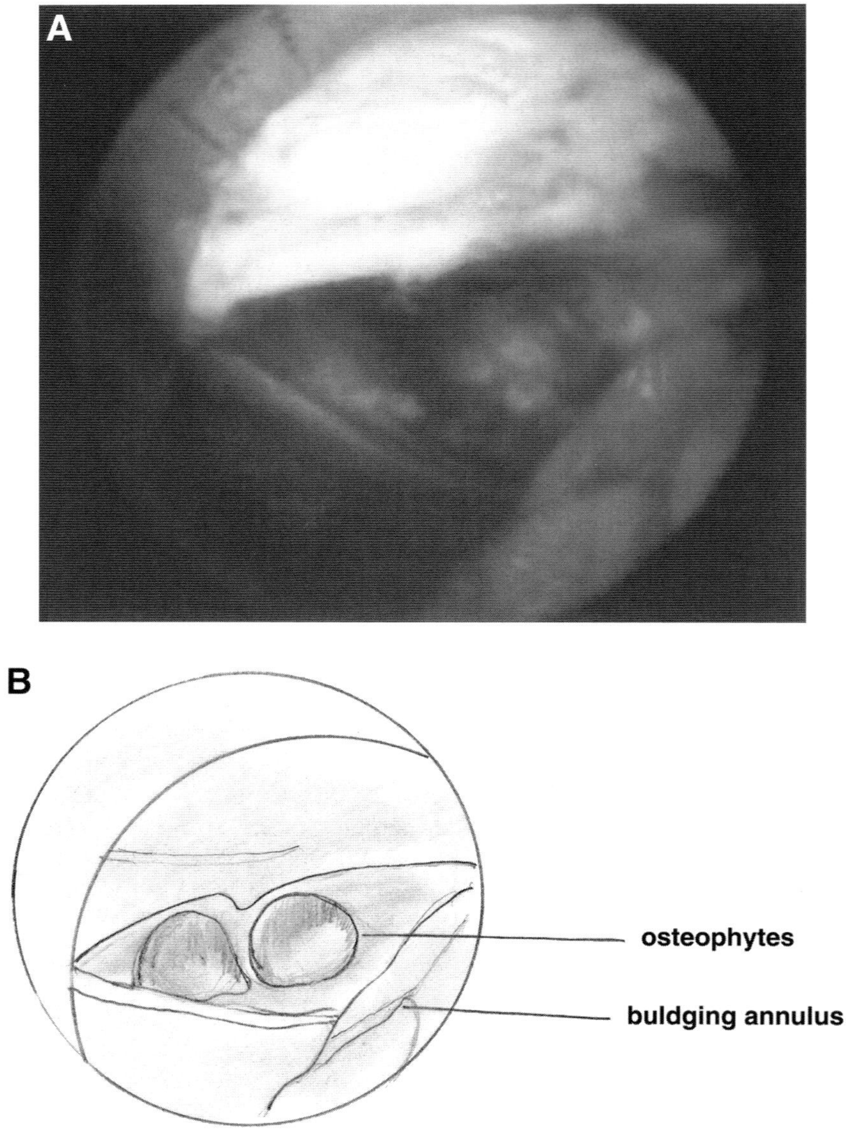

Fig. 3. **(A)** Intraoperative arthroscopic view of lateral recess of patient shown in Fig. 1. Note how the osteophytes that are arising from the vertebral body of the proximal segment contribute to the development of root canal stenosis. **(B)** The fibers of the bulging annulus are seen distal to the above osteophytes.

MANAGEMENT OF DYSESTHESIA

The operating surgeon has the responsibility to prepare and warn the patient of potential development of dysesthesia following surgery. This reduces or prevents the undue anxiety that invariably accompanies this organic disorder. In our experience, intraoperative injection of diluted fentanyl solution around the nerve root ganglia at the onset of the operative procedure reduces the incidence of development of postoperative dysesthesia.

Following proper positioning of the patient and insertion of an 18-gage needle into the foramen, a mixture of 1 cc of fentanyl and 3 cc of saline solution is injected into the foramen. Within a few minutes following the injection, the surgeon may proceed with positioning of the cannulated obturator and working cannula, and completion of the operative procedure. Bathing of the root ganglia in the fentanyl solution will have a tendency to alter the sensitivity of the root ganglia to external stimulation. Fentanyl-induced antinociceptive effect is supraspinally mediated. It interacts with opioid receptors that are present in the dorsal ganglia and dura and the central nervous system *(18)*.

In addition, it is advisable to inject a diluted solution of a steroid compound into the foramen prior to withdrawal of the instruments. Postoperatively the majority of patients respond favorably to the use of oral nonsteroidal anti-inflammatory medications and analgesics within 4–6 wk. However, when the presenting symptoms are severe, under a strict sterile environment, the patient is positioned prone on the operating room table and the 18-gage needle is reinserted into the foramen according to the previously described steps. Injection of the steroid compound around the nerve root ganglia invariably provides relief and enhances recovery time.

REFERENCES

1. Sachs B, Fraenkel J. Progressive ankylotic rigidity of the spine (spondylose rhizomelique). J Nerv Ment Dis 1900;27:1–15.
2. Epstein JA, Epstein BS, Rosenthal AD, et al. Sciatica caused by nerve root entrapment in the lateral recess: the superior facet syndrome. J Neurosurg 1972;36:584–589.
3. Hoyland JA, Freemont JA, Jayson MIV. Intervertebral foramen venous obstruction: a cause of periradicular fibrosis? Spine 1989;14:538–568.
4. Olmarker K, Rydevik B, Holm S. Edema formation in spinal nerve roots induced by experimental graded compression: an experimental study on the pig cauda equina with special reference to differences in effects between rapid and low onset of compression. Spine 1989;14:569–573.
5. Parke WW. The significance of venous return impairment in ischemic radiculopathy and myelopathy. Orthop Clin North Am 1991;22:213–222.
6. Kambin P, Nixon JE, Chait A, et al. Annular protrusion: pathophysiology and roentgenographic appearance. Spine 1988;13:671–675.
7. Kambin P, McCullen G, Park W, et al. Minimally invasive arthroscopic spinal surgery. Instruct Course Lect 1997;46:143–161.
8. Schaffer JL, Kambin P. Minimally invasive spine surgery. Textbook Rheumatol Update 1994;9:2–12.
9. Kirkaldy-Willis WH, Paine KW, Cauchois J, McIvor G. Lumbar spinal stenosis. Clin Orthop 1974;99:30–50.
10. Yamada H, Oya M, Okada T, Shiozawa Z. Intermittent cauda equina compression due to narrow spinal canal. J Neurosurg 1972;37:83–88.
11. Kambin P, Casey K, O'Brien E, Zhou L. Transforaminal arthroscopic decompression of lateral recess stenosis. J Neurosurg 1996;84:462–467.
12. Kambin P. Arthroscopic treatment of spinal pathology, in Operative Arthroscopy, 2nd ed. (McGinty JB, Casperi RB, Jackson RW, Poehling GG, eds.), Lippincott-Raven, Philadelphia, 1996, pp. 1227–1233.

13. Chiu J. Transforaminal endoscopic micro decompression of herniated lumbar discs and spinal stenosis. 22nd International Course for Percutaneous and Endoscopic Spinal Surgery, Jan 2004; ISMISS/SICOT, Zurich, Switzerland.
14. Knight MTN, Goswami A, Patko JT. Endoscopic foraminoplasty : a prospective study on 250 consecutive patients with independent evaluation. J Clin Laser Med Surg 2001;19:73–81.
15. Burton CV, Kirkaldy-Willis WH, Yong-Hing K, et al. Causes of failure of surgery on the lumbar spine. Clin Orthop 1981;157:191–199.
16. Ray CT. Transfacet decompression with dowel fixation: a new technique for lumbar lateral spinal stenosis. Acta Neurochir Suppl 1988;43:48–54.
17. Kambin P, O'Brien E, Zhou L. Arthroscopic microdiscectomy and selective fragmentectomy. Clin Orthop 1998;347:150–167.
18. Jaffe RA, Rose MA. A comparison of local anesthetic effect of Meperidine Fentanyl and Sufentanil on dorsal root axons. Anesth Analg 1996;83:776–781.

7

Role of Epidural and Radicular Veins in Chronic Back Pain and Radiculopathy

Wesley W. Parke, PhD

INTRODUCTION

Although the pattern and major components of the human medullary arterial supply were widely known by the end of the nineteenth century, the details of the associated venous circulation were generally ignored. Despite Brechet's *(1)* quite accurate description and later depiction of the complexity of the spinal venous system, published in 1835 (Fig. 1), the ubiquity and variability of its ramifications evidently discouraged further consideration beyond the comprehension that the veins collectively served as collateral channels to the caval and azygos systems. Another factor that may have contributed to the general disregard of the anatomical particulars of these channels may have been related to their structural delicacy. The thinness and transparency of their walls render them almost invisible during conventional cadaver dissections unless they show postmortem evidence of congestion or are specifically filled with a contrast medium. Clemens *(2)* noted that these vessels were quite pliable, which permitted considerable distension under collateral load. Thus, the Queckenstedt maneuver, which tests the patency of the spinal subarachnoid space by compression of the jugular or intra-abdominal veins, causes an increase in cerebrospinal fluid (CSF) pressure by an external compression from the expansion of the collaterally loaded epidural plexus. Clemens also postulated that a passive congestion of the spinal cord was prevented by minute valves in the proximal sources of the radicular veins that drain the spinal cord, a unique situation considering that none of the other sinus veins possess valves. After Batson *(3)*, in the mid–20th century, emphasized this fact by demonstrating the extensive multidirectional flow allowed in these vessels and its significance as a route of metastatic transport of neoplastic cells, interest in the form and function of the spinal vein dramatically increased. Thus, a closer inspection of the initially assumed random entanglement of these vessels eventually yielded the following fairly consistent underlying pattern. This pattern shows several (usually four or more) major longitudinal epidural channels that connect a circumferentially coursing series of vessels that are segmentally arranged in relation to the intervertebral foramina through which they communicate with a segmentally equivalent perivertebral plexus (Fig. 2). The intervertebral connecting branches usually consist of a superior set that exits the foramen embracing

From: *Arthroscopic and Endoscopic Spinal Surgery: Text and Atlas: Second Edition*
Edited by: P. Kambin © Humana Press Inc., Totowa, NJ

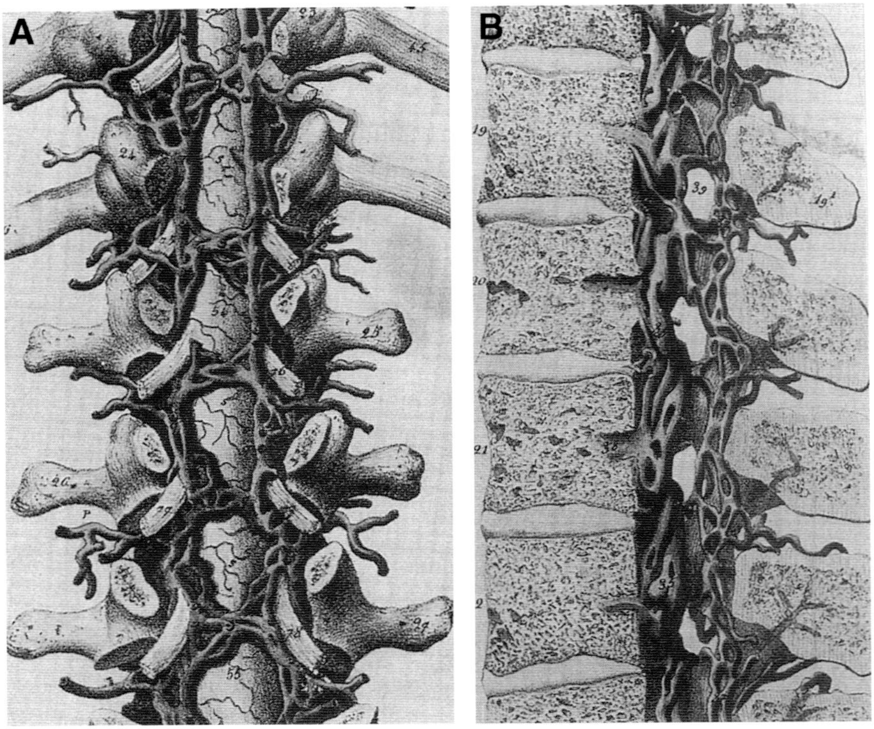

Fig. 1. **(A)** Posterior and **(B)** lateralviews of spinal epidural venous plexus taken from a hand-colored copy of Brechet's original work (published ca. 1835, courtesy of Scott Memorial Library, Jefferson Medical College).

the dorsal root ganglion (DRG) and the exiting nerve roots (Fig. 3), and an inferior set closely related to the pedicle of the inferior foraminal margin.

The contempory experimentally and clinically derived consensus maintains that much of the spinal neurogenic pain associated with degenerative changes in the vertebral osseous and soft-tissue components involves a compressive radiculomedullary ischemia. It was understandable that earlier investigations of the mechanical factors thought to be responsible for this would be approached through studies of the more readily injectable arterial components almost exclusively. The term *neuroischemia* was then primarily regarded as an impairment of the arterial flow because the extent and pervasive distribution of venous channels appeared to guarantee an unlimited, trouble-free access to efferent vascular drainage.

Shortly after publications by Parke and associates *(4,5)* established the basic patterns of the radicular blood supply, clinical observations indicated that the thin-walled low-pressure side of the radiculomedullary circulation may play an unsuspected predominant role in the etiology of intradural spinal ischemias. It then became evident that the efferent vascular channels may be directly affected by the spatial encroachments of degenerative vertebral tissues and/or be compromised by extravertebral changes in the venous resistance consequent to general circulatory problems. Regarding the former, Magnaes *(6)* quantitated some of the compressive effects of spinal stenosis on the

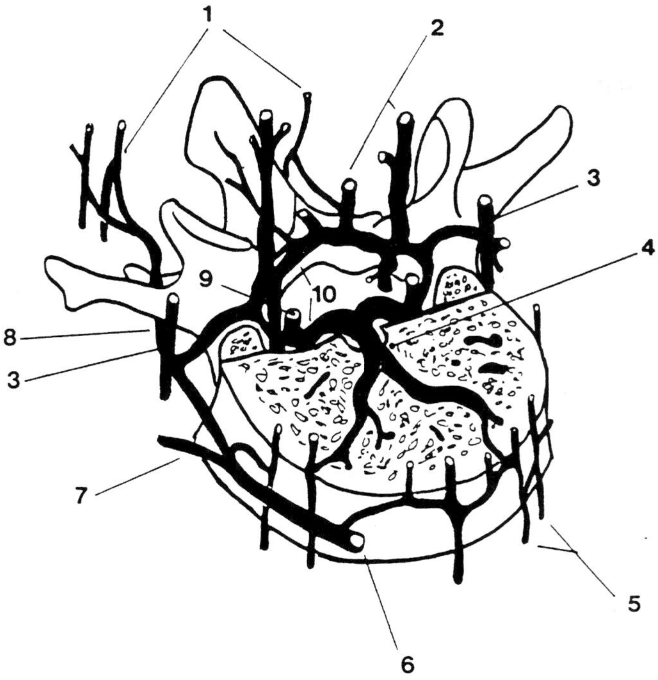

Fig. 2. Schema showing various venous relations of a lumbar vertebra: 1, dorsal external vertebral plexus; 2, dorsal epidural plexus; 3, ascending lumbar veins; 4, basivertebral vein; 5, ventral external vertebral plexus; 6, lumbar segmental vein; 7, muscular vein from posterior abdominal wall; 8, circumferential channels of epidural plexus; 9, ventral longitudinal vein; 10, segmental circumferential epidural.

lumbosacral roots. In noting that the typical L4–L5 stenosis, which often involves a spondylolithesis compounded by facet joint and ligamentum flavum hypertrophies, may restrict the flow of the CSF distal to the level of the lesion, he measured the resulting "spinal block" pressure. This he defined as the amount of elevation in CSF pressure consequent to an infusion caudal to the stenosis that was required to force the fluid past the block (Fig. 4).

In a series of 42 patients with clinical and myelographic indications of a central lumbar stenosis, Magnaes *(6)* was able to determine a pathological degree of pressure on the cauda equina in 67% of cases. He concluded that the block pressure was the main mechanical factor responsible for paresis and pain because it was highest during the spinal extension of standing and walking and exceeded the mean arterial pressure in several cases. Magnaes also noted a frequent spontaneous elevation in CSF pressure in the caudal dural sac during spinal extension and walking but considered this a subordinate factor. Unfortunately, Magnaes's work was too early to appreciate that it was the venous side of the radicular circulation that was most labile to compressive factors, and his publication appeared 2 yr before Rydevik et al. *(7)* demonstrated the nutritional aspects of CSF circulation. In retrospect, it is now apparent that pressures well below those approaching the mean arterial pressure could have a great effect on the radicular circulation by producing a resistance to venous

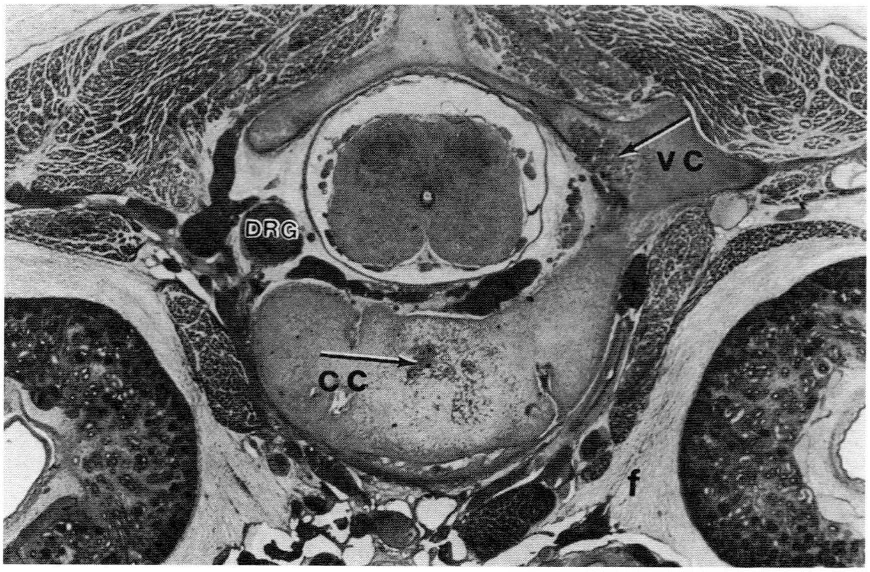

Fig. 3. Vertebra of human fetus (38-mm crown-rump length) showing centers of ossification (CC and VC) and, by virtue of obliquity of the cut, left intervertebral foramen. Terminal congestion fills part of the epidural and perivertebral plexus, showing foraminal veins embracing the DRG. Perirenal fascia (f) is indicated.

drainage. In addition, the spinal block impedes the free replenishment of the CSF in the caudal dural sac and further deprives the lower root sections of this source of metabolic turnover through a stagnation of the confined Venous Hypertension lower sac fluids.

VENOUS HYPERTENSION

Clinical investigators have recorded the exacerbation of neurogenic pain in cases in which spinal stenosis has been associated with venous hypertension. LaBan *(8)* and LaBan and Wesolowski *(9)* noted that patients with diminished right heart compliance and spinal stenosis may eventually show neurogenic pain even in static recumbent situations. They attributed this to an increased external pressure on the already sensitized roots by the distension of the epidural sinuses. Kaiser et al. *(10)* visualized through computed tomography (CT) the obstructive production of this epidural venous stasis by a spinal stenosis and its venous engorgement. Because the spinal canal, like the cranial cavity, is a relatively nondistensible container, there is a limited allowance for spatial encroachment before neurological elements are compressed. In a spinal stenosis, the roots are already chronically restricted by the circumferential degenerative hypertrophies, but because the epidural venous sinuses also share this compromised space, it is not difficult to conceptualize that their distension, owing to increased cardiopulmonary resistance in the caval venous return, would provide an additional insult to a chronic situation. Because this pain is not immediately manifest when the patient reclines but gradually increases with prolonged recumbency, often to be initiated after the onset of sleep, LaBan *(8)* postulated the existence of a "venous creep." This implies that the thin epidural sinus walls respond to the increased pressure by a delayed gradual distension that amplifies the epidural expansive pressure. More recently, Madsen and Heros *(11)* and Parke *(12)*

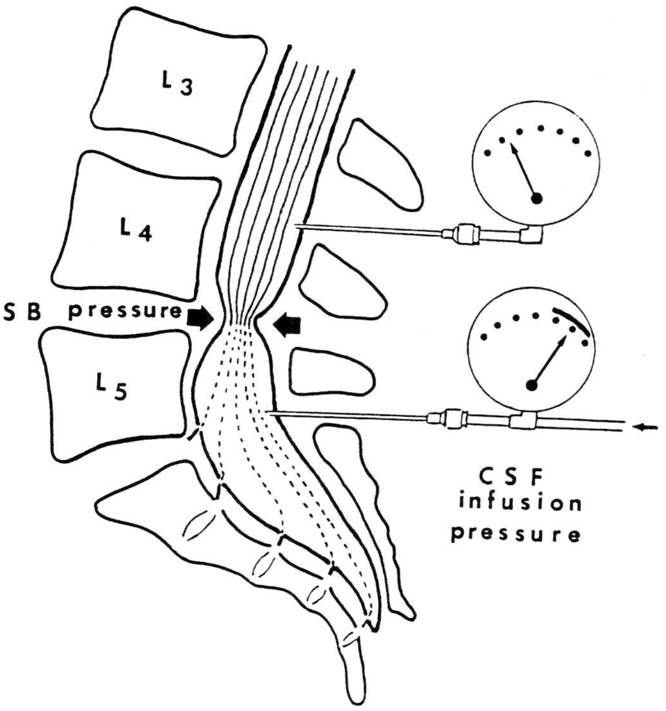

Fig. 4. Schema derived from data provided by Magnaes *(6)* showing how he determined "spinal block" (SB) pressure through infusion into lower dural sac. The degree of pressure required to force the fluid past the spinal block determined the SB pressure.

have shown that "arterialization" of spinal veins by anomalous arteriovenous shunts in the region of the conus medullaris also exacerbates the neurogenic pain in patients with spinal stenosis. They hypothesized that a variable combination of increased mechanical constriction by dilated epidural veins and the direct increased resistance to the radicular circulation by venous hypertension contributed to initiation of the pain. Aboulker et al. *(13)* recorded cases of caval anomalies in which the impeded venous return produced symptoms of cord and root ischemias, and they concluded that epidural venous hypertension alone may produce radicular and/or cord symptoms without adjunct stenotic compressions.

A graphic depiction of the venous compromise by degenerative encroachments is provided in Fig. 5, in which the left side of the schema shows the consequences of segmental constrictions (spinal stenoses), and the right side indicates how such a situation may be further exacerbated by extravertebral hypertensions similar to those dual supply of Intradural roots reported by LaBan and colleagues *(8,9)*.

DUAL SUPPLY OF INTRADURAL ROOTS

Because the very long intradural roots of the lumbosacral spinal nerves were without access to the frequent collateral support characteristic of peripheral nerves and were initially believed to be supplied only from their distal ends, they were subjected to a series of studies in an attempt to provide a basic knowledge of the pathophysiology of nerve

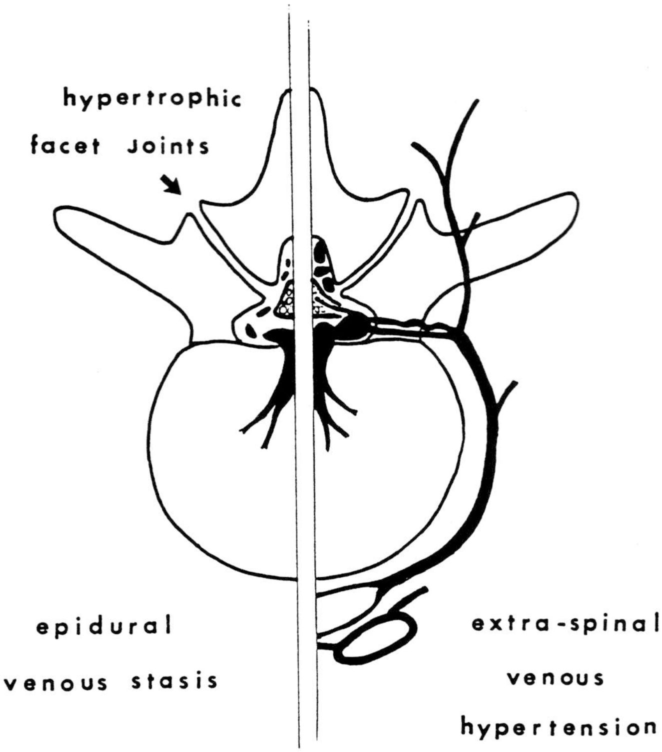

Fig. 5. Schema showing confined spatial relationships of epidural venous sinuses in stenotic section of lumbar spinal canal. The left side indicates how the compromised space may restrict the venous flow at that level. The right side shows how extraspinal venous hypertension may engorge sinuses and provide additional pressure on dura and contained roots.

root nutrition. Subsequently, the injection studies of Parke et al. *(4)* and Parke and Watanabe *(5)*, using a series of graduated pressure injections, showed that the roots receive an arterial supply from both ends through equivalent groups of longitudinally coursing peri- and intraradicular arteries that maintain a rather consistant caliber until they anastomose in the midsections of the radicular fascicles. An additional important finding was the occurrence of numerous and relatively large normal arteriovenous anastomoses throughout the length of each root (Fig. 6A,B). These vascular shunts apparently serve to protect the functional integrity of the radicular circulation in the event of focal compressions. Of particular significance to the knowledge of root metabolism were the contemporary investigations of Rydevik et al. *(7)*, who, using isotopically labeled methyl glucose, demonstrated that approx 50% of the root nutrition is derived from ambient CSF, a fact that necessitates the gauzelike architecture of the pia-arachnoid sheath.

A study of chronically compressed roots by Watanabe and Parke *(14)* indicated that the involved site of compression was most likely metabolically deprived. It had been strongly indicated that the radicular pain associated with nerve distortions is somehow related to the resulting ischemia because the reduction in oxygen intake in patients with neurogenic claudication exacerbates their symptoms and shortens their "claudication

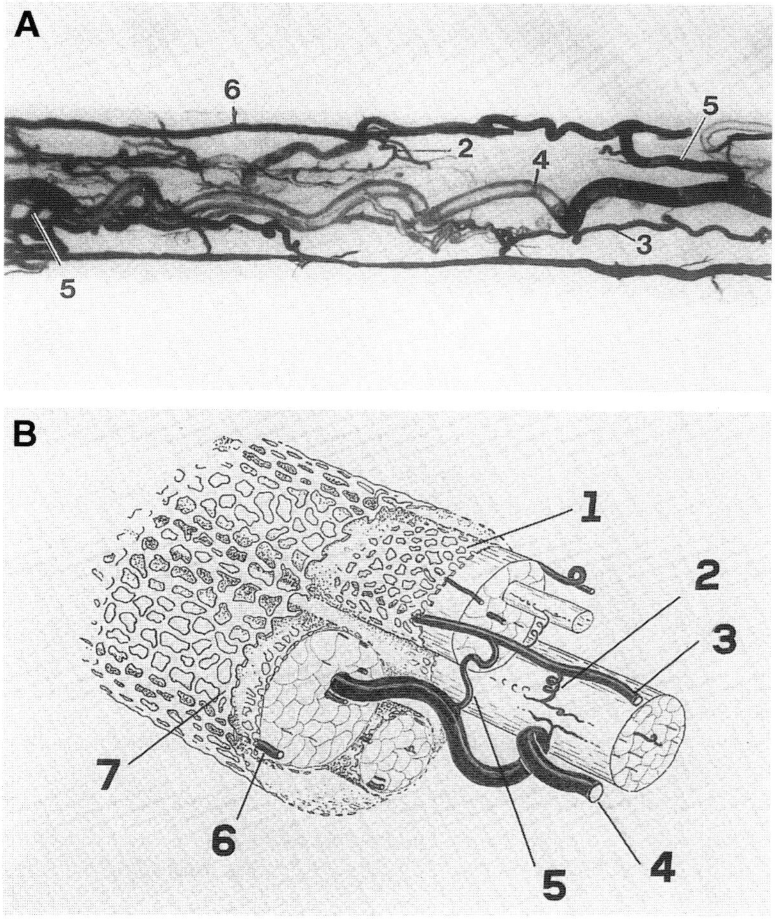

Fig. 6. (A) Low-power (×20) transillumination photomicrograph of L4 nerve root showing injected arteries and gas-filled veins demonstrating course of these intraradicular vessels and frequent arteriovenous anastomotic shunts. **(B)** Graphic compilation of structure and vasculature of typical lumbosacral nerve root. (From ref. *5*.) The numbers in both (A) and (B) are common to equivalent structures: 1, fascicular pia; 2, inter- and intrafascicular arteries; 3, longitudinal radicular artery; 4, large radicular vein (does not course with artery); 5, arteriovenous anastomosis; 6, collateral radicular artery; 7, gauzelike pia-arachnoid that permits free percolation of CSF to assist root metabolism.

time" when walking *(15)*. However, Watanabe and Parke *(14)* found that the arterial phase of the vasa radiculorum appears to be well compensated and maintains some continuity despite a severe compression provided that the pressure had developed slowly over several years. Further study then indicated that it is the venous side of the radicular circulation that is more vulnerable (Fig. 7).

VASCULAR PATTERN OF INTRADURAL ROOTS

Contrary to some preexisting concepts, vascular and neuronal analyses now indicate that the intradural roots are part of the central nervous system (CNS), and that the relationship of the arteries to the veins more resembles that found in the brain than in the peripheral nerves. This is shown by the fact that the radicular veins do not accompany the arterial

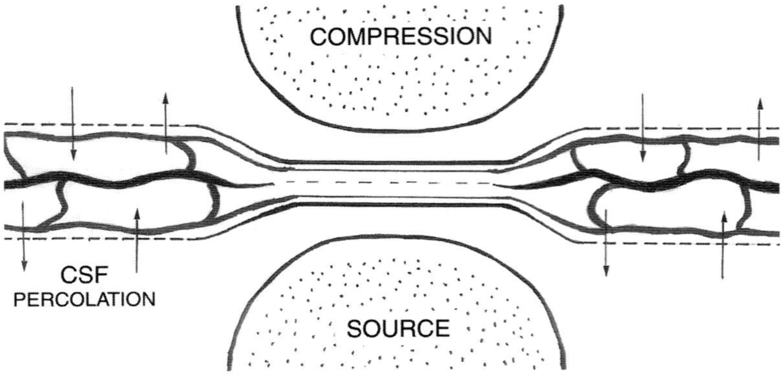

Fig. 7. Schema illustrating role of arteriovenous anastomoses in maintaining vascular function in compressed root. Note that the anatomoses ensure the afferent-efferent cycle of the blood flow up to both sides of the compression point.

pattern of distribution but are fewer and run a separate and usually deeper more central course. Being thin walled, they are more susceptible to the spatial distortions imposed by degenerative changes in the dimensions of the spinal canal and intervertebral foramina and show a complete interruption in the chronically compressed nerve root.

Nerve root distortion is a consistent finding in neurogenic claudication and sciatica, but studies of both nerve roots and peripheral nerve have shown that although compression alone may disrupt most nerve functions, it usually does not cause pain *(16–18)*. There is currently a consensus that some degree of intrinsic irritation or inflammation must develop before nerve distortion, by itself, may elicit pain. Studies of graded and intermittent pressures on nerve roots in the pig cauda equina have revealed that the resulting nutritional disruption in the affected nerve, by both impedance of CSF percolation and interruption of the vascular channels, leads to visible edema and venous congestion *(19)*. It is this irritated and inflammed segment that becomes hypersensitive and elicits pain with additional or prolonged insults. In 1998, Takata et al. *(20)* noted that compressed roots were evident in CT myelograms owing to their edematous enlargement. Subsequently, a detailed study by Kobayashi et al. *(21)* showed that compression disrupts a type of blood-nerve barrier unique to the radicular microvessels and permits abnormal extravasations that produce edema.

A single-level stenosis may exist without marked claudication, which has led to the assumption that a double level of nerve root compression is more likely to be symptomatic *(21,22)*. The previously mentioned shunt function concept indicates that the radicular vascular pattern with its frequent and effective series of arteriovenous anastmoses allows for some circulatory compensation for single-point compressions (Fig. 8). However, a two-point compression would vascularly isolate the intermediate root segment and lead to changes consequent to obvious metabolic deprivation (Fig. 9). A two-point compression relative to a spinal stenosis may only involve a single nerve root wherein the superior level of compression results from the stenotic constriction (of it and other roots) and a herniated nucleus pulposis provides a second lower foraminal compression with the development of the irritable edematous condition in the individual root between these points, or there can be two levels of stenotic constriction that would affect all the roots between the levels. In the latter situation, the intervening isolated dural sac could provide conditions analogous to a compartment syndrome *(23)*.

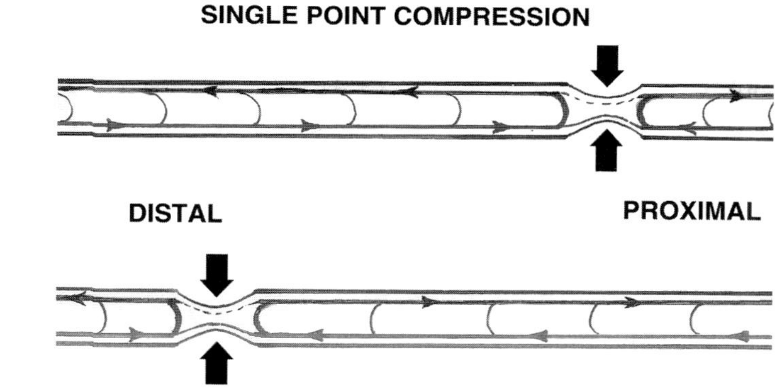

Fig. 8. Illustration depicting advantage of both a proximal and distal source to radicular circulation that allow flow from either end to supply any root segment from above or below a single point of pressure.

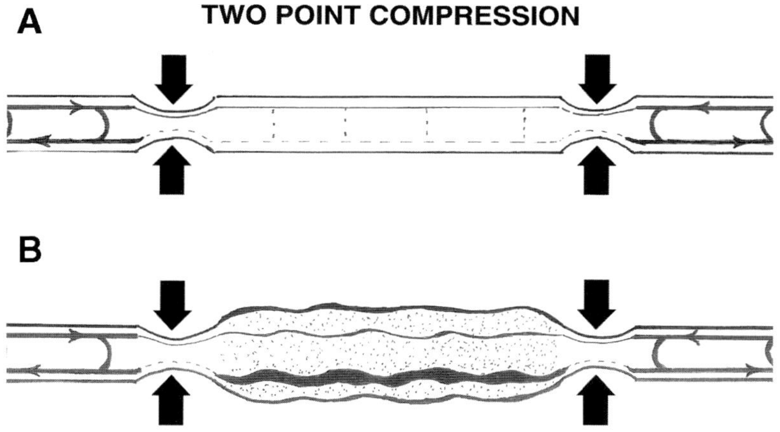

Fig. 9. **(A)** Illustration depicting problem of two-point pressures on long nerve root. The intervening longer segment between the compressions may become almost completely nutritionally isolated and dependent only on the CSF metabolic exchange. **(B)** Illustration showing that vascular deprivation likely leads to changes in vascular permeability with its consequent edema and root sheath fibrosis.

ANIMAL EXPERIMENTAL STUDIES

The best demonstrations of the venous lability of the radiculomedullary circulation have been provided by studies involving experimental compressions of the lumbosacral roots in the dog *(22)* and in the pig *(16,19,24)*. In these studies, it was noted that an obvious venous congestion was a major consistent feature associated with the site of the experimental compression. Both research groups used graduated stages of constriction, and the dog model was reported to show little alteration in neurologic function until a 50% constriction had been attained. In the pig model, however, Olmarker and colleagues *(16,19,24)* recorded the graduations of pressure in millimeters of mercury injected into compressing balloons, and they remarked on how little pressure was required to induce a venous congestion that they believed could eventually lead to alterations in nerve function. Both groups noted that the venous congestion soon induced an intraneurial edema. This radicular edema cannot be readily equated to the lymphedema found in the peripheral systems because the spinal roots, like the rest of the CNS, possess no lymphatics, since they are able to discharge their extracellular proteins directly into the CSF. Olmarker and colleagues *(16,19,24)* noted that the edema formed more rapidly following rapid compression than in slow compression and concluded that it results from alterations in the permeability of the microvessels. This may cause the microvessels to leak macromolecules into the endoneurial spaces and alters the nutritional access to the axons, impairing function of the nerves *(25)*.

SLOW VS RAPID COMPRESSION

Both the findings of Watanabe and Parke *(14)* and Delmarter et al. *(22)* showed a marked loss in the number of neuronal fibers in severely constricted roots. However, the rapidly induced experimental compressions evidently produced a more immediate and drastic neurological deficit than did the 5- to 10-yr periods required to produce the 75% constrictions noted in the Parke and Watanabe case. It was also recorded that beyond the 50% constriction in the roots of dogs, the arteries were interrupted, whereas in the observed 75% constriction of the gradual, long-term compression of the human roots, the arteries remained intact *(14)*. Thus, there is a strong indication that very slowly developing degenerative stenotic compressions may allow sufficient time for arterial and neuronal compensations and substitutions to preserve the more essential functions and may thus mask the severity of the condition, despite the loss of a great amount of larger, well-myelinated fibers and the irreversible loss of muscular strength. This was well illustrated by the fact that the patient in the Parke and Watanabe case, despite a neurogenic claudication, was able to walk into the hospital without assistance a few days before his death from cardiovascular failure, and with only about 25% of the original nerve fibers supplying his leg musculature.

VASCULARITY OF DORSAL ROOT GANGLION

Contemporary accounts of radiculomedullary circulation provide little or no mention of the vascular distribution to the DRG *(26–28)*, despite the fact that Bergmann and Alexander *(29)* published a well-detailed treatment of the subject several decades before most investigations of intrinsic radicular circulation were conducted. The lack of a general awareness of this work may be attributed to the fact that its publication preceded the development of sufficient interest and background (an informational matrix that historians conveniently label with the German word Fragestellung) necessary to emphasize its clinical significance. Unfortunately, Bergmann and Alexander *(29)* relied only on pen-and-ink drawings to corroborate their verbal descriptions of the major vessels, and a mental reconstruction from their injected microscopic series of cross-sections to determine the finer intraganglionic vasculature.

More recent studies have concentrated on the functional aspects of DRG circulation with a greater regard for the measurable physiological reactions than for the morphological intricacies of the vascular pattern. This apparent neglect of the probable roles of the vascular peculiarites of the DRG may originate partly in the recognition that much of the vessel architectonics of the entire human radiculomedullary circulation is unique to the large primate species, and that the functional generalizations derived from various experimental animals are demonstrably more reliable than the morphological ones *(30)*. Recently, Parke and Whalen *(31)* were able to provide transilluminated photomicrographs of the finely injected dorsal root ganglia of human perinatal cadavers and venous injections of adult human specimens. From these it was determined that the vessel distributions from a few lower-level ganglia described by Bergmann and Alexander *(29)* could be generalized to derive a pattern of distribution that is characteristic of the DRG in all levels of the various vertebral regions, and the arterial ramifications could be summarized in a single description (Fig. 10A). In essence, it was shown that the nuclear parenchyma is highly vascularized primarily from vessels entering the proximal and distal poles of each ganglion. These, through predominantly longitudinal derivatives that course parallel to the long axis of the ganglion, supply the cordlike arrangements of the neuronal nuclei with a dense capillary bed. A secondary, finer network of arteries that is also mostly derived from the proximal and distal polar sources forms a fine reticular system over the surface of the ganglion. This periganglionic plexus communicates with the deeper vessels by a network of centripetally coursing fine channels. The distal and proximal polar arteries are derived from the epidural branches of the intersegmental vertebral arteries, as indicated in the generalized illustration of the "generic" DRG arterial vasculature shown in Fig. 10A.

Injections of the cadaver segmental veins was a limited success, because the numerous open channels of the dissected segments failed to provide the closed system necessary to develop adequate pressures. Nevertheless, the results indicated the existence of a consistent periganglionic venous plexus that receives the major efferent blood flow from the interior of the DRG parenchyma. This supports the observations that Bergmann and Alexander *(29)* derived from their histological sections.

In 1977, Howe et al. *(32)* published a physiologically based study showing that, unlike the lack of ectopic impulses generated by the compression of normal nerve roots, prolonged periods of repetitive nerve firings followed a brief acute compression of the normal DRG. In an excellent article, Yoshizawa et al. *(33)* provided evidence that the blood flow volume in the dorsal root of dogs is less than that of the gray matter of the cord and the peripheral nerves, whereas the DRG blood flow volume is approximately twice that of the nerve root and similar to the blood flow in the gray matter of the cord. By using the hydrogen clearance method, they were able to show that the DRG blood flow was reduced 40–45% by a compression of 60 g on the distal side of the ganglion, and 10–15% by equivalent pressure on the proximal side.

Rydevik et al. *(23)* recorded the endoneurial pressures within the normal rat dorsal nerve root and its DRG and observed it to be higher than the internal fluid pressure within the animal's sciatic nerve, with a reading of 3.7 cm of water. They then noted that it rose to as high as 9.6 cm of water subsequent to a mechanical deformation. Because miniature compartment syndromes have been shown to exist after compression of a peripheral nerve *(34)*, it was concluded that such a high-pressure elevation in the DRG would likely affect the nutrition of the neuron cells, and a long-standing edema could result in DRG endoneurial fibrosis. Although Rydevik et al. *(23)* recognized that

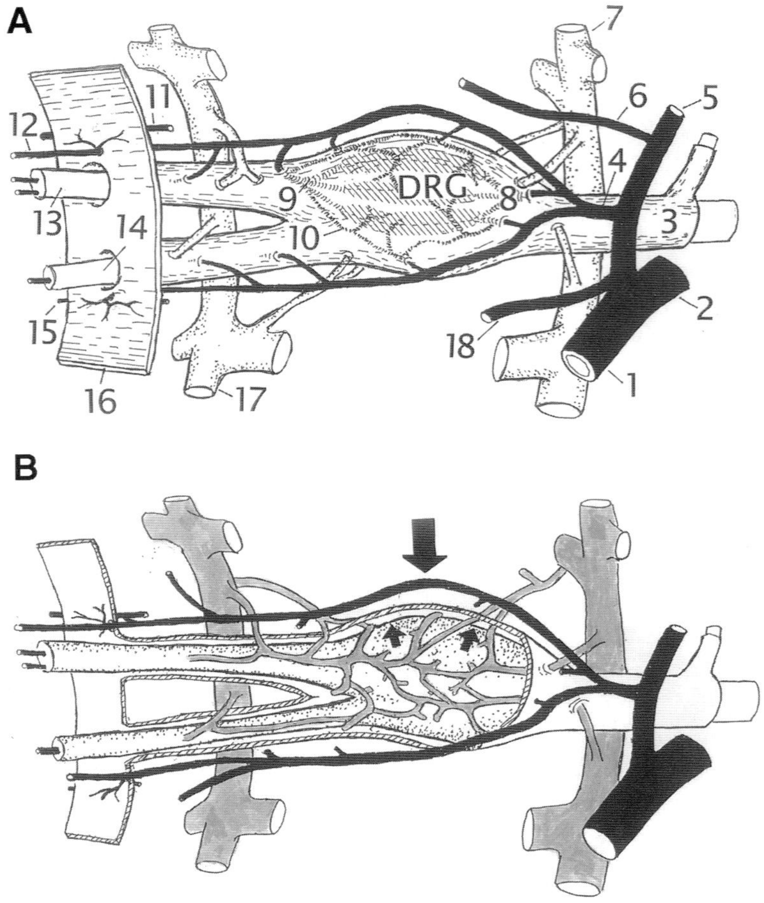

Fig. 10. **(A)** Labeled schema of "generic" DRG with its regional vascular and dural relations: 1, segmental artery; 2, lumbar, intercostal, or cervical artery; 3, spinal nerve; 4, radiculomedullary branch of segmental artery; 5, dorsal branch of segmental artery; 6, internal artery to lamina; 7, paravertebral venous plexus; 8, distal polar DRG arteries; 9, proximal polar DRG arteries; 10, periganglionic arterial plexus; 11, meningeal segmental artery; 12, medullary artery to dorsolateral spinal artery; 13, dorsal nerve root; 14, ventral nerve root; 15, smaller inconsistent meningeal intersegmental artery; 16, spinal dura; 17, epidural venous plexus; 18, dorsal artery to vertebral bodies and their ligaments. **(B)** This schema duplicates the anatomical relations labeled in (A), but the periganglionic venous plexus has been reconstructed to emphasize its vulnerable position adjacent to the fibrous dura where external pressures (large arrow) or edematous internal pressures (small arrows) could readily create a venostasis leading to a DRG compartment syndrome. (Adapted from ref. *31*.)

the increase in pressure within the closed fibrous dural compartment of the DRG would impede normal vascular flow, they did not relate it to any predisposing characteristic of the vascular pattern.

The demonstrable fact that when a mechanical pressure is applied to an endoneurial and/or perineurial vascular system a venostasis is achieved at a significantly lower pressure than that required to stop the arterial flow indicates that this greater lability of the efferent side of the system may be more responsible for ischemic neuropathies than was previously supposed.

Regarding the intrinsic vascularity of the human DRG as described and illustrated here, it is obvious that the structural arrangement of the vessels presents an inherent vulnerability to compressive factors. Weinstein *(35)* made a functional allusion that the DRG could be regarded as the "brain" of the motion segment unit. This metaphor may be taken one step further with respect to the DRG's circulation. Like the cerebral vascularity, the main arterial supply of the DRG cellular masses tends to immediately run deep and central to reach their functional position in the parenchyma. The efferent veins, as in the cerebral cortical tissues, generally run a separate centrifugal course and rise to the surface to collect in a periganglionic plexus that is distributed countercurrent to the much finer, but equivalently located, periganglionic arterial plexus.

An analysis of the unique structural arrangement of the vascularity of the human DRG in relation to its relatively unyielding fibrous adnexa, as graphically rendered in Fig. 10B, shows that by the structure and position of the major venous drainage, the human DRG is remarkably predisposed to the development of a classic compartment syndrome. The total effect of an external mechanical compression may be complex. In an acute phase, the compression would force the dural capsule to impede directly the immediately underlying efferent flow in the periganglionic plexus and thus resist the normal afferent nutrition to the deeper parenchymal constituents. By subsequent alterations in the vascular permeability, a resulting endoneurial edema would reflexly push the periganglionic venous plexus against its unyielding fibrous container and create a more chronic venostasis *(36)*. A prolonged maintenance of this condition could lead to endoneurial fibrosis, increased sensitivity, and repetitive ectopic firing of the contained neural elements.

CONCLUSION

The information discussed herein should be instructive when considering surgical approaches to the spine. The judicious necessity of a surgical intervention automatically admits that the involved segmental region has been subject to a spatial encroachment that may have already affected the efferent vascular blood flow to the foraminal venous channels. Therefore, the extensive use of electrocautery just to achieve a clearer field should obviously be avoided. The operative field reductions inherent in the more minimal approaches, especially those using percutaneous instrumentation, may provide some marked advantages. The most prominent of these would be a mitigation of both the extent of required venostasis and the undesirable consequences resulting from the inadvertent manipulation of the DRG.

REFERENCES

1. Brechet G. Essai sur les Veines der Rachis, Mequigon-Morvith, Paris, 1819.
2. Clemens HJ. Die Venesysteme der menschlichen Wirbelsaule, Walter de Gruyter, Berlin, 1961.
3. Batson OV. The function of the vertebral veins and their role in the spread of metastasis. Am Surg 1940;112:138–145.
4. Parke WW, Gammell K, Rothman RH. Arterial vascularization of the cauda equina. J Bone Joint Surg 1981;63(A):53–62.

5. Parke WW, Watanabe R. The intrinsic vasculature of the lumbosacral spinal nerve roots. Spine 1985;10:508–515.
6. Magnaes B. Clinical recording of pressure on the spinal cord and cauda equina: parts 1 and 2. J Neurosurg 1982;57:48–63.
7. Rydevik B, Holm S, Brown MD, et al. Diffusion from the cerebrospinal fluid as a nutritional pathway for spinal nerve roots. Acta Physiol Scand 1990;138:247, 248.
8. LaBan MM. "Vespers curse" night pain—the bane of hypnos. Arch Phys Med Rehabil 1984;65:501–504.
9. LaBan MM, Wesolowski DF. Night pain associated with diminished cardiopulmonary compliance. Am J Phys Med Rehabil 1988;67:155–160.
10. Kaiser MC, Capesius P, Roilgen A, et al. Epidural venous stasis. Neuroradiology 1984;26: 435–438.
11. Madsen JR, Heros RC. Spinal arteriovenous malformations and neurogenic claudication. J Neurosurg 1988;57:793–797.
12. Parke WW. The significance of venous return impairment in ischemic radiculopathy and myelopathy. Orthop Clin North Am 1991;22:213–221.
13. Aboulker J, Bar D, Marsault C, et al. L'hypertension vieneuse intra-rachidienne par anomalies multiples du system cave: une cause majeure de souffrance medullaire. Chirurgerie 1977;103:1004–1015.
14. Watanabe R, Parke WW. Vascular and neural pathology of lumbosacral spinal nerve roots in spinal stenosis. J Neurosurg 1986;64:64–70.
15. Evans JG. Neurogenic intermittant claudication. BMJ 1964;2:985–987.
16. Olmarker K, Rydevik B, Holm S. Edema formation in spinal nerve roots induced by experimental graded compression. Spine 1989;14:569–573.
17. Pedowitz RA, Rydevik BL, Hargrens AR, et al. Neurophysiologic and histologic changes induced by acute graded compression of the pig cauda equina. Paper presented at the International Society for the Study of the Lumbar Spine, Miami, FL, 1998.
18. Rydevik B, Hannson TH, Garfin SR. Pathophysiology of cauda equina compression. Semin Spine Surg 1989;1:139–142.
19. Olmarker K, Rydevik B, Holm S, Bagge U. Effects of experimental graded compression on blood flow in spinal nerve roots: a vital microscopic study on the porcine cauda equina. J Orthop Res 1989;7:817–823.
20. Takata K, Inuoe S, Takahashi K, Ohtsuka Y. Swelling of cauda equina in patients who have herniation of a lumbar disc. J Bone Joint Surg 1998;70A:361–368.
21. Kobayashi S, Yoshizawa H, Hichiya Y, et al. Vasogenic edema induced by compression injury to the spinal nerve root. Spine 1993;18:1410–1424.
22. Delmarter LB, Bohlman HH, Dodge LD, Biro C. Experimental lumbar spinal stenosis. J Bone Joint Surg (Am) 1990;72:110–120.
23. Rydevik BL, Myers RR, Powell HC. Pressure increase in the dorsal root ganglion following mechanical compression: closed compartment syndrome in nerve roots. Spine 1989;14:574–576.
24. Olmarker K, Rydevik B, Hansson T, et al. Compression induced changes in the nutritional supply of the porcine cauda equina. J Spinal Disord 1990;3:25–29.
25. Myers RR, Murakami H, Powell HC. Reduced nerve blood flow in edematous neuropathies: a biomechanical mechanism. Microvasc Res 1986;32:145–151.
26. Corbin JL. Anatomie et Pathologie Arterielles de la Moelle, Masson et Cie, Paris, 1961.
27. Crock HV, Yoshizawa H. The Blood Supply of the Vertebral Column and Spinal Cord in Man, Springer-Verlag, New York, 1977.
28. Lazorthes G, Gouaze A, Zadwh JO, et al. Arterial vascularization of the spinal cord. J Neurosurg 1971;35:253–262.
29. Bergmann L, Alexander L. Vascular supply of the spinal ganglion. Arch Neurol Psychiatry 1941;46:761–782.

30. Parke WW. Point of view (a cautionary discussion on the necessity, advantage and pitfalls of animal models in research). Spine 1995;20:765.
31. Parke WW, Whalen JL. The vascular pattern of the dorsal root ganglion and its probable bearing on a compartment syndrome. Spine 2002;27:347–352.
32. Howe JF, Loeser JD, Calvin WH. Mechanosensitivity of dorsal root ganglia and chronically injured axons: a physiological basis for radicular pain of nerve root compression. Pain 1977;3:25–41.
33. Yoshizawa H, Kobayashi S, Hachia Y. Blood supply of nerve roots and dorsal root ganglia. Orthop Clin North Am 1991;22:195–211.
34. Lundborg GI, Myers R, Powell H. Nerve compression injury and increased endoneurial pressure: a miniature compartment syndrome. J Neurol Neurosurg Psychiatry 1983;46: 1119–1124.
35. Weinstein JN. Part B: Basic Science Perspectives. In: New Perspectives in Low Back Pain (Frymoyer JW, Gordon SL, eds.), American Academy of Orthopedic Surgeons, Park Ridge, IL;1989 pp. 57–110.
36. Hoyland JA, Freemont AJ, Jayson MIV. Intervertebral foramen venous obstruction: a cause of periradicular fibrosis. Spine 1989;14:538–568.

8

Diagnostic and Therapeutic Percutaneous Transpedicular Approaches to the Spine

Alexander G. Hadjipavlou, MD, George M. Kontakis, MD, Ioannis Gaitanis, MD, and Michael Tzermiadianos, MD

TRANSPEDICULAR BIOPSY

Historical Review and Rationale for the Procedure

Open biopsy advocates prefer transpedicular biopsy (TPB) because it maximizes tissue retrieval, thus providing the highest diagnostic success rate. Open biopsy is especially relied on after failed needle biopsy or in selected presumed primary bone or cartilaginous tumors *(1)*. However, the complications and morbidity associated with an open surgical procedure provided incentive for the development of closed needle biopsy techniques.

Historically, preference for closed biopsy of the spine developed because it was claimed to be less invasive, less morbid, and more cost-effective than open biopsy. Closed biopsy has also become increasingly accurate as techniques and image modalities have evolved. Local anesthesia and an outpatient setting contribute to enhanced cost-effectiveness. Local anesthesia also allows nerve root monitoring during biopsy. Consequently, percutaneous biopsy of spinal lesions has become the biopsy technique of choice, but not without potential complications, such as nerve injury, bleeding, pneumothorax, and inadequate amount of tissue retrieval for diagnosis *(2–5)*.

The reported diagnostic success rates of closed needle biopsy of the spine are variable and decrease significantly with primary bone tumors *(2,3,6,7)* and tumors with complex architecture and cell pleomorphism (such as giant cell tumors, aneurysmal bone cyst, osteoblastoma, osteosarcoma, or chondrosarcoma) *(8,9)*. Crush artifacts, one of the problems created by small needles *(3)*, predisposes conventional closed biopsy to an inferior success rate *(6,10)*. Fyfe et al. *(10)* reported a cadaveric study in which biopsy specimens with tissue core diameters ≥2 mm enhanced diagnostic accuracy. Because the pedicle accommodates biopsy instruments that retrieve tissue core diameters >2 mm, the diagnostic success rate of a percutaneous TPB should approach the success rate of an open procedure. Larger tissue core diameters also avoid the diagnostic problems created by crush artifacts. Therefore, there was room for improvement and a transpedicular approach was developed as an alternative to the other biopsy methods for vertebral lesions involving the sacrum and thoracic, lumbar, and seventh cervical vertebral *(11,12)*.

Enthusiasm regarding surgery involving the vertebral pedicle is reflected by the ever-increasing information regarding transpedicular fixation *(13)*, morphology *(14–21)*, biomechanics *(22)*, fracture management *(13,23)*, and hemiepiphysiodesis *(24)*.

From: *Arthroscopic and Endoscopic Spinal Surgery: Text and Atlas: Second Edition*
Edited by: P. Kambin © Humana Press Inc., Totowa, NJ

Transpedicular fixation techniques have continued to increase in popularity since their inception *(25,26)*. The pedicular channel also has been used for fracture reduction *(27,28)*, external skeletal fixation *(29)*, decompression *(30)*, thoracic discectomy *(31)*, bone grafting *(26)*, and methylmethacrylate insertion *(26)*.

Despite increasing knowledge of vertebral morphometry and experience with transpedicular fixation, it was a long time before the pedicle was popularized as a channel for percutaneous vertebral needle biopsy.

The use of the pedicular channel for open biopsy is not a new idea. In 1928, von Lackum (as reported by Duncan and Ferguson *(32)* in 1936) performed a transpedicular curettage of a vertebral body giant cell tumor in an 8-yr-old girl. In 1933, Capener *(33)* described an anterolateral decompression in which the pedicle was removed to access lesions in the vertebral body. In 1949, Michele and Krueger *(34)* described a transpedicular approach as one of four posterior approaches to the vertebral body. It was not until 1979 that Travaglini *(35)* reintroduced this technique in the English literature.

The belated development of this technique may be attributed to three explanations. First, the proximity of the pedicle to neural elements deterred closed biopsy attempts because of fears of injuring these vital structures. Second, appreciation of the biopsy potential of vertebral body lesions through the pedicle has been limited *(36)*. Third, the larger tissue samples retrievable with open biopsy made open procedure (with radiographic guidance when indicated) the "gold standard" to which all other biopsy procedures had to be compared.

In 1983, Roy-Camille et al. *(13)* first described an open (TPB) technique used in a series of 47 patients. In 1990, Rengachary described a transpedicular technique that included a hemilaminectomy, a partial facetectomy, and a partial pediculectomy *(19)*. Also in 1990, Fidler and Niers *(37)* reported one case of an open TPB. In 1991, Renfrew *(7)* reported percutaneous TPBs in six patients using computed tomography (CT). We have reported the technique of TPB as an efficacious, safe, and cost-effective method *(12,38–43)*. In most cases, it can be performed under local anesthesia, with fluoroscopic guidance.

The Percutaneous Transpedicular Biopsy Technique

The percutaneous procedure requires a high-resolution image intensifier and a radiolucent operating table that can be precisely tilted. The transverse pedicle width and the pedicle angle in the axial plane are determined from preoperative CT images. The operating table is canted until the pedicular angle in the axial plane is perpendicular to the floor and the X-ray beam is collinear with the sagittal pedicular angle determined from lateral views of the vertebral body. A "bull's-eye" view of the pedicle should be obtained. This procedure is analogous to obtaining perfect circles during distal interlocking procedures of intramedullary femoral nail. Local anesthesia is obtained by injecting plain 1% lidocaine hydrochloride along the intended biopsy tract and infiltrating the posterior primary ramus as it emerges from the junction of the transverse process and superior facet of the corresponding joint and adjacent superior and inferior facet joints. After insertion of the guide pin, the physician makes a small stab wound incision about 1 cm long to allow the passage of a modified Kambin dilator *(44)* (5.35-mm diameter; Smith & Nephew) over the guide pin until it reaches bone (Fig. 1). Following this, a cannulated modified Kambin sleeve (6.4-mm diameter; Smith & Nephew) is passed over the dilator and guide pin until it abuts the cortical margins of the pedicle (Fig. 2). The use of a cannulated sleeve prevents clogging of the bone biopsy instrument with

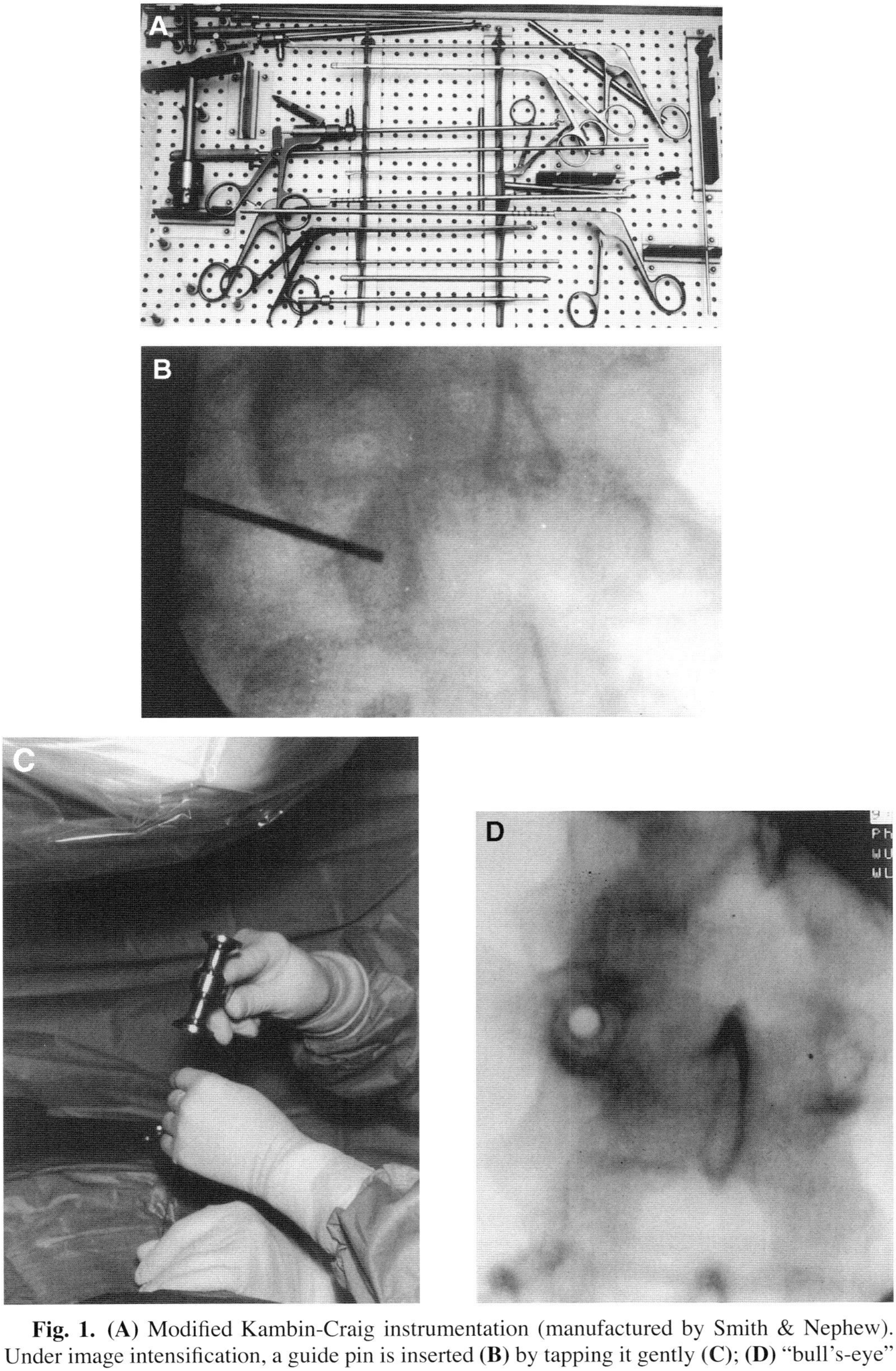

Fig. 1. (A) Modified Kambin-Craig instrumentation (manufactured by Smith & Nephew). Under image intensification, a guide pin is inserted **(B)** by tapping it gently **(C)**; **(D)** "bull's-eye" view into the pedicle.

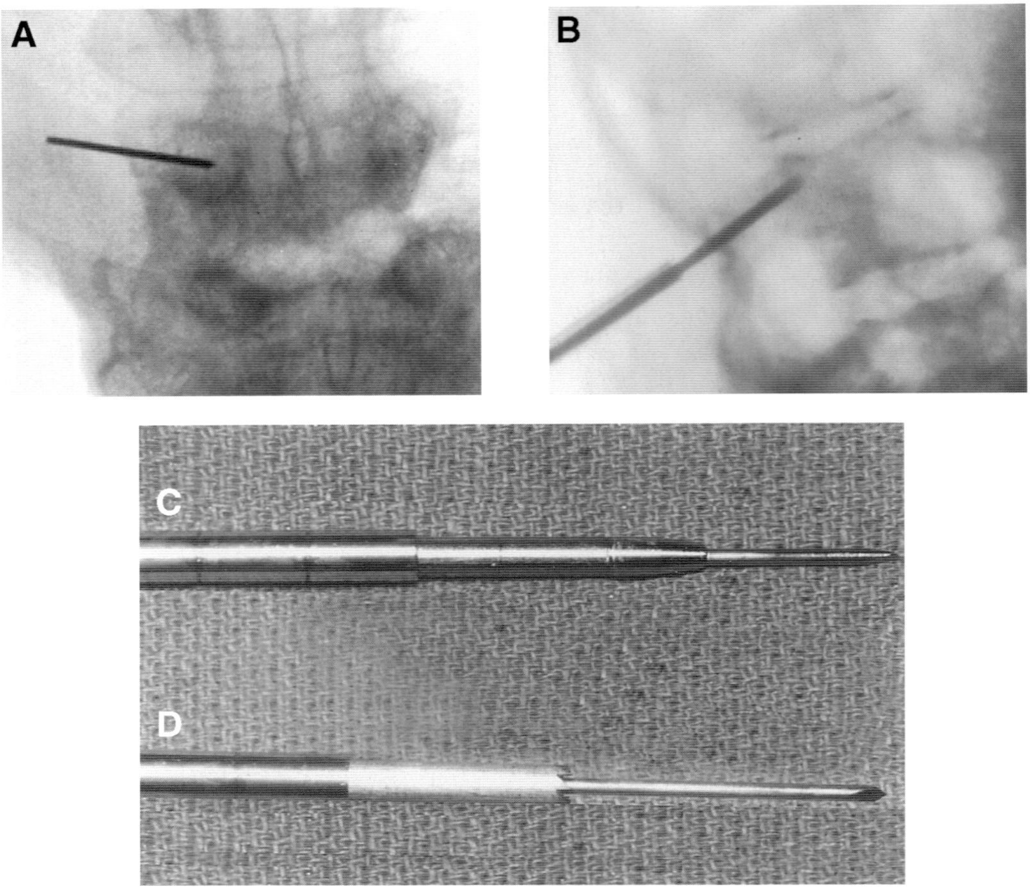

Fig. 2. **(A,B)** The pin is angled to the lesion intended for biopsy. Next a dilator **(C)** is passed over the guide pin to dissect the soft tissues, and a cannulated sleeve is inserted over the dilator until it reaches the pedicle. The dilator is then removed, and the toothed cutting biopsy tool **(D)** is inserted into the sleeve over the guide pin. (Partially reproduced with permission from ref. *40*.)

subcutaneous tissue or muscle fibers and also facilitates the insertion of the instrument for discectomy. Next, the physician removes the dilator and advances a toothed, modified Craig biopsy tool (3.2- or 5.15-mm diameter; Smith & Nephew) over the guide pin into the target. This tool has a larger diameter than the conventional Craig needle biopsy and a knob to attach a torque device that will facilitate manual introduction of the biopsy tool. The larger lumen allows passage of various instruments through the biopsy tool. It is important that the surgeon remove simultaneously the Steinmann pin and the biopsy tool. This method allows the successful removal of a core of bone or pathological tissue, because the specimen is impacted between the guide pin and the bone biopsy instrument *(12,40)* (Fig. 3).

We have demonstrated in the laboratory and in the clinical setting that retrieval of osteopenic bone and pathological soft tissue is enhanced as tissue is impacted between the biopsy cutting core tool and the guide pin. This expedience holds securely the biopsy specimen within the cutting core tool. Sufficient space also exists for insertion of instruments at various angles and directions to increase tissue sampling and access any vertebral

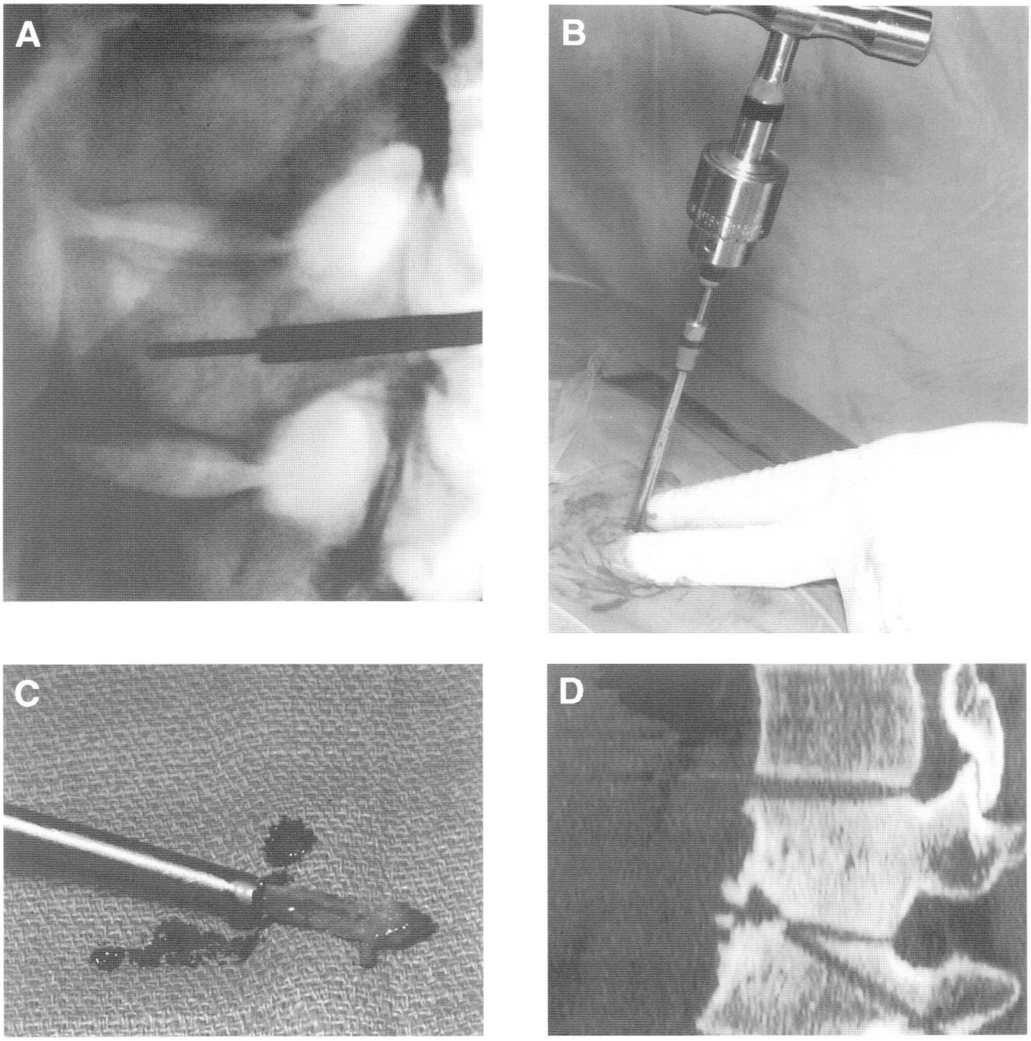

Fig. 3. Lateral radiograph demonstrating toothed biopsy cutting tool as it is inserted into vertebral body over guide pin **(A)** using a T-handle torque device **(B)**. As the cutting biopsy tool is being inserted, tissue is impacted between the guide pin and the biopsy tool and held firmly inside the tool. This expedience facilitates retrieval of tissue **(C,D)**. (Partially reproduced with permission from ref. *40*.)

body lesion. The integrity of the inferior and the medial cortical walls of the pedicle must be preserved in order to prevent any spread of hematoma, infection, or tumor inside the spinal canal. Additional tissue can be retrieved using curettes or biopsy forceps through the cannulated sleeve after removal of the guide pin (Fig. 4). The cannulated sleeve also facilitates insertion of hemostatic agents such as Surgicel (Johnson & Johnson Medical) or methylmethacrylate bone cement. The use of bone wax for hemostasis is not recommended because it does not pack well within the pedicle via the cannulated sleeve. Drains for 24 h are used only in cases of infection or benign conditions. If a drain is inserted, the patient must return on the first postoperative day for removal of the drain. We do not advocate drainage in the presence of malignancy.

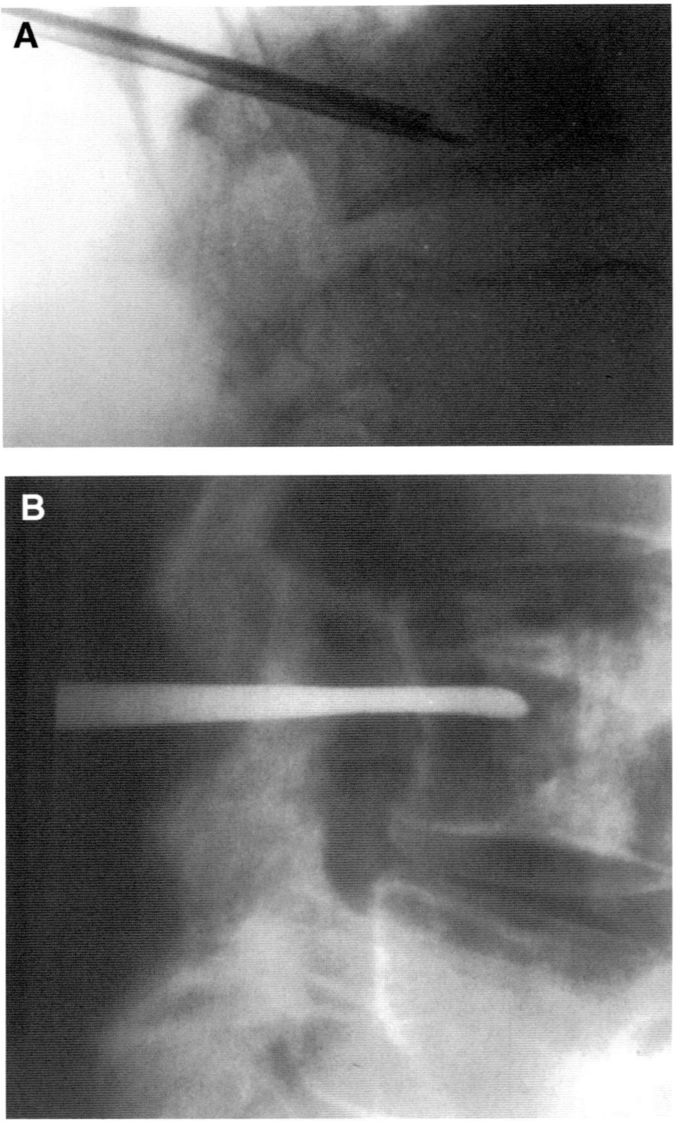

Fig. 4. The biopsy tool can be repositioned in different directions. **(A)** Further biopsy specimens can be removed by means of **(B)** curettage or **(C,D)** biopsy forceps.

Discussion

As graphed by Misenhimer et al. *(17)*, average cancellous pedicle width (transverse inside diameter) from T1 to L5, measured by sounding, ranges from slightly more than 1 mm at T4 to slightly less than 6 mm at L5. Because a biopsy needle that will retrieve a tissue core diameter larger than 2 mm has an outside diameter of nearly 3 mm, adequate space exists in most pedicles for transpedicular retrieval of substantial tissue specimen.

A transverse inner pedicle diameter that measures <3 mm is not a contraindication for percutaneous TPB. According to Zindrick et al. *(21)*, the average transverse outside

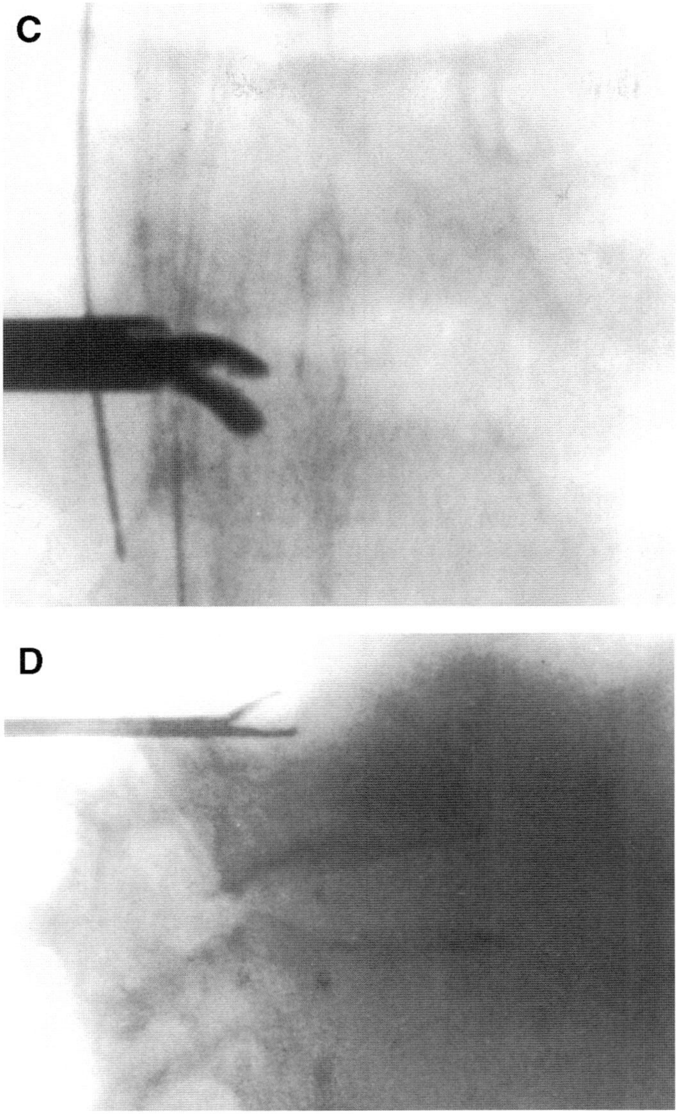

Fig. 4. *(Continued)*

diameters of the pedicular isthmus in the fifth thoracic vertebra is 4.5 mm and in the fifth lumbar vertebra is 18 mm. The narrowest pedicle diameter is 5 mm at T5 thoracic level, and the inside pedicle diameter measures <3 mm *(45)*. Band-saw cuts through the frontal plane of the vertebral pedicle demonstrated that this is neither circular nor elliptic but egg shaped, with the narrow end superior and the wider end inferior. Furthermore, we have confirmed that the pedicle is mostly cancellous bone with a thin shell of cortical bone *(12)*. Finally, the nerve root courses medial to the medial wall of the pedicle and inferior to the inferior wall of the pedicle, whereas the dural sacs lie immediately adjacent to the medial wall of the pedicle. Percutaneous TPB can safely be performed by cutting through the lateral wall extrapedicularly and avoiding

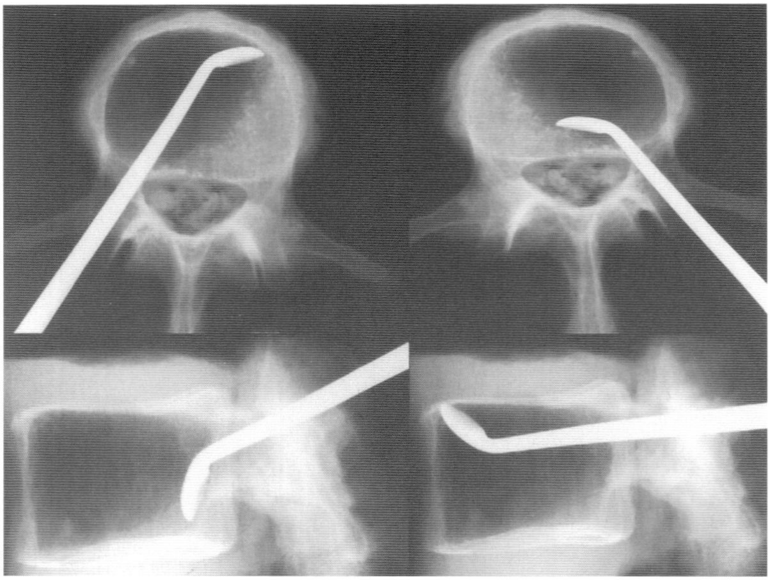

Fig. 5. In the laboratory, we have shown that through pedicular channels, bone can be retrieved from any region of the vertebral body. (Partially reproduced with permission from ref. *12*.)

violation of the medial pedicular wall. Inserting bone biopsy instruments through this area is minimally problematic. Caution should be taken not to violate the foramen, which provides nutrient vessels to vital nerve tissue structures.

Not only will the pedicle accommodate a variety of biopsy instruments, but the pedicle also will provide access to any vertebral body lesion. In our laboratory study, we have shown that instruments passed through one vertebral pedicle can access more than 50% of the volume of the vertebral body, including tissue directly anterior to the spinal canal (Fig. 5). Furthermore, this volume is accessible without performing a laminectomy, facetectomy, or pediculectomy, as described by others *(46)*. Additional tissue can be obtained by performing multiple passes at various angles. Greater latitude for angling instruments exists in the sagittal plane than in the axial plane, because sagittal pedicle diameter is greater than transverse diameter. The volume of tissue retrievable through the pedicle supports use of the percutaneous transpedicular technique for routine biopsy of vertebral body lesions. In cadaveric specimens, an experimental study showed that a 2-mm trephine does not obtain suitable bone core for histological examination, whereas the amount of samples obtained with a 3.5-mm trephine is adequate for histopathological examination *(47)*.

Fidler and Niers *(37)* recommended an open transpedicular approach over a percutaneous procedure. They claim that the open approach facilitates block excision of tissue and prevents dissection of hematoma and damage to the pedicular wall. Violation of the pedicular wall may potentially contaminate the epidural space or the paravertebral structures. However, using the percutaneous technique as we have described, these potential complications can be avoided and the patient can be spared the morbidity and cost associated with an open surgical procedure *(12)*.

Renfrew et al. *(48)* recommended CT-guided percutaneous TPB of the spine. This was based on the fact that the proximity of neural elements to the pedicle makes transpedicular biopsy under fluoroscopy a hazardous procedure. However, high-resolution image intensifiers display sufficient details of vertebral elements so as to allow protection of the medial and inferior walls of the pedicle during biopsy, thus avoiding injury to the neural elements. In our series, there were no advantages of CT guidance over image intensification *(12)*. Cost-effectiveness is an advantage of image intensification over CT. Moreover, in the presence of spinal deformities, image intensification is easier to maneuver.

Negative results can be encountered as a consequence of technical errors. We believe that pitfalls owing to faulty biopsy instrumentation retrieval techniques can be avoided.

Failures can be encountered when the guide pin technique is not used while retrieving the biopsy tool (Fig. 6). We encountered no diagnostic problems with crush artifact despite crowding the biopsy tool with a guide pin. Impaction of tissue between the needle and guide pin facilitates tissue retrieval in osteopenic bone and friable soft-tissue lesions. Another pitfall can be encountered when the pedicle is sclerotic and the lesion in the vertebral body is lytic. In this situation, dense bone from the pedicle is packed into the biopsy cannulated instrument and clogs the cutting tool, which makes almost impossible any further retrieval of pathological soft tissue from the vertebral body. This problem prompted us to modify the technique by removing vertebral tissue in sequence. The surgeon first creates an empty tunnel in the pedicle by removing a core of bone. Then the surgeon reinserts the empty biopsy tool through the empty pedicle into the pathological friable tissue, and, thus, the tool can retrieve a specimen for biopsy unimpeded (Fig. 7).

The reported complications of this procedure were minor and the incidence ranged from 0 to 5.6% *(40,42,49–53)*. In our series *(40)*, we had one technical complication—a retained piece of drainage tube in the pedicle—which was easily retrieved via the percutaneous transpedicular tract, previously created, using a biopsy forceps under local anesthesia. Serious bleeding, which can be encountered in hypervascular tumors, is easily manageable by plugging the pedicle with either methylmethacrylate bone cement or Surgicel *(40)*. To avoid spillage of malignant tumor tissues into the surrounding area, we also advocate the use of methylmethacrylate cement to plug the pedicular entrance (Fig. 8). In cases of infection, drainage for suction irrigation can be left *in situ*. The reported diagnostic accuracy of PTB ranges from 89 to 99% *(40,49,51–55)*. In our series of 86 procedures, the diagnostic accuracy was 95%. All diagnostic failures (four cases) occurred in the first 54 patients of our series *(40)*. In the subsequent patients, our success rate was 100% *(42)*. When technical pitfalls are avoided, the diagnostic success rate of TPB is equivalent to that of open biopsy techniques and with significantly less morbidity (Figs. 9–18).

In conclusion, we recommend the percutaneous TPB technique over open biopsy or closed posterolateral biopsy for its safety, minimal morbidity, simplicity, diagnostic accuracy, and cost-effectiveness. The caliber of the pedicle accommodates biopsy instruments that are able to access any vertebral body lesion and retrieve sufficient tissue for diagnosis. In addition, the use of local anesthesia provides a reliable monitor of nerve root function. Bleeding is also easily controlled. Furthermore, the technique can extend to the upper thoracic levels including the C7 vertebra, provided a high-resolution image intensifier is available.

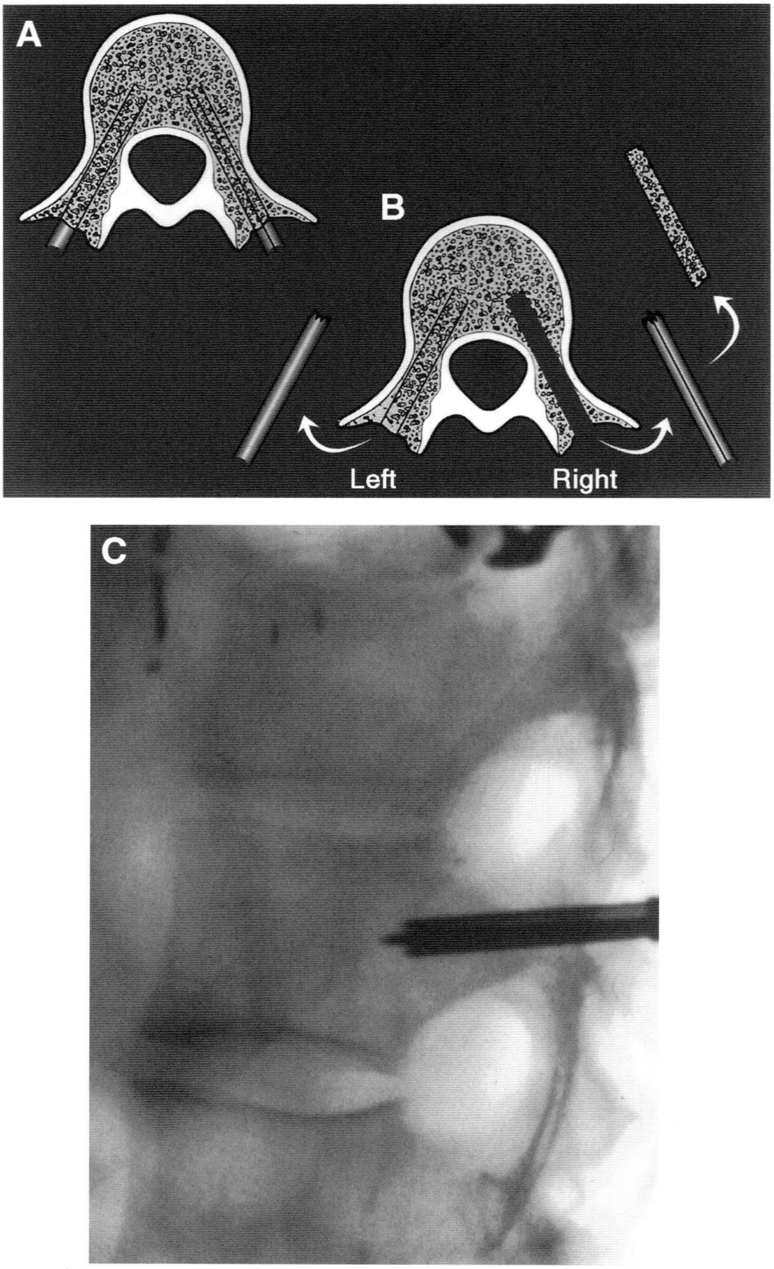

Fig. 6. (A,B) This drawing demonstrates that removal of biopsy specimens through the right pedicle is greatly facilitated by removing the guide pin of the biopsy cutting tool and the guide pin simultaneously. **(B,** right) Tissue is packed between the biopsy cutting tool and the guide pin. Using this technique, we have never failed to retrieve vertebral tissue, neither in the laboratory nor in the clinical setting **(C)**. However, if the guide pin technique is not used, the core, cut by the biopsy tool, might not remain inside the biopsy instrument (especially if the tissue is osteopenic or friable) when the instrumentation is removed (see left pedicle). (Partially reproduced with permission from ref. *40*.)

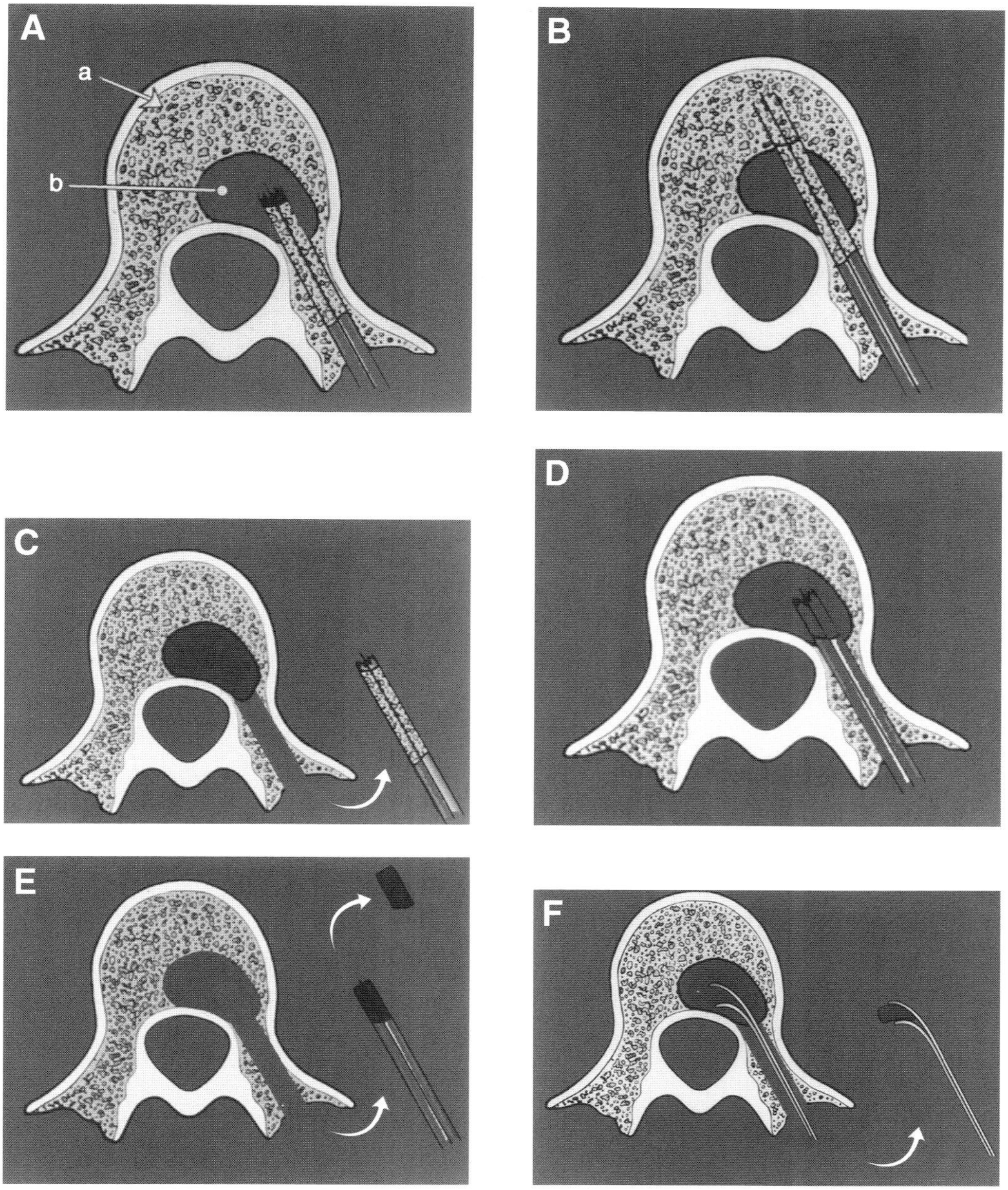

Fig. 7. **(A)** Bone from the pedicle can clog the tip of the biopsy cutting tool and, thus, may not allow friable tissue from a lytic lesion (b) to enter the biopsy tool. **(B)** Further insertion of the biopsy cutting tool may even crush a soft-tissue lesion against hard bone. **(C)** First a core of bone is removed from the pedicle. **(D)** Then the empty biopsy cutting tool should be reinserted through the open pedicular channel, to retrieve soft tissue unimpeded **(E)**. **(F)** Further specimens of friable soft tissue can be removed by mean of biceps forceps. (Modified with permission from ref. *40*.)

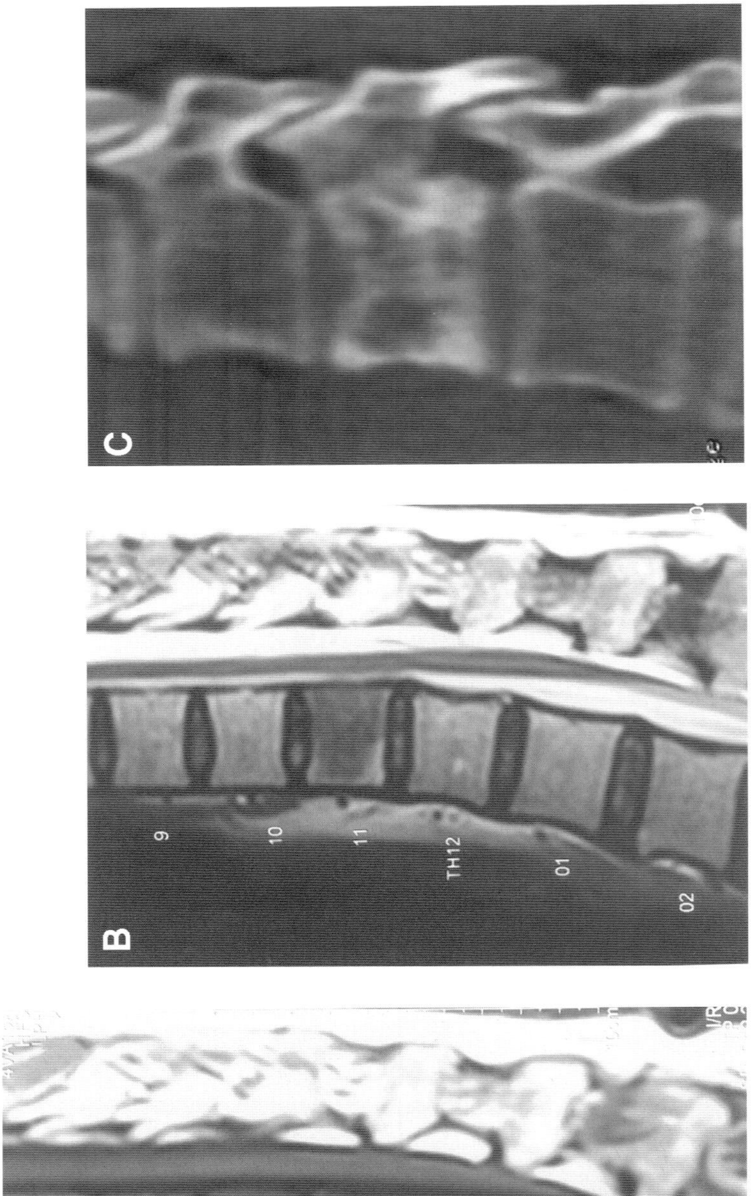
A
B
9
10
11
TH12
01
02
C

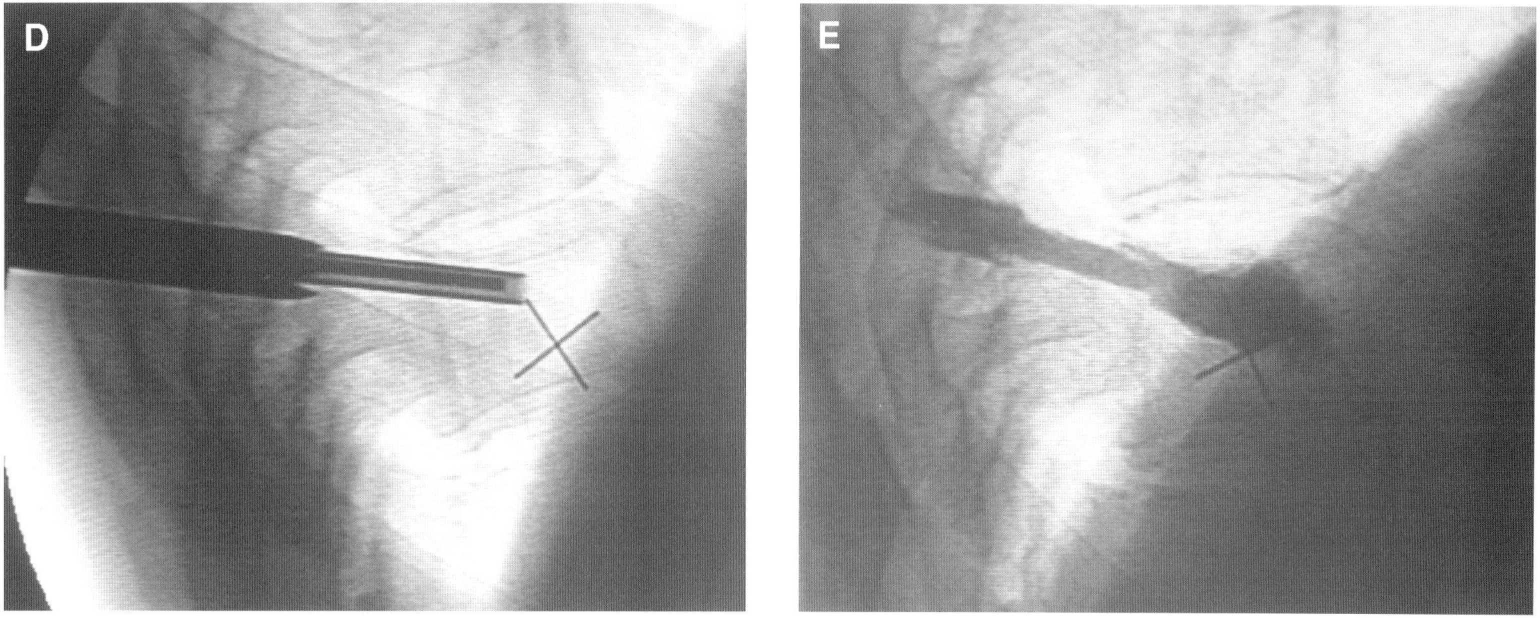

Fig. 8. **(A)** T1 A-weighted image shows a low signal intensity, and **(B)** T2-weighted image shows a high signal intensity of a metastatic mixed lesion as seen on CT scan (lateral reformat). **(D,E)** After transpedicular biopsy, some bleeding was encountered, and this was controlled by inserting PMMA bone cement into the lytic component of the tumor and the pedicle. Postoperatively the patient was pain free.

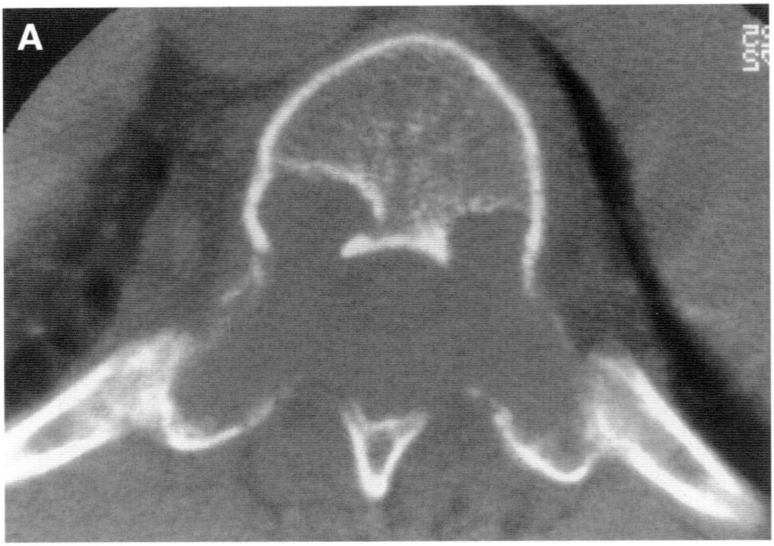

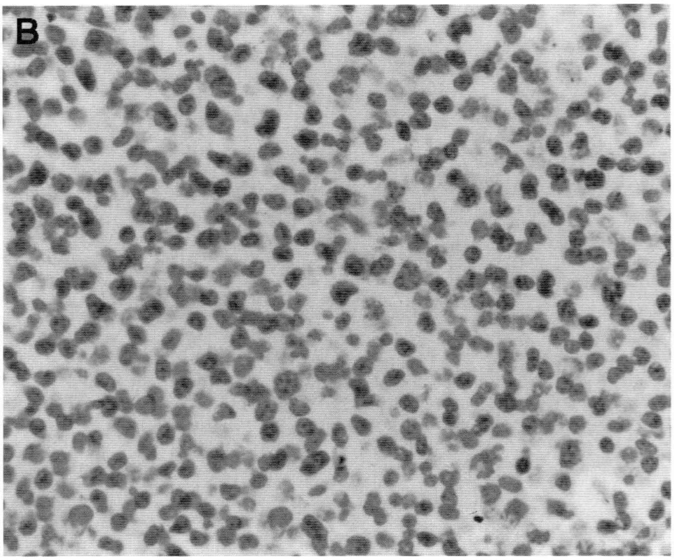

Fig. 9. An axial CT scan of the T12 vertebra shows that it is affected with **(A)** solitary myeloma and **(B)** its histology. A lateral radiograph demonstrates **(C)** pathological fracture of L3 vertebra and **(D)** biopsy-revealed lymphoma.

MANAGEMENT OF PYOGENIC SPONDYLODISCITIS

Historical Review and Rationale for the Procedure

Because MRI has shown that the pathological lesion involves the disc and the two adjacent vertebral bodies *(56)*, the term *spondylodiscitis* is preferred. The natural history of uncomplicated spondylodiscitis is self-limiting healing. However, a variable degree of bone destruction frequently takes place during the infectious process *(57)*. Depending on the degree of bone destruction, it is not uncommon for the spine to heal

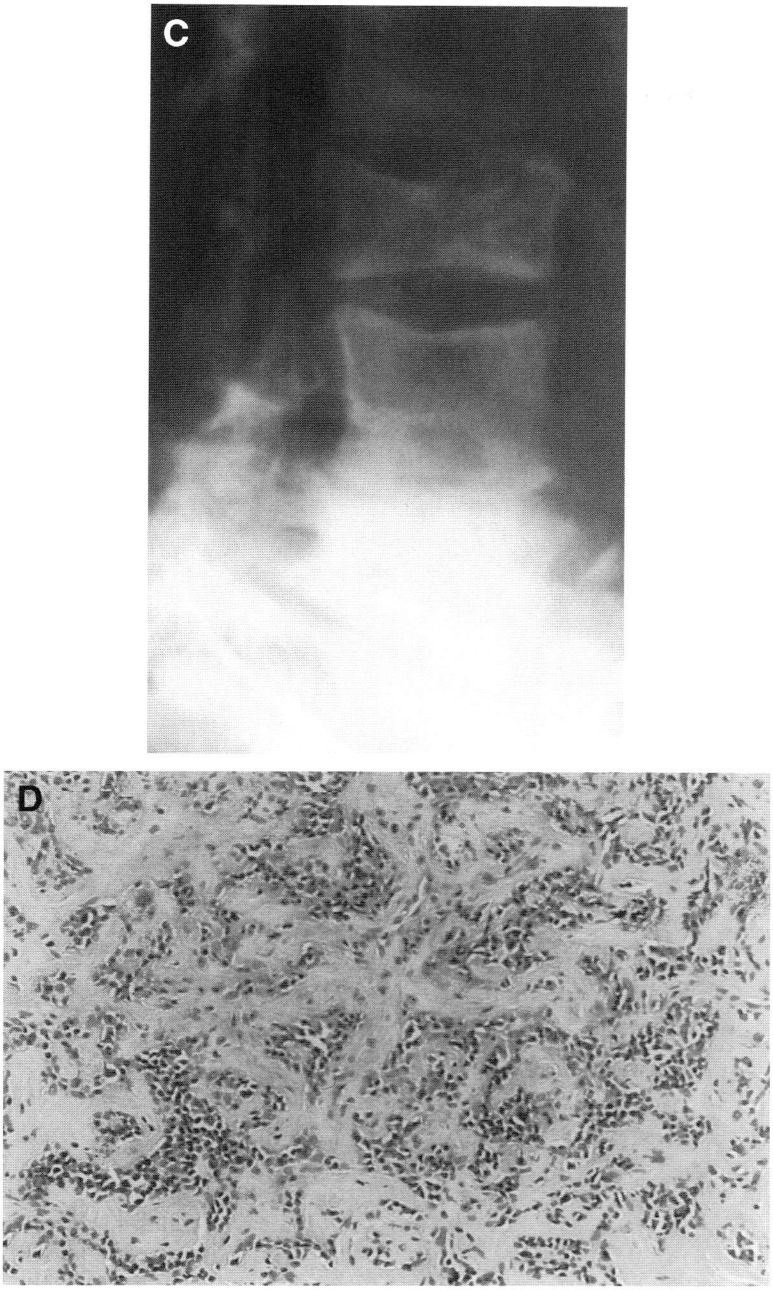

Fig. 9. *(Continued)*

in a kyphotic deformity, which, in turn, may predispose to mechanical low-back pain *(58)*. Reports have indicated that mechanical low-back pain is frequently associated with conservative treatment of vertebral osteomyelitis *(59)*. Early diagnosis is crucial for management of this condition *(60–62)*, because delayed treatment also may result in serious neurological complications *(63)*.

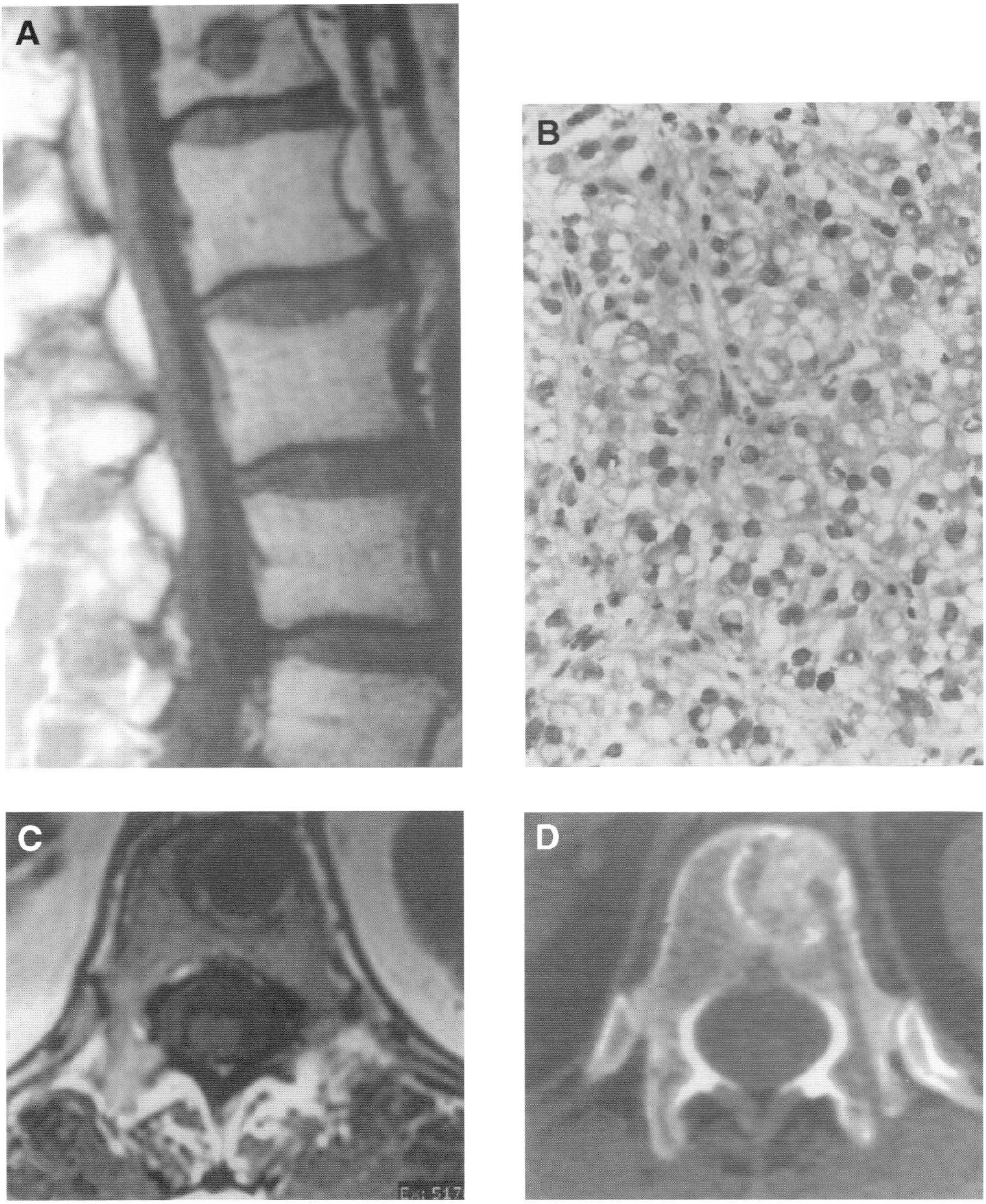

Fig. 10. **(A)** T1 A-weighted magnetic resonance imaging (MRI) image of a lytic lesion is shown. **(B)** TPB revealed renal cell carcinoma. **(C)** An axial T1-weighted MRI image of a blastic lesion is shown. **(D)** An axial CT scan shows the removed biopsy core. **(E)** Histological examination revealed osteoblastoma.

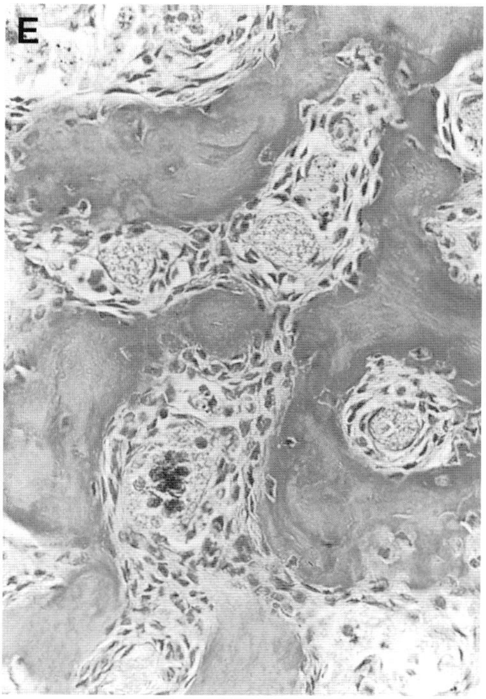

Fig. 10. *(Continued)*

The treatment of joint infections typically includes surgical debridement, irrigation, and prolonged antibiotic therapy *(64–69)*. Gradually, the percutaneous arthroscopic approach has superseded open arthrotomy *(70,71)*. A similar concept has been applied successfully to the treatment of pyogenic spondylodiscitis. Percutaneous discectomy, by means of a nucleotome, can evacuate infected disc material as an alternative to open surgery *(72–74)*. However, reports are scanty and only two or three patients are referred to in each report.

Fraser et al. *(75)* showed experimentally that during the natural course of discitis, granulation tissue from the subchondral bone would invade the intervertebral disc, resorb the disc space, and heal the infection. Intradiscal invasion of vascular granulation tissue was present in our histopathological studies *(76)*. Successful treatment of discitis entails spontaneous fusion. However, the spine very often may either fail to fuse, developing pseudoarthrosis, or fail to heal in good alignment, resulting in kyphotic deformity. Both conditions may predispose to chronic low-back pain. Spontaneous interbody fibrous or bony fusion occurs in 6–24 mo *(77,78)*. However, according to Frederickson et al. *(79)*, spontaneous ankylosis occurs in only 35% of patients. Therefore, it seems reasonable to assume that any medical manipulation that accelerates the natural healing process may prevent these complications *(38,41)*. Although the published data are not from prospective randomized studies, there is good evidence in the studies to support this concept. Transpedicular drainage of Pot's abscess, as an adjunct to posterior stabilization, was performed successfully to speed up the process of healing *(80)*.

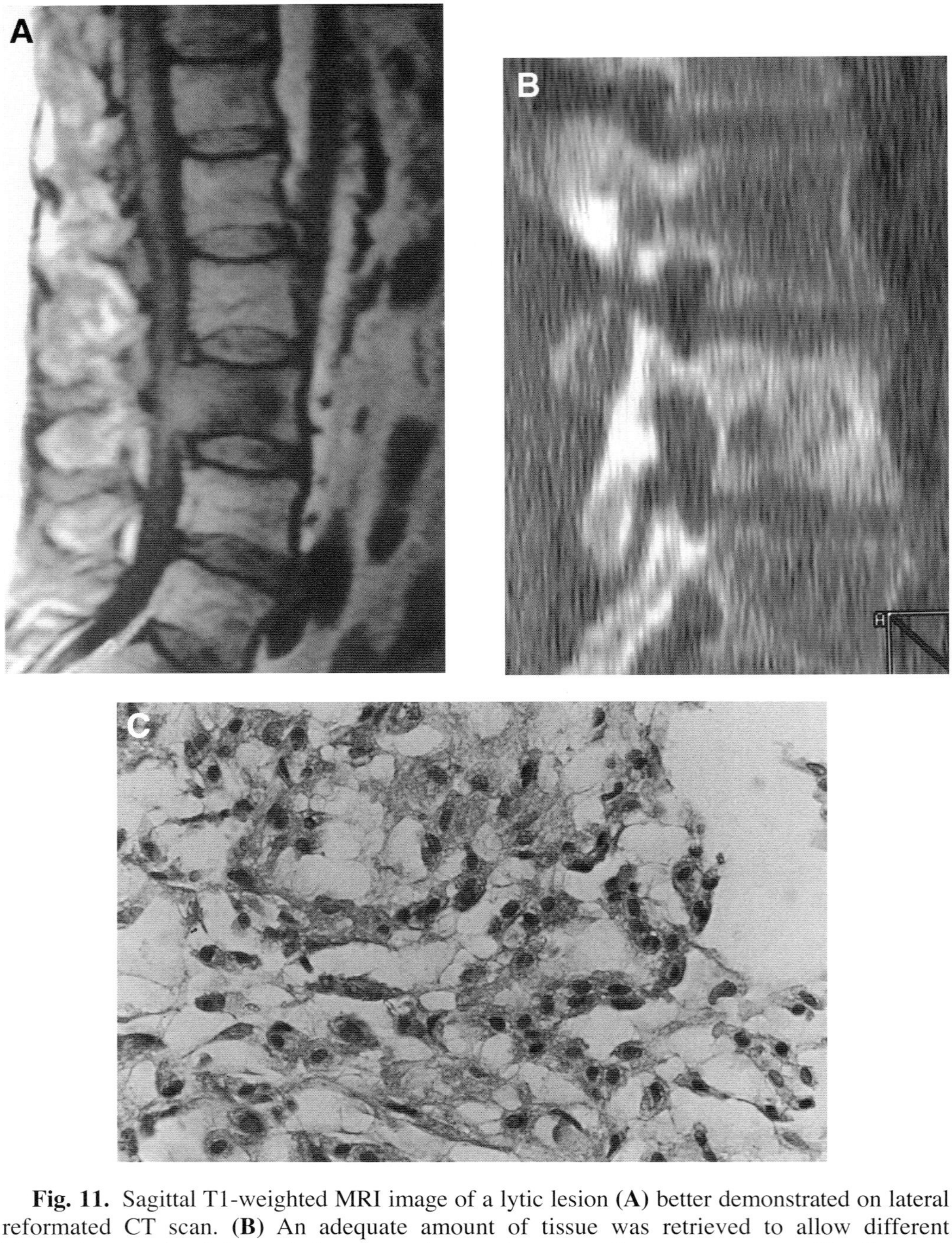

Fig. 11. Sagittal T1-weighted MRI image of a lytic lesion **(A)** better demonstrated on lateral reformated CT scan. **(B)** An adequate amount of tissue was retrieved to allow different histopathological staining techniques in order to enhance the diagnostic accuracy. The diagnosis was chordoma. **(C)** Typical physalipherous cells; **(D)** cluster epithelioid cells; **(E)** S1 100 protein stain; **(F)** Vimentin stain.

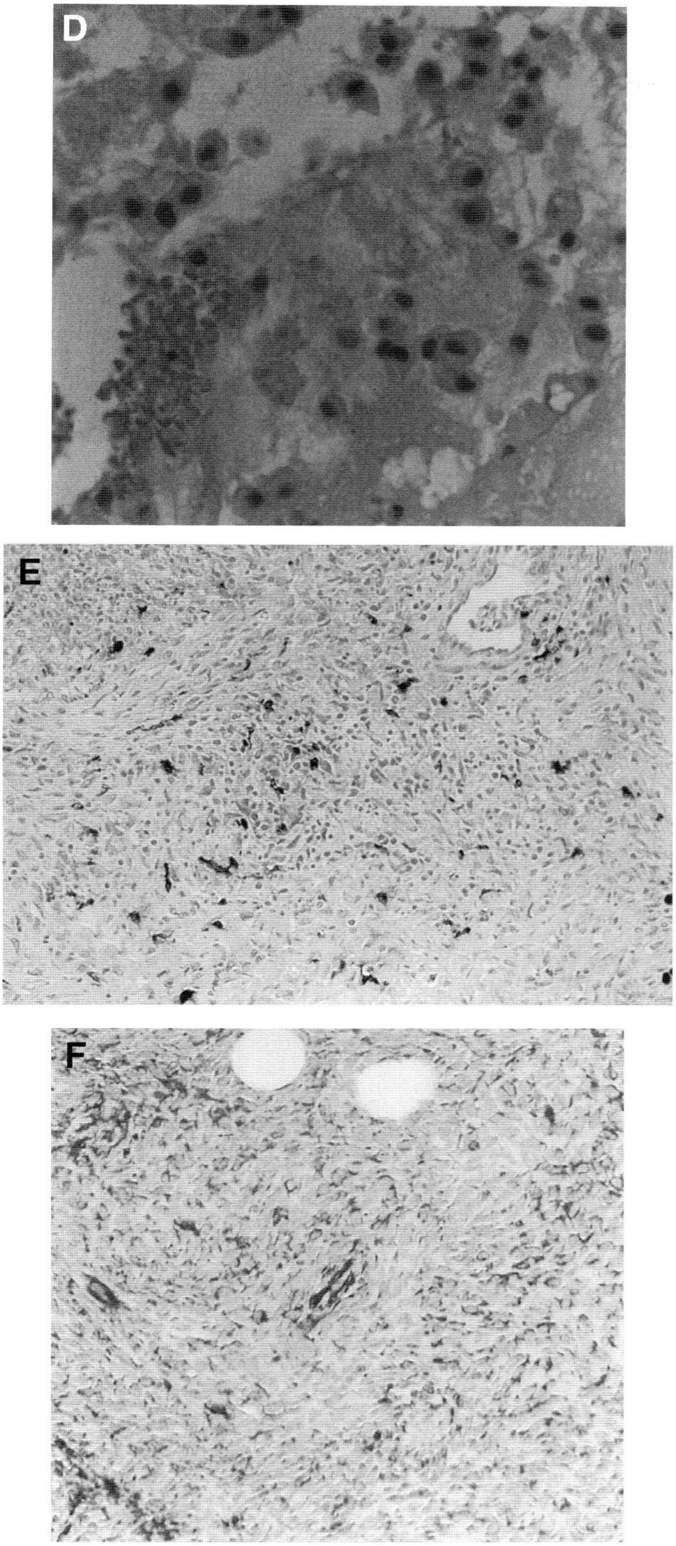

Fig. 11. *(Continued)*

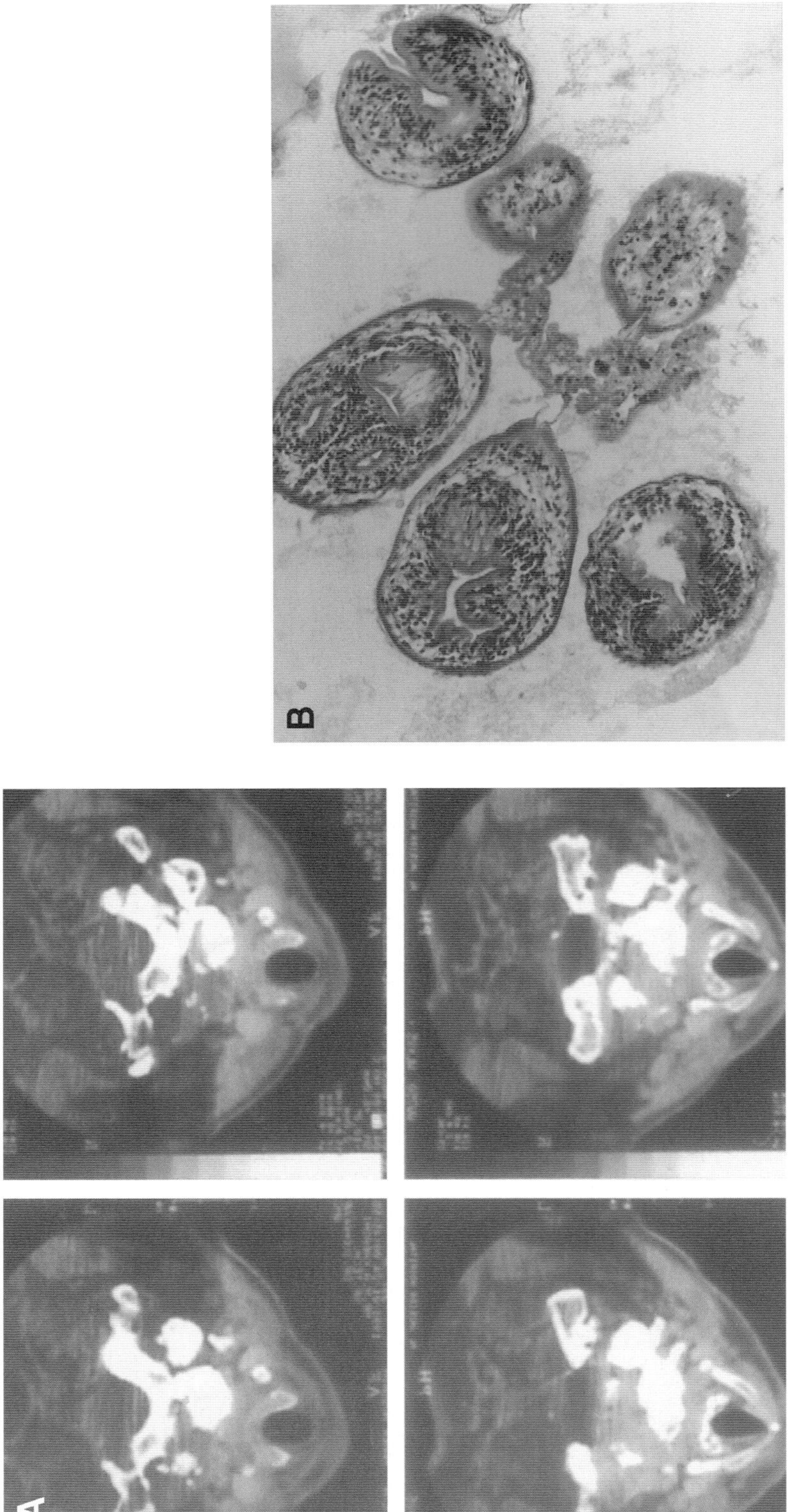
A
B

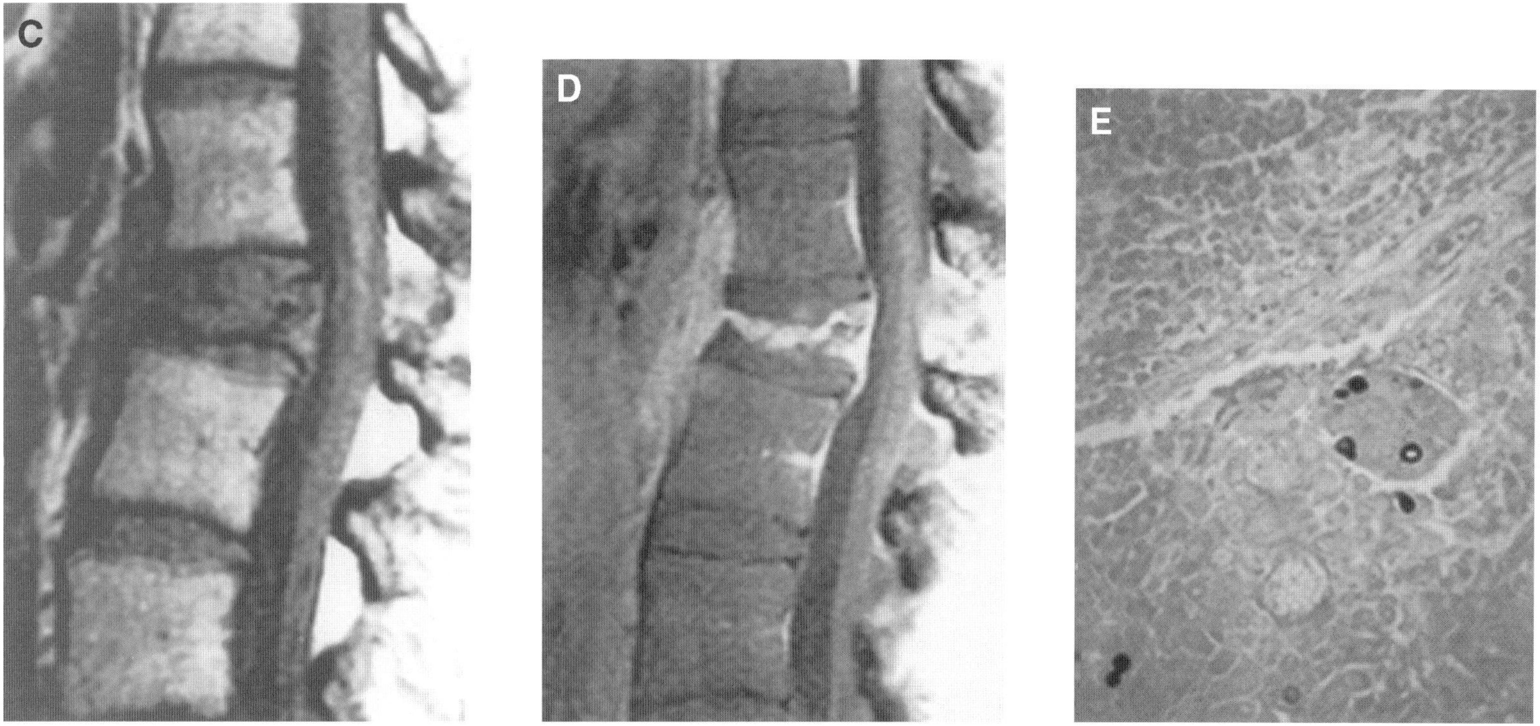

Fig. 12. Hydatid disease as seen on **(A)** axial CT scan and **(B)** its histology. T1- and T2-weighted MRI images demonstrating spondylodiscitis **(C, D)** caused by blastomycosis as seen on histology **(E)**.

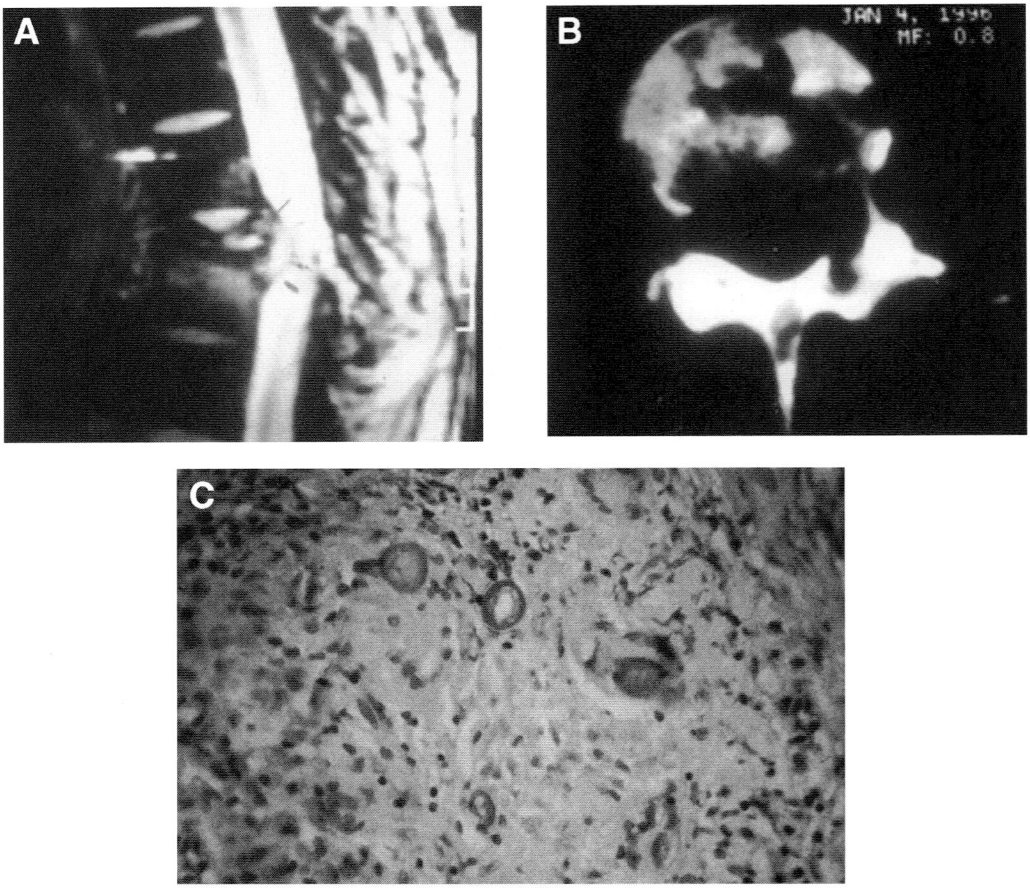

Fig. 13. **(A)** T2-weighted MRI image and **(B)** axial CT scan showing an osteolytic lesion of a thoracic vertebral body. **(C)** TPB revealed coccidiomycosis.

The objective of transpedicular discectomy is to accelerate the natural course of healing by evacuating the bulk of the offending infected disc and, conceivably, by opening channels through the subchondral bone to speed the process of disc invasion by the reparative granulation tissue. For these reasons, and because we had considerable experience in using the technique of the transpedicular route for vertebral biopsies, we decided to design a transpedicular approach for discectomy in pyogenic spondylodiscitis *(41–43,81)*.

The Percutaneous Transpedicular Discectomy Technique

Local or general anesthesia is suitable for percutaneous transpedicular discectomy, depending on the severity of pain. The patient is prone, either on a fluoroscopic table in the radiology suite or on an operating table in the surgical suite, as for a TPB procedure. The target for the pin is the pedicle that is caudal to the affected disc. The tip of the guide pin should be in the center of the pedicle bull's-eye on fluoroscopic view.

Using an image intensifier, the technician obtains a lateral view to determine cephalad angulation of the Steinmann pin in the sagittal plane; this approach is necessary for

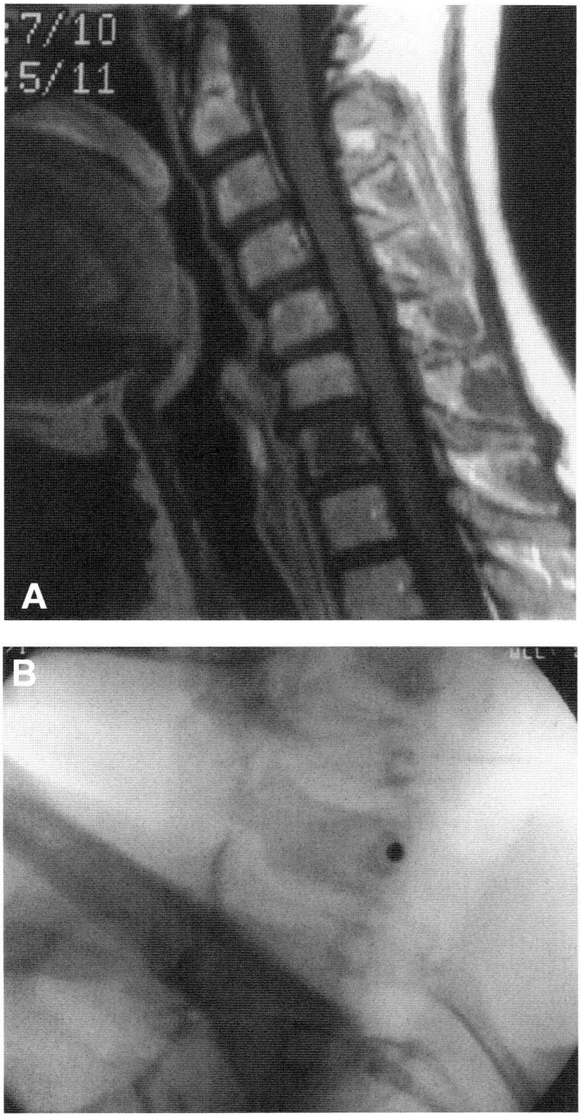

Fig. 14. (A) Sagittal T1-weighted MRI image showing a metastatic lesion. Needle biopsy failed. TPB bull's-eye **(B)** through the osteoblastic pedicle of the C7 vertebra **(C)** revealed an osteoblastic reactive bone with nidus of malignancy (a metastatic lesion from cancer of the breast [**D**]). **(E)** A CAT scan demonstrates the biopsy track. Usually needle biopsy fails in osteoblastic lesions. **(F)** An axial CT of a chondral lesion is shown. **(G)** TPB revealed chondrosarcoma.

reaching the center of the affected disc without violating the confinements of the pedicle. The physician then holds the Steinmann pin firmly in this position and gently taps it with a mallet until its tip reaches the inner annulus along the posterior portion of the disc. Under no circumstances should the pin violate the inferior border of the pedicle, because the pin can damage the exiting nerve root. Avoiding an approach through the more cephalad pedicle prevents this danger. Image intensifier views in the oblique and

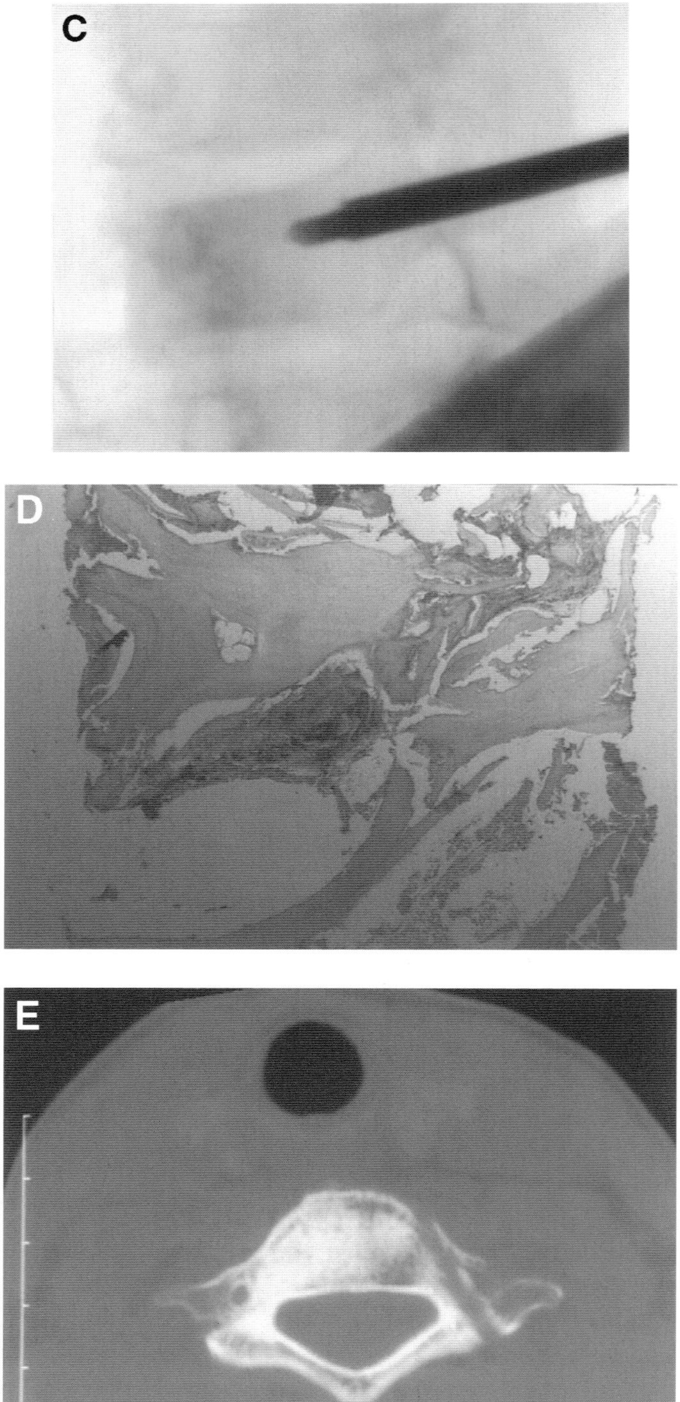

Fig. 14. *(Continued)*

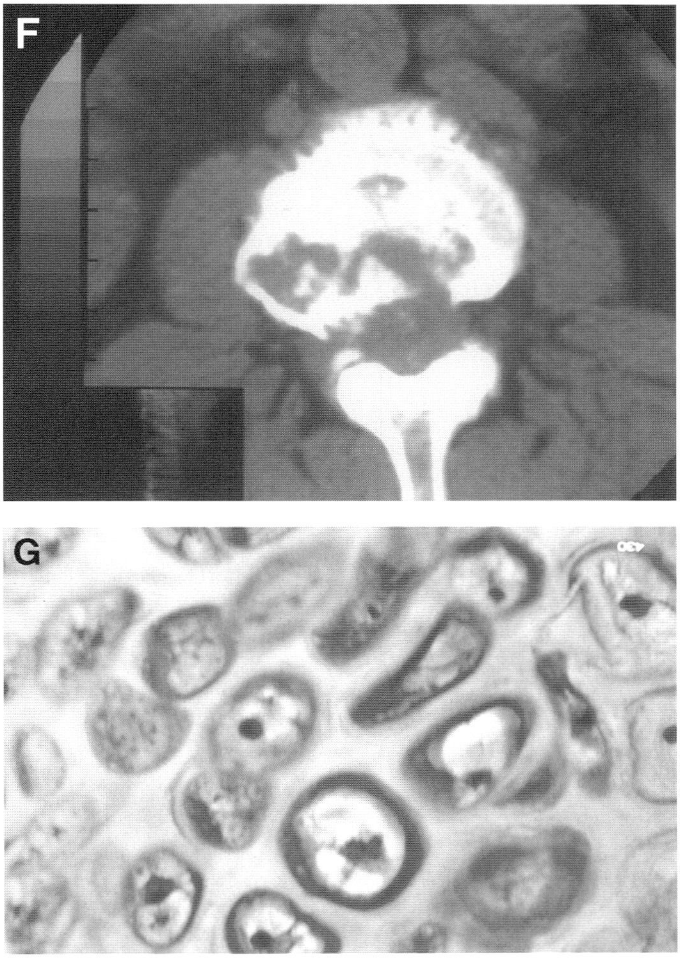

Fig. 14. *(Continued)*

lateral planes may be used to assess the progress of the pin and thus ensure the integrity of the pedicle and the track of the guide pin.

This procedure has three phases. The first phase is similar to the TBP approach. In the second phase, discectomy is performed by means of tissue forceps. A modified Kambin discectomy forceps (Smith & Nephew), which is inserted through the cannulated sleeve, allows extraction of additional tissue from the disc. These tissue samples are sent for pathohistological and bacteriological studies. Repositioning of the Steinmann pin through the pedicular tract allows direction of the biopsy instrument to a different part of the disc. By moving the biopsy forceps into these different positions, an adequate discectomy can take place in a piecemeal fashion (Fig. 19). The set is equipped with one straight and two different angled Kambin flexible discectomy forceps.

The third phase of the procedure involves suction aspiration through the use of a flexible automated nucleotome (Surgical Dynamics, Alameda, CA) (Fig. 20). The flexible automated nucleotome enters through the skin sleeve and the pedicular channel into

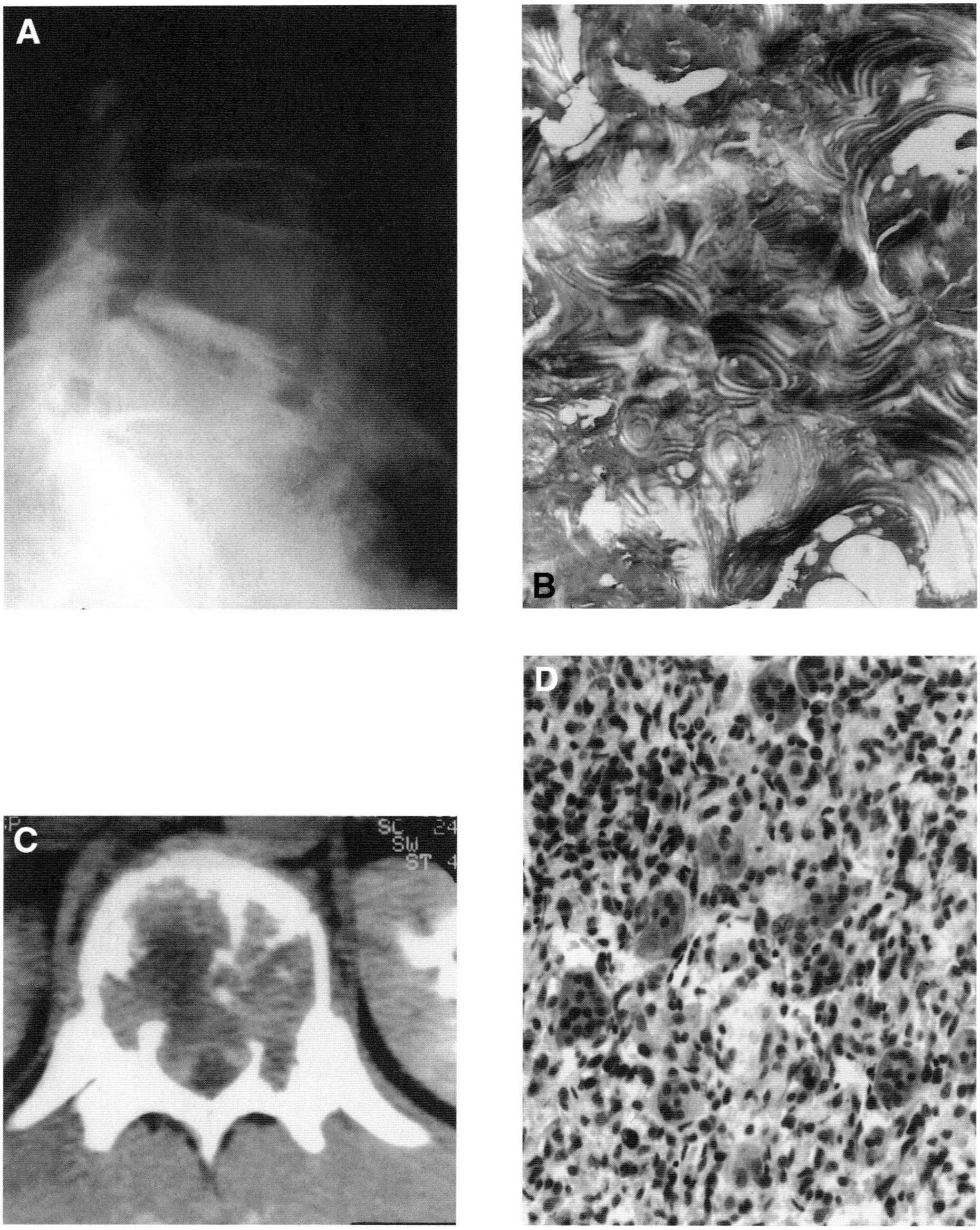

Fig. 15. **(A)** A lateral radiograph of an L5 vertebral lesion is shown. **(B)** TPB revealed Paget disease of bone. **(C)** An axial CT scan image of an osteolytic lesion is shown. **(D)** TPB revealed a giant cell tumor.

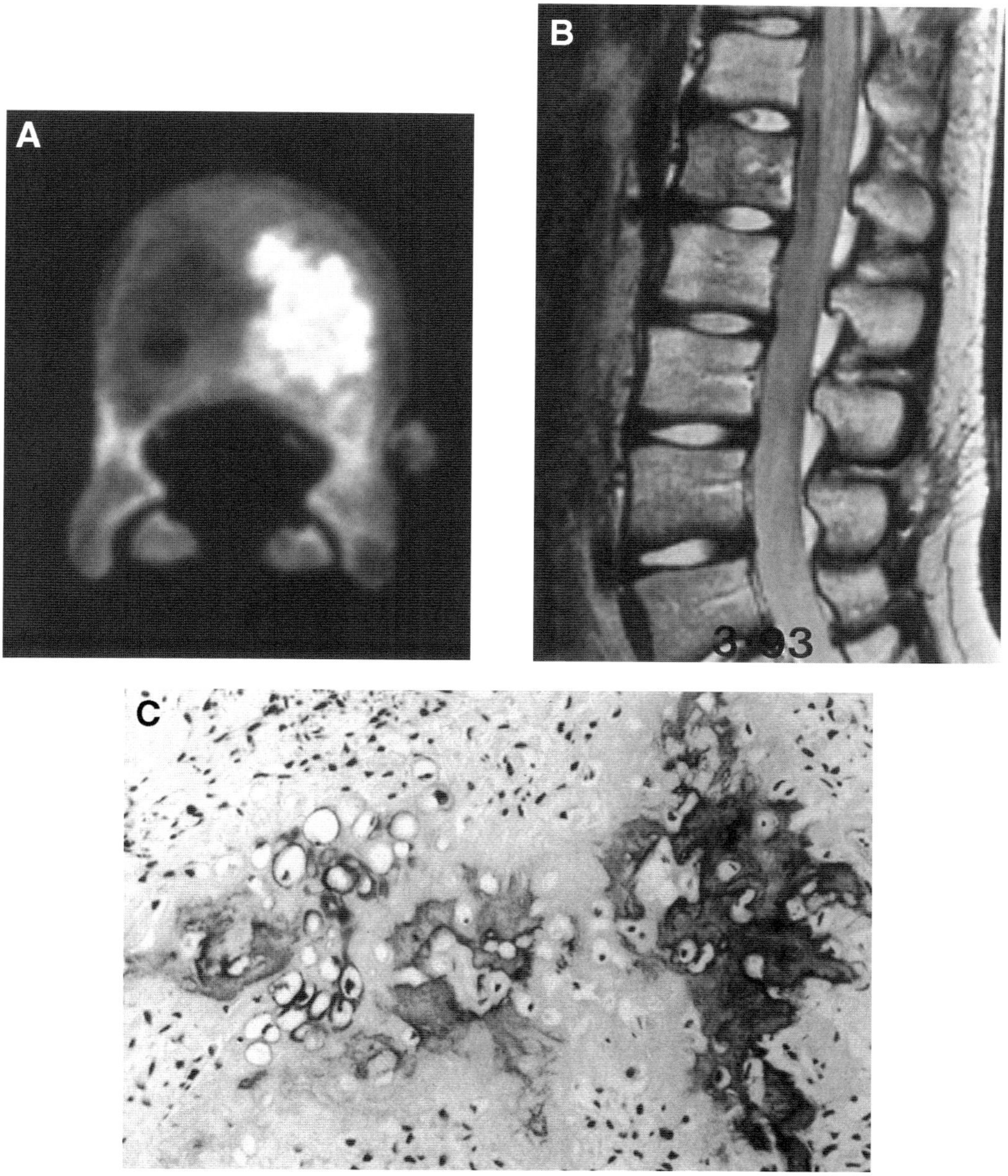

Fig. 16. **(A)** Axial CT scan image of osteoblastic lesion; **(B)** sagittal spin echo MRI. **(C)** TPB revealed osteosarcoma.

the vertebral body and disc space. The tip of the nucleotome is flexible to a maximum angulation of 90° in order to permit excision of different parts of the disc. The whole procedure is performed under fluoroscopic guidance. After completion of the discectomy, 10 French metal braided sheaths (Arrow International, Reading, PA) go through the pedicular channels into the discs for irrigation and drainage. These sheaths are attached to suction from a vacuum draining bag (Snyder Hemovac, Zimmer Patient

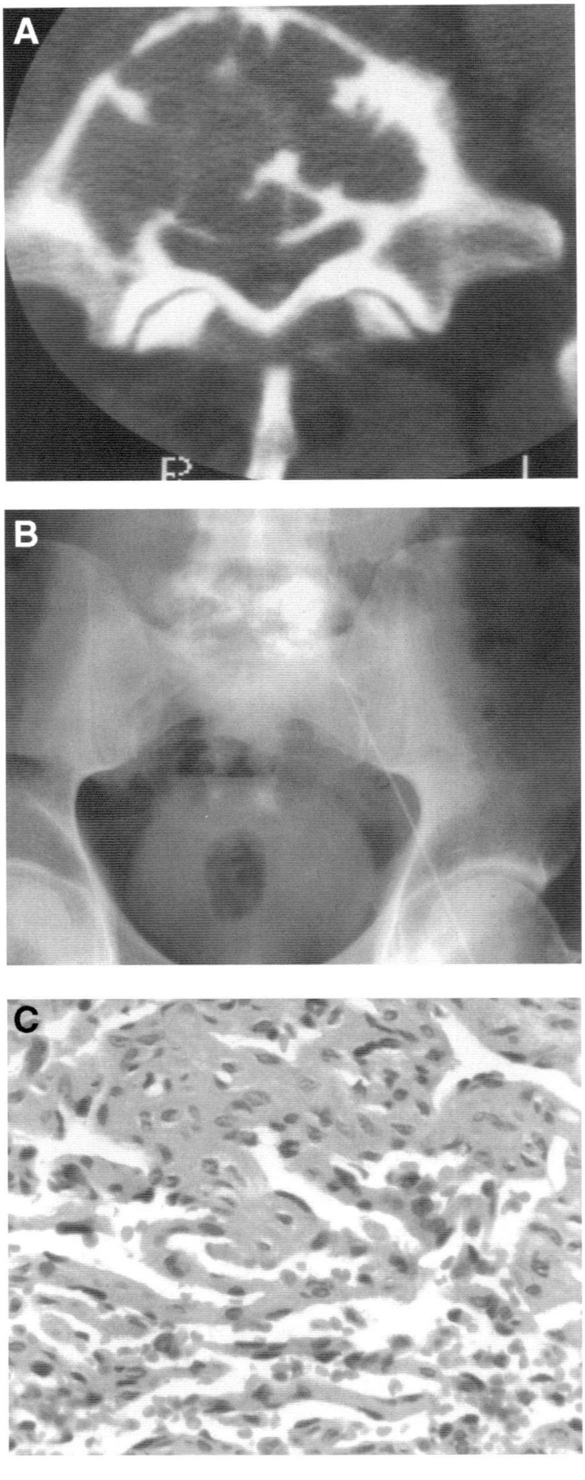

Fig. 17. Axial CT scan of (**A**) an osteolytic vascular lesion as seen on (**B**) arteriogram. (**C**) TPB revealed hemangioendotheliosarcoma.

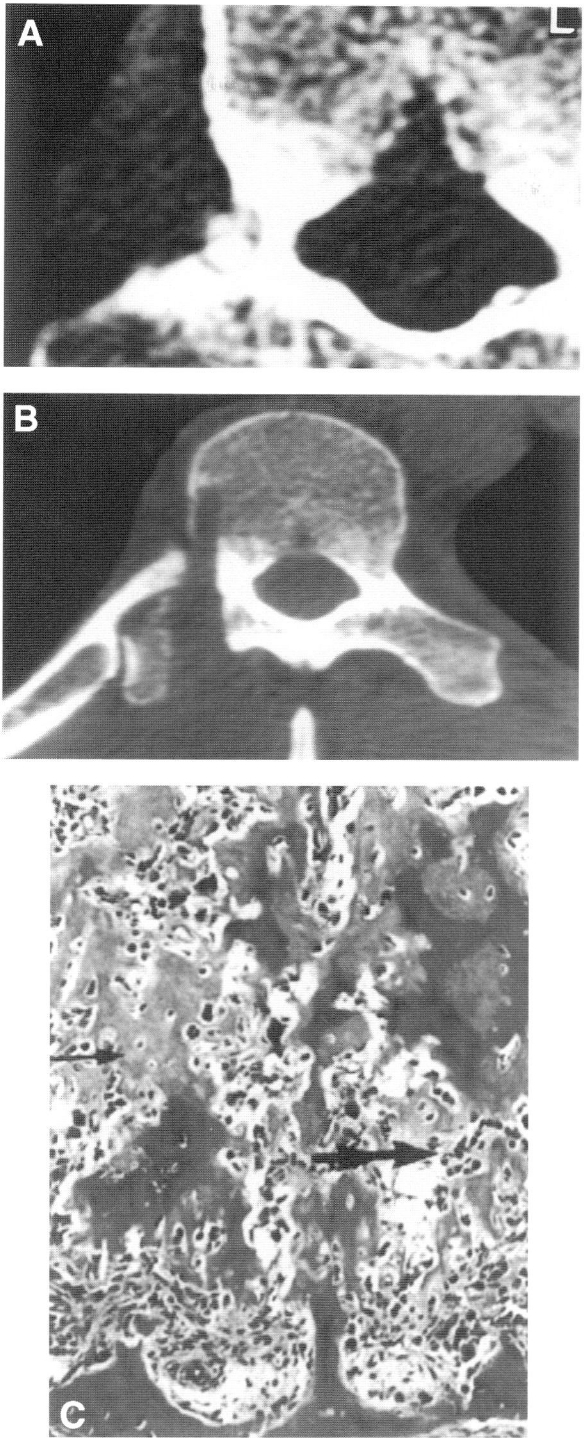

Fig. 18. (A) Axial CT scan demonstrating a painful osteoid osteoma of pedicle. TPB cored out the whole osteoid osteoma **(B)** as seen in **(C)**. This biopsy was diagnostic and therapeutic. Three years postoperatively the patient was free of pain.

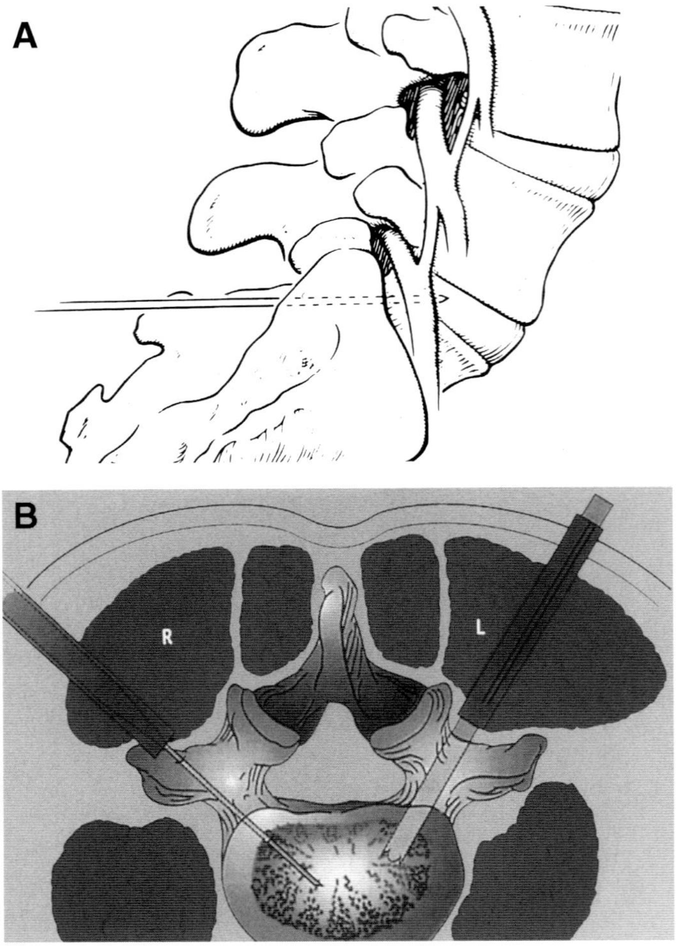

Fig. 19. **(A, B** [right]**)** Diagrammatic demonstration of a guide pin into intervertebral disc (A, lateral lumbosacral view). A 2-mm Steinmann pin is introduced percutaneously rostrally angled through the pedicle, which is caudal to the affected disc, and advanced to the disc (right side). **(B,** left**)** Axial view of diagrammatic demonstration of pin into disc, with dilator and external sleeve abutting against pedicle. The toothed biopsy cutting tool removes a core of bone from the pedicle and vertebral body to allow easy passage of the dissection forceps **(C)**. The external sleeve allows easy percutaneous passage of the discectomy instrumentation **(D)**. (Modified with permission from ref. *41*.)

Care Division, Dover, OH). Irrigation takes place by instilling a solution of 2 g of cefazolin (Ancef; Smith-Kline Beecham, Philadelphia, PA) and 10 mL of saline. Eventually, culture results will dictate the choice of antibiotics.

Discussion

Percutaneous transpedicular discectomy for spondylodiscitis is a technically safe surgical procedure and is feasible in the thoracic as well as the lumbar spine. The

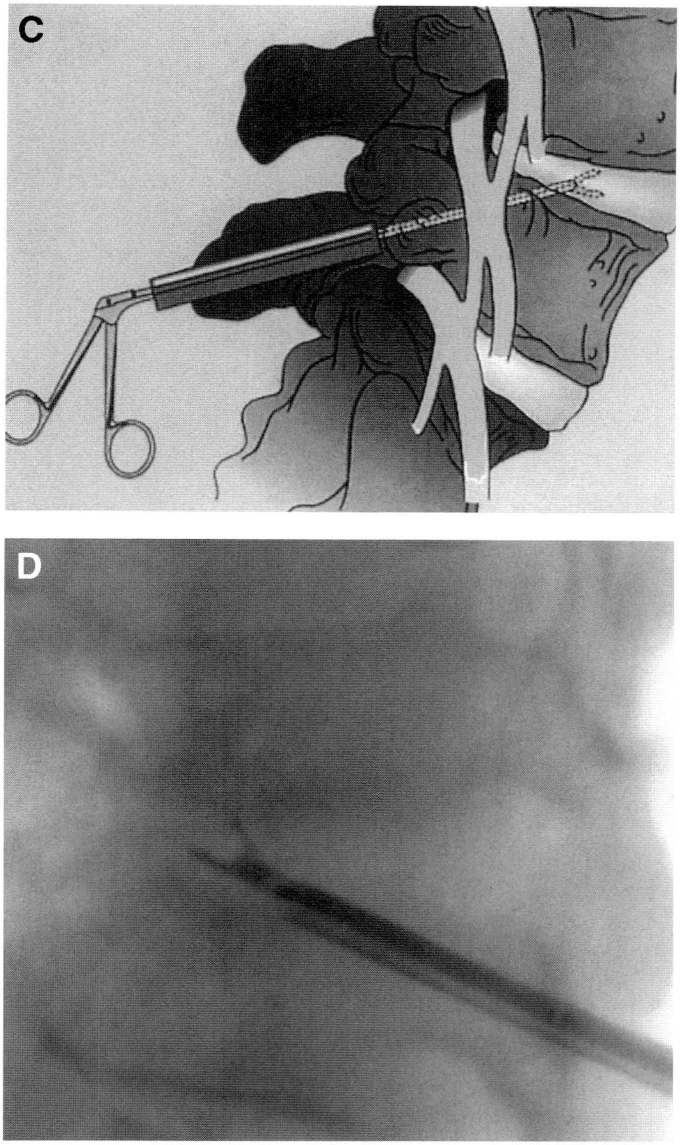

Fig. 19. *(Continued)*

transpedicular tract allows the use of relatively large instruments for aggressive decompression without concern about possible spinal cord, nerve root, or vascular injuries. Our technique advocates bilateral access with channels measuring 5.15 mm, which allow the passage of relatively large discectomy forceps and an automated nucleotome. We strongly urge that access of the intended discectomy level be from the more caudally placed adjacent pedicle. Access through a more cephalad pedicle has the potential of penetrating the inferior borders of the pedicle and damaging the exiting nerve root.

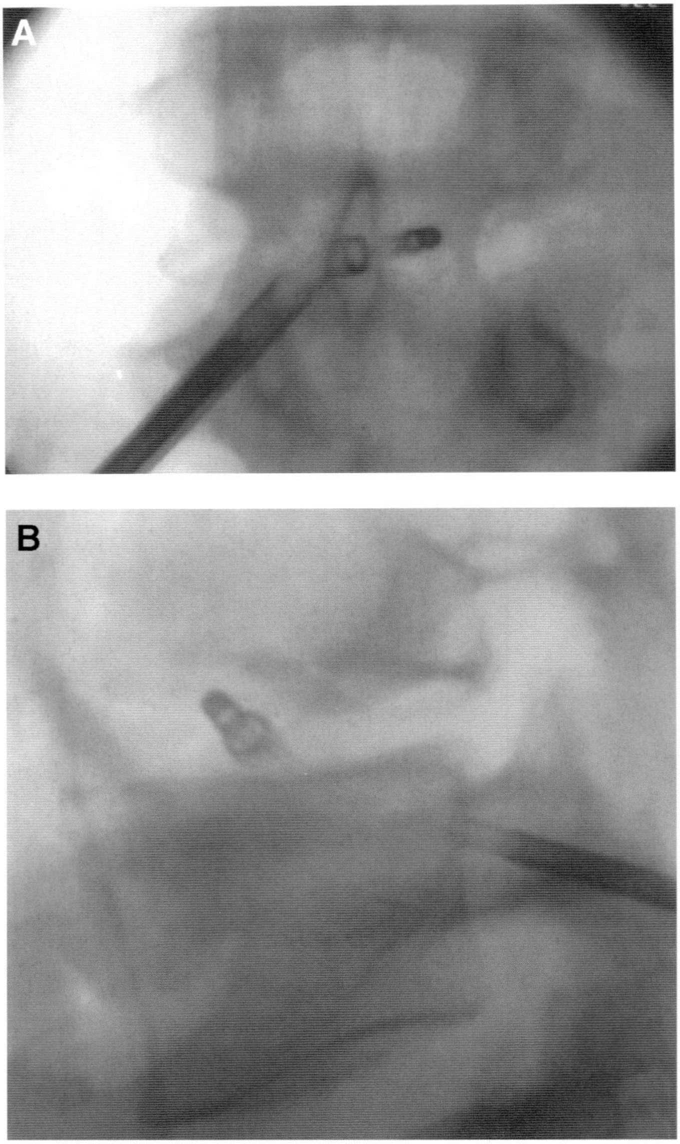

Fig. 20. (**A**) AP and (**B**) lateral radiograph demonstrating flexible nucleotome within disc space during the procedure, debulking infected disc and evacuating pus and necrotic material. (**C**) Appearance of nucleotome in action on one side and discectomy by means of Kambin discectomy forceps on right side. (**D**) Axial CT scan of vertebral body demonstrating drain tube transversing pedicle. (Partially reproduced with permission from ref. *38*.)

We also strongly recommend that the procedure take place under fluoroscopic guidance, aiming the guide pin a bull's-eye into the pedicular center or just superior to the pedicular equator. The procedure also allows the installation of Hemovac tubes (Zimmer Health Care Division, Dover, OH) for drainage and antibiotic irrigation. Although the procedure can be done safely and effectively under local anesthesia, we advocate

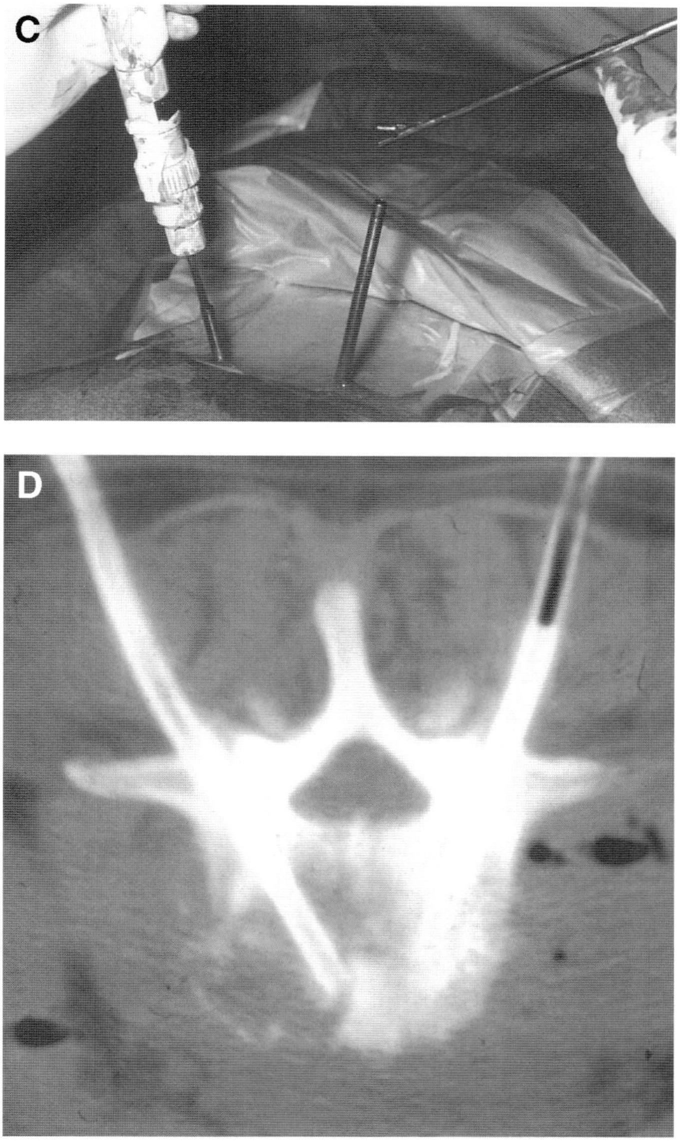

Fig. 20. *(Continued)*

general anesthesia because of severe pain in most patients with spondylodiscitis. Local anesthesia is useful in high-risk septic patients or those with other serious medical conditions. Immediate response after transpedicular discectomy is usually observed in 75% of unselected patients *(41,43,81)*. With proper indications, as we have practiced ever since the publication of the original article, we have achieved almost a 95% success rate (Figs. 21 and 22).

Percutaneous transpedicular discectomy is ineffective for the treatment of spondylodiscitis with severe neurological deficit caused by large epidural inflammatory tissue

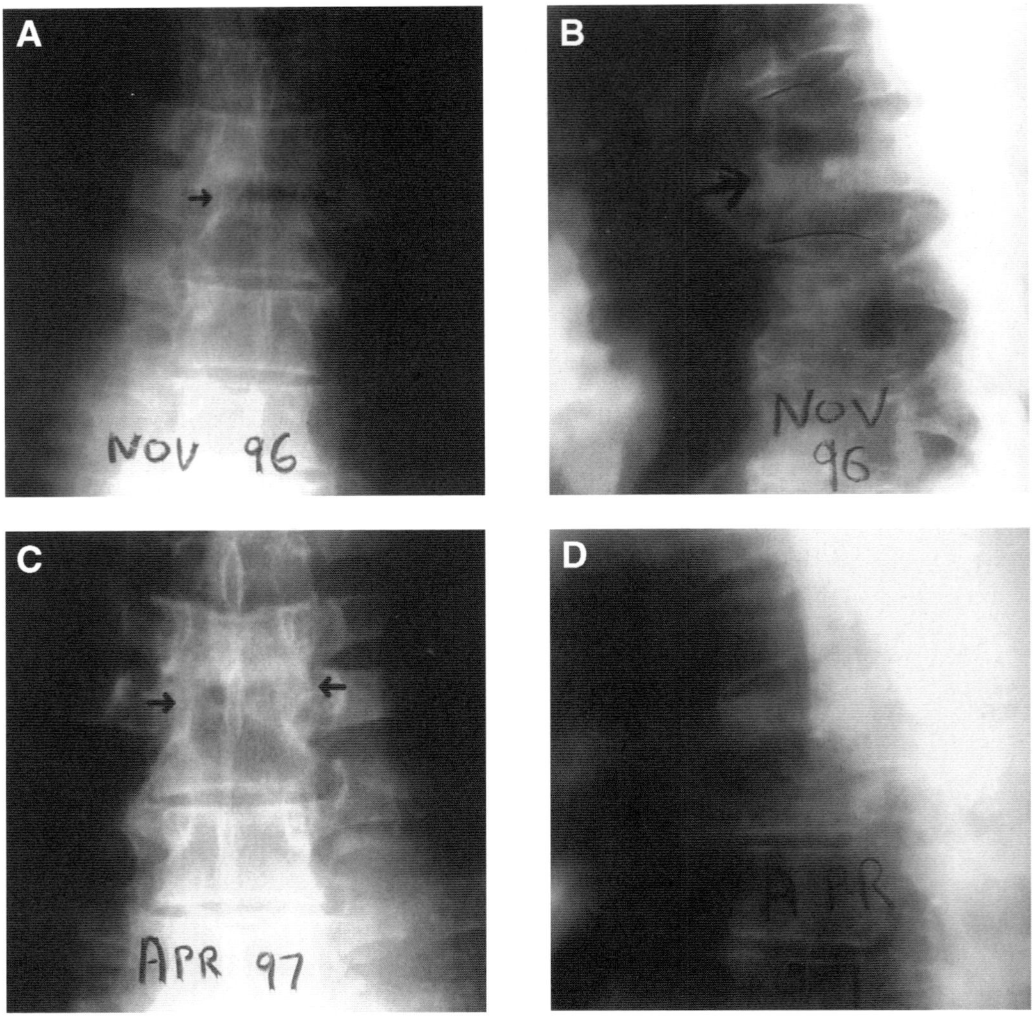

Fig. 21. (**A**) AP and (**B**) lateral view of spondylodiscitis of T4–T5 region treated by percutaneous transpedicular discectomy. (**C,D**) Five months later there was a complete bony ankylosis. (Reproduced with permission from ref. *41*.)

compressing the neural elements. Therefore, percutaneous transpedicular discectomy is contraindicated for the treatment of any spinal epidural abscess, or when there is neurocompression of the cord or the conus medullaris in the thoracic or thoracolumbar spine by inflammatory granulation tissue.

In conclusion, percutaneous transpedicular discectomy is safe and highly effective during the early stages of spondylodiscitis, when bone destruction is not extensive. It is ineffective in the presence of infected disc herniation, foraminal stenosis, and excessive bone destruction with spinal deformity. This procedure is contraindicated when there is spinal epidural abscess and neurocompression by deformity, inflammatory tissue, or a combination thereof.

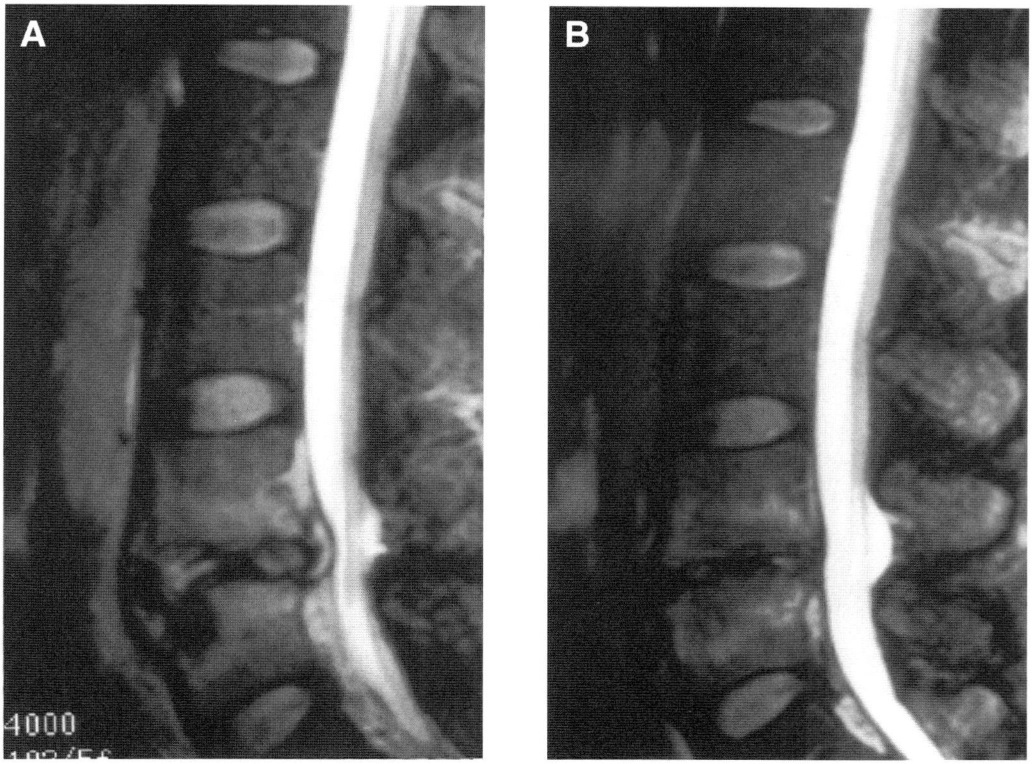

Fig. 22. **(A)** A sagittal T2-weighted MRI image of the lumbar spine in a 38-yr-old woman demonstrates changes typical of spondylodiscitis with a small epidural component. **(B)** A sagittal T2-weighted MRI image 2 mo postoperatively, showing resolution of the infection without kyphosis. The discectomy accelerated the natural process of healing and prevented kyphotic deformity. (Reproduced with permission from ref. *38*.)

REFERENCES

1. Mirra JM, Eckardt JJ, Rosen G. Biopsy considerations, in Bone Tumors: Clinical, Radiologic and Pathologic Correlations (Picci P, Gold RH, eds.), Lea & Febiger, Philadelphia, 1989, pp. 31–34.
2. Kattapuram SV, Khurana JS, Rosenthal DI. Percutaneous needle biopsy of the spine. Spine 1992;17:561–564.
3. Kattapuramm SV, Rosenthal DI. Percutaneous biopsy of skeletal lesions. Am J Roentgenol 1991;157:935–942.
4. Metzger CS, Johnson DW, Donaldson WF. Percutaneous biopsy in the anterior thoracic spine. Spine 1993;18:373–378.
5. Murphy WA, Destouet JM, Gilula LA. Percutaneous skeletal biopsy 1981: a procedure for radiologists—results, review and recommendations. Radiology 1981;139:545–549.
6. Kattapuram SV, Rosenthal DI. Percutaneous needle biopsy of the spine, in Tumors of the Spine: Diagnosis and Clinical Management (Sundaresan N, Schmidek HH, Schiller Al, Rosenthal DI, eds.), WB Saunders, Philadelphia, 1990, pp. 46–51.
7. Robertson RC, Ball RP. Destructive spine lesions: diagnosis by needle biopsy. J Bone Joint Surg 1935;17:749–758.
8. Laredo JD, Bard M. Current status of musculoskeletal interventional radiology. Radiol Clin North Am 1994;32:377–398.

9. Tehranzadch J, Freiberger RH, Glielman, B. Closed skeletal needle biopsy review of 120 cases. Am J Roentgenol 1983;140:113–115.
10. Fyfe IS, Henry APJ, Mulholland RC. Closed vertebral biopsy. J Bone Joint Surg (Br) 1983;65:140–143.
11. Kornblum MB, Wesolowski DP, Fischgrund JS, Herkowitz HN. Computed tomography–guided biopsy of the spine: a review of 103 patients. Spine 1998;23:81–85.
12. Stringham DR, Hadjipavlou A, Dzioba RB, Lander P. Percutaneous transpedicular biopsy of the spine. Spine 1994;19:1985–1991.
13. Roy-Camille R, Saillant G, Mamoudy P. Biopsie du corps vertebral par voie posterieure transpediculaire. Rev Chir Orthop 1983;69:147–149.
14. Banta CJ, King AG, Dabezies EJ, Liljeberg RL. Measurement of effective pedicle diameter in the human spine. Orthopedics 1989;12:939–942.
15. Berry JL, Moran JM, Berg WS, Steffee AD. A morphometric study of human lumbar and selected thoracic vertebrae. Spine 1987;12:363–367.
16. Krag MH, Weaver DL, Beynnon BD, Haugh LD. Morphometry of the thoracic and lumbar spine related to transpedicular screw placement for surgical spinal fixation. Spine 1988;13:27–32.
17. Misenhimer GR, Peek RD, Wiltse LL, Rothman SLG, Widell EH. Anatomic analysis of pedicle cortical and cancellous diameter as related to screw size. Spine 1989;14:367–372.
18. Olsewski JM, Simmons EH, Kallen FC, Mendel FC, Severin CM, Berens DL. Morphometry of the lumbar spine: anatomical perspectives related to transpedicular fixation. J Bone Joint Surg (Am) 1990;72A:541–549.
19. Schmidek HH, Gomes FB, Seligson D, McSherry JW. Management of acute and stable thoracolumbar with and without neurologic deficit. Neurosurgery 1980;7:30–35.
20. Whitecloud TS, Skalley TC, Cook SD, Morgan EL. Roentgenographic measurement of pedicle screw penetration. Clin Orthop 1989;245:57–68.
21. Zindrick MR, Wiltse LL, Doornik A, et al. Analysis of the morphometric characteristics of the thoracic and lumbar pedicles. Spine 1987;12:160–166.
22. Yamagata M, Hiroshi K, Shohei M, et al. Mechanical stability of the pedicle screw for the lumbar spine. Spine 1992;17:551–554.
23. Greenfield RT, Grant RG, Bryant D. Pedicle screw fixation in the management of unstable thoracolumbar spine injuries. Orthop Rev 1992;6:701–706.
24. King AG, MacEwen GD, Bose WJ. Transpedicular convex anterior hemiepiphysiodesis and posterior arthrodesis for progressive congenital scoliosis. Spine 1992;17:S291–S294.
25. Steffee AD, Biscup RS, Sitowski DJ. Segmental spine plates with pedicle screw fixation: a new internal fixation device for disorders of the lumbar and thoracolumbar spine. Clin Orthop 1986;203:45–53.
26. Steffee AD. Segmental spine plates with pedicle screw fixation. Clin Orthop 1986;103: 45–53.
27. Olerud S, Karlstrom G, Sjostrom L. Transpedicular fixation of thoracolumbar vertebral fractures. Clin Orthop 1988;227:44–51.
28. Roy-Camille R, Saillant G, Mazel CH. Plating of thoracic, thoracolumbar, and lumbar injuries with pedicle screw plates. Orthop Clin North Am 1986; 17:147–159.
29. Magerl FP. Stabilization of the lower thoracic and lumbar spine with external skeletal fixation. Clin Orthop 1984;189:125–141.
30. Hardaker WT, Cook WA, Friedman AH, Fitch RD. Bilateral transpedicular decompression and Harrington rod stabilization in the management of severe thoracolumbar burst fractures. Spine 1992;17:162–171.
31. Patterson RH Jr, Arbit E. A surgical approach through the pedicle to protruded thoracic discs. J Neurosurg 1978;48:768–772.
32. Duncan GA, Ferguson AB. Benign giant-cell tumor of the fourth lumbar vertebra: a case report. J Bone Joint Surg (Am) 1936;3:769–772.

33. Capener N. The evolution of lateral rachiotomy. J Bone Joint Surg (Br) 1954;36:173–176.
34. Michele JM, Krueger FJ. Surgical approach to the vertebral body. J Bone Joint Surg (Am) 1949;31:873–878.
35. Travaglini F. Tumours of the vertebral body: transpedicular biopsy with posterior surgical stabilization. Bull Hosp Joint Dis 1979;40:1–12.
36. Stoker DJ, Kissin CM. Percutaneous vertebral biopsy: a review of 135 cases. Clin Radiol 1985:36:569–577.
37. Fidler MW, Niers BBAM. Open transpedicular biopsy of the vertebral body. J Bone Joint Surg (Br) 1990;72:884, 885.
38. Arya S, Crow WN, Hadjipavlou AG, Nauta HJW, Borowski AM, Vierra LA, Walser E. Percutaneous transpedicular management of discitis. JVIR 1996; 7:921–927.
39. Borowski AM, Crow WN, Hadjipavlou AG, Chaljub G, Mader J, Cesani F, vanSonnenberg E. Percutaneous management of pyogenic spondylodiscitis. AJR 1998;170:1587–1592.
40. Hadjipavlou AG, Arya S, Crow WN, Maggio WW, Lander P, Nardone EM, Eyal A. Percutaneous transpedicular biopsy of the spine. J Intervent Radiol 1996;11:103–108.
41. Hadjipavlou AG, Crow WN, Borowski A, Mader JT, Adesokan A, Jensen R. Percutaneous transpedicular discectomy and drainage in pyogenic spondylodiscitis. Am J Orthop 1998;188–197.
42. Hadjipavlou AG, Kontakis GM, Gaitanis I, Katonis PG, Lander P, Crow WN. Effectiveness and pitfalls of percutaneous transpedicular biopsy of the spine. Clin Orthop 2003;411:54–60.
43. Hadjipavlou AG, Mader JT, Necessary JT, Muffoletto AJ. Hematogenous pyogenic spinal infections and their surgical management: Spine 2000;25:1668–1679.
44. Kambin P (ed). Arthroscopic Microdiscectomy: Minimal Intervention in Spinal Surgery, Williams & Wilkins, Baltimore, 1990.
45. Saillant G. Etude anatomique des pedicules vertebraux: application chirurgicale. Rev Chir Orthop 1976;62:151–160.
46. Ball RP. Needle (aspiration) biopsy. J Tenn State Med Assoc 1934;27:203–207.
47. Ward JC, Jeanneret B, Oehlschlegel C, Magerl F. The value of percutaneous transpedicular vertebral bone biopsies for histologic examination: results of an experimental histopathologic study comparing two biopsy needles. Spine 1996;21:2484–2490.
48. Renfrew DL, Whitten CG, Wiese JA, el-Khoury GY, Harris KG. CT-guided percutaneous transpedicular biopsy of the spine. Radiology 1991;180:574–576.
49. Hsu WC, Lim KE. Computed tomography–guided percutaneous transpedicular biopsy of the thoracic spine. Chang Gung Med J 2001;24:368–375.
50. Jho HD. Endoscopic microscopic transpedicular thoracic discectomy: technical note. J Neurosurg 1997;87:125–129.
51. Minart D, Vallee JN, Cormier E, Chiras J. Percutaneous coaxial transpedicular biopsy of vertebral body lesions during vertebroplasty. Neuroradiology 2001;43:409–412.
52. Moller S, Kothe R, Wiesner L, Werner M, Ruther W, Delling G. Fluoroscopy-guided transpedicular trocar biopsy of the spine—results, review and technical notes. Acta Orthop Belg 2001;67(5):488-499.
53. Pierot L, Boulin A. Percutaneous biopsy of the thoracic and lumbar spine: transpedicular approach under fluoroscopic guidance. Am J Neuroradiol 1999;20:23–25.
54. Ashizawa R, Ohtsuka K, Kamimura M, Ebara S, Takaoka K. Percutaneous transpedicular biopsy of thoracic and lumbar vertebrae—method and diagnostic validity. Surg Neurol 1999;52(6):545–551.
55. Jelinek JS, Kransdorf MJ, Gray R, Aboulafia AJ, Malawer MM. Percutaneous transpedicular biopsy of vertebral body lesions. Spine 1996;21:2035–2040.
56. Dagirmanjian A, Schils J, McHenry M, Modic MT. MR imaging of vertebral osteomyelitis revisited. Am J Roentgenol 1996;167:1539–1543.
57. Ambrose GB, Alpert M, Neer CS. Vertebral osteomyelitis: a diagnostic problem. JAMA 1966;197:619–622.

58. Waldvogel RA, Papageorgiou PS. Osteomyelitis: the past decade. N Engl J Med 1980;303: 360–370.
59. Ottolenghi CE. Aspiration biopsy of the spine: technique for the thoracic spine and results of twenty-eight biopsies in this region and overall results of 1050 biopsies of other spinal segments. J Bone Joint Surg 1969;51A:1531–1544.
60. Post MJD, Sze G, Quencer RM, et al. Gadolinium enhanced MR in spinal infection. J Comput Assist Tomogr 1990;14:721–729.
61. Sklar EML, Post MJD, Lebwohl NH. Imaging of infection of lumbosacral spine. Neuroimaging 1993;3:577–590.
62. Wisneski RJ. Infectious disease of the spine: diagnostic and treatment considerations. Orthop Clin North Am 1991;22:491–501.
63. Eismont FJ, Bohlman HH, Soni PL, et al. Pyogenic and fungal vertebral osteomyelitis with paralysis. J Bone Joint Surg 1983;65A:19–29.
64. Emery SE, Chan DP, Woodward HR. Treatment of hematogenous pyogenic vertebral osteomyelitis with anterior debridement and primary bone grafting. Spine 1989;14:284–291.
65. Estherhai JL Jr, Gelb I. Adult sepric arthritis. Orthop Clin North Am 1991;22:503–514.
66. Krodel A, Sturz H, Siebert CH. Indication for and results of operative treatment of spondylitis and spondylodiscitis. Arch Orthop Trauma Surg 1991;110:78–82.
67. Lane JG, Falahaee MH, Wojtys EM, et al. Pyarthrosis of the knee: treatment considerations. Clin Orthop 1990;252:198–204.
68. Lee TC, Lu K, Yang LC, Huang HY, Liang CL. Transpedicular instrumentation as an adjunct in the treatment of thoracolumbar spine tuberculosis with early stage bone destruction. J Neurosurg 1999;91:163–169.
69. Taylor TKF, Dooley BJ. Antibiotics in the management of postoperative disc space infections. Aust NZ J Surg 1978;48:74, 75.
70. Jackson RW. The septic knee arthroscopic treatment. Arthroscopy 1985;1:194–197.
71. Ivey M, Clark R. Arthroscopic debridement of the knee for septic arthritis. Clin Orthop 1985;199:201–206.
72. Gebhard JS, Brugman JL. Percutaneous discectomy for the treatment of bacterial discitis. Spine 1994;19:855–857.
73. Onik G, Shang Y, Maroon JC. Automated percutaneous biopsy in postoperative diskitis: a new method. AJNR 1990;1:391–393.
74. Vu WY, Siu C, Tong PC, et al. Percutaneous suction aspiration for osteomyelitis: report of two cases. Spine 1991;16:198–202.
75. Fraser RD, Osti OL, Vernon-Roberts B. Iatrogenic discitis: the role of intravenous antibiotics in prevention and treatment: an experimental study. Spine 1989;14:1025–1032.
76. Lucio E, Adesokan A, Hadjipavlou AG, Crow WN, Adegboyega PA. Pyogenic spondylodiskitis. Arch Pathol Lab Med 2000;124:712–716.
77. Garcia A, Grantham SA. Hematogenous pyogenic vertebral osteomyleitis. J Bone Joint Surg 1960;42A:429–436.
78. Sapico FL, Montgomerie JZ. Pyogenic vertebral osteomyelitis: report of nine cases and review of the literature. Rev Infect Dis 1979;1:754–756.
79. Frederickson B, Yuan H, Olans R. Management and outcome of pyogenic vertebral osteomyelitis. Clin Orthop 1978;131:160–167.
80. Guven O, Yalgin S, Karahan M, Esemenli T. Transpedicular drainage of Pot's abscess: a report of two cases. Am J Orthop 1995;24:421–425.
81. Crow WN, Borowski AM, Hadjipavlou AG, Walser EM, Arya S, Calme MB, Amps J, Jensen R, Somisetty S, Alford B, Adesokan A. Percutaneous transpedicular automated nucleotomy for debridement of infected discs. JVIR 1998;9:161–165.

9

Selective Endoscopic Discectomy™

Twelve Years of Experience

Anthony T. Yeung, MD

INTRODUCTION

More than 12 yr have passed (1991) since I learned and adopted arthroscopic microdiscectomy (AMD) from pioneer endoscopic spine surgeon Parviz Kambin, who, along with Sadahisa Hijikata, first established the technique for percutaneous nucleotomy in the early 1970s. A cadaver dissection of the traditional posterior anatomy of the lumbar spine compared with the foraminal anatomy clearly illustrates the feasibility and advantages of the foraminal approach to the lumbar disc (Fig. 1A,B). Kambin's AMD technique evolved gradually to allow for more dorsal placement of the cannula to effect posterolateral fragmentectomy and resection of the posterior annulus for stenosis, and it made possible the removal of extruded and sequestered herniated discs *(1–4)* (Fig. 2). Hijikata *(5)* also recently reviewed his 12 yr of experience with endoscopic discectomy. In 1996, a new design of the operating spine endoscope adding multichannel irrigation and complementary instrumentation (Fig. 3) *(6)* allowed further development of endoscopic spine surgery to include the treatment of annular tears causing discogenic back pain *(7,8)*. Advanced techniques of foraminoplasty for central and lateral recess stenosis followed *(9–12)*. The third-generation system design change to the Yeung Endoscopic Spine Surgery (YESS) system gave me more flexibility to maneuver the endoscope and improved ability to probe spinal anatomy in a conscious patient *(13)*. Continued evolution of this technique afforded me the ability to better evaluate the pathological process causing the patient's discogenic back pain. Conditions previously not considered surgical, such as annular tears, were evaluated and managed successfully through the endoscope. Synovial facet cysts, inflammatory membranes containing neoneurogenesis, osteophytosis impinging on sensitive nerves, anomalous furcal nerves, autonomic nerves, and conditions irritating the dorsal root ganglion (DRG) of the exiting nerve were identified as sources of discogenic pain and sciatica.

From 1991 to 2004, I treated more than 2300 patients with discogenic pain, degenerative conditions of the lumbar spine, and the whole spectrum of disc herniations including extruded and sequestered fragments *(14,15)*. The success rate in the first 500 patients was 432 of 500 (86%) good/excellent results according to the modified MacNab criteria *(11)*.

From: *Arthroscopic and Endoscopic Spinal Surgery: Text and Atlas: Second Edition*
Edited by: P. Kambin © Humana Press Inc., Totowa, NJ

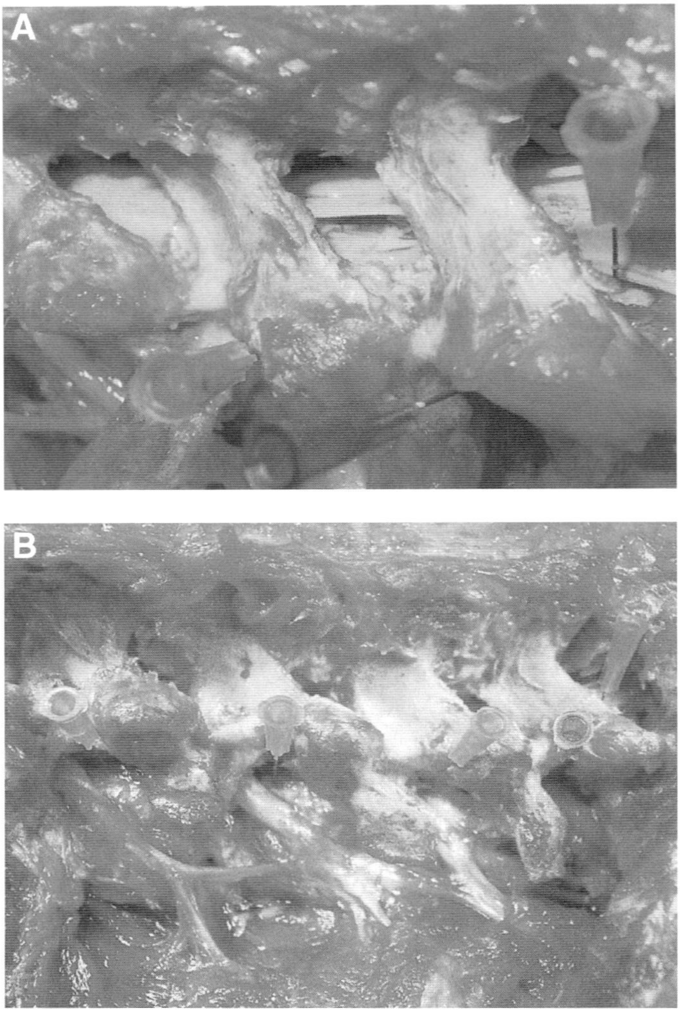

Fig. 1. (A) Anatomy of the posterior port provides easier access to the posterior disc and spinal canal at L5-S1 (blue hubbed needle), but with planning, most contained disc herniations can be removed posterolaterally. **(B)** Anatomy of posterolateral foraminal port from L2-S1. Only in the L5-S1 disc space is access to the spinal canal restricted because of the pelvis and the relatively wide facet (gray hubbed needle in the L5-S1 disc). High lumbar disc herniations from L1 to L3 are easier to reach endoscopically through the posterolateral foraminal portal. L4-L5 provides ample room for either approach. Note the furcal nerve branches entering the psoas muscle.

A subsequent retrospective study of 219 consecutive patients with radiculopathy secondary to large intracanal noncontained lumbar disc herniations demonstrated a satisfactory outcome in 204 (93.1%) patients based on modified MacNab criteria, but the rate was even higher (94.8%) when patients were asked to respond to a study patient-based outcome questionnaire *(16)*. In this chapter, I review my 12 yr of experience evolving from Kambin's AMD into the treatment of discogenic back pain and sciatica by selective endoscopic discectomy.

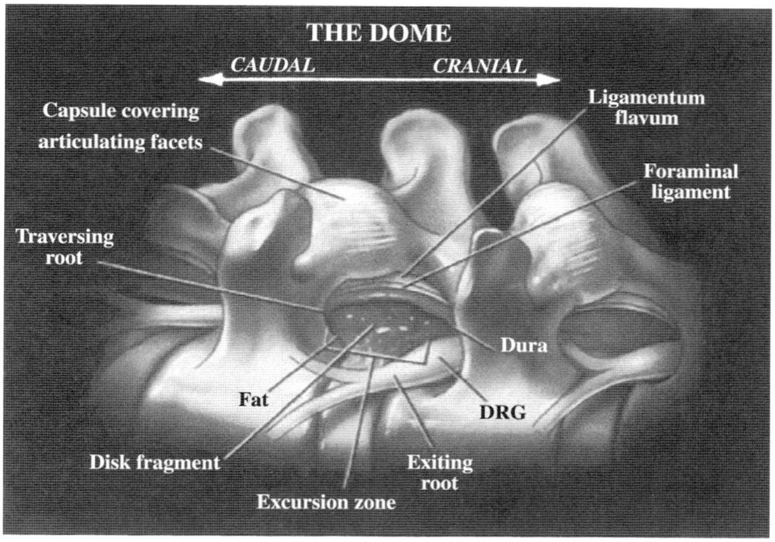

Fig. 2. The dome. Spinal structures in the foramen accessible to visualization and surgical intervention and probing via the posterolateral approach include the annulus, disc, pedicle, facet, and epidural space. This approach also visualizes neurocompression in the "hidden zone" of the lateral recess, a common cause of failed back surgery syndrome (FBSS). (Courtesy of Hal Matthews, MD.)

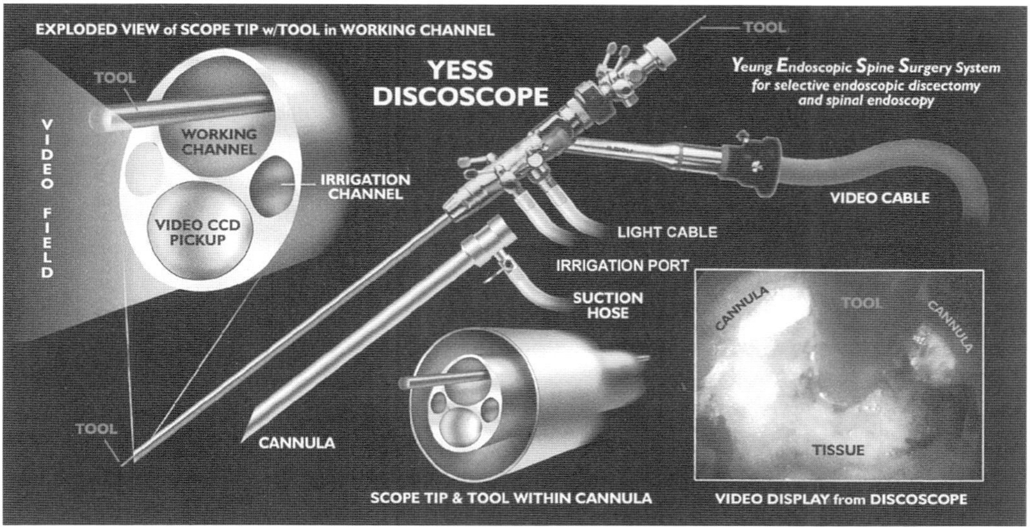

Fig. 3. Yeung spine scope system. YESS discoscope and partial instrument set. The spinal endoscope is designed with multichannel irrigation and a cannula system that allows access to targeted areas while protecting sensitive nerves. (From ref. *15.*)

ROLE OF EVOCATIVE CHROMODISCOGRAPHY

At Kambin's 1991 course, Prof. Hans Joerg Leu described the use of indigocarmine dye to stain and label the nucleus pulposus (NP). To maintain the ability to recognize structural anatomy, it was necessary to dilute the dye to a 10% solution to effect differential tissue

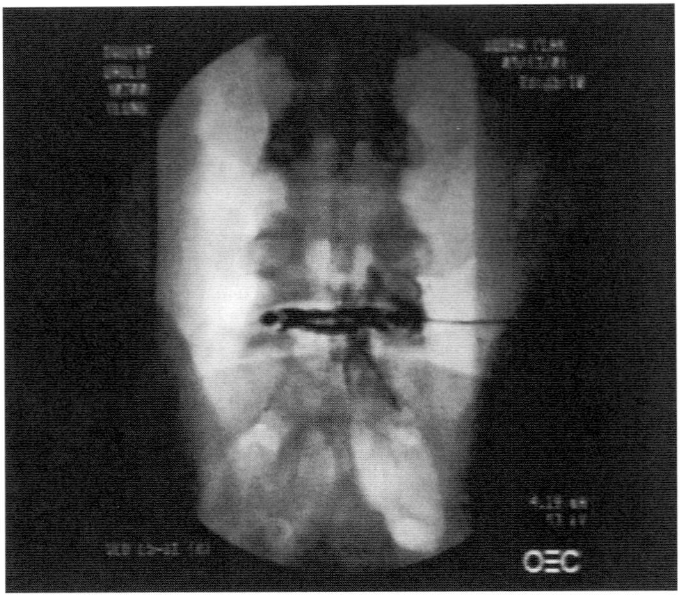

Fig. 4. This intraoperative discogram in a patient with a papacentral herniated nucleus pulposus (HNP) by magnetic resonance imaging (MRI) not only confirmed the patient's concordant back pain and sciatica, but the leakage of contrast to the traversing and exiting nerves alerted the surgeon to look for extruded disc fragments and grade V annular tears, especially in the lateral zone.

staining that did not overwhelm the NP with stain. I adopted this adjunctive technique initially to help with a visualized nuclectomy *(17)*. With differential staining, it was easier to recognize NP from annulus and from facet capsule. The epidural space with its epidural vessels and fat was simple to recognize. When pain was reproduced by discography, the clinical improvement in the patient's back pain correlated well with concordant pain reproduction. The use of discography also helped predict whether the herniation was extruded or contained, and the nuclear material was clearly stained for easier endoscopic extraction *(18)* (Fig. 4). I trademarked evocative chromodiscography™ as an integral part of spinal endoscopy. The process of removing the indigocarmine dye-labeled nucleus was trademarked selective endoscopic discectomy™ and this technique is the focus of this chapter *(15)* (Fig. 5).

The literature on discography is currently considered controversial only because of the high interobserver variability by discographers in reporting the patient's subjective pain as well as the ailing patient's ability to give a clear response, especially if the pain response is altered by the use of analgesics or sedation during the procedure. Although much of the literature that contributes to the controversy of discography points out the pitfalls of depending on discography, the majority of the literature supports its use by clinicians who know how to use it. The surgeon who is accomplished in endoscopic spine surgery prefers to do the discography himself or herself in order to decrease the interobserver variability in interpreting the patient's response. When a discographer compares his or her own assessment of the patient's pain response with the report of another discographer, there can be some variability in diagnosis and interpretation. This variability may result in unpredictable treatment results. The incidence of "false-positive" discograms,

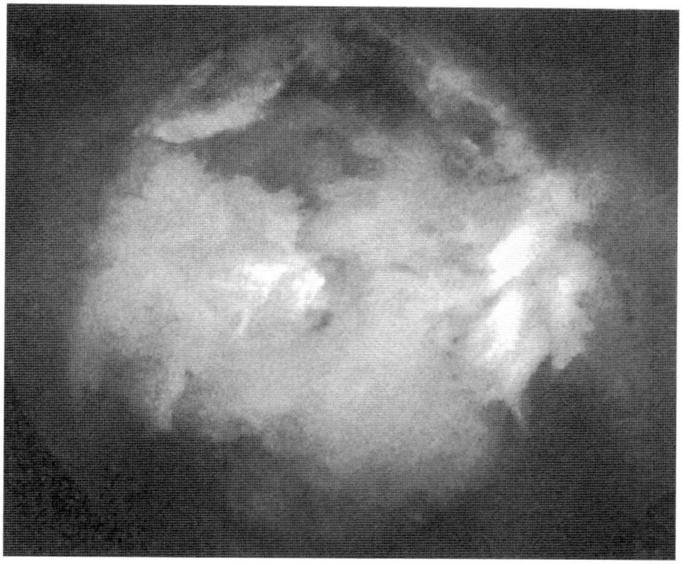

Fig. 5. NP stained with indigocarmine dye. The indigocarmine dye stains the NP light blue, helping the endoscopic surgeon target the stained nucleus for extraction. Here, the herniation has extruded past the unstained annulus. Removal of the extruded herniation will expose the traversing nerve in the epidural space.

however, can be significantly decreased in the hands of an experienced endoscopic surgeon. False-positive discography should really be false interpretation of positive discography results. The experienced endoscopic surgeon learns to correlate the patient's response to the discogram pattern of the painful disc that is being treated. There is good correlation of discograms with different types of annular tears and disc herniations. The surgical result can then be predicted on the basis of the visualized condition. For example, the discogram can be used to predict the presence of a collagenized disc fragment vs a soft herniation; the extrusion of a disc fragment as a noncontained herniation; or the presence of the type, grade, and location of a painful vs nonpainful annular tear. Discography is used by the surgeon as a means of further identifying concordant discogenic pain in clinical situations in which the patient's clinical presentation is matched with MRI findings. Controversy in the literature has arisen because of the lack of a good spectrum of therapeutic surgical treatments once the pain is confirmed, and because of the plethora of articles pointing out the pitfalls of false interpretation *(19,20)*.

ROLE OF ELECTROTHERMAL THERAPY

Prior to my adoption of AMD, I was using the potassium-trideuterium-phosphate (KTP) laser for laser disc decompression. When I combined the two techniques for nuclectomy, the laser provided hemostasis and better visualization *(21–24)*. I observed that patients with disc protrusions but with predominant back pain who were not candidates for traditional transcanal surgery found relief of their back pain with KTP-assisted AMD. The staining of the disc provided a chromophore that enhanced the efficacy of the KTP laser *(25)*. In 1993, I tested a unipolar electrode by Ellman and introduced to me by

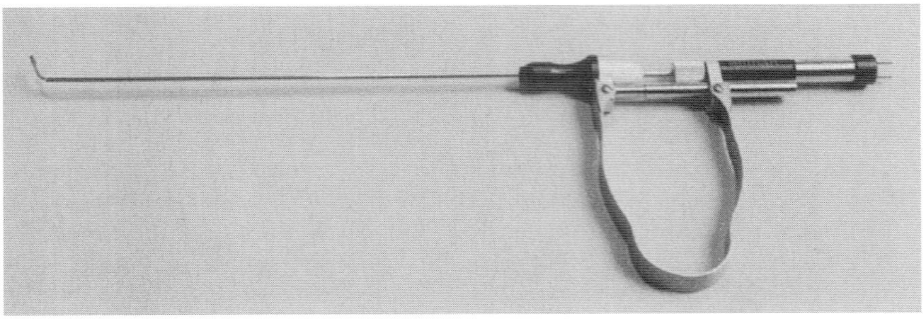

Fig. 6. Ellman Bipolar Triggerflex Probe. This bipolar flexible device has provided effective hemostasis as well as electrothermal shrinkage of disc tissue and annular tears under visualized control. It offers better control of the energy source by its bipolar design.

Dr. Peter Morrison. Later, an electrode made by Smith and Nephew was used with the Ellman unit and the new working channel endoscope. In a retrospective 2- to 4.5-yr follow-up study of my first 100 patients by Farouq Al-Hamdan, a spine fellow under Alex Hadjipavlou, it was documented that the use of the KTP laser as an adjunct to AMD relieved back pain as well as leg pain in 65% of the patients. The overall good/excellent result by MacNab criteria was 89% for sciatica. The KTP laser was initially used to provide hemostasis and better visualization, but its side effect of laser thermal annuloplasty prompted an International Review Board (IRB) study using a temperature-controlled flexible probe by Oratec in lieu of the laser.

In 1998, an IRB-approved study commenced at St. Luke's Medical Center to evaluate the efficacy of electrothermal treatment in the process of arthroscopic microdiscectomy for herniated discs. This study, sponsored by Oratec, using a temperature-controlled flexible probe, provided a better tool to contract annular defects caused by the disc herniation and ablating granulation tissue in annular tears. The patient's response to this application of electrothermal energy provided information that electrothermal treatment of the disc was effective in decreasing discogenic back pain, but the fluctuations in temperature control caused me to switch to a bipolar flexible probe *(26,27)*. Oratec investigated the intradiscal electrothermal (IDET) catheter in the same time period. I now use a bipolar flexible probe by Ellman designed specifically for thermal annuloplasty that has proven to be as effective as the Oratec probe, but with a more established and accepted use of electrothermal energy in spine surgery *(27)* (Fig. 6).

Rauschning's cryosections of normal and pathoanatomy have more recently demonstrated inflammation in and around the sensitive DRG and identified granulation tissue in annular tears *(28,29)* (Figs. 7 and 8). It is also well known that although a spinal structure is capable of pain, spinal pathology on imaging studies does not always correlate with the debilitating pain that is resistant to conservative management *(30)*. What may be very painful in one person may be well tolerated or painless in another. Evocative discography has been shown to be helpful in identifying the disc as a pain generator in axial back pain and sciatica *(18,31–37)*, and electrothermal treatment of the disc is demonstrated to be effective in decreasing discogenic back pain.

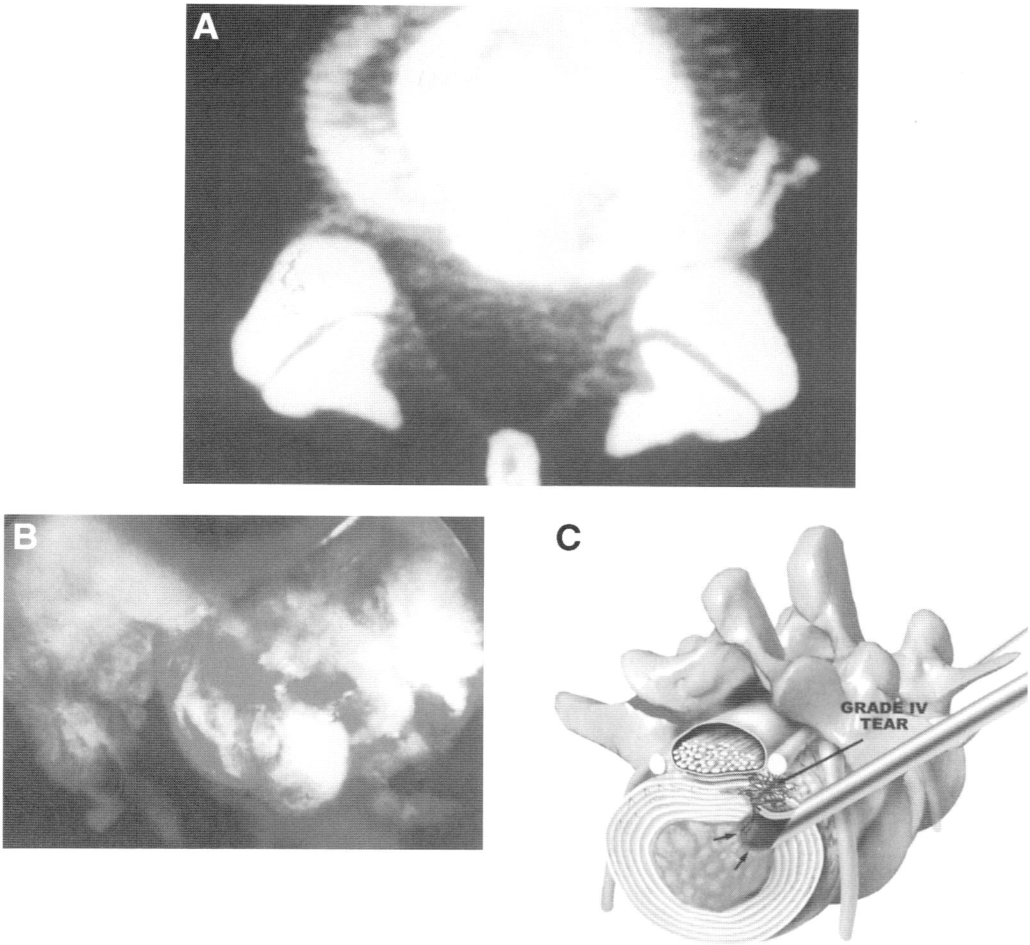

Fig. 7. **(A)** Annular tears. This computed tomography (CT) discogram outlines a foraminal HNP and far-lateral annular tear that will irritate the DRG of the exiting nerve. Endoscopic visualization of the foramen may reveal the presence of an inflammatory membrane, extruded NP, and granulation tissue. **(B)** Granulation tissue and inflammation surrounding small disc fragment in foramen. Grade V annular tears open into the epidural space or psoas muscle, allowing the ingrowth of nerves and capillaries and creating an inflammatory response, which, if next to a spinal nerve or the DRG, can cause pain out of proportion to what may be anticipated from traditional imaging studies. Tears in this area will also result in groin pain by irritating the psoas muscle and genital-femoral nerve. Patients with annular tears who obtain pain relief from foraminal epidural blocks may experience more lasting relief of 2 or more years with selective endoscopic discectomy and thermal annuloplasty. **(C)** Bipolar radiofrequency treatment of annular tears under direct visualization. Interpositional disc material should be removed from the annular layers to treat the annular tear effectively. **(D)** Preoperative endoscopic view of grades V annular tear demonstrating granulation tissue in tear. **(E)** Postoperative view of annulus after thermal modulation with Ellman Bipolar Triggerflex Probe.

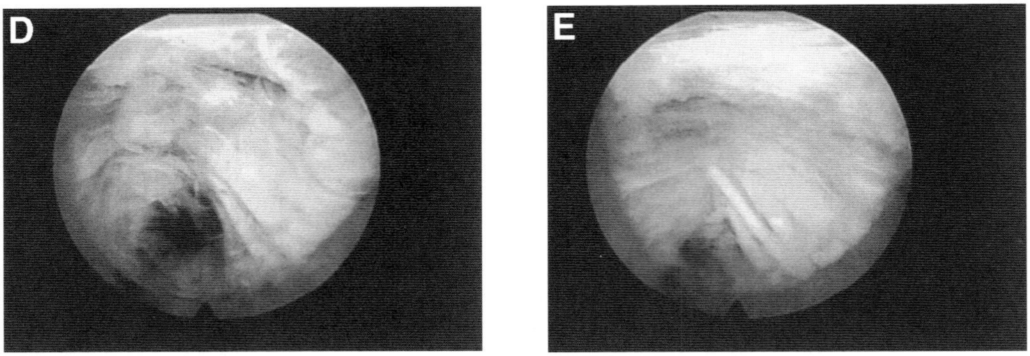

Fig. 7. *(Continued)*

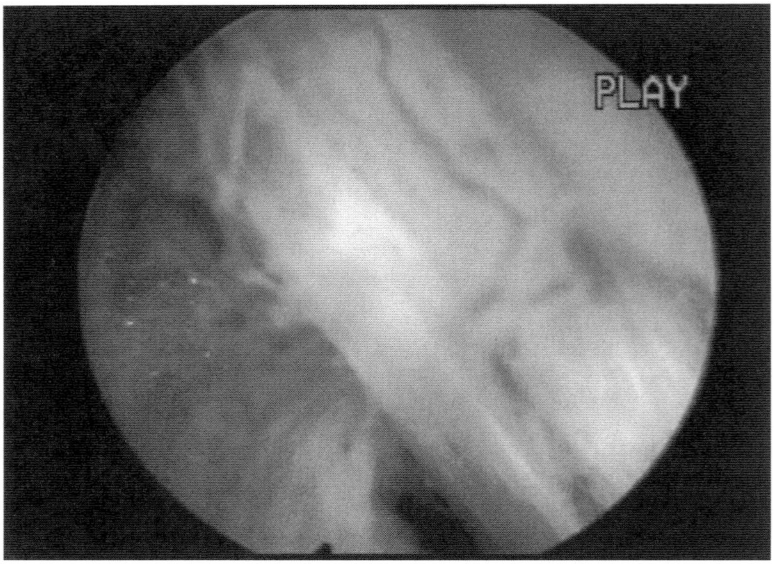

Fig. 8. Exiting nerve. The exiting nerve is in the "hidden extraforaminal zone" that is irritated by far-lateral annular tears and disc herniations that escape detection by MRI and transcanal surgical exploration. It contains the DRG, which, when sensitized by the inflammatory byproducts of a degenerative disc, is responsible for the "nondermatomal" distribution in patients with chronic sciatica. The presence of fat around the exiting nerve is a more sensitive indication of lateral recess stenosis than findings on MRI or CT myelogram.

ROLE OF THE LASER

Laser technology also evolved to become more user friendly. The first laser to be approved by the Food and Drug Administration was the KTP laser, a laser in the blue/green wavelength spectrum that was effective for soft-tissue ablation, but the bright light limited its use when direct visualization was desired *(22)*. The Holmium:yttrium-aluminum-garnet (YAG) laser was effective for the ablation of soft tissue as well as bone. Current designs now include a side-firing irrigated probe and a straight fiber that can be delivered through a curved guide that will angle the laser beam up to 45°. The laser has opened the door for the removal of osteophytes and lateral stenosis that cause neuropathic pain in patients who

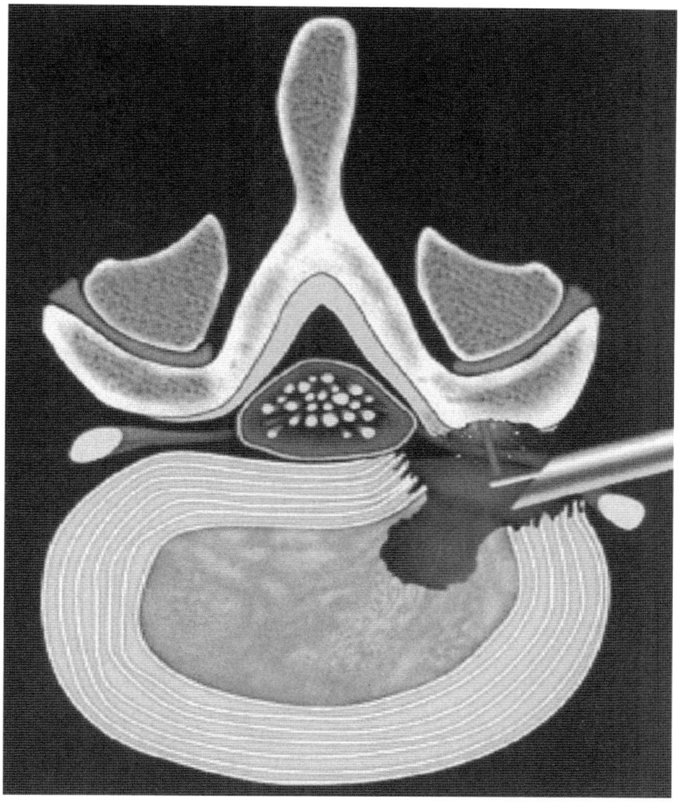

Fig. 9. Role of laser in foraminoplasty. Side-firing laser (Trimedine) or end-firing laser fibers (Lisa) directed by a flexible cannula are used for precise foraminoplasty of the lateral recess.

have no other surgical options *(15)*. Figures 9 and 10 demonstrate the use of the laser in foraminoplasty.

ADJUNCTIVE THERAPY WITH CHYMOPAPAIN

Chymopapain is the only minimally invasive technique that has been validated with two large double-blind studies and numerous cohort studies that found it effective for the treatment of contained disc herniations. I have used chymopapain to assist the extraction of large noncontained disc herniations that extrude past the outer annular fibers, with a good/excellent result by MacNab criteria 10% higher than when no chymopapain was used *(38)*. If the height of the herniation is greater than the base on MRI, it is likely that the herniated nucleus is collared by the annulus, making it more difficult to remove from within the disc. Chymopapain-treated NP is soft and slippery, making mechanical removal easier. If chymopapain extravasates along the course of the contrast agent used for discography, it will theoretically denature and treat the extruded fragment to make it less inflammetogenic. The extruded fragment is also exposed to phagocytosis and eventual absorption if exposed to the epidural vasculature. In more than 500 surgical cases of chymopapain-assisted selective endoscopic discectomy, I have never had any complications from the use of chymopapain. Because of the absence of complications when used in conjunction with endoscopic disc removal, I

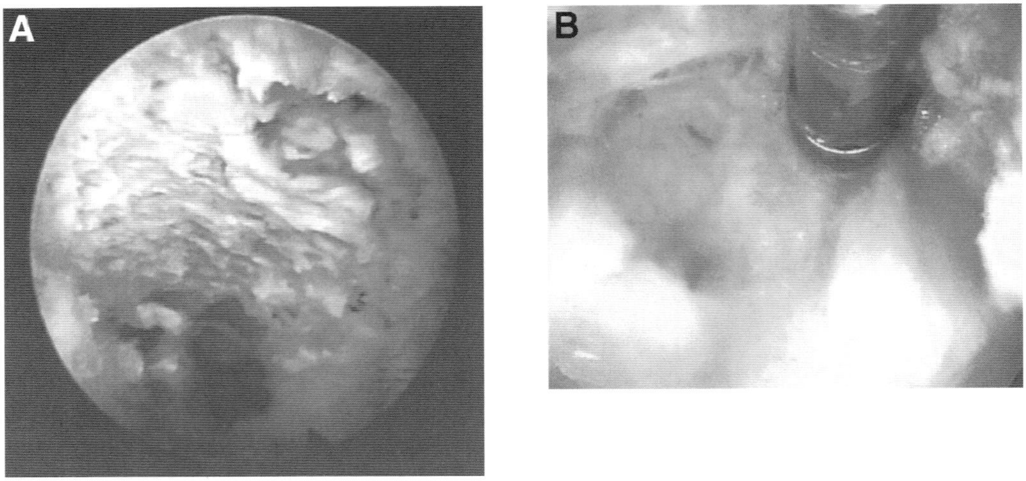

Fig. 10. (**A**) Postoperative endoscopic view of foraminoplasty of superior articular facet at L5-S1; (**B**) postoperative view of decompressed exiting nerve after foraminoplasty.

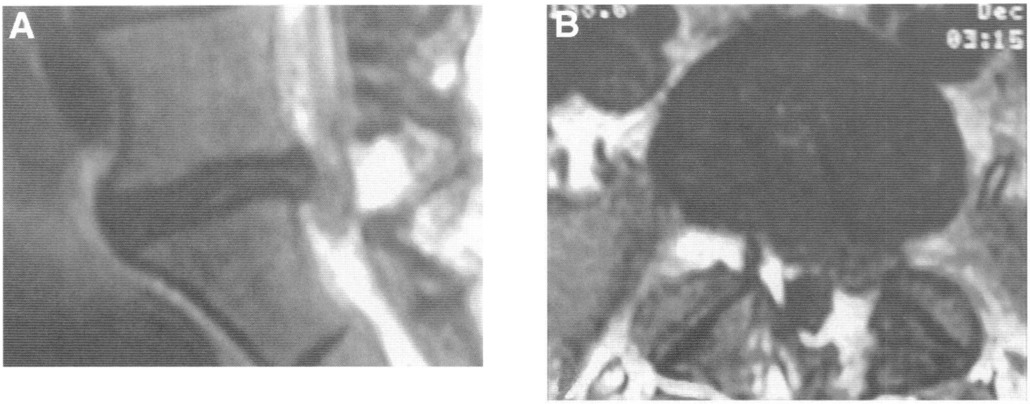

Fig. 11. (**A**) Chymopapain-assisted selective endoscopic discectomy. (**B**) Preoperative MRI of extruded fragment in horizontal disc at L5-S1 that is anatomically difficult to reach. By using chymopapain, the results of endoscopic removal have been demonstrated to be improved by 10% overall, by reducing the rate of residual HNP or recurrent HNP.

now do not find it necessary to test routinely for antibodies to chymopapain with the Chymofast test unless the patient requests it (Figs. 11–13).

NEUROMONITORING

In 100 consecutive cases, I studied neuromonitoring to determine whether sensory/motor complications could be reduced. I specifically studied whether neuromonitoring by continuous electromyogram (EMG) or somatosensory evoked potentials (SSEP) would affect the incidence of dysesthesia or help predict decompression of the nerve *(39)*. Although an increase in conduction velocity was identified when a mechanically compromised nerve was decompressed, I concluded that neuromonitoring was no more effective than monitoring the patient for intraoperative pain when a dilute solution of lidocaine (0.5%) was used. There was no difference in the dysesthesia or complication rate of the 100 cases vs a

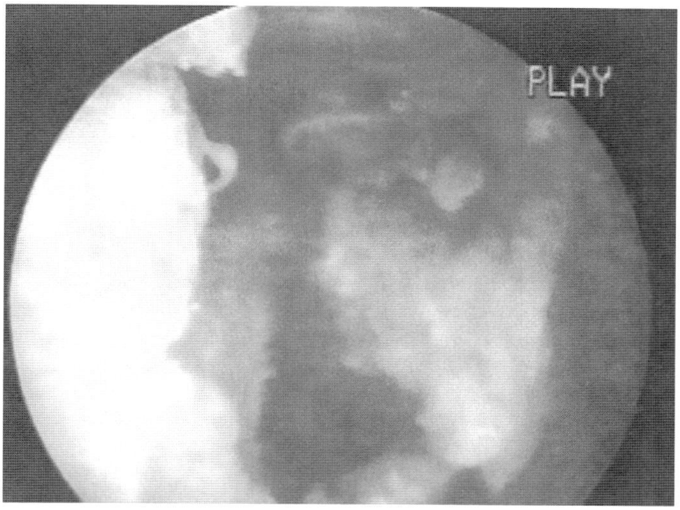

Fig. 12. An extruded fragment labeled by indigocarmine and pretreated by chymopapain allowed for easier manual extraction. The chymopapain loosened the fragment, making it easier to remove, aided by suction on the working channel of an endoscope.

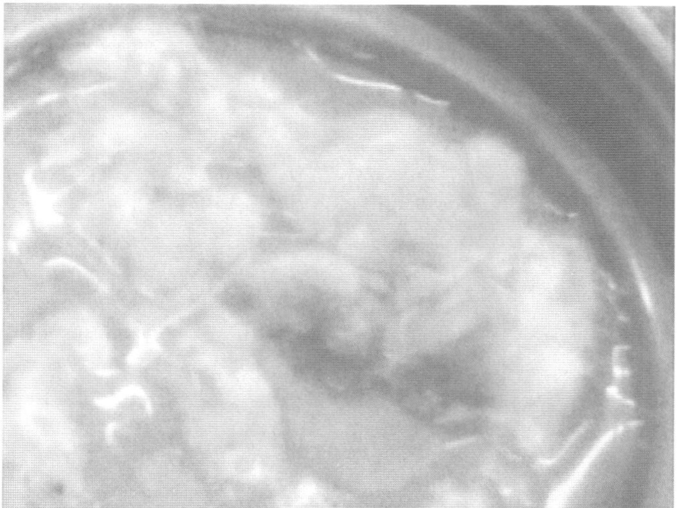

Fig. 13. Chymopapain-treated NP. Note the differential staining of the extracted nuclear material. Unstained collagenized disc was extracted from the epidural space where the indigocarmine dye did not reach. By visualizing the decompressed foramen, successful relief of leg pain was immediate postoperatively.

matched number of patients who had no neuromonitoring. Although neuromonitoring may give the novice surgeon a greater sense of security early in his or her endoscopic practice, analysis of the results of the prospective study of 100 consecutive patients did not shown

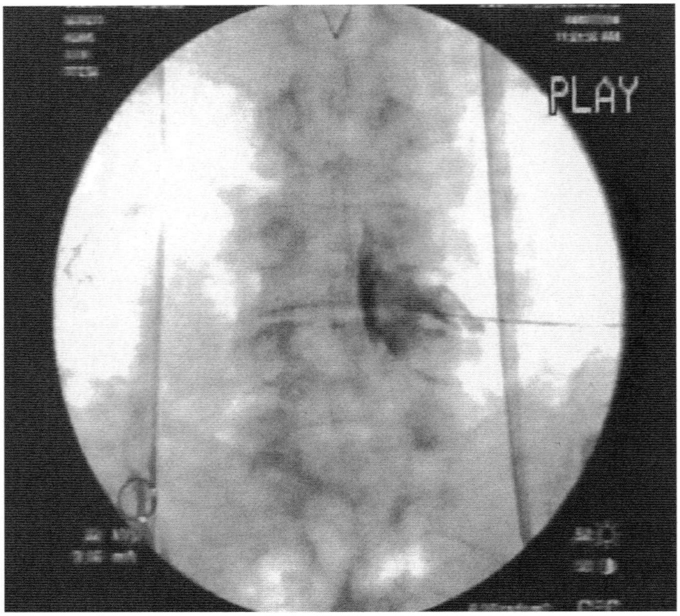

Fig. 14. Foraminal epidurograms. Foraminoepidurography is a new technique for foraminal needle placement from the far-lateral skin portal mimicking surgical access to the epidural space that allows the surgeon to produce an epidurogram that complements the MRI by outlining the position of the traversing and exiting nerves in the foramen. This information provides the surgeon with additional information preoperatively and serves as a "practice run" for surgery.

neuromonitoring to be any more useful for avoiding complications than patient feedback on pain during the procedure.

FORAMINOGRAPHY AND THERAPEUTIC INJECTIONS

The efficacy of endoscopic lumbar disc surgery can be enhanced by surgeons performing than own discography and foraminal injections. Foraminal epidurography and foraminal therapeutic injections are correlated with identification of pathoanatomy in the lumbar spine (Figs. 14–17). Surgeons use information gleaned from these injection procedures to better select patients for surgical interventional techniques that the they have incorporated into their endoscopic surgical practice. Patients with disc protrusions, annular tears, and foraminal stenosis may get temporary relief with the therapeutic injection, but if the response is short-lived, additional information gathered by performing the epiduralgram will help guide surgeons when they must consider the technical feasibility of using the same or similar portal for the insertion of the operating cannulas. By performing epidurograms, surgeons can obtain additional information of the anatomy of the foramen, the outline of the traversing and exiting nerves, and the therapeutic response afforded by the epidural injection *(37)*. Injection at L5-S1 will also help surgeons with preoperative planning if surgery is eventually required.

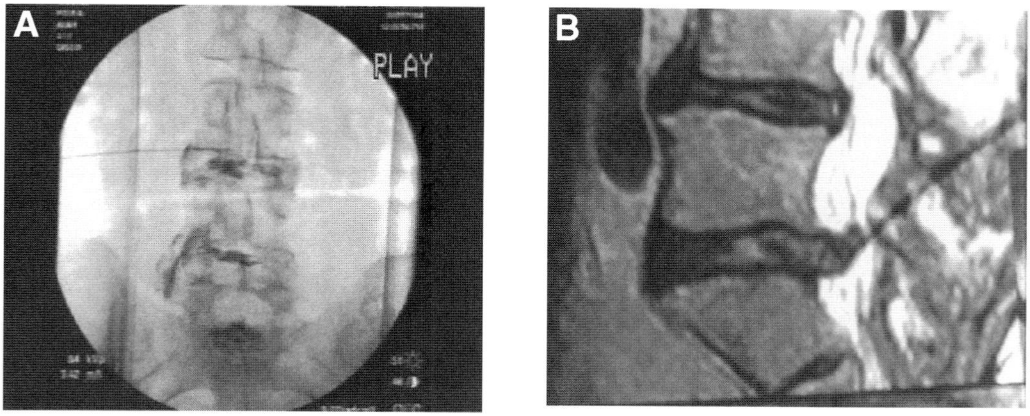

Fig. 15. **(A)** Anatomical limitations at L5-S1. The narrow pelvis in this patient limited access to the disc, but it was still possible to insert a needle into the disc for discography. Depending on the type of disc protrusion, the endoscopic surgeon will have a better idea about the prognosis of the surgical procedure contemplated. If this patient had an extruded disc herniation, it would be better to opt for the transcanal approach. **(B)** Horizontal L5-S1 disc. The pelvis becomes an even greater obstacle at L5-S1 if the disc is horizontal, which makes it much more difficult to get into the epidural space. Removal of the lateral facet could overcome this obstacle. Good preoperative planning is enhanced by foraminoepidurography.

PRESENT APPLICATIONS AND FUTURE TRENDS

Indications

Any pathological lesion that is accessible, is visible, is treatable, or requires endoscopic confirmation through the foramen may ultimately become an indication for diagnostic and therapeutic endoscopy. Patient selection for pain and radiculopathy from disc herniation is similar to selection criteria for traditional spine procedures. Endoscopic surgical indications, however, may be dictated by the limitations of the endoscopic procedure itself with respect to the patient's anatomy or the surgeon's skill and experience with endoscopic spine surgery. At L5-S1, anatomical restrictions may cause the surgeon to opt for the posterior transcanal approach (Fig. 15A,B). For herniations from T10 to L4, the foraminal approach provides excellent access to the disc and epidural space. As the experience of the surgeon increases, previous contraindications become relative, depending partly on the surgeon's ability to endoscopically visualize, probe, and access the pathological lesion. Restrictions are dictated only by anatomical considerations in accessing the patient's spinal pathology and the rationale for the endoscopic procedure itself. As the surgeon's experience increases, former contraindications become relative, depending on the surgeon's experience, and his or her ability to address the spinal condition to be treated. The three zones within reach of the spine endoscope transforaminally are illustrated in Fig. 16.

Inclusion Criteria

Discogenic pain as determined by evocative discography implicates the disc as a pain generator. Symptomatic disc herniation is the obvious indication, limited only by the accessibility of endoscopic instruments to the herniated fragment. The ideal lesion

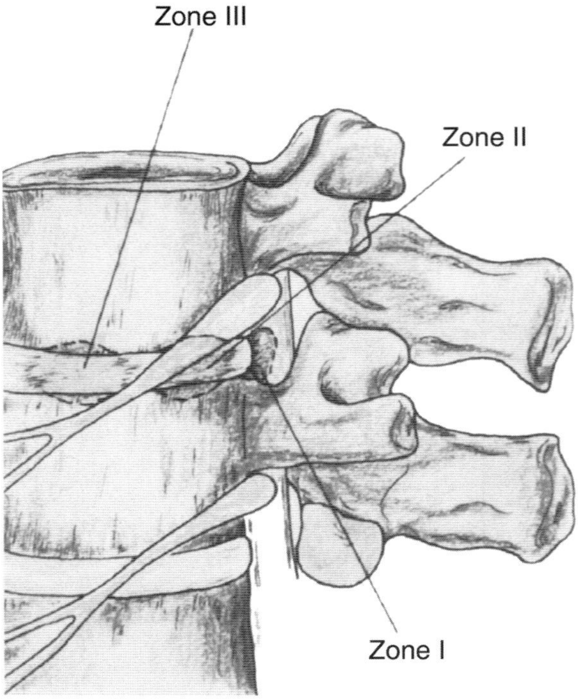

Fig. 16. Three zones on foramen accessible by endoscope. Zones II and III are not usually visualized by surgeons using the transcanal approach unless they are experienced in the paramedical approach to the lateral recess.

for endoscopic discectomy is a far-lateral, extraforaminal disc herniation. Traditional approaches to far-lateral disc herniations are more difficult, requiring a paramedian incision through very vascular tissue. The exiting nerve and the DRG are at risk of neuropraxia in both approaches *(28,29)*. Although a traditional spine surgeon can access the lateral zone of the disc with a paramedian incision, it is easier to access the extraforaminal zone through the foramen. A typical foraminal view of NP extruded past the posterior annulus is shown in (Fig. 17). Through this approach to the disc, endoscopic excisional biopsy and disc space debridement are also ideal for surgically debriding infectious discitis (Fig. 18). Currently treated with immobilization and parenteral antibiotics, discitis is much more effectively treated when augmented by endoscopic excisional biopsy and debridement. The surgeon will not have to be overly concerned about creating dead space for the inflamed or infected disc material to spread into the dead space created by a posterior approach. The clinical results are dramatic, and tissue biopsy is more accurate than needle aspiration in identifying the cause of discitis. Even sterile discitis will benefit from intradiscal debridement and irrigation.

Foraminal stenosis in selected patients will respond to foraminoplasty by endoscopic techniques. Lateral recess stenosis is one cause of FBSS that can absolutely be diagnosed and treated by foraminal decompression *(40)*. The pathoanatomical finding may be osteophytosis tethering the exiting nerve at the superior vertebral end plate and/or

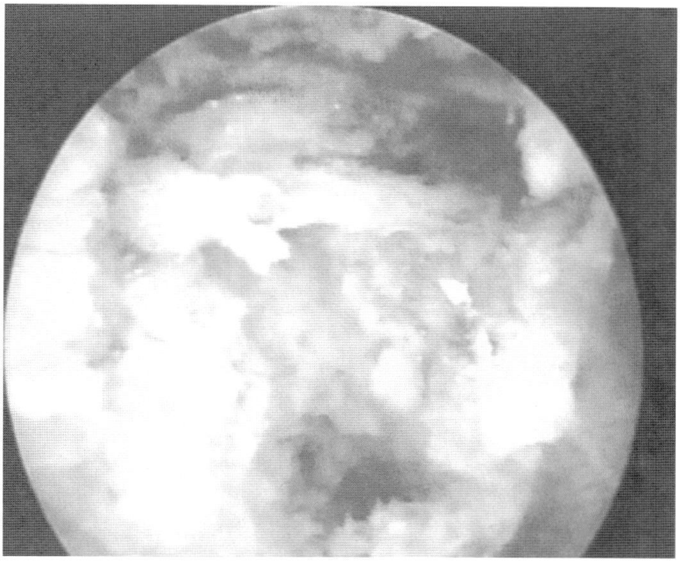

Fig. 17. Foraminal view of HNP. The indigocarmine-stained disc tissue has extruded past the posterior longitudinal ligament in this foraminal HNP at L4-L5.

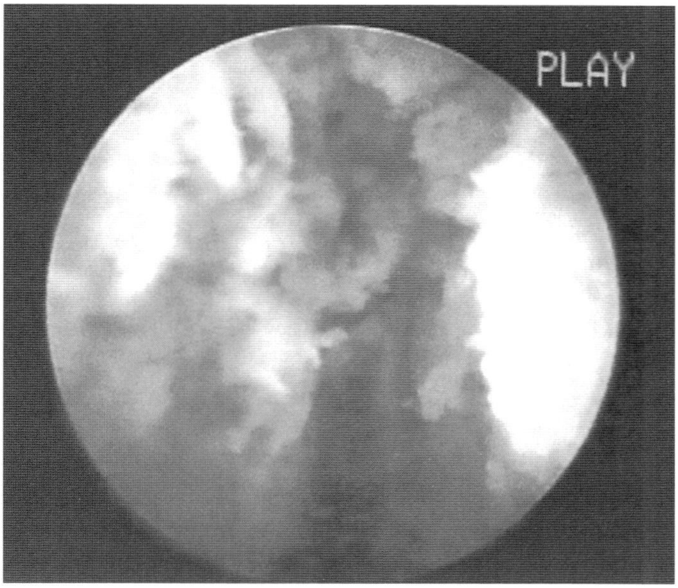

Fig. 18. Discitis. Intradiscal view of discitis after debridement. Usual findings of inflammatory disc material and loose end-plate cartilage are readily removed from the disc space. Pain relief is immediate, and abundant tissue is available for laboratory analysis.

stenosis and lack of fat around the exiting nerve (Fig. 19). Although trephines, rasps, and burrs can be used, the Ho:YAG side-firing laser is feasible as a visually controlled soft-tissue and bone ablation device. The cannula chosen for this task has an open side channel that will protect the exiting nerve while the laser is used to dissect the tethering

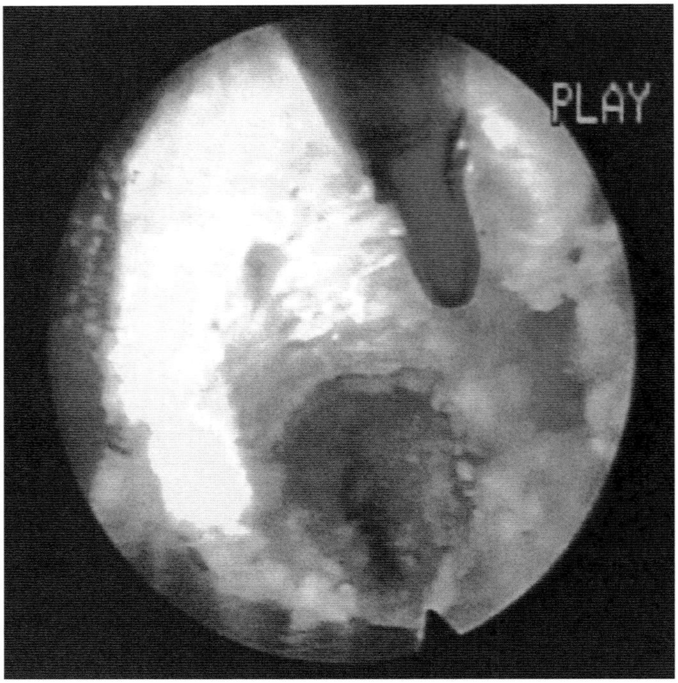

Fig. 19. Dissecting exiting nerve. In lateral recess stenosis, the scarred exiting nerve is released with a bare laser fiber. This picture demonstrates lateral recess stenosis as the most common cause of FBSS.

osteophyte and scar tissue from the nerve. Endoscopic foraminoplasty has not been shown to cause increased instability even in spondylolisthesis. When mild degenerative spondylolisthesis is present, the disc bulge can be successfully treated by selective discectomy and thermal annuloplasty when there is a sciatic component to the patient's complaint. The technique is most useful for lateral recess stenosis, a condition responsible for atypical leg pain rather than true intermittent claudication of central spinal stenosis. In central spinal stenosis, when there is concomitant posterior disc protrusion, decompression of the spinal canal can be effectively accomplished by resecting the bulging annulus in a collapsed disc, thus lowering the floor of the foramen. In isthmic spondylolisthesis, when there is more leg than back pain, this is usually owing to impingement on the exiting nerve by the pseudoarthrosis at the pars defect. The goal is then to decompress the compromised exiting nerve by elevating the dome formed by the inferior facet and lamina without further destabilizing the spinal segment.

Exclusion Criteria

Except for pregnancy, there are no absolute exclusion criteria, only relative contraindications depending on the skill and experience of the surgeon. Spinal endoscopy and spinal probing can be used for diagnostic purposes in extremely difficult or confusing clinical situations. Therefore, if endoscopy is helpful for diagnostic purposes, exclusion criteria may depend mainly on the accessibility of the spinal pathology and the endoscopic skills of the surgeon. The risks and benefits of the procedure must be weighed against the need to use this fluoroscopically guided procedure under local anesthesia or sedation.

Future Considerations

The spine scope will eventually be used for any condition for which visual inspection of the foramen is desired. I have used spinal endoscopy for the following reasons: to inspect a spinal nerve that is suspected of being irritated by orthopedic hardware adjacent to the pedicle, to remove suspected recurrent or residual disc herniations that do not show up on imaging studies, to decompress the lateral recess by foraminoplasty, to remove osteophytes and facet cysts that cause unrelenting sciatica, and to locate painful lateral annular tears or small disc herniations not evident on physical examination or MRI. In single- and multilevel discogenic pain, for which the patient has no viable options, endoscopic discectomy and thermal annuloplasty have been successful for treating chronic lumbar discogenic pain. A minority of patients may continue to have significant back pain, and a few may feel worse, but in the context of a progressive degenerative condition, the results are encouraging and will give most patients relief while awaiting the development of newer procedures such as nucleus replacement, total disc replacement, and minimally invasive stabilization procedures of the posterior spinal column.

Current Imaging Methods

In my experience, imaging studies are only about 70% accurate and specific for predicting pain. Conditions such as lateral annular tears, rim tears, end-plate separation, small subligamentous disc herniations, intranuclear herniations, anomalous nerves, and miscellaneous discogenic conditions are cumulatively missed approx 30% of the time. These conditions can be diagnosed by means of spinal endoscopy. Tears that are in the lateral and anterior aspect of the disc are routinely missed on MRI studies. Very small disc herniations that protrude past the outer fibers of the annulus are also missed because the fragment may be flattened against the posterior longitudinal ligament or nerve, appearing on the MRI as a thickened or bulging annulus, but really containing a subligamentous herniation. When the nerve root is "swollen" or enlarged, MRI is not always capable of distinguishing it from a conjoined nerve or a nerve with an adherent fragment of disc. When the disc tissue is in direct contact with the nerve, the nerve can be irritated and a painful inflammatory membrane forms. Even an epidural venous plexus that is inflamed can contribute to back pain and sciatica. Anomalous nerve branches known as furcal nerves are never seen on MRI but can be visualized with spinal endoscopy of the foramen.

When an inflammatory membrane is present, the patient's pain pattern can be confusing. Diagnostic spinal endoscopy has confirmed "nondermatomal" pain in scores of patients with proximal thigh, buttock, and groin pain at levels distal to the root origin of the anatomical area.

Technique

Accessing the foramen is simplified and standardized by drawing coordinates on the patient's skin to determine the optimal skin window and annular window for positioning the surgical instruments toward the center of the disc (Fig. 20). Reference points are the anatomical center of the disc, the superior facet of the inferior vertebra, and the skin window. The needle trajectory must also be in a line of inclination between the end plates of the adjacent vertebrae. Adjustments in the trajectory will be made to accommodate individual anatomical considerations and the pathology to be accessed.

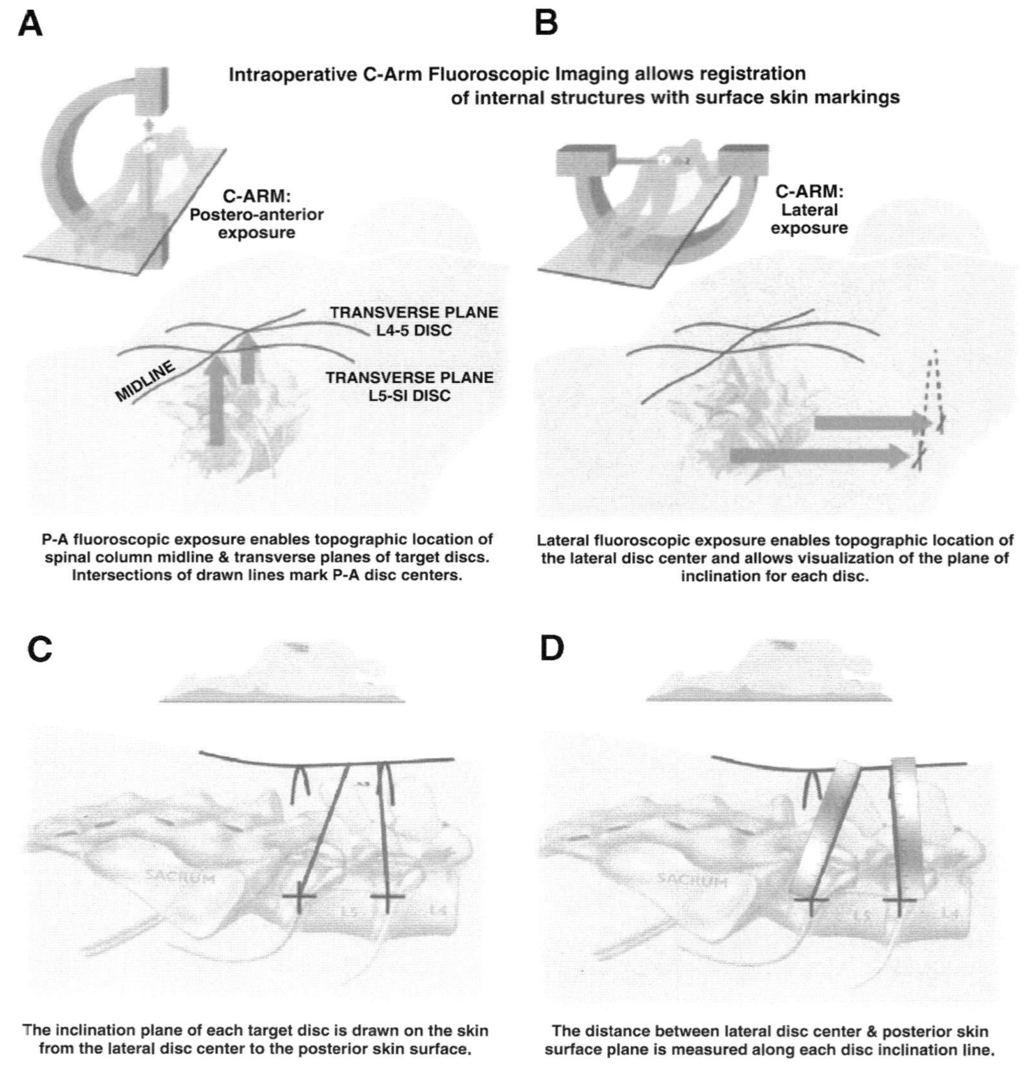

Fig. 20. YESS technique determination of optimal instrument path using the Yeung instrumentation trajectory protocol. Interoperative C-arm fluoroscopic imaging allows registration of internal structures with surface skin markings. **(A)** Posteroanterior fluoroscopic exposure enables topographic location of spinal column midline and transverse planes of target discs. Intersections of the drawn lines mark posteroanterior disc centers. **(B)** Lateral fluoroscopic exposure enables topographic location of the lateral disc center and allows visualization of the plane of inclination for each disc. **(C)** The inclination plane of each target disc is drawn on the skin from the lateral disc center to the posterior skin surface. **(D)** The distance between the lateral disc center and the posterior skin surface plane is measured along each disc inclination line. **(E,F)** This distance is then measured from the midline along the respective transverse plane line for each disc. At the end of this measure, a line parallel to midline is drawn to intersect each disc inclination line. This intersection marks the skin entry point of "skin window" for each target disc. Needle insertion at this point toward the target disc at an angle of 25–30° to the surface skin plane will determine the path of all subsequent instrumentation.

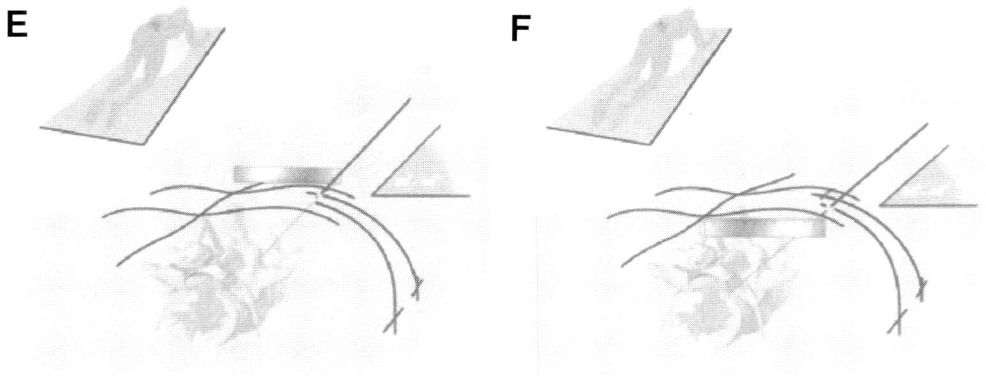

The distance is then measured from the midline along the respective transverse plane line for each disc. At the end of this measure a line parallel to midline is drawn to intersect each disc inclination line. This intersection marks the skin entry point or "skin window" for each target disc. Needle insertion at this point toward the target disc at an angle 30-25 degrees to the surface skin plane will determine the path of all subsequent instrumentation.

Fig. 20. *(Continued)*

Once the optimal trajectory is established, the cannulas are inserted to allow for endoscopic surgery under direct visualization.

Endoscopic spine surgery has a very high learning curve but is within the grasp of every endoscopic surgeon with proper training. As with any new procedure, the complication rate is higher during the learning curve, and it may vary according to the skill and experience of each surgeon. The endoscopic technique, because of its approach, may pose additional risk for iatrogenic injury, but it is possibly safer than traditional surgery because the patient is awake and able to provide immediate input to the surgeon when pain is generated. Those surgeons who can master the technique to the extent that they prefer endoscopic surgery over traditional surgery for the same condition will have the ability to perform the surgery without causing the patient undue pain. For most disc herniations and discogenic pain, experienced endoscopic spine surgeons will opt for the endoscopic approach as the treatment of choice for their patients.

The future of endoscopic spine surgery is extremely bright. There will soon be an explosion of new imaging systems, endoscopes, and endoscopic instruments. Refined techniques and image-guided systems may help diminish the learning curve. Coupled with advancements in tissue regeneration and enhancement of tissue healing, and the trend toward tissue healing instead of removal, regeneration over healing, and arthroplasty instead of fusion, the spine surgeon may no longer have to consider spine surgery as paradoxical. As a treatment modality, it will no longer be considered a last resort in a desperate patient. There will be a paradigm shift in the way clinicians view and approach patients with back pain, especially when endoscopic spine surgery is further validated with outcome studies and becomes routinely available.

REFERENCES

1. Kambin P. Arthroscopic microdiscectomy. Spine J 2003;.3(3 Suppl):60S–64S.
2. Kambin P, Casey K, O'Brien E, Zhou L. Transforaminal arthroscopic decompression of lateral recess stenosis. J Neurosurg 1996;84(3):462–467.

3. Kambin P, O'Brien E, Zhou L, Schaffer JL. Arthroscopic microdiscectomy and selective fragmentectomy. Clin Orthop 1998;(347):150–67.
4. Kambin P, Savitz MH. Arthroscopic microdiscectomy: an alternative to open disc surgery. Mt Sinai J Med 2000;67(4):283–287.
5. Hijikata S. Percutaneous nucleotomy. A new concept technique and 12 years' experience. Clin Orthop 1989(238):9–23.
6. Yeung AT. Spinal endoscopy with a multichannel, continuous irrigation, discoscope with integrated inflow and outflow ports (poster presentation), in North American Spine Society Annual Meeting, New York, 1997.
7. Yeung AT. Arthroscopic electro-thermal surgery for discogenic low back pain: a preliminary report, in International Intradiscal Therapy Society Annual Meeting, San Antonio, 1998.
8. Yeung AT. Classification and electro-thermal treatment of annular tears. in American Back Society Annual Meeting December 12, Las Vegas, 1998.
9. Yeung AT. Minimal access surgery for degenerative conditions of the lumbar spine, in 3rd Congress Meeting of the Chinese Speaking Orthopedic Society and Annual Congress of the Chinese Orthopedic Association, Taipei, Taiwan, 1999.
10. Yeung AT. Minimally invasive disc surgery with the yeung endoscopic spine system (YESS). Surg Technol Int 2000;VIII:267–277.
11. Yeung AT. The evolution of percutaneous spinal endoscopy and discectomy: state of the art. Mt Sinai J Med 2000;67(4):327–332.
12. Yeung AT. Selective discectomy with the yeung endoscopic spine system, in The Practice of Minimally Invasive Spinal Technique, (Savitz MH, Chiu J, Yeung AT, eds.); AAMISMS Education LLC, New City, NY:2000, pp. 115–122.
13. Yeung AT. Patho-anatomy of discogenic pain, in Minimally Invasive Spine Update, 1999. Disney Magic Cruise Nov 5–8.
14. Yeung AT, Tsou PM. Posterolateral endoscopic excision for lumbar disc herniation: surgical technique, outcome, and complications in 307 consecutive cases. Spine, 2002;27(7):722–731.
15. Yeung AT, and Yeung CA. Advances in endoscopic disc and spine surgery: foraminal approach. Surg Technol Int 2003;11:253–261.
16. Tsou PM, and Yeung AT. Transforaminal endoscopic decompression for radiculopathy secondary to intracanal noncontained lumbar disc herniations: outcome and technique. Spine J 2002. 2(1):41–48.
17. Yeung AT. The value of an intra-operative discogram: its role in arthroscopic microdiscectomy, in International Intradiscal Therapy Society Annual Meeting and San Francisco Spine Institute Course, 1995.
18. Yeung AT. The role of provocative discography in endoscopic disc surgery, in The Practice of Minimally Invasive Spinal Technique, (Savitz MH, Chiu J, Yeung AT, eds.) AAMISMS Education LLC, New City, NY:2000, pp. 231–236.
19. Carragee EJ, Tanner CM, Khurana S, et al. The rates of false-positive lumbar discography in select patients without low back symptoms. Spine 2000;25(11):1373–1380; discussion, 1381.
20. Carragee, EJ,Tanner CM, Yang B, Brito JL, Truong T. False-positive findings on lumbar discography: reliability of subjective concordance assessment during provocative disc injection. Spine 1999;24(23):2542–2547.
21. Yeung AT. Enhancement of KTP/532 LDD and AMD procedures with a vital dye, in AAOS Annual Meeting Scientific Exhibit, 1992.
22. Yeung AT. Considerations for use of the KTP laser for disc decompression and ablation, in Spine: State of the Art Reviews, 1993.
23. Yeung AT. Enhancement of KTP/532 LDD and AMD procedures with a vital dye, in International Intradiscal Therapy Society March 10–14, Phoenix, 1993.
24. Yeung AT. Enhancement of KTP/532 laser disc decompression and arthroscopic microdiscetomy with a vital dye, in AAOS Audio Video Program, AAOS 61st Annual Meeting, 1994.

25. Yeung AT. Laser as an adjunct to arthroscopic microdiscectomy, in North American Spine Society Annual Meeting, New York, 1997.
26. Yeung AT, Gore SA. Evolving methodology in treating discogenic back pain by selective endoscopic discectomy (SED). J Minimally Invasive Spinal Tech 2001;1:8–16.
27. Yeung AT, Morrison PC, Felts MS, Carter JL. Intradiscal thermal therapy for discogenic low back pain, in The Practice of Minimally Invasive Spinal Technique, (Savitz MH, Chiu J, and Yeung AT eds.), AAMISMS Education LLC, New City, NY:2000.
28. Yeung AT. Macro-and micro-anatomy of degenerative conditions of the lumbar spine (best paper presentation award), in International Intradiscal Therapy Society 16th Annual Meeting, 2003.
29. Yeung AT. Rauschning's anatomy for minimally invasive spine surgery, in Spine Across the Sea 2003, July 27–31, 2003.
30. Modic MT, Masaryk TJ, Ross JS, Carter JR. Imaging of degenerative disk disease. Radiology 1988;168(1):177–186.
31. Aprill C, Bogduk N. High-intensity zone: a diagnostic sign of painful lumbar disc on magnetic resonance imaging. Br J Radiol 1992;65(773):361–369.
32. Aprill CN. Diagnostic Disc Injection, in The Adult Spine: Principles and Practice Frymoyer JW, ed. Lippincott-Raven, Philadelphia, 1996, pp. 539–562.
33. Bini W, Yeung AT, Calatayud V, Chaabant A, Seferlis T. The role of provocative discography in minimally invasive selective endoscopic discectomy. Neurocirugia (Austr), 2002. 13(1): p. 27–31; discussion, 32.
34. Guyer RD, Ohnmeiss DD. Lumbar discography. Spine J 2003;3(3 Suppl): p. 11S–27S.
35. Guyer RD, Ohnmeiss DD. Lumbar discography: position statement from the North American Spine Society Diagnostic and Therapeutic Committee. Spine 1995;20(18): p. 2048–2059.
36. Yeung AT. Evocative lumbar discography: treatment of multi-level cases, in 1st World Congress American Academy of Minimally Invasive Spinal Medicine and Surgery, 2000.
37. Yeung AT. Discography, foraminal epidurography and therapeutic foraminal injections: its role in endoscopic spine surgery, in International 22nd Course for Percutaneous Endoscopic Spinal Surgery and Complementary Techniques, 2004.
38. Yeung AT. Intra-operative chemonucleolysis as an adjunct to arthroscopic microdiscectomy, in International Intradiscal Therapy Society Annual Meeting, 1997.
39. Yeung AT, Porter J, Merican C. SEP as a sensory integrity check in selective endoscopic discectomy using the Yeung endoscopic spine system, in 2nd World Congress American Academy of Minimally Invasive Spinal Medicine and Surgery, 2001.
40. Yeung AT. Failed back surgery syndrome, in The Practice of Minimally Invasive Spinal Technique, (Savitz MH, Chiu J, Yeung AT, eds.), AAMISMS Education LLC, 2000 pp. 293–296.

10

Minimally Invasive Posterior Fusion and Internal Fixation With the Atavi® System

Richard D. Guyer, MD and Terry P. Corbin, BS

INTRODUCTION

Although interest in minimally invasive posterior internal fixation and fusion has recently exploded, it is not because the technical developments are also recent. The foundations of these procedures were laid more than 60 yr ago, when the first endoscopes were used to examine patients' spinal nerves within the cauda equina *(1)*. From that beginning, the evolution was slow until several technological advances facilitated a safe and effective procedure with a reasonable learning curve.

The major milestones in this evolution are provided in Table 1 and are discussed in this chapter. The trend toward minimally invasive spinal surgery must be credited first to Lyman Smith, the developer of chymopapain for chemonucleolysis *(2)*. Although chemonucleolysis has been proven to have limitations, the initial interest generated has led to many other minimally invasive discectomy approaches, including mechanical techniques by Kambin *(3)* and Hijikata *(4)*, automated percutaneous discectomy *(5)*, and laser techniques *(6,7)*. Dr. Parviz Kambin made numerous contributions to the advancement of this field. In particular, he defined the "triangular working zone" for posterolateral approaches to the disc *(8)*. He also first used sequentially larger dilators to minimize the trauma of introduction of larger cannulae for more sophisticated intradiscal and foraminal procedures *(9,10)*. He developed a cannula with a side port through which an endoscope could be inserted for visualizing tools and anatomical structures (Fig. 1), and he later used an endoscope with a field of view at a 70° angle to the long axis of the cannula to view the surgical field.

As the pioneers refined the mechanical discectomy techniques, especially with the addition of endoscopic visualization *(11)*, the possibility of interbody fusion became a reality. Kambin *(9)* developed a technique using a powered reamer to decorticate the end plate. He subsequently reported that the fusion rate was only 57%, leading him to investigate the use of internal fixation to supplement interbody fusion *(12)*.

Several clinicians developed pedicle screw internal fixation approaches, following the early work of Magerl *(13)*, who used external fixation via screws into the pedicles to

From: *Arthroscopic and Endoscopic Spinal Surgery: Text and Atlas: Second Edition*
Edited by: P. Kambin © Humana Press Inc., Totowa, NJ

Table 1
Milestones in Evolution of Minimally Invasive Posterior Fusion

Year	Innovator	Milestone
1938	Pool	First report of endoscope use to visualize dorsal nerve roots
1955	Ottolenghi, Craig	Developed posterolateral approach for percutaneous transpedicular biopsy of vertebral body
1963	Smith	Beginning of minimally invasive spine surgery trend as a result of publication on chemonucleolysis
1968	Wiltse	Muscle-splitting approach
1983	Kambin	Muscle dilators used to prepare path for cannula
1987	Goldthwaite, White	Described pioneering efforts to decorticate transverse processes percutaneously
1987	Kambin	Triangular working zone defined for posterolateral approaches to the disc defined
1991	Kambin	Performs laminotomy through a cannula with endoscopic visualization
1991	Kambin	Performs endoscopic-assisted lumbar interbody fusion with percutaneous pedicle screw internal fixation
1994	Goldthwaite et al.	Patent application filed describing foraminotomy procedure performed through cannula with endoscopic visualization
1999	Knirk et al.	Validates concept of pedicle screw placement through Endius FlexPosure retractor in cadavers
2001	Jahng et al.	Confirms accurate pedicle screw placement possible through FlexPosure in sheep
2004	Winer et al.	Describes patient benefit of Atavi technique for posterolateral fusion with pedicle screw internal fixation

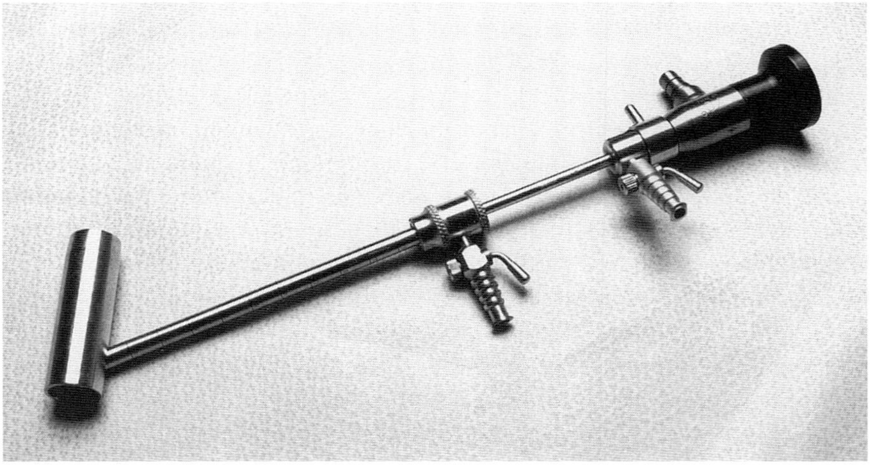

Fig. 1. Kambin cannula with endoscope in side port.

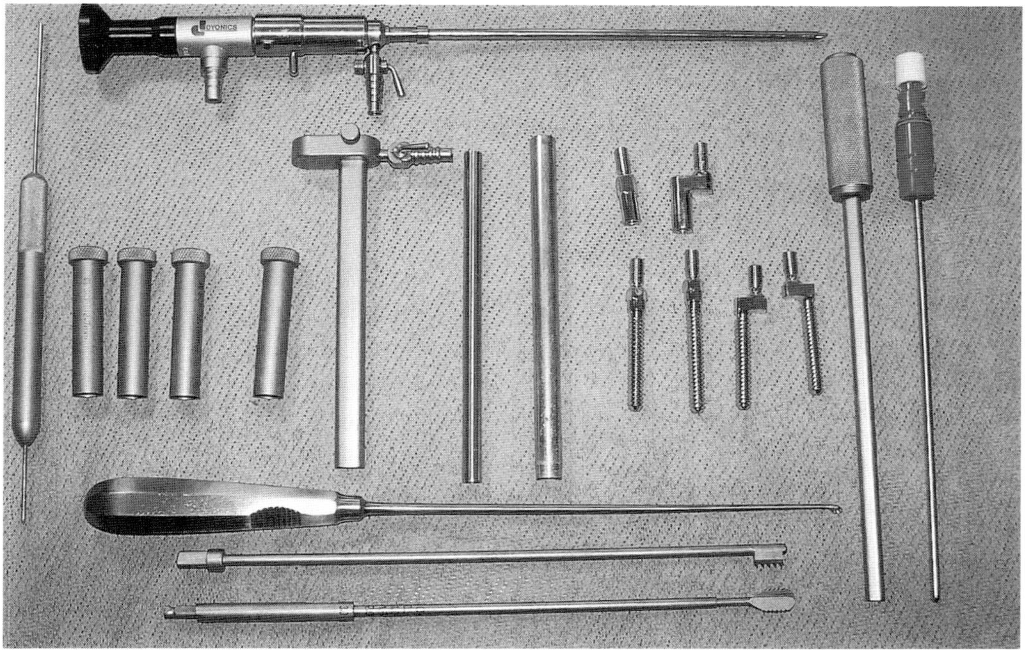

Fig. 2. Kambin instrument set for percutaneous interbody fusion and pedicle screw internal fixation.

temporarily stabilize the spine while interbody graft consolidated. Leu et al. *(14)* also used external fixation, inserted percutaneously, to make the procedure less invasive. Kambin used subcutaneous plates to connect the pedicle screws; the internal fixation hardware was removed in a second procedure approx 8 mo after implantation. He reported a 90% fusion rate using this construct *(12)*. The Kambin instrument set is illustrated in Fig. 2; a fluoroscopic image of the pedicle screws and further description of the Kambin procedure is included in Chapter 5.

Kambin achieved a good fusion rate with his technique, but there are limitations to this approach. Regan and Guyer *(15)* described the significant learning curve associated with procedures based on the Kambin anthroscopic microdiscectomy (AMD) techniques. The Kambin fusion approach requires a second surgery, as well. To avoid the need for a second surgery, Goldthwaite and White *(16)* used a different approach based on AMD: a percutaneous posterolateral fusion. They did not use internal fixation in their initial work, speculating that fusion could be enhanced with osteoinductive factors to obviate internal fixation.

Although it has been more than 16 yr since this speculation, growth factors such as rhBMP-2 are not yet available for use in posterolateral fusions. In 1996, Boden et al. *(17)* confirmed the feasibility of posterolateral decortication and graft placement through an endoscope working channel in an animal model for growth factor research. The initial clinical studies of rhBMP-2 for posterolateral fusion have been slowed by changes to the carrier needed to keep the growth factor from leaking out of the fusion bed. Because no

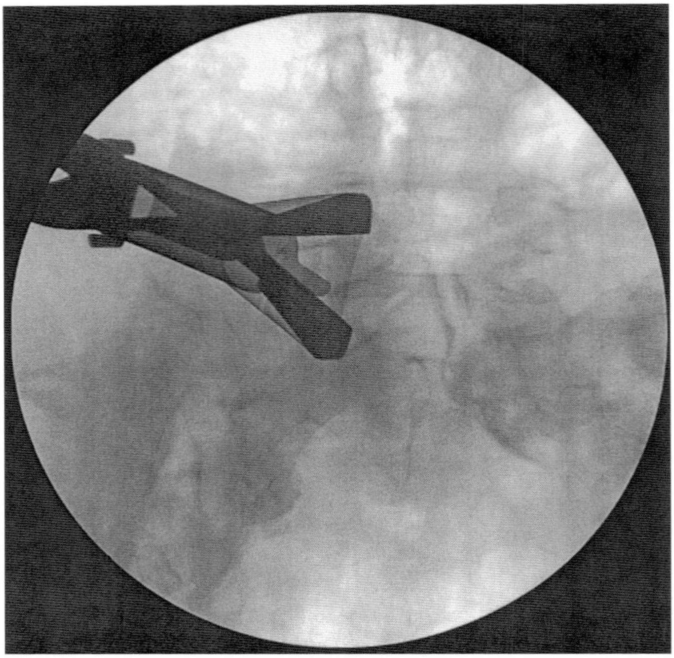

Fig. 3. FlexPosure retractor in position and expanded.

osteoinductive material is available to speed up and increase the likelihood of posterior lumbar fusions, internal fixation is still an important part of the spine surgeon's armamentarium.

THE ENDIUS ATAVI® MINIMALLY INVASIVE INTERNAL FIXATION CONCEPT

Endius developed an adjunct to the Kambin minimally invasive fusion technique that offers significant benefits. Its paradigm was to improve the available working space and visualization in the hope that this would reduce the learning curve associated with arthroscopic fusion. This was accomplished by designing the FlexPosure® retractor, which has an expanding skirt (Fig. 3). The original application was discectomy and decompression, but the early users quickly steered the development effort toward fusion and internal fixation. Fusion using the FlexPosure retractor is termed an Atavi procedure by its developers.

With the FlexPosure skirt expanded, there is sufficient space for a one- or two-level pedicle screw placement. Recently, oval retractors have been introduced, with fixed dimensions of 24 × 30 mm at the top, expanding to 40 × 80 mm at the bottom of the skirt. These retractors are used with the components given in Table 2 to perform the complete array of one- and two-level spine procedures.

Knirk and Osuna *(18)* conducted the first test of the FlexPosure retractor for delivery of internal fixation hardware. They demonstrated feasibility of accurate pedicle screw placement in cadavers. This was followed by an in vivo demonstration of feasibility in

Table 2
Major Components of the Endius Atavi System

	Description/use
Instrument/equipment	
FlexPosure retractor	Retractor with fixed dimension at top and expanding skirt at bottom
MDS microdebrider with Bipolar sheath	Shaver with Bipolar outer sheath; used for soft-tissue removal (including nucleotomy) with simultaneous hemostasis
Flex Arm®	Holds FlexPosure retractor and endoscope; easily repositioned with vacuum release button
Endoscope/camera	Endoscope features 30° view; high-resolution three-chip camera
Decompression instruments	Family of instruments optimized for use in minimally invasive decompression; includes angled Kerrisons, osteotomes, curettes, probes
Internal fixation implants	
Wave frame plate fixation system	Simple titanium plate-pedicle screw system for single-level posterolateral fusions
TiTLE rod fixation system	State-of-the-art titanium top-loading rod and pedicle screw system for one- and two-level fusions; unique features incorporated for MIS approach
MiCOR precision bone allograft	Used in MiLIF™ lumbar interbody fusion procedure

a sheep model by Jahng et al. *(19)*. Only 6% of the screws in this study were misplaced despite the small size of sheep pedicles.

Based on these results, in late 2000 several centers started a human study to evaluate the procedure and equipment. Shortly thereafter, hemostasis was improved with the addition of a bipolar sheath for the MDS™ microdebrider, which is used for soft-tissue removal. At the same time, a three-chip camera and a scope retractor mount were introduced, improving the arthroscopic image. These improvements reduced the incidence of procedures converted to open surgery owing to difficulties with visualization.

The preliminary study report *(20)* demonstrated that the theoretical advantages of minimally invasive fusion were achieved with this procedure. The average blood loss was only 280 mL, and the average hospital stay was 3.5 d. These are considerably lower than for comparable open surgery cases compiled by one of the investigational sites. In this early series, the longer-term outcomes were also good: the fusion rate was 88% and the average improvement in the Oswestry Disability Index was from 52 to 23 at 3 mo follow-up. Similarly, the visual analog 11-point pain scale score dropped from an average of 7.4 preop to 2.6 at 3 mo.

Most of these improvements were obtained in the first 6 wk, which again suggests that the theoretical benefits of minimally invasive fusion are being achieved. This rapid improvement is attributed to less damage to paraspinal muscles during the procedure. Kim and Fox *(21)* noted that multifidus intramuscular pressure is 30–40 torr (mmHg) lower

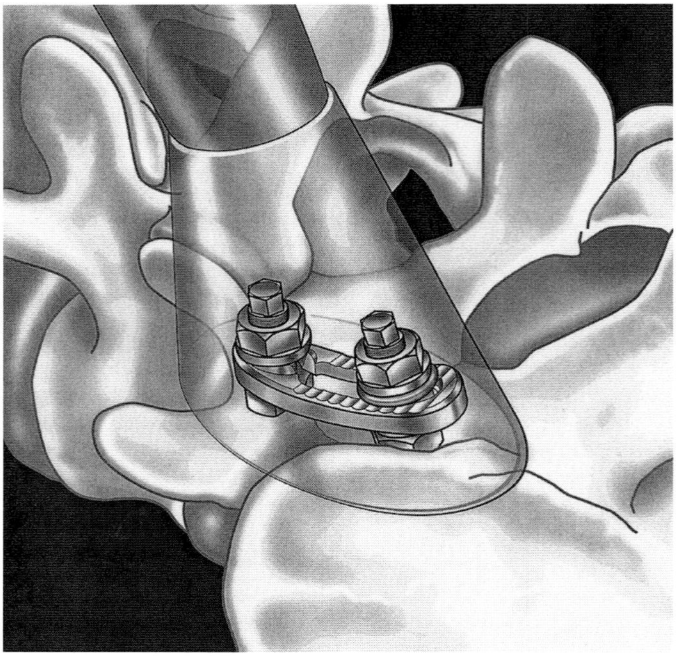

Fig. 4. Wave frame internal fixation system.

in Atavi fusions than in open cases. This results in muscle that looks healthier at closure and has less atrophy and edema *(22)*. The net is less postoperative pain and better function for the patient. Preserving the multifidus is particularly important because it contributes more than two-thirds of the stiffness of the lumbar spine—resistance to flexion/extension, lateral bending, and rotation *(23)*.

The original internal fixation system used in this feasibility study was called the Diamond Plate. This construct required assembly of two screws, four washers, one plate, and two nuts within the 21 × 35 mm operative field in the retractor. The Wave® Frame was introduced to simplify the technique; this plate has integral washers for easier assembly (Fig. 4). The FlexPosure retractor was recently expanded into a family with several new members:

- A 21-mm-diameter FlexPosure that expands to 25 × 40 mm.
- A 24-mm-diameter FlexPosure that expands to 30 × 63 mm, sufficient for a two-level posterolateral fusion with pedicle screw internal fixation.
- Two oval FlexPosure retractors with top dimensions of 24 × 30 mm, opening at the bottom to 40 × 50 or 40 × 80 mm, sufficient for a three-level fusion.

During the study any necessary spinal stenosis decompression was performed through a small midline incision. Subsequently, Hartjen et al. *(24)* have developed instruments and techniques for decompression through the FlexPosure retractor, eliminating the need for an additional incision. Endius has introduced a new visualization method by providing a mount for the FlexPosure that has an integrated surgical light. In this mode, procedures can be conducted under direct vision through loupes or an operating microscope (Fig. 5). This feature is particularly useful for decompression around the nerve roots. The depth perception afforded by the binocular vision adds to procedure safety. For the new user, the transition from an open technique to Atavi with direct vision is very easy.

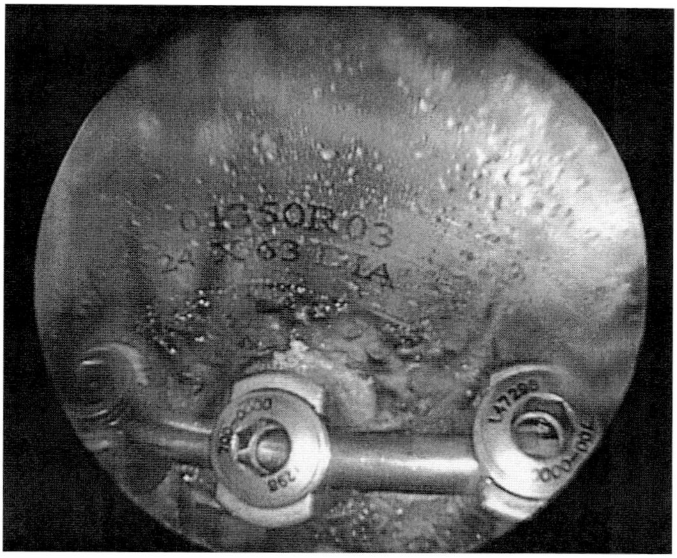

Fig. 5. TiTLE rod and pedicle screw system, endoscope view.

Two other improvements have been made to the internal fixation capabilities of the Atavi procedure. In September 2002, Endius introduced the TiTLE titanium rod and screw system (Fig. 5). This is a low-profile top-loading system optimized for assembly in minimally invasive fusion techniques. A notable feature is the friction in the multiaxial tulip; the tulip stays in position so that rod placement is easier. This system includes a complete set of instruments for distraction and compression. Whereas the Wave Frame plate was only available for single-level fusions, the TiTLE system can be used to make constructs up to three levels with pedicle screws at each level.

The most recent addition to the Atavi line is the MiCOR™ allograft block. These crescent-shaped implants are useful for minimally invasive interbody fusion procedures. A number of traditional posterior or lateral approaches to the interbody space can be accomplished through the FlexPosure retractor with the MiCOR graft and TiTLE internal fixation hardware *(22)*.

The Atavi procedure incorporates the muscle-splitting approach to the lumbar spine first espoused by Wiltse et al. (25). With the refinements introduced over the last 4 yr, all of the procedures described in Wiltse and Spencer's subsequent review (26) can be performed: decompression of lateral herniations and spinal stenosis, fusion, and pedicle screw internal fixation. Because the Atavi procedure is useful in most indications for lumbar spine surgery, the new user can overcome the learning curve and stay proficient relatively easily. With the addition of the oval FlexPosure retractor, the learning curve is markedly diminished (Fig. 6).

ATAVI PROCEDURE COMPARED TO EMERGING MINIMALLY INVASIVE FUSION/INTERNAL FIXATION TECHNIQUES

In addition to the Atavi procedure, several other approaches to minimally invasive posterior fusion with internal fixation have been described in the literature. In 2000, Muller et al. *(27)* described a "keyhole" approach for endoscopically assisted internal

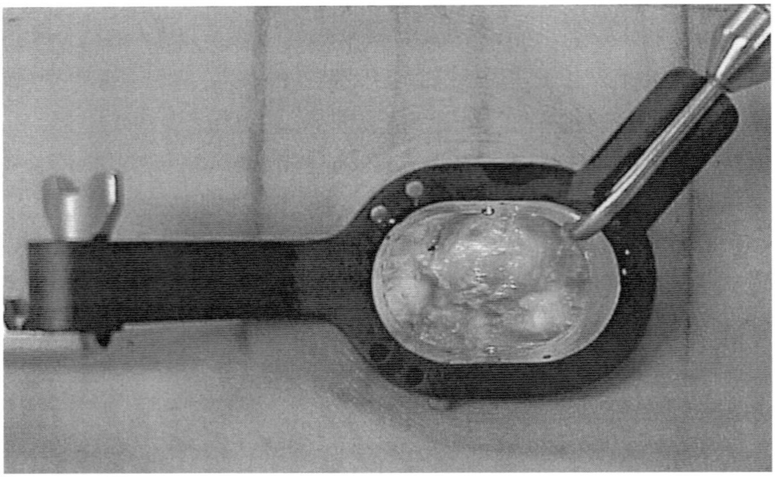

Fig. 6. Oval FlexPosure retractor with direct vision.

fixation. They used ports developed for thoracoscopic surgery for introducing the pedicle screws. The screws were connected by rods bluntly tunneled between the screws. The initial results in cadavers and a small number of patients demonstrated feasibility and screw placement accuracy of 93%. A limitation of the equipment used was the relative lack of room in the port when the endoscope was in position; the endoscope was removed when the screws were inserted. The ports must be removed to pass the rod between the screws, a blind procedure.

Foley et al. *(28)* described an internal fixation technique called the Sextant procedure by its manufacturer, Medtronic Sofamor Danek. This equipment is used to percutaneously insert pedicle screws and accurately connect them with rods. The primary application is internal fixation to supplement an anterior lumbar interbody fusion or posterior lumbar interbody fusion; there is no provision for posterolateral fusion. Like the Muller technique, the Sextant procedure involves blind tunneling for the rod passage with no provision for hemostasis in the muscle. A total of six small incisions are needed for a one-level fusion. Internal fixation for a two-level fusion can be provided by placing screws in the end vertebrae, skipping the intervening vertebra.

Spinal Concepts recently introduced the Pathfinder system for minimally invasive posterior internal fixation (Fig. 7). The system is similar to the Sextant approach in that it allows accurate blind placement of the rod through the pedicle screws. Rather than the multiple small incisions for Sextant patients, Pathfinder patients have one larger incision over the pedicles on each side. The surgical field is limited with the Pathfinder technique, similar to working through the early Kambin straight cannula.

Both the Sextant and the Pathfinder techniques depend heavily on intraoperative fluoroscopy in contrast to the Atavi approach, which allows placement of pedicle screws through either direct or endoscopic visualization.

CONCLUSION

The Endius Atavi system has incorporated the advantages of the Wiltse muscle-sparing paraspinal approach to the lumbar spine and the Kambin arthroscopic technique with a

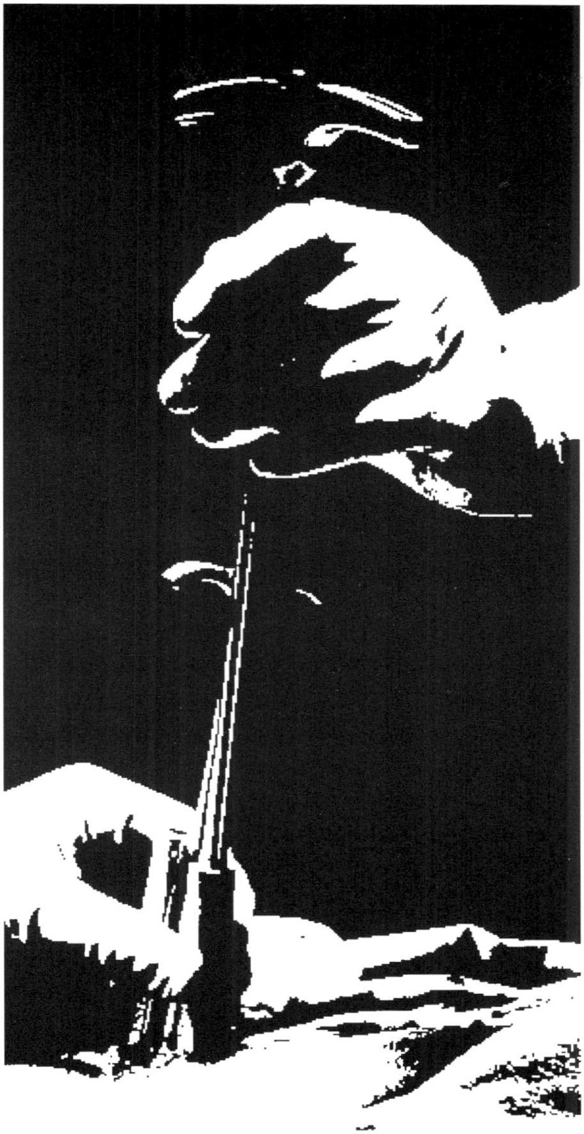

Fig. 7. Spinal Concepts Pathfinder equipment for internal fixation.

unique expanding retractor as the foundation for a family of products for minimally invasive lumbar spinal surgery. With the addition of the oval FlexPosure retractor, the learning curve is markedly reduced, and the larger surgical field allows application of similar techniques to open surgery. Although the equipment is new and the clinical follow-up is relatively short, there appears to be significant benefit for the patient in terms of reduced rehabilitation time and postoperative pain. The system can be used for most lumbar spine surgical procedures, which justifies the investment of time in learning the nuances.

REFERENCES

1. Pool JL. Myeloscopy: diagnostic inspection of the cauda equina by means of the endoscope. Bull Neurol Inst NY 1938;7:178–189.
2. Smith L, Garvin PJ, Gesler RM, Jennings RB. Enzyme dissolution of the nucleus pulposus, Nature 1963;198:1311–1312.
3. Kambin P, Gellman H. Percutaneous lateral discectomy of the lumbar spine: a preliminary report. Clin Orthop 1983;174:127–132.
4. Hijikata S. Percutaneous discectomy: a new treatment method for lumbar disk herniation. J Toden Hosp 1975;5:5–13.
5. Onik G, Helms C, Ginsburg L, et al. Percutaneous lumbar discectomy using a new aspiration probe. AJR 1985;144:1137–1140.
6. Ascher PW, Holzer P. Laser denaturation of the nucleus pulposus of herniated intervertebral discs, Arthroscopic Microdiscectomy: Minimal Intervention in Spinal Surgery (Kambin P, ed.), Urban & Schwarzenberg, Baltimore, 1991, pp. 137–140.
7. Sherk HH, Black J, Rhodes A, et al. Laser discectomy. Clin Sports Med 1993;12:569–577.
8. Kambin P, Brager M. Percutaneous posterolateral discectomy: anatomy and mechanism. Clin Orthop 1987;223:145–154.
9. Kambin P. Posterolateral percutaneous lumbar interbody fusion, Arthroscopic Microdiscectomy: Minimal Intervention in Spinal Surgery (Kambin P, ed.), Urban & Schwarzenberg, Baltimore, 1991, pp. 117–121.
10. Kambin P. Endoscopic spinal surgery past and future. Video presentation of endoscopic laminotomy and foraminotomy. Presented at the annual meeting of the International Society for Minimally Invasive Spinal Surgery, January 1991, Zurich, Switzerland.
11. Schreiber A, Suezawa Y. Transdiscoscopic percutaneous nucleotomy in disc herniation. Orthop Rev 1986;15:35–38.
12. Kambin P. Arthroscopic lumbar intervertebral fusion, in The Adult Spine: Principles and Practice, 2nd ed. (Frymoyer JW, Ducker T, Hadler N, et al., eds.), Lippincott-Raven, New York, 1997, pp. 2037–2047.
13. Magerl F. Stabilization of the lower thoracic and lumbar spine with external skeletal fixation. Clin Orthop 1984;189:125–141.
14. Leu H, Hauser R, Schreiber A. Percutaneous lumbar spine fusion. Acta Orthop Scand Suppl 1993;251:116–119.
15. Regan JJ, Guyer RD. Endoscopic techniques in spinal surgery. Clin Orthop 1997;335: 122–139.
16. Goldthwaite N, White AH. Toward percutaneous spine fusion, in Lumbar Spine Surgery: Technique & Complications, Mosby, St. Louis, 1987, pp. 512–522.
17. Boden SD, Moskovitz PA, Morone MA, Toribitake Y. Video-assisted lateral intertransverse process arthrodesis: validation of a new minimally invasive lumbar spinal fusion technique in the rabbit and nonhuman primate (rhesus) models. Spine 1996;21:2689–2697.
18. Knirk J, Osuna R. Endoscopically assisted posterolateral fusion with pedicle screw instrumentation: feasibility study. Paper presented at the North American Spine Society, Chicago, 1999.
19. Jahng TA, Fu TS, Cunningham BW, Dmitriev AE, Kim DH. Endoscopic instrumented posterolateral lumbar fusion with Healos and recombinant human growth/differentiation factor-5. Neurosurg 2004;54:171–180.
20. Winer M, Goodwin C, Hartjen C, Davison, T. Minimally invasive spine surgery with pedicle screw internal fixation; the Endius Atavi™ system, in Emerging Spine Surgery Technologies (Corbin TP, Connolly PJ, Boden SD, Yuan HA, Bao Q-B, eds.), Quality Medical Publishing, St. Louis, in press.
21. Kim KD, Fox A. The Atavi™ approach to minimally invasive spine surgery, in Surgical Techniques in Spinal Instrumentation (Kim DH, Vaccaro AR, Fessler RG, eds.), Thieme, New York, in press.

22. Winer MH, Alamin TF. Minimally invasive lumbar interbody fusion with pedicle screw internal fixation: the Endius Atavi™ system in The Practice of Minimally Invasive Spinal Technique, 2nd (Savitz MH, ed.), AAMISMS Education LLC, Richmond, VA, in press.
23. Wilke HJ, Wolf S, Claes LE, Arand M, Wiesend A. Stability increase of the lumbar spine with different muscle groups: a biomechanical in vitro study. Spine 1995;20:192–198.
24. Hartjen C, Martin R, Sweeney T. Technique for Decompression During Endoscopic Posterolateral Fusion Surgery, Endius, 2002.
25. Wiltse LL, Bateman JG, Hutchinson RH, Nelson WE. The paraspinal sacrospinalis-splitting approach to the lumbar spine. J Bone Joint Surg Am 1968;50:919–926.
26. Wiltse LL, Spencer CW. New uses and refinements of the paraspinal approach to the lumbar spine. Spine 1988;13:696–706.
27. Muller A, Gall C, Marz U, Reulen HJ. A keyhole approach for endoscopically assisted pedicle screw fixation in lumbar spine instability. Neurosurg 2000;47:85–95.
28. Foley KT, Holly LT, Schwender JD. Minimally invasive lumbar fusion. Spine 2003;28: S26–S35.

11
Vertebral Augmentation for Osteoporotic Compression Fractures

Daisuke Togawa, MD, PhD
and Isador H. Lieberman, MD, MBA, FRCS(C)

INTRODUCTION

Osteoporosis is a systemic disease currently afflicting approx 44 million Americans; this figure will increase as the population ages. It results in progressive bone mineral loss and concurrent changes in bony architecture that leave bone vulnerable to fracture, often after minimal or no trauma. The spine is the most common site of osteoporotic fracture, with vertebral compression fracture (VCF) occurring in 20% of people over the age of 70 yr, and up to 50% of women 80 yr and older *(1,2)*. Overall, 700,000 people per year in the United States suffer a VCF, exceeding even the frequency of hip fractures *(3)*. Osteoporotic VCFs have been shown to be associated with up to a 30% age-adjusted increase in mortality *(4)*. The cost to society of managing osteoporotic VCF patients in the United States in 1995 was $746 million *(5)*. Possible acute complications of vertebral fracture include cord compression, urinary retention, and ileus *(6)*. Long-term consequences include considerable pain (reported in 35% of detectable VCFs) *(7)* as well as pulmonary compromise (a 9% loss in predicted forced vital capacity with each vertebral fracture) *(8)*. Other chronic sequelae include deconditioning, deformity, insomnia, and depression, resulting in substantial physical, functional, and psychosocial impairment *(8,9)*.

Nonoperative Management of VCFs

Two-thirds of patients with acute, painful VCFs experience pain improvement regardless of the treatment applied. Traditional, nonoperative management includes bed rest, analgesics, and bracing. This type of medical management, however, fails to restore spinal alignment, and the lack of mobility itself can result in secondary complications, including worsening osteoporosis, atelectasis, pneumonia, deep vein thrombosis, decubitus ulcer, and pulmonary embolism. An alternative approach is supervised ambulatory mobility by a physiotherapist plus hydrotherapy *(10)*. In one-third of patients, severe pain, limited mobility, and poor quality of life persist despite appropriate nonoperative management. Whether the pain has resolved or not, no patient after a VCF spontaneously achieves a realigned spine, corrected sagittal contour, or restoration of vertebral height.

From: *Arthroscopic and Endoscopic Spinal Surgery: Text and Atlas: Second Edition*
Edited by: P. Kambin © Humana Press Inc., Totowa, NJ

Operative Management of VCFs

Historically, the only alternative to nonoperative management of symptomatic vertebral fractures was open surgical decompression (anterior or posterior decompression and stabilization via internal fixation hardware and bone grafting), and this was usually reserved for those patients with gross spinal deformity or neurological impairment (<0.5%) *(6)*. This surgical caution came about because of the adverse risk/benefit ratio in this elderly population with poor bone quality and multiple comorbid conditions.

Percutaneous vertebroplasty (PVP) is a minimally invasive method that involves the percutaneous injection of polymethyl methacrylate (PMMA) into a collapsed vertebral body to stabilize the vertebra. Originally developed for osteolytic metastasis, myeloma, and hemangioma, the procedure resulted in quick, effective pain relief and a low complication rate *(11–13)*. PVP is now also increasingly used for the treatment of osteoporotic vertebral fractures *(9)*. However, PVP does not expand the collapsed vertebra, potentially locking the spine in a kyphotic posture. In addition, the PMMA bone filler has associated problems (epidural leakage, thermal necrosis, inability to integrate with bone, handling difficulties, toxicity to patient and operator) *(2,14)*.

Kyphoplasty is an advanced minimally invasive technique with a number of potential advantages over PVP, including lower risk of cement extravasation and better restoration of vertebral body height *(15)*. A cannula is introduced into the vertebral body, followed by insertion of an inflatable bone tamp, which, when deployed, reduces the compression fracture and restores the vertebral body toward its original height, while creating a cavity to be filled with bone cement. The cement augmentation is therefore done with more control into the low-pressure environment of the preformed cavity with viscous, partially cured cement.

PERCUTANEOUS VERTEBROPLASTY

Background

Percutaneous vertebral augmentation (vertebroplasty, or PVP) was first reported by Galibert and colleagues in 1984 and initially involved augmentation of the vertebral body with PMMA to treat a hemangioma. PVP was reportedly not performed in the United States until 1994. Originally targeted for osteolytic metastasis, myeloma, and hemangioma, PVP resulted in early appreciable pain relief and a low complication rate *(13,16)*. Its indications subsequently expanded to osteoporotic vertebral collapse with chronic pain, and then further to include treatment of asymptomatic vertebral collapse and even prophylactic intervention for at-risk vertebral bodies *(17)*. Nevertheless, the treatment of acute fractures in ambulatory patients and prophylactic treatment remain controversial *(18)*. In fact, vertebral augmentation itself is somewhat controversial, with questions concerning a lack of defined indications, expected complications, outcome measures, and the need for long-term follow-up data *(2)*.

An open question in PVP is the mechanism of pain relief. The most intuitive explanation involves simple mechanical stabilization of the fracture. However, another possibility is the analgesic result from local chemical, vascular, or thermal effects of PMMA on nerve endings in surrounding tissue *(9,19)*. Supporting this concept is the lack of correlation between cement volume and pain relief *(20,21)*. Further evidence against an effect resulting solely from mechanical stabilization is the fact that PVP typically does not restore lost vertebral body height and therefore does not correct altered biomechanics *(1,18)*.

Technique

Injection of opacified PMMA is performed via a transpedicular or paravertebral approach under continuous fluoroscopic guidance to obtain adequate filling and to avoid PMMA leakage. For complex or high-risk cases, computed tomography (CT) and fluoroscopic guidance are sometimes combined *(11,18)*. In routine cases, PVP can be performed under local anesthesia with slight sedation in less than 1 h *(1)*, although general anesthesia is sometimes required because pain may intensify during cement injection *(9)*. Preceding PMMA injection, intraosseous venography is often used to determine the filling pattern and identify sites of potential PMMA leakage (outline the venous drainage pattern, confirm needle placement within the bony trabeculae, and delineate fractures in the bony cortex). However, some clinicians have dispensed with routine venography *(1)*.

Contraindications to vertebroplasty include coagulopathy, absence of facilities to perform emergency decompressive surgery in the event of a complication, and extreme vertebral collapse (>65–70% reduction in vertebral height) *(9)*.

Results

From 1985 to March 2004, 329 articles on PVP were published in peer-reviewed journals. Vertebroplasty data from more than 1000 patients have been reported in several case series *(1,11,13,18,22–34)*. The longest reported follow-up is 3 yr, although the first article on vertebroplasty was published in 1987. Reportedly, pain has been reduced in 70–90% of patients. There have been no reported cement failures, and only two reported cases of fracture progression in the treated vertebral bodies (caused by inadequate cement fill). Barr et al. *(18)* reported the results of 47 patients treated with vertebroplasty with an average follow-up of 18 mo. Their article outlines marked to complete pain relief in only 63% of patients with osteoporotic VCFs. Vertebroplasty, however, does not address the spinal deformity. In addition, this technique requires a high-pressure cement injection using low-viscosity cement, thus increasing the risk of cement leaks through the fracture clefts or the venous sinuses. Evans et al. *(26)* reported their retrospective results of 245 cases with an average follow-up of 7 mo. In thier study, pain score was significantly decreased and the ability to participate in an active daily lifestyle was significantly improved following vertebroplasty *(26)*.

Complications

The principal risk of PVP, which involves the forced injection of low-viscosity PMMA cement into the closed space of the collapsed vertebral body, is cement extravasation. Extravasation rates are as high as 65% when used to treat osteoporotic fractures *(13,28)*. The likelihood is greater when using cement with a liquid rather than paste consistency, or with higher PMMA volume *(25)*. However, in most settings, the majority of extravasations have no clinical relevance, at least in the short term *(1)*.

The consequence of an extravasation depends on its location. In epidural or foraminal extravasation, nerve root compression and radiculopathy is the major risk. This occurred in 11 of 274 patients (4%) treated by Deramond et al. *(11)*. Three of those patients required surgical nerve root decompression. Other clinicians have described a

5% rate of radiculopathy as well *(6,20,35)*. Extravasation into perivertebral veins can cause cement embolism to the lungs; deaths attributed to cement embolism have been documented. However, two reported deaths attributed to pulmonary embolism were felt to be unrelated to the procedure; no cement material was detected by chest X-ray of the first patient *(9,36)*, and the second pulmonary embolism arose from deep venous lower-extremity thrombosis *(11)*. On the other hand, extravasation into adjacent disks or paravertebral tissue, although common, generally produces no symptoms and carries little clinical significance; many such extravasations can be avoided by careful needle positioning *(11)*.

Other operative and long-term complications of PVP are specific to PMMA as a filler *(1,17,37)*. The physician may work with PMMA in large batches in order to keep it liquid and to extend the working time for vertebroplasty. However, its high polymerization temperature (86–107°C within cement core) *(38)* can damage adjacent tissue, including the spinal cord and nerve roots *(14)*, leading to an inflammatory reaction and transitory exacerbation of pain *(9)*. When injecting PMMA monomer, physician vigilance and caution is required. Absorption of PMMA monomer during the injection can induce hypotension by virtue of its cardiotoxic and arrythmogenic properties *(39)*. Placing a material in the spine affords proximity and access to the chest and the heart. Therefore, vertebral augmentation with PMMA demands meticulous attention to technique.

Overall, the risk of complications that carry clinical significance following PVP for osteoporotic vertebral fracture is felt to be 1–3%, and most potential complications can be avoided with good technique *(11)*.

KYPHOPLASTY

Background

Kyphoplasty is an advanced surgical technique that has evolved from a marriage of vertebroplasty with balloon angioplasty. It has a number of potential advantages, including lower risk of cement extravasation and better restoration of vertebral body height. A cannula is introduced into the vertebral body, via a transpedicular or extrapedicular route, followed by insertion of an inflatable bone tamp, which, when deployed, reduces the compression fracture and restores the vertebral body toward its original height. This then creates a cavity to be filled with bone cement. The cement augmentation can now be completed with more control into the low-pressure environment of the preformed cavity with viscous, partially cured cement. Using a cannula for bone filler with a steel stylet as a plunger enables the operator to apply cement at considerably higher viscosity than is possible with injection through a 5-cc syringe and an 11-gage needle. Both the higher cement viscosity and controlled fill reduce the risk of cement extravasation. Filling is performed under continuous lateral fluoroscopic guidance similar to vertebroplasty. The procedure can be performed under general anesthesia or local with intravenous sedation; most patients are able to return home the same day as the procedure.

Technique

With the patient under general or local anesthesia in prone position on a radiolucent spinal frame (Fig. 1A), two C-arms are positioned for anteroposterior and lateral fluoroscopic images (Fig. 1B). Once positioned, the C-arms and patient are not moved, to ensure repeatable images throughout the case. Two 3-mm incisions are made at the

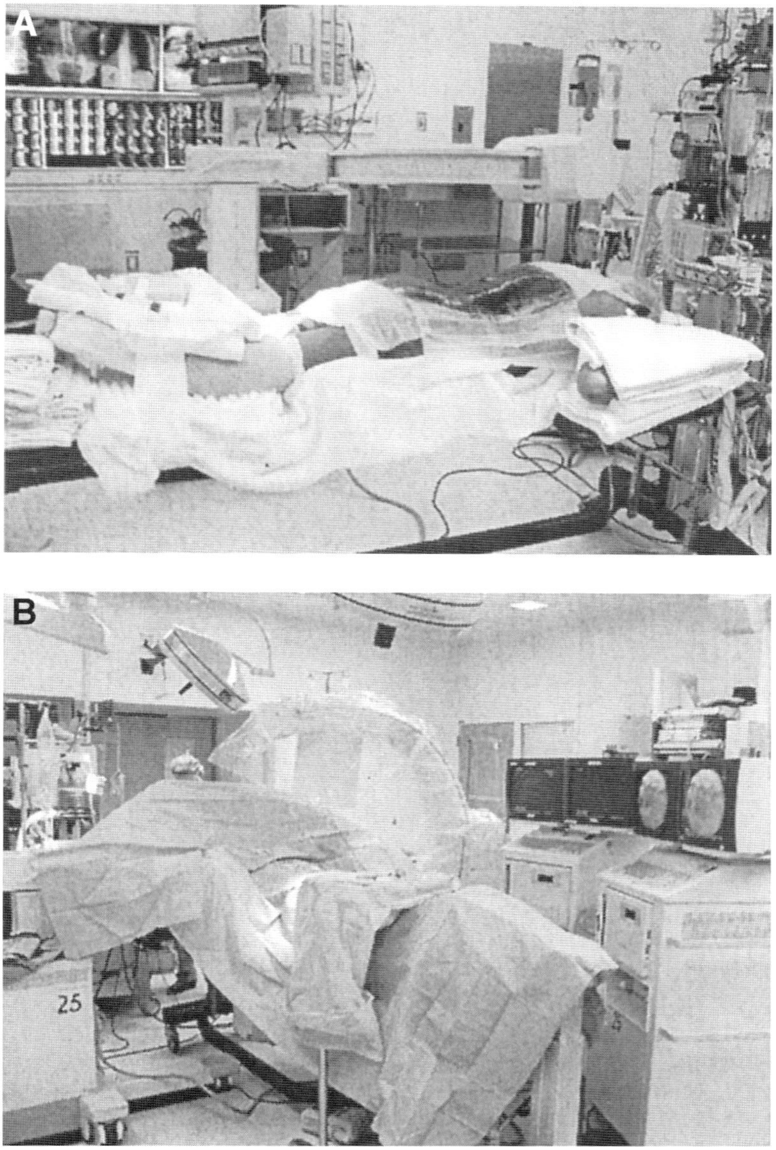

Fig. 1. **(A)** Patient and **(B)** operation room setup.

vertebral level parallel to the pedicles in both planes. Then a guide wire or biopsy needle is advanced into the vertebral body via a transpedicular or extrapedicular approach, depending on the fracture configuration and the patient's anatomy. The guide wire is exchanged for the working cannula using a series of obturators. Once the working cannula is positioned, the surgeon reams out a corridor to accommodate the inflatable bone tamp (IBT) and positions the IBT under the collapsed end plate. To deploy the IBT, inflation proceeds slowly under fluoroscopy until maximum fracture reduction is achieved or the balloon reaches a cortical wall (Fig. 2). At this point the surgeon deflates and removes the IBT, mixes the cement, prefills the cement cannulae,

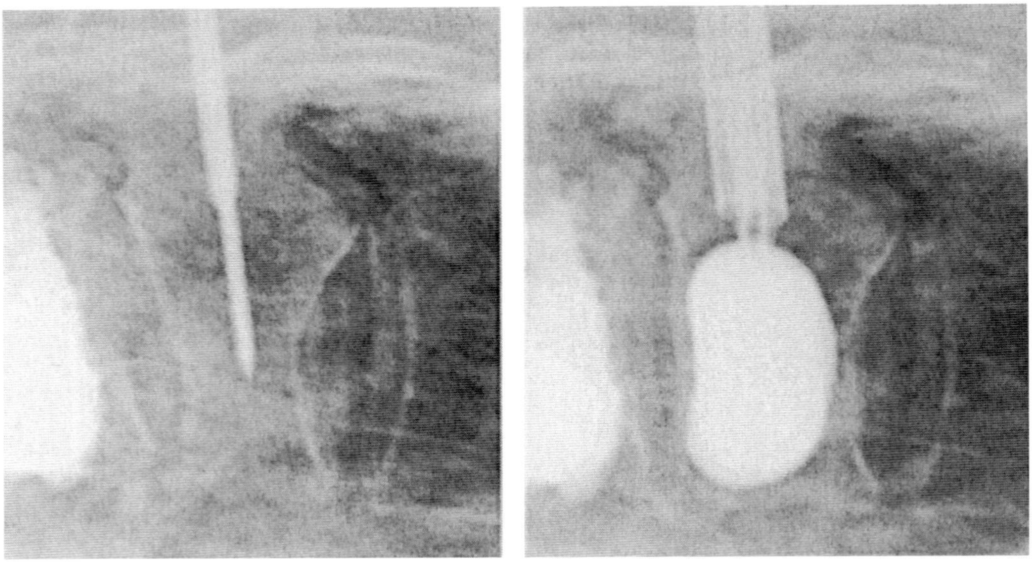

Fig. 2. Fracture reduction using IBT.

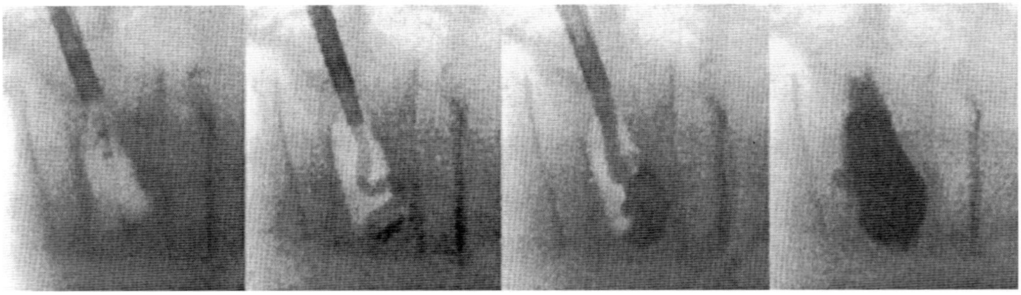

Fig. 3. Cement deposition.

and allows the cement to partially cure in the cement cannulae. Once partially cured, PMMA is slowly extruded into the vertebral body through each pedicle under continuous lateral fluoroscopic guidance (Fig. 3). This technique permits a controlled fill. In most instances, the volume of cement can slightly exceed that of the bone cavity to interdigitate filler from the central bolus with the surrounding bone. Once filling is complete and the cement has hardened, the surgeon removes the cannula and closes the 3-mm incisions.

Results

In our ongoing Institutional Review Board-approved study *(15,40,41)*, more than 900 consecutive kyphoplasty procedures were performed in more than 300 patients between April 1999 and February 2004. The mean age was 69 yr (range: 35–89 yr). The mean duration of symptoms was 7 mo. Outcome data were obtained by administering the Short Form-36 health survey (SF-36), and visual analog scale (VAS) for pain rating.

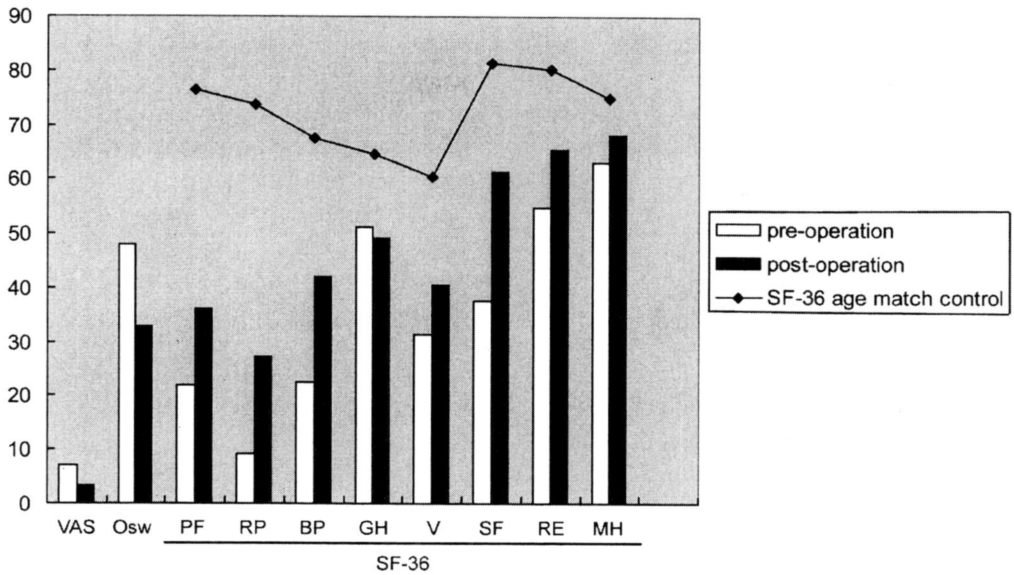

Fig. 4. SF-36 scores from ongoing Institutional Review Board-approved study. VAS, visual analog pain score; Osw, Oswestry disability index; PF, physical function; RP, role physical; BP, bodily pain; GH, general health; V, vitality; SF, social function; RE, role emotional; MH, mental health.

Additionally, the patients underwent detailed neurological and radiographical examinations pre- and postoperatively. Perioperative and clinical follow-up revealed that the procedure was well tolerated, with improvement in pain and early mobilization. The levels treated ranged from T3 to L5 with 47% of the vertebrae at the thoracolumbar junction. Length of stay ranged from 0.5 to 9 d (mean: 1.1 d). In our experience, no clinically significant cement leaks and no perioperative complications were attributable to the IBT or tools. Pre- and postoperative SF-36 data are available on more than 230 (72%) patients with follow-up ranging from 1 wk to 59 mo (mean: 14 mo). SF-36 scores improved in every category, statistically significant in all but the general health modality (Fig. 4). Physical function improved from 22.0 to 36.0 ($p \leq 0.0001$). Role physical improved from 9.3 to 27.3 ($p \leq 0.0001$). Bodily pain improved from 22.4 to 41.9 ($p \leq 0.0001$). Vitality improved from 31.4 to 40.7 ($p \leq 0.0001$). Social function improved from 37.7 to 61.2 ($p \leq 0.0001$). Role emotional improved from 54.8 to 65.5 ($p = 0.030$). Mental health improved from 63.1 to 68.0 ($p < 0.001$). General health did not change significantly, with a score from 51.3 to 49.2 ($p = 0.067$). The VAS scores improved from a preoperative level of 7.0 to an initial postoperative level of 3.2 ($p < 0.0001$). At last follow-up examination, the value had not changed significantly, with a score of 3.4 ($p < 0.0001$).

Ledlie and Renfro *(42)* reported functional and radiographic outcomes in the first 96 kyphoplasty patients with 133 fractures. Their follow-up period was a minimum of 12 mo, and the mean patient age at the time of surgery was 76 yr (51–93 yr). Regarding pain as rated by the patient using a 10-point VAS, the mean score was decreased to 1.4 at the 1-yr follow-up, whereas the mean preoperative VAS score was 8.6. Ambulatory status was also improved postoperatively. More than 90% (27/29, with 1-yr follow-up) of the patients were ambulatory at 1 yr, whereas only 35% (28/79) of the patients were ambulatory preoperatively.

Phillips et al. *(43)* also recently reported their early radiographic and clinical results of kyphoplasty. In their study, 29 patients with 61 fractures between T6 and L5 were evaluated. The mean age of the patients was 70 yr. Their clinical information including pain relief, improvement in activity, and satisfaction with the surgical procedur, as well as their sagittal spinal alignment on the standing radiographs, was assessed and followed up to 1 yr. Average pain scores were significantly decreased to 2.6 and 0.6 at 1 wk and 1 yr, respectively, whereas average pain score was 8.6 preoperatively.

In addition to good clinical results, height restoration by kyphoplasty has been reported in several studies. Our initial results showed height restoration in 70% of 70 fractured vertebrae treated with kyphoplasty. In patients in whom the vertebral fractures were reduced by kyphoplasty, vertebral height was increased by a mean of 46.8%.

Garfin et al. *(44)* reported in a prospective multicenter series that the average anterior and midline height were 83 ± 14 and 76 ± 14% before treatment, respectively, but were increased to 99 ± 13 and 92 ± 11% after treatment, respectively. In vertebral bodies with 15% or more of the estimated height lost, the average anterior and midline height were 68 ± 12 and 64 ± 13% before treatment, respectively, but improved to 84 ± 14 and 90 ± 12% after treatment, respectively *(44)*.

Ledlie and Renfro *(42)* reported from radiographic measures anterior and midline points of the fractured vertebrae using the two nearest normal vertebrae as reference points. At 1 yr, the anterior vertebral height was 85% of the predicted height and midline height was 89%, whereas their preoperative heights were 66 and 65%, respectively.

Phillips et al. *(43)* also reported that local kyphosis improved by a mean of 14° in patients with reducible fractures.

Complications

In our series of patients *(15,40)*, cement extravasation was seen in <10% of cases. No problems were identified clinically as a result of these extravasations immediately after surgery or at final follow-up. In one patient, a myocardial infarction occurred as a result of fluid overload during the procedure.

In a separate prospective multicenter series reported by Garfin and Reilley *(45)*, there were six major complications out of 600 cases associated with the kyphoplasty procedure. Four of these complications (0.75%) were neurological *(45)*. These were directly attributable to surgeon error and breach of technique.

To date, no reports of primary or secondary infection of the cement mantle have been published. In our series of more than 300 patients, we had no primary infections. We did, however, encounter one hematogenous infection 2 yr after the kyphoplasty in a patient receiving multiple blood and platelet transfusions for Waldenström's macroglobulinemia.

Ledlie and Renfro *(42)* reported that asymptomatic cement leaks were noted in 9% of vertebral bodies treated, but no device- or procedure-related complications were reported.

Phillips et al. *(43)* reported that asymptomatic cement leaks were observed in 6 of 61 (9.8%) vertebral fractures. In this series as well, there were no clinical consequences attributable to the bone tamp or cement deposition.

VERTEBROPLASTY vs KYPHOPLASTY

Although both vertebroplasty and kyphoplasty provide excellent pain relief, kyphoplasty has the potential to improve spine biomechanics and decrease the risk of cement extravasation. PVP usually will not expand the vertebral body or regain normal spine alignment. Hiwatashi et al. *(46)* reported an increase in vertebral body height after vertebroplasty to measure the vertebral heights in preoperative magnetic resonance imaging (MRI) and postoperative CTs. The heights of 85 vertebral bodies in 37 patients were measured before and after vertebroplasty in this study. The results showed an average increase in vertebral body height of 2.5 mm anteriorly, 2.7 mm centrally, and 1.4 mm posteriorly. However, the investigators did not distinguish height corrections from the positioning, and it is still unclear how much was corrected by the procedure itself. In addition, the significance of this methodology to measure the height between MRI and CT is uncertain. Preliminary data indicate that kyphoplasty may restore near-normal height, preventing kyphosis that leads to respiratory and digestive problems. Restoration of height and sagittal alignment may also work to protect vulnerable vertebral levels above or below the site(s) treated by minimizing force transfer.

The vertebroplasty technique is much more prone to cement leaks than kyphoplasty, because the PMMA is injected in a liquid state and will take the path of least resistance through any cracks in surrounding bone. In administering vertebroplasty, the operator injects the liquid cement, typically pausing or stopping once a leak becomes evident. On the other hand, in kyphoplasty, the expanded balloon creates a cavity and pushes bone to the edges of the cavity, thus sealing off potential fissures and cracks. Greater placement control is possible in a kyphoplasty, in which the operator can fill the cavity with a more viscous cement to the point at which the cement bolus reaches and interdigitates with the bony margins. The initial kyphoplasty findings show lower rates of cement extravasation compared with published results of vertebroplasty series, supporting the hypothesis that filling with high-viscosity cement into a previously formed cavity may be an improvement over the injection of low-viscosity liquid cement into the unreduced vertebral body.

CONCLUSION

Osteoporotic VCFs pose a significant clinical problem including spinal deformity, pain, reduced pulmonary function and mobility, as well as an overall increase in mortality in the elderly. Traditional medical and surgical options in many cases prove inadequate.

PVP is a relatively noninvasive technique that has gained increased acceptance over the last decade in the treatment of symptomatic osteoporotic vertebral fractures. The available clinical studies describe pain relief achieved in >90% of symptomatic osteoporotic fractures, with only infrequent, mostly minor, complications. Some of the drawbacks of PVP stem from the use of PMMA, because of its toxicity and poor handling characteristics, rather than from the procedure itself.

Kyphoplasty is a modification of PVP that may add a margin of safety by virtue of a lower observed incidence of cement leakage. Kyphoplasty has been shown to be worthwhile in acute vertebral fractures to predictably restore vertebral height and to facilitate a controlled fill of the vertebral body. Favorable outcomes in early trials appear to imply that kyphoplasty permits early mobilization, which has the potential to decrease mortality.

Considering the greater mortality that is associated with osteoporotic compression fractures, early mobilization in patients with vertebral fractures is of prime importance.

The next logical step beyond treatment of evident vertebral fractures is prophylactic augmentation. Prevention of osteoporotic vertebral fractures with a combination of pharmacologics and timely reinforcement of at-risk osteoporotic vertebrae is the ultimate goal aside from prevention of osteoporosis itself. It is here that new osteoconductive synthetic composites will figure more prominently as an emerging alternative to cement. Advances in minimally invasive surgical techniques, imaging, and synthetic engineering are rapidly changing the treatment protocols available for osteoporotic compression fracture.

REFERENCES

1. Heini PF, Walchli B, Berlemann U. Percutaneous transpedicular vertebroplasty with PMMA: operative technique and early results. A prospective study for the treatment of osteoporotic compression fractures. Eur Spine J 2000;9:445–450.
2. Einhorn TA. Vertebroplasty: an opportunity to do something really good for patients. Spine 2000;25:1051, 1052.
3. Riggs BL, Melton LJ 3rd. The worldwide problem of osteoporosis: insights afforded by epidemiology. Bone 1995;17:505S–511S.
4. Kado DM, Browner WS, Palermo L, Nevitt MC, Genant HK, Cummings SR. Vertebral fractures and mortality in older women–a prospective study: Study of Osteoporotic Fractures Research Group. Arch Intern Med 1999;159:1215–1220.
5. Ray NF, Chan JK, Thamer M, Melton LJ 3rd. Medical expenditures for the treatment of osteoporotic fractures in the United States in 1995: report from the national osteoporosis foundation. J Bone Miner Res 1997;12:24–35.
6. Bostrom MP, Lane JM. Future directions: augmentation of osteoporotic vertebral bodies. Spine 1997;22:38S–42S.
7. Cooper C, Atkinson EJ, O'Fallon WM, Melton LJ 3rd. Incidence of clinically diagnosed vertebral fractures: a population-based study in Rochester, Minnesota, 1985–1989. J Bone Miner Res 1992;7:221–227.
8. Leech JA, Dulberg C, Kellie S, Pattee L, Gay J. Relationship of lung function to severity of osteoporosis in women. Am Rev Respir Dis 1990;141:68–71.
9. Cotten A, Boutry N, Cortet B, Assaker R, Demondion X, Leblond D, Chastanet P, Duquesnoy B, Deramond H. Percutaneous vertebroplasty: state of the art. Radiographics 1998;18:311–320; discussion 320–313.
10. Patel U, Skingle S, Campbell GA, Crisp AJ, Boyle IT. Clinical profile of acute vertebral compression fractures in osteoporosis. Br J Rheumatol 1991;30:418–421.
11. Deramond H, Depriester C, Galibert P, Le Gars D. Percutaneous vertebroplasty with polymethylmethacrylate: technique, indications, and results. Radiol Clin North Am 1998;36:533–546.
12. Chiras J, Depriester C, Weill A, Sola-Martinez MT, Deramond H. [Percutaneous vertebral surgery: Technics and Indications]. J Neuroradiol 1997;24:45–59.
13. Jensen ME, Evans AJ, Mathis JM, Kallmes DF, Cloft HJ, Dion JE. Percutaneous polymethylmethacrylate vertebroplasty in the treatment of osteoporotic vertebral body compression fractures: technical aspects. Am J Neuroradiol 1997;18:1897–1904.
14. Deramond H, Wright NT, Belkoff SM. Temperature elevation caused by bone cement polymerization during vertebroplasty. Bone 1999;25:17S–21S.
15. Lieberman IH, Dudeney S, Reinhardt MK, Bell G. Initial outcome and efficacy of "kyphoplasty" in the treatment of painful osteoporotic vertebral compression fractures. Spine 2001;26:1631–1638.
16. Galibert P, Deramond H, Rosat P, Le Gars D. [Preliminary note on the treatment of vertebral angioma by percutaneous acrylic vertebroplasty]. Neurochirurgie 1987;33:166–168.

17. Bai B, Jazrawi LM, Kummer FJ, Spivak JM. The use of an injectable, biodegradable calcium phosphate bone substitute for the prophylactic augmentation of osteoporotic vertebrae and the management of vertebral compression fractures. Spine 1999;24:1521–1526.
18. Barr JD, Barr MS, Lemley TJ, McCann RM. Percutaneous vertebroplasty for pain relief and spinal stabilization. Spine 2000;25:923–928.
19. Mathis JM, Petri M, Naff N. Percutaneous vertebroplasty treatment of steroid-induced osteoporotic compression fractures. Arthritis Rheum 1998;41:171–175.
20. Cotten A, Dewatre F, Cortet B, Assaker R, Leblond D, Duquesnoy B, Chastanet P, Clarisse J. Percutaneous vertebroplasty for osteolytic metastases and myeloma: effects of the percentage of lesion filling and the leakage of methyl methacrylate at clinical follow-up. Radiology 1996;200:525–530.
21. Dean JR, Ison KT, Gishen P. The strengthening effect of percutaneous vertebroplasty. Clin Radiol 2000;55:471–476.
22. Cotten A, Duquesnoy B. Vertebroplasty: current data and future potential. Rev Rhum Engl Ed 1997;64:645–649.
23. Cortet B, Cotten A, Boutry N, Dewatre F, Flipo RM, Duquesnoy B, Chastanet P, Delcambre B. Percutaneous vertebroplasty in patients with osteolytic metastases or multiple myeloma. Rev Rhum Engl Ed 1997;64:177–183.
24. Weill A, Chiras J, Simon JM, Rose M, Sola-Martinez T, Enkaoua E. Spinal metastases: indications for and results of percutaneous injection of acrylic surgical cement. Radiology 1996;199:241–247.
25. Martin JB, Jean B, Sugiu K, San Millan Ruiz D, Piotin M, Murphy K, Rufenacht B, Muster M, Rufenacht DA. Vertebroplasty: clinical experience and follow-up results. Bone 1999;25:11S–15S.
26. Evans AJ, Jensen ME, Kip KE, DeNardo AJ, Lawler GJ, Negin GA, Remley KB, Boutin SM, Dunnagan SA. Vertebral compression fractures: pain reduction and improvement in functional mobility after percutaneous polymethylmethacrylate vertebroplasty retrospective report of 245 cases. Radiology 2003;226:366–372.
27. Cohen JE, Lylyk P, Ceratto R, Kaplan L, Umanskyt F, Gomori JM. Percutaneous vertebroplasty: technique and results in 192 procedures. Neurol Res 2004;26:41–49.
28. Cortet B, Cotten A, Boutry N, Flipo RM, Duquesnoy B, Chastanet P, Delcambre B. Percutaneous vertebroplasty in the treatment of osteoporotic vertebral compression fractures: an open prospective study. J Rheumatol 1999;26:2222–2228.
29. Cyteval C, Sarrabere MP, Roux JO, Thomas E, Jorgensen C, Blotman F, Sany J, Taourel P. Acute osteoporotic vertebral collapse: open study on percutaneous injection of acrylic surgical cement in 20 patients. Am J Roentgenol 1999;173:1685–1690.
30. Maynard AS, Jensen ME, Schweickert PA, Marx WF, Short JG, Kallmes DF. Value of bone scan imaging in predicting pain relief from percutaneous vertebroplasty in osteoporotic vertebral fractures. Am J Neuroradiol 2000;21:1807–1812.
31. Grados F, Depriester C, Cayrolle G, Hardy N, Deramond H, Fardellone P. Long-term observations of vertebral osteoporotic fractures treated by percutaneous vertebroplasty. Rheumatology (Oxf) 2000;39:1410–1414.
32. Kim AK, Jensen ME, Dion JE, Schweickert PA, Kaufmann TJ, Kallmes DF. Unilateral transpedicular percutaneous vertebroplasty: initial experience. Radiology 2002;222:737–741.
33. Kaufmann TJ, Jensen ME, Schweickert PA, Marx WF, Kallmes DF. Age of fracture and clinical outcomes of percutaneous vertebroplasty. Am J Neuroradiol 2001;22:1860–1863.
34. Ryu KS, Park CK, Kim MC, Kang JK. Dose-dependent epidural leakage of polymethylmethacrylate after percutaneous vertebroplasty in patients with osteoporotic vertebral compression fractures. J Neurosurg 2002;96:56–61.
35. Kuivaniemi H, Tromp G, Prockop DJ. Mutations in collagen genes: causes of rare and some common diseases in humans. FASEB J 1991;5:2052–2060.

36. Padovani B, Kasriel O, Brunner P, Peretti-Viton P. Pulmonary embolism caused by acrylic cement: a rare complication of percutaneous vertebroplasty. Am J Neuroradiol 1999;20:375–377.
37. Cunin G, Boissonnet H, Petite H, Blanchat C, Guillemin G. Experimental vertebroplasty using osteoconductive granular material. Spine 2000;25:1070–1076.
38. Leeson MC, Lippitt SB. Thermal aspects of the use of polymethylmethacrylate in large metaphyseal defects in bone: a clinical review and laboratory study. Clin Orthop 1993:239–245.
39. Phillips H, Cole PV, Lettin AW. Cardiovascular effects of implanted acrylic bone cement. Br Med J 1971;3:460, 461.
40. Coumans JV, Reinhardt MK, Lieberman IH. Kyphoplasty for vertebral compression fractures: 1-year clinical outcomes from a prospective study. J Neurosurg 2003;99:44–50.
41. Dudeney S, Lieberman IH, Reinhardt MK, Hussein M. Kyphoplasty in the treatment of osteolytic vertebral compression fractures as a result of multiple myeloma. J Clin Oncol 2002;20:2382–2387.
42. Ledlie JT, Renfro M. Balloon kyphoplasty: one-year outcomes in vertebral body height restoration, chronic pain, and activity levels. J Neurosurg 2003;98:36–42.
43. Phillips FM, Ho E, Campbell-Hupp M, McNally T, Todd Wetzel F, Gupta P. Early radiographic and clinical results of balloon kyphoplasty for the treatment of osteoporotic vertebral compression fractures. Spine 2003;28:2260–2265.
44. Garfin SR, Yuan HA, Reiley MA. New technologies in spine: kyphoplasty and vertebroplasty for the treatment of painful osteoporotic compression fractures. Spine 2001;26:1511–1515.
45. Garfin SR, Reilley MA. Minimally invasive treatment of osteoporotic vertebral body compression fractures. Spine J 2002;2:76–80.
46. Hiwatashi A, Moritani T, Numaguchi Y, Westesson PL. Increase in vertebral body height after vertebroplasty. Am J Neuroradiol 2003;24:185–189.

12

Principles of Transthoracic, Transperitoneal, and Retroperitoneal Endoscopic Techniques in the Thoracic and Lumbar Spine

Geoffrey M. McCullen, MD and Hansen A. Yuan, MD

INTRODUCTION

Endoscopes are rigid, straight, or angled systems that provide visualization, light, and magnification to anatomical areas, thereby avoiding larger open incisions. The endoscope consists of optical fibers and a light source. Each fiber delivers a separate piece of visual information to a camera and a video-integrated system. The camera processes the multiple image components into picture elements known as "pixels." To increase picture quality and clarity, the number of optical fibers and pixels would have to be increased. Given the size constraints of an endoscope, an increase in the number of optical fibers would require a decrease in fiber size. However, if the fiber becomes too small, the capacity to transmit light is significantly impeded. Presently, the maximum number of pixels in a camera system given the size constraints of the straight 10-mm-diameter thoracic or lumbar endoscope is 30,000. Zero and 30° angled scopes are most commonly used.

Imaging advances have assisted the safe implementation of minimally invasive strategies. In laparoscopic interbody fusions, the exact midline of the disc must be identified using a true anteroposterior fluoroscopic image with symmetrical pedicles and flat end plates. Radiation safety precautions should be followed to minimize the risks while working under fluoroscopy. Frameless stereotaxy, developed in 1992, was initially designed for intracranial use. The technique links the anatomy to a preoperatively acquired image. In endoscopic approaches, navigational systems have been difficult to apply because of problems with registration (precisely correlating anatomical landmarks with image reference points). External landmarks are not reliable as implanted fiducials for registration. A frame attached to a pedicle screw (placed percutaneously) can serve as a stable, fixed reference. A computed tomography (CT) scan is subsequently performed. Registration, using the geometry of the frame as fiducials, has been successful when used with endoscopic spine surgery *(1,2)*.

Intraoperative nerve monitoring can assess for nerve compression or irritability. Mechanically elicited electromyograph activity recorded in the muscles innervated by the lumbar nerve roots can alert the surgeon to nerve proximity.

From: *Arthroscopic and Endoscopic Spinal Surgery: Text and Atlas: Second Edition*
Edited by: P. Kambin © Humana Press Inc., Totowa, NJ

ADVANTAGES OF ENDOSCOPIC TECHNIQUES

The principal purpose of endoscopic techniques is to approach the spine through portals rather than larger skin incisions. At the target site, the same operative procedure is performed using an endoscopic approach as is performed using an open approach. Benefits include decreased soft-tissue disturbance, leading to lesser postoperative scarring and pain as well as reduced ultimate healing time. In addition, the entire operating team is able to watch the monitor during the procedure.

DISADVANTAGES OF ENDOSCOPIC TECHNIQUES

Spinal endoscopic procedures are technically demanding and require a dedicated effort to safely overcome the "learning curve." The vascular or thoracic surgeon and the spine surgeon should train together in the laboratory before performing live surgery on humans. The surgeon should always be prepared to convert the case to an open procedure with open laparotomy and thoracotomy instruments and vascular instruments close at hand.

THORACOSCOPIC SPINAL PROCEDURES (*SEE* TABLE 1)

In 1807, in Frankfurt, Germany, Bozzini was the first recorded individual to use an endoscope. Known as the "*lichtleiter*," this device used candle illumination to examine body orifices *(3)*. Lens and light amplification improvements followed. Throughout the 1920s, Jacobaeus, in Sweden, was the first to perform both laparoscopic and thoracoscopic procedures in humans *(4,5)*. He used a cystoscope and a heated platinum lighting loop. Thoracoscopic intrapleural pneumolysis was performed on patients with tuberculosis.

With improvements in medical management of tuberculosis, interest in thoracic endoscopic approaches waned from 1960 to 1990. In the early 1990s, renewed interest was experienced in thoracoscopy for the inspection and treatment of pleural diseases and for endoscopic pulmonary resection. During these procedures, excellent visualization of the thoracic spine was recognized. Thoracoscopic spine procedures began with the drainage of an intervertebral disc abscess *(6,7)*.

Similar to open thoracotomy, the majority of thoracoscopic procedures are performed in the lateral decubitus position requiring a dual lumen endotracheal tube for selective lung ventilation. Thoracoscopic spine surgery indications include anterior release of large (>80°) and fixed (corrects to <60° with push-prone views) scoliotic curves, Scheuermann's kyphosis >90° that fails to correct to <50° with hyperextension, anterior fusion in skeletal immaturity to decrease the incidence of postoperative crank-shaft, decompressive discectomy, and corpectomy. Endoscopic anterior instrumentation has been developed and is still evolving. Problems encountered include obtaining safe bicortical screw purchase and difficulties performing compression or distraction and rod rotation.

The recent introduction of the prone position for thoracoscopic spinal procedures offers benefits including a more familiar orientation, gravity-assisted retraction, gravity-assisted correction of kyphosis, elimination of the need for repositioning, and use of a standard single-lumen endotracheal tube *(8,9)*. Simultaneous posterior exposure and prone thoracoscopic release has been reported *(10)*.

Principles of Technique

With thoracoscopy, it is possible to visualize from T4 to L1 and thoracoscopic right or left approaches are possible. Compared to open procedures, thoracoscopic techniques cause less acute and chronic postoperative pain/intercostal neuralgia and improve pulmonary function *(11,12)*. In addition, improved shoulder girdle strength and range of motion *(12)*, decreased cost, and reduced hospital stay have been reported with the thoracoscopic technique *(11,13)*.

Thoracoscopic procedures are usually contraindicated in those patients who have undergone multiple anterior thoracic procedures with expected scar and adhesions. Patients with neuromuscular deformity and a history of pneumonia or empyema often have thick pleural adhesions. Those patients with significant restrictive lung disease will be unable to tolerate single-lung ventilation.

Lateral thoracoscopy requires single-lung ventilation, a double-lumen endotracheal tube, and high airway pressures. Correct placement of the double-lumen endotracheal tube followed by confirmation with fiberoptic bronchoscopy is necessary. The tube can dislodge, or tracheal tears may occur when turning the patient from supine to the lateral position.

When approached from the convex side of a scoliotic curve, single-lung ventilation must occur in the smaller lung on the concave side of the curve. Large scoliotic curves (>90°) result in a smaller chest cavity, limiting the space available to perform the endoscopic procedure successfully *(12)*. Patients with right idiopathic scoliosis have a more posterior aorta *(14)*. Whereas an open thoracotomy approach allows circumferential exposure of the spine so that a finger can be placed around the opposite side to protect the far-side vasculature during placement of screws, with thoracoscopic fusion such protection is not possible.

Prone thoracoscopy uses double-lung ventilation, with decreased tidal volumes and increased respiratory rate. There is less anesthetic preparation time with prone vs lateral thoracoscopy *(8,9)*. Postoperative oxygen requirements are decreased with double-lung vs single-lung ventilation *(9)*. The lateral position must be used for discectomy above T4 using an axillary portal anterior to the pectoralis major.

Intercostal neuralgia after thoracoscopy is not uncommon, occurring in approx 7% of cases *(15)*. Softer, flexible trocars have helped reduce the development of intercostal neuralgia. The sixth or seventh intercostal space is the safest region for entry for the first thoracic port. All subsequent port placements should be performed under direct visualization. Perforation of the diaphragm and parenchymal lung injury are best avoided by directly visualizing all instruments when introduced into the chest cavity.

With endoscopic instrumentation, screw pullout at the cephalad screw is usually the result of poor screw placement and unicortical purchase. Long screw tips adjacent to the aorta on the contralateral side are a cause for concern. Tension pneumothorax can occur secondary to overadvancement of a guide wire during cannulated screw instrumentation *(16)*.

Results

Thoracoscopic procedures have been compared with open procedures in clinical and laboratory studies. In the laboratory, thoracoscopic discectomy for release/fusion is equal to the open technique in the percentage of disc removal (76% for open, 68% for thoracoscopic) *(17)* and in the adequacy of the biomechanical release *(18)*. In scoliosis anterior release/fusion, the percent curve correction, blood loss, and complication rate are similar when comparing open and endoscopic methods *(9,12,19)*. The endoscopic technique is 28% more expensive, reflecting the cost of the expensive disposable tools *(20)*. Thoracoscopic release requires a 50% longer operating time compared to open thoracotomy *(14)*. The "learning curve" demonstrates improvement in operating times, with early thoracoscopic release taking 29 min/disc level, improving to 22 min/level with experience *(20)*. Thoracic disc excision for radicular and myelopathic patients has demonstrated a 70% clinical success rate, with a mean operative time of 173 min, blood loss of 259 cc, and average hospital stay of 4 d *(21)*.

LUMBAR TRANSPERITONEAL AND RETROPERITONEAL ENDOSCOPIC SPINAL PROCEDURES

In 1901, Ott *(22)* used a cystoscope to visualize structures within the pelvis. In 1902, Kelling *(23)* was the first to induce pneumoperitoneum in dogs. Oxygen followed by CO_2, was used for insufflation. In 1938, Veress developed the insufflation needle that bears his name and is still in use today.

In 1991, Obenchain and Cloyd described transperitoneal laparoscopic lumbar discectomy *(24)* (*see also* Table 2). Performed in a supine position, the technique is used to access the L4-L5 and L5-S1 levels. Laparoscopic instrumentation with BAK cylindrical interbody devices (Sulzer Spine Tech, Minneapolis, MN) was first reported in 1995 *(25)*. Typically three or four 1-cm portal sites are prepared: one or two for retraction, one for working instruments, and one for the endoscope. The posterior peritoneum is opened. Blunt dissection in the retroperitoneal space is performed in order to avoid injury to the parasympathetic plexus. Laparoscopic approaches to the L5-S1 level have been commonly performed because this space is below the bifurcation. The L4-L5 level can be difficult to expose when the level is above the bifurcation and the iliolumbar vein must be identified, ligated, and divided in order to retract the great vessels from left to right.

A balloon-assisted endoscopic retroperitoneal gasless (BERG) technique allowing the use of conventional instruments and avoiding the complications of CO_2 insufflation has been described *(26)*. The patient is placed in the supine position with a radiolucent support placed under the patient's left flank. An incision is made midway between the iliac crest and the costal margin along the midaxillary line. The external and internal oblique muscles are dissected bluntly. The transversus abdominus muscle is entered, exposing the retroperitoneal fat. Blunt finger dissection is used followed by introduction of a dissecting balloon. An endoscope is placed through the cannula into the balloon while the balloon is being inflated, allowing visualization of the expanding retroperitoneal space and close observation of the "receding line" of the peritoneum. A 2-cm incision is made 2 cm off the anterior abdominal midline. Dissection continues until the balloon is identified. A fan-shaped retractor is placed and is used to elevate the anterior abdominal wall. A retractor is used to displace the peritoneum and intra-abdominal contents medially. The balloon is deflated. The endoscope is used to visualize in a gasless working cavity.

The endoscopic retroperitoneal approach was first developed for urological surgical procedures and adapted for lumbar spine interbody fusion *(27)*. The procedure can be performed using gas insufflation, balloon insufflation (gasless), or a combination of the two techniques. A lateral decubitus positioning is utilized. A 2- to 3-cm incision is created at the intended level (L2-L5) that is centered on a line between the eleventh rib and the anterior superior iliac spine. Blunt dissection is performed through the muscles using an endoscopic trocar until the fat of the retroperitoneal space is identified. A dissection

Table 1
Thoracoscopic Spinal Endoscopy

Advantages	Disadvantages	Options
Improved visualization	Large (>90°) scoliosis curves creating smaller available "working space"	Lateral positioning: double-lumen endotracheal tube, single-lung ventilation
Less tissue dissection to accomplish approach	Inability to perform circumferential exposure for far-side tissue protection	Prone positioning: double-lung ventilation, simultaneous anterior/ posterior procedures
Similar discectomy extent and release capability when compared to open thoracotomy	Difficult but improving anterior instrumentation	

balloon is placed and inflated until a retroperitoneal cavity has been created. The balloon is removed and either CO_2 insufflation (to a pressure of 5 mmHg) or a self-retaining retractor system is placed. Typically, three ports are used: retraction, endoscope, and working instruments.

Principles of Technique

In transperitoneal laparoscopy, insufflation is required for visualization. To maintain pneumoperitoneum, the use of suction is limited. CO_2 insufflation can cause hypercapnia, elevation of the peak pulmonary pressures and mean arterial pressure, and CO_2 embolism (secondary to decreased diaphragm movements and increased CO_2 absorption). Despite a Trendelenburg positioning and the use of multiple ports, the small bowel mobilization and retraction remains a problem. Vascular mobilization can be even more difficult. Routine preoperative magnetic resonance imaging or CT scanning can be used to classify vascular anatomy *(28)*. If the bifurcation of the great vessels is above the L4-L5 disc space, a laparoscopic approach to L4-L5 is technically more feasible. Otherwise, the iliolumbar vein should be identified, mobilized, and ligated for exposure to the L4-L5 level.

Previous intra-abdominal or retroperitoneal operative interventions may create scar that adversely affects tissue mobilization and visualization. Laparoscopic procedures are unable to visualize the neural elements and to directly address spinal canal stenosis. Fusion for internal disc derangement with tall discs is a relative contraindication because it is more difficult to obtain adequate disc distraction. The larger interbody devices that would be required for fusion of tall disc spaces cannot be delivered through existing devices that would maintain pneumoperitoneum.

Retroperitoneal, lateral disc exposure can be used for access to L4-L5 and above *(2)*. Lateral endoscopic retroperitonoscopy has a reduced risk of small-bowel adhesions and autonomic plexus dysfunction *(27)*. Performed in the lateral decubitus position, this procedure allows the intra-abdominal contents to "fall away" from the spine. In the retroperitoneal endoscopy, the peritoneum is left intact, decreasing the postoperative complications related to manipulation of the bowel and disruption of the peritoneum. In addition, the intact peritoneum serves as a retractor aiding in the control of the bowel.

Table 2
Laparoscopic Spinal Procedure

Advantages	Disadvantages	Options
Anterior interbody fusion	Typically requires CO_2 insufflation; elevated mean arterial pressure, hypercapnia, embolism, unrecognized venous bleeding	Prone: transperitoneal, retroperitoneal gasless (BERG), L4-L5 and L5-S1; complications: vessel mobilization, retrograde ejaculation, ureteral injury
	No direct canal decompressive capability	Lateral: retroperitoneal, L4-L5 to L2-L3; complications: psoas, genitofemoral, and lumbosacral plexus injuries
	Interbody graft size/shape limitations	

With lateral retroperitoneal laparoscopy, the psoas is often very large and difficult to mobilize. A muscle-splitting approach through the psoas may lead to injury of the genitofemoral nerve or elements of the lumbosacral plexus. A transpsoas dissection at L5-S1 would risk the L4 and L5 nerve roots, the femoral nerve, and the obturator nerve and, therefore, is not recommended. The psoas muscle can be split more anteriorly than the dorsal fourth of the lumbar vertebral body from the cranial third of the L3 vertebral body and above. When the psoas is split at the caudal two-thirds of L3 or at L4 there is a risk of injury to the genitofemoral nerve *(29)*.

Results

In a study comparing transperitoneal laparoscopic vs mini-open approach, the complication rate was 20% in laparoscopic vs 4% in mini-open *(30)*. Sixteen percent of the transperitoneal laparoscopic approaches have been considered "inadequate," allowing one rather than two cages to be placed *(30)*. Approximately 10% of laparoscopic procedures have required conversion to open for repair of vessel lacerations or to close tears in the peritoneum *(31,32)*. There is no significant difference between minilaparotomy and transperitoneal laparoscopic approach when comparing analgesia requirements, time to resuming oral intake, or length of hospitalization *(30,33)*. Laparoscopy costs more ($1374/case on average) *(28)*. Laparoscopic operative time averages 167 min for single level and 215 min for multiple levels *(28)*.

Laparoscopic complications include vascular and peritoneal/visceral injuries. During laparoscopy, the insufflation pressure should be decreased to 10 mmHg or less during stages within the case to check for areas of venous bleeding that could otherwise go unrecognized at case completion. Retrograde ejaculation rate among males is high after lumbosacral laparoscopy—16–25% *(28,31)*—compared with a 6% rate with mini-open *(34)*. Avoiding monopolar electrocautery and limiting the degree of dissection along the left side of the aorta and the left iliac artery may help to minimize the risk of ejaculatory dysfunction *(28)*. Ureteral injury has been reported *(35)*. During transperitoneal laparoscopy, the sigmoid colon mesentery is approached from the right. The right ureter, traveling over the right iliac artery, must be identified before making the posterior peritoneum incision. In lateral endoscopic transpsoas approaches, a 30% rate of transient paresthesia in the groin/thigh region has been reported *(2)*.

CONCLUSION

Endoscopic spinal procedures are a relatively recent addition to the spine surgeon's armamentarium. The techniques offer the surgeon an enhanced visualization of the operative target site with less skin, soft tissue, and muscle disruption. Although there are definite benefits, these procedures are technically challenging and there are associated risks.

As new modalities are developed, care should be directed to prevent inventing new indications to justify the technique. The core indications for surgical intervention should not change. A "learning curve" should be expected and preparations made for it. Endoscopic technology will continue to evolve by merging it with biomedical advancements in robotics and image guidance systems.

REFERENCES

1. Bergey D, Regan J. Lateral endoscopic transpsoas spinal fusion: review of technique and clinical outcomes in a consecutive series. Spine J 2003;3:166S.
2. Brody F, Rosen M, Tarnoff M, Leberman I. Laparoscopic lateral L4-5 disc exposure. Surg Endosc 2002;16(4):650–653.
3. Bush RB, Leonhardt H, Bush IV, Landes RR. Dr. Bozzini's Lichtleiter: a translation of his original article (1806). Urology 1974;3:119–123.
4. Jacobeaus JC. Possibility of the use of the cystoscope for investigation of serious cavities. Munch Med Wochenschr 1920;57:2090–2091.
5. Jacobeaus JC. The cauterization of adhesions in pneumothorax treatment of tuberculosis. Surg Gynecol Obstet 1921;32:493–500.
6. Mack MJ, Regan JJ, Bobechko WP, et al. Application of thorascopy for diseases of the spine. Ann Thorac Surg 1993; 56:736–738.
7. Regan JJ, Mack MJ, Picetti G. A technical report of video-assisted thorascopy (VATS) in thorascopic spinal surgery: preliminary description. Spine 1995;20:831–837.
8. King AG, Mills TE, Loe WA Jr, Chutkan NB, Revels TS. Video-assisted thorascopic surgery in the prone position. Spine 2000;25 (18):2403–2406.
9. Succato DJ, Elerson E. Positioning for anterior thorascopic release and fusion: prone versus lateral. Spine 2003;E 28(18):2176.
10. Lieberman IH, Salo PT, Orr RD, Kraetschmer B. Prone position endoscopic transthoracic release with simultaneous posterior instrumentation for spinal deformity. Spine 2000;25(17):2251–2257.
11. Dickman CA, Detweiler PW, Porter RW. Endoscopic spine surgery. Clin Neurosurg. 2000;46:526–553.
12. Newton PO, Marks M, Faro F, et al. Use of video-assisted thoracoscopic surgery to reduce perioperative morbidity in scoliosis surgery. Spine 2003;28:S249–S254.
13. Han PP, Kenny K, Dickman CA. Horacoscopic approaches to the thoracic spine: experience with 241 surgical procedures. Neurosurgery 2002;51:88–95.
14. Succato DJ, Duchene C. MRI analysis of the position of the aorta relative to the spine: a comparison between normal patients and those with idiopathic scoliosis. J Bone Joint Surg 2003;85A:1461–1469.
15. McAfee PC, Regan JR, Zdeblick T, et al. The incidence of complications in endoscopic anterior thoracic and lumbar spinal reconstructive surgery. Spine 1995;20:1624–1632.

16. Roush TF, Crawford AH, Berlin RE, Wolf RK. Tension pneumothorax as a complication of video-assisted thorascopic surgery for anterior correction of idiopathic scoliosis. Spine 2001;26(4):448–450.
17. Huntington CF, Murrell W, Betz RR, et al. Comparison of thoracoscopic and open thoracic discectomy in a live ovine model of anterior fusion. Spine 1998;23(15):1699.
18. Wall EJ, Bylski-Austrow DI, Shelton FS, Crawford AH, Kolata RJ, Baum DS. Endoscopic discectomy increases thoracic spine flexibility as effectively as open discectomy: a mechanical study in a porcine model. Spine 1998;23(1):9–16.
19. Huang EY, Acosta JM, Gardocki, RJ, et al. Thoracoscopic anterior spinal release and fusion: evolution of a faster, improved approach. J Pediatr Surg 2002;37(12):1732–1735.
20. Newton PO, Shea KG, Granlund KF. Defining the pediatric spinal thoracoscopy learning curve: sixty-five consecutive cases. Spine 2000;25(8):1028–1035.
21. Anand N, Regan JJ. Video-assisted thorascopic surgery for thoracic disc disease: classification and outcome study of 100 consecutive cases with a two year minimum follow-up. Spine 2002;27(8):871–879.
22. Ott DV. Illumination of the abdomen. J Akusk Ahensk Boliez 1901;15:1045–1049.
23. Kelling G. Uberoesophagoskopie, gastoskopie and kalioskope. Munch Med Wochenschr 1902;52:21.
24. Obenchain TG. Laparoscopic lumbar discectomy. J Laparoendosc Surg 1991;1:145–149.
25. Zucherman JF, Zdeblick TA, Bailey SA, Mahvi D. Hsuk Y, Kohrs D. Instrumented laparoscopic spinal fusion: preliminary results. Spine 1995;20:2029–2034.
26. Thalgott JS, et al. Balloon-assisted endoscopic retroperitoneal gassless (BERG) lumbar discectomy and fusion, 15th Annual Meeting of the Joint Section on Disorders of the Spine and Peripheral Nerves, Orlando, 1999.
27. McAfee PC, Regan JJ, Geis WP, Fedder IL. Minimally invasive anterior retroperitoneal approach to the lumbar spine: emphasis on the lateral BAK. Spine 1998;23:1476–1484.
28. Kleeman TJ, Michael Ahn U, Clutterbuck WB, et al. Laparoscopic anterior lumbar interbody fusion at L4-5. Spine 2002; 27:1390–1395.
29. Moro T, Kikuchi S, Konno S, Yaginuma H. An anatomic study of the lumbar plexus with respect to retroperitoneal endoscopic surgery. Spine 2003;28(5):423–428.
30. Zdeblick TA, David SM. A prospective comparison of surgical approach for anterior L4-5 fusion: laparoscopic versus mini anterior lumbar interbody fusion. Spine 2002;25 (20):2682–2687.
31. Escobar E, Transfeldt E, Garvey T, Ogilvie J, Graber J, Schuttz L. Video-assisted versus open anterior lumbar spine fusion surgery: a comparison of four techniques and complications in 135 patients. Spine 2003;28(7):729–732.
32. Regan JJ, Yuan H, McAfee PC. Laparoscopic fusion of the lumbar spine: minimally invasive spine surgery. A prospective multicenter study evaluating open and laparoscopic lumbar fusion. Spine 1999;24:402–411.
33. Rodriguez HE, Connolly MM, Dracopoulos H, Geisler FH, Pobielski FJ. Anterior access to the lumbar spine: laparoscopic versus open. Am Surg 2002;68(11):982–983.
34. Kaiser MG, Haid RW Jr, Subach BR, Miller JS, Smith CD, Rodts GE Jr. Comparison of mini-open versus laparoscopic approach for anterior lumbar interbody fusion: a retrospective review. Neurosurgery 2002;51:97–105.
35. Guingrich JA, McDermott JC. Ureteral injury during laparoscopy-assisted anterior lumbar fusion. Spine 2000;25(12):1586–1588.

13

Use of Laser in Minimally Invasive Spinal Surgery and Pain Management

John C. Chiu, MD, DSc and Martin H. Savitz, MD, PhD

INTRODUCTION

Arthur L. Schawlow and Charles H. Townes are credited with the invention of the laser—light amplification by stimulated emission of radiation—dating back to 1958 with the publication of "Infrared and Optical Lasers." The work of Schawlow and Townes traced back to the 1940s, when there was an attempt to create a device for studying molecular structure *(1)*. Extending the research from microwaves to the infrared region of the spectrum required a series of mirrors to focus the shorter wavelengths. In 1960, a patent was granted for the laser. Townes was awarded the Nobel Prize in Physics in 1964, and Schawlow in 1981 *(2)*.

Numerous applications in medicine have been adapted to the specialties of ophthalmology, plastic surgery, urology, vascular surgery, general surgery, gynecology, neurosurgery, and orthopedics. Ascher *(1)* in Germany was one of the first investigators to employ the CO_2 and neodymium lasers in neurosurgery. His experience with hemostasis and vaporization in the resection of tumors of the brain and spine was extensive.

LASER DISCECTOMY

In 1985, Ascher *(3)* applied laser technique to disc surgery. Measurements of the intradiscal pressure were made before and after laser discectomy with a saline manometer in order to document objectively the pathophysiological effect. In 1990, Yonezawa et al. *(4)*, in Japan, used the neodymium:yttrium-aluminum-garnet (Nd:YAG) laser through a double-lumen needle with a bare quartz fiber. The tip-type pressure transducer was similarly able to record the preoperative and postoperative intradiscal pressure. In 1992, Davis *(5)* employed the potassium-trideuterium-phosphate (KTP) laser for lumbar disc ablation and considered the success rate (32 of 40 patients, or 80%) equivalent to the results obtained by Onik *(6)* with his nucleotome and automated percutaneous lumbar discectomy. Again in 1992, Choy et al. *(7)* reported percutaneous laser discectomy (PLD) with the Nd:YAG laser; 333 cases of herniated, nonsequestered lumbar discs were diagnosed by computed tomography (CT) and/or magnetic resonance imaging (MRI). The success rate at an outpatient surgical facility was 78.4% over a 5-yr period,

From: *Arthroscopic and Endoscopic Spinal Surgery: Text and Atlas: Second Edition*
Edited by: P. Kambin © Humana Press Inc., Totowa, NJ

Table 1
Studies of PLDs From 1994 to 1999

Authors/ref.	Year	Laser	Cases
Ohnmeiss et al. *(13)*	1994	Nd:YAG	204
Simons et al. *(14)*	1994	Nd:YAG	150
Schatz and Talalla *(15)*	1995	Nd:YAG	500
Liebler *(16)*	1995	Nd:YAG	333
		KTP	117
Siebert et al. *(17)*	1996	Nd:YAG	180
Casper et al. *(18)*	1996	Ho:YAG	50
Nerubay et al. *(19)*	1997	CO_2	50
Pedachenko et al. *(20)*	1998	Nd:YAG	273
Hellinger *(8)*	1999	Nd:YAG	2535

and the follow-up was 12–62 mo (average: 26 mo). One-third of repeat MRIs showed a moderate decrease in disc herniation. Kambin *(8)* reported the effects of the CO_2, Nd:YAG, and holmium (Ho).YAG lasers on the nucleus pulposus in cadaveric discs in 1991. Sherk et al. *(9)*, beginning in 1993 and continuing to the present, have performed laser discectomy on a series of patients.

Between 1994 and 1999, nine series of PLDs were reported (Table 1), totaling more than 4300 patients. The overall success rate was about 80%. Hellinger *(10)* operated on 38 thoracic disc herniations. Isolated postoperative complications including transient foot drop, permanent traumatic neuropathies, pleuritis, pneumothorax, and complex regional pain syndrome *(11)* were <1% *(12)*.

A variety of wave configurations and powers created a 1.5-cm^3 defect in the center of the disc. Adjoining tissue was studied histologically for possible thermal effect *(8)*. Thermocouples were placed in adjacent nerve roots, end plates, and posterior longitudinal ligaments to record temperature changes. Intradiscal pressure measurements were also made before and after laser ablation. All of the lasers caused minimal temperature elevations to 102°F in the nerve roots. Histological slides confirmed that the free-beam Nd:YAG caused an excessive thermal change in the end plates and nerve roots. Further findings included the fact that 1200–1500 J of laser energy diminished the intradiscal pressure by 25–50%. The free-beam CO_2 was not practical because the laser could not easily be delivered into the disc space. The Nd:YAG contact fiber and the Ho:YAG fiber were readily inserted through a needle, and both delivered effective amounts of laser energy.

The published advantages of PLD *(21–25)* include simplicity of minimally invasive technique, small caliber of instruments, documented reduction in intradiscal pressure, low rate of complication, and no spinal instability. Blind laser nucleolysis through a posterolateral approach *(26,27)* has a number of limitations and disadvantages: minimal flexibility, inability to reach subligamentous fragments, no documentation of area of vaporization of collagenized nucleus, and lack of control of thermal spread to nerve root and end plates. Blind PLD, like automated percutaneous lumbar discectomy, occupies an important place in the history of minimally invasive surgery and is still

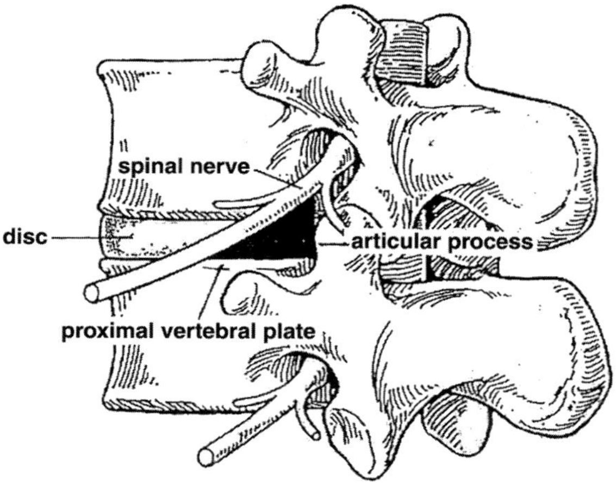

Fig. 1. The triangular working zone represents ample access for a percutaneous approach to lumbar disc space.

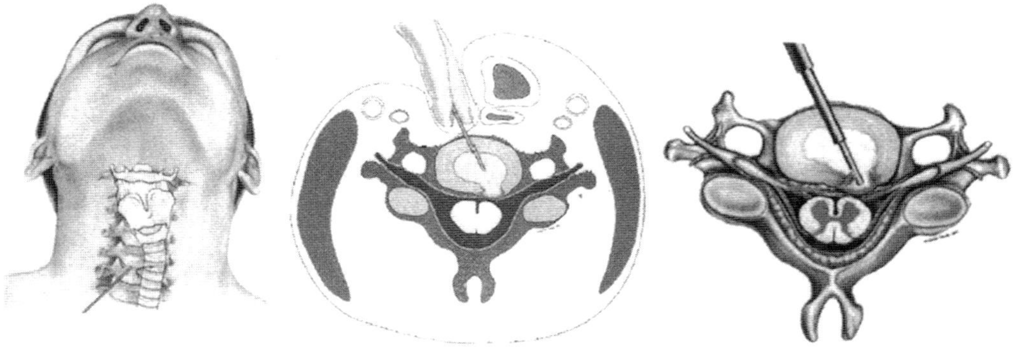

Fig. 2. Drawing of anterior approach to cervical disc and insertion of spinal needle followed by nucleotome *(28)*.

performed by some spinal surgeons. Most minimally invasive spinal surgeons prefer mechanical removal of disc material following proper positioning of instruments in the triangular working zone (Fig. 1) *(6)* (*see* Chapter 4). Other surgeons use both instruments and laser modulation under endoscopic control *(28–32)* (Fig. 1). Monitoring the thermal effects of the laser on neural tissue mitigates almost all complications. The use of the laser can also be extended and expanded under direct visualization.

Interventional procedures on the spine in cases of discogenic pain syndromes should not merely be measured by their success rate but also by the resulting amount of postoperative complications *(21–25)*. Particular attention should be devoted to sequelae resulting from spinal interventions including injections in close proximity to the spine. Nerve blocks or paravertebral infiltrations can result in disasters such as paraplegia *(24,25)*. During October and November of 1989, Siebert and colleagues *(15–17)* (abdominal position) and Hellinger *(21)* (lateral position) introduced nonendoscopic percutaneous laser disc decompression and nucleotomy with the Nd:YAG laser in Germany, after Ascher *(1)* and Choy

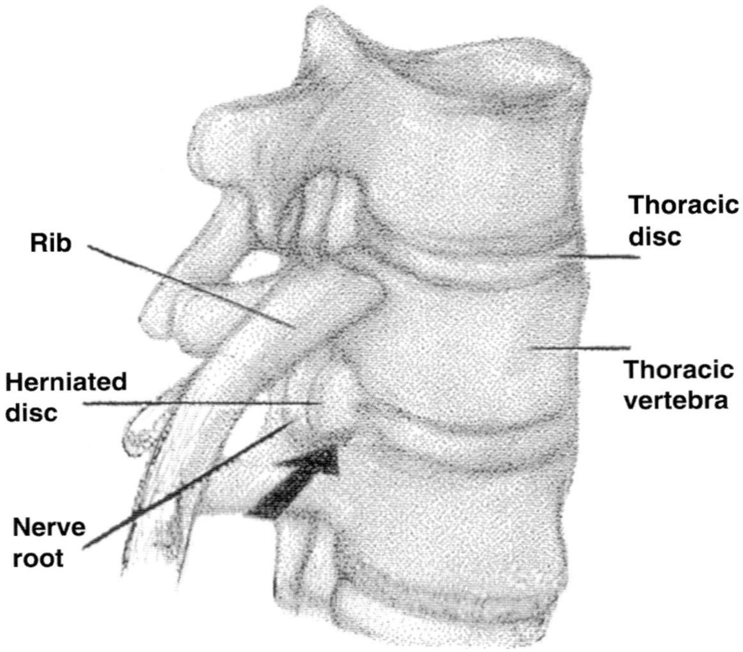

Fig. 3. The arrow represents the posterolateral approach to thoracic disc space.

et al. *(29,30)* had undertaken the first global attempts in 1986. Topological elaboration of the cervical spine (Fig. 2) and the thoracic spine soon followed (Fig. 2 and 3). Complications of PLD have included paraspinal hematoma, perforation in the peripheral ileum, vasovagal reactions, intradiscal abscess, worsening of preexisting foot drop, postoperative cholangitis, and postoperative cerebrovascular accident *(21–25)*.

LASER FACET RHIZOTOMY

Lumbar facets or zygapophyseal joints are synovial arthroses richly innervated with nerve endings from the medial branch of the posterior primary ramus *(33)*. Osteoarthritis of the lumbar facet joint is a common cause of disabling low-back pain. Facet joint arthritis on MRI and CT scan does not necessarily correlate with symptoms. Some patients can have extensive facet arthritis on imaging study and be clinically asymptomatic, whereas other patients can have subtle evidence of arthritis radiologically with classic symptoms of arthritis clinically *(34)*. Many patients report referred sciatica as well. Currently, the treatment options include apophyseal joint nerve blocks for short-term relief and facet joint denervation for long-term relief by cryotherapy or radiofrequency. The results of facet rhizotomy have been variable, with a significant number of patients requiring repeat procedures or experiencing inadequate relief of pain.

Few reports of laser-assisted lumbar facet rhizotomy have appeared in the literature *(35)*. By means of a 17-gage needle (Fig. 4), the Ho:YAG straight-firing laser probe (Trymedine, Irvine, CA) was directed at the medial branch of the dorsal ramus, the nerve that gives rise to the articular branches at each level. Each facet joint receives its nerve supply from multiple segments above and below *(34)*. The laser probe was also directed

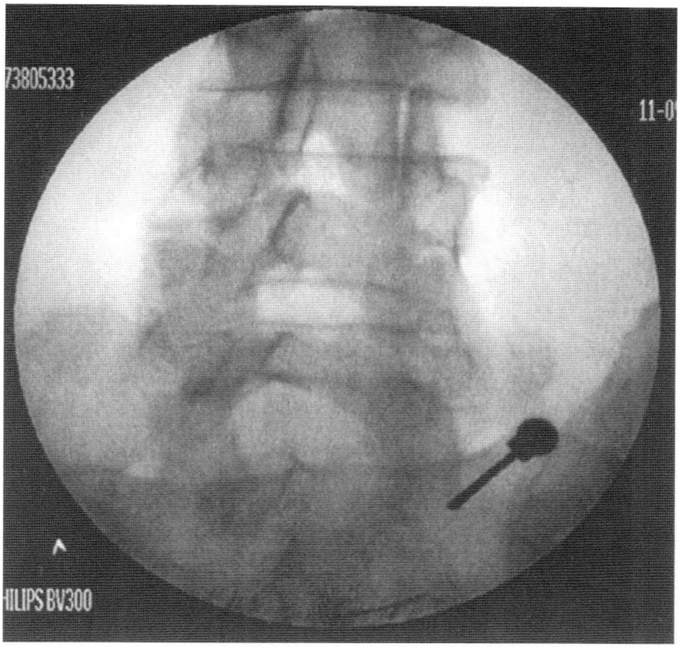

Fig. 4. Fluoroscopic view of needle placed on facet at L5-S1.

onto the facet joint to thermocoagulate the finer capsular branches with a total of 500 J of energy. There was a significant difference in pain relief between patients with unoperated backs vs patients who had undergone prior spinal surgery. Laser has the advantage of thermocoagulating a relatively larger area in the vicinity of the probe tip than a radiofrequency probe. More recently, Katzman *(36)* reported arthroscopic laser-assisted facet joint denervation. A large number of patients who failed to be relieved by radiofrequency facet rhizotomy experienced marked relief of pain following the laser procedure.

ENDOSCOPIC LASER FORAMINOPLASTY

With accumulated experience with endoscopically assisted mechanical and laser lumbar discectomy *(37)*, the need for a method to decompress more effectively the lateral recess and intervertebral neural foramen from very large or extruded disc protrusions, recurrent discs, scar tissue, and spondylitic spurs became evident *(38)*. The most frequently seen lumbar spinal disc disease in the elderly is spinal and lateral foraminal stenosis *(39)*. Lateral stenosis may be congenital or degenerative when secondary to acute disc disease and spinal trauma. Transforaminal Microdecompressive Endoscopic Assisted Discectomy and Foraminoplasty (TF-MEAD) (Fig. 5) is a new system of more aggressive mechanical instrumentation and laser application.

Positioning of a Steerable Spinoscope (Karl Storz Endoscopy, Culver City, CA) with a flexible tip that can bend up to 90° and rotate to reach 360° is checked throughout the procedure by fluoroscopy in two planes (Fig. 6). At the involved nerve root distribution, sterile needle electrodes are placed for continuous intraoperative neurophysiological electromyograph monitoring *(40)*. If a pain provocation test and discogram were not

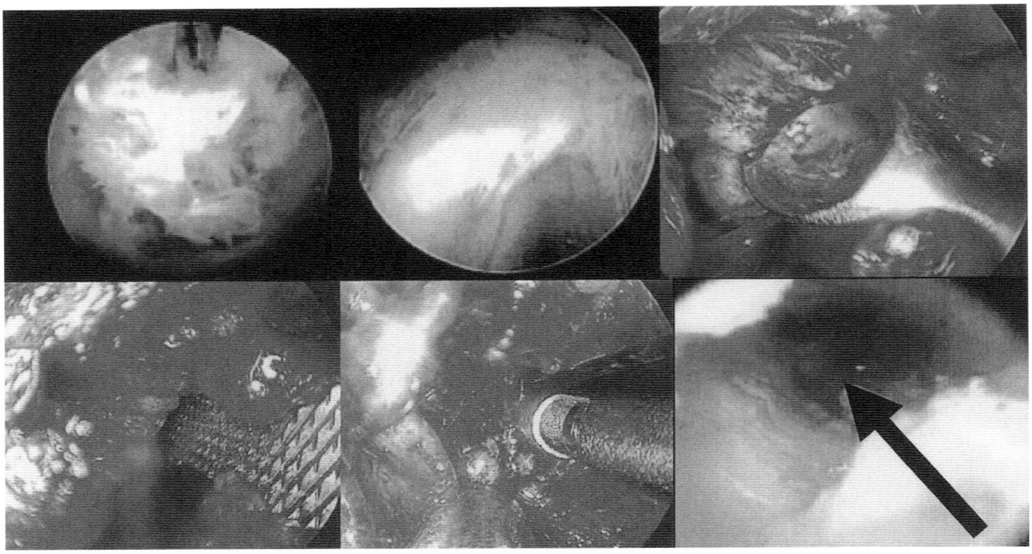

Fig. 5. Endoscopic view of lumbar mechanical decompressive foraminoplasty and discectomy: **(A)** disc removal with cutter forceps; **(B)** removal of disc fragment below nerve; **(C)** curette for osteophytic decompression; **(D)** rasp for osteophytic decompression; **(E)** bone punch, rongeur for foramen decompression; **(F)** postforaminoplasty disk defect (arrow).

done preoperatively, they are done at the outset. Under fluoroscopy the extended side of the appropriate cannula is turned to face the nerve root for retraction and protection. The cannula retractors have various duck bill extensions. Larger, more aggressively toothed trephines are then inserted and rotated to cut through annulus, disc protrusion, spur, or spondylitic bar. A slim rongeur, spinal disc forceps, or pituitary forceps and curettes can aid in decompressing the foramen and the lateral recess (Fig. 5). Biting forceps, a discectome, and an Ho:YAG laser with continuous irrigation are used consecutively to perform intradiscal discectomy. A lower-energy nonablative laser is applied for shrinking and tightening of the disc (laser thermodiskoplasty) *(41,42)*. Laser thermodiskoplasty can also cause sinovertebral neurolysis or denervation. The discectome is employed to remove charred debris from use of the laser.

The disc space and neural foramen can be directly visualized and examined by endoscopy to confirm adequate disc decompression and to perform further decompression when necessary. If the foramen is compromised, the depth of insertion of the endoscope is adjusted; the nerve root is again protected by the duck bill extension; and spurs are removed with curettes, bone punches, and Kerrison rongeurs. TF-MEAD effectively treats spinal pathology at multiple levels and bilaterally. Many elderly patients suffering symptoms caused by lateral spinal stenosis and disc problems can be successfully treated.

LASER SYMPATHECTOMY

Two common syndromes in which sympathetic pain appears are causalgia and reflex sympathetic dystrophy. True causalgia follows partial injury to a major nerve trunk such as

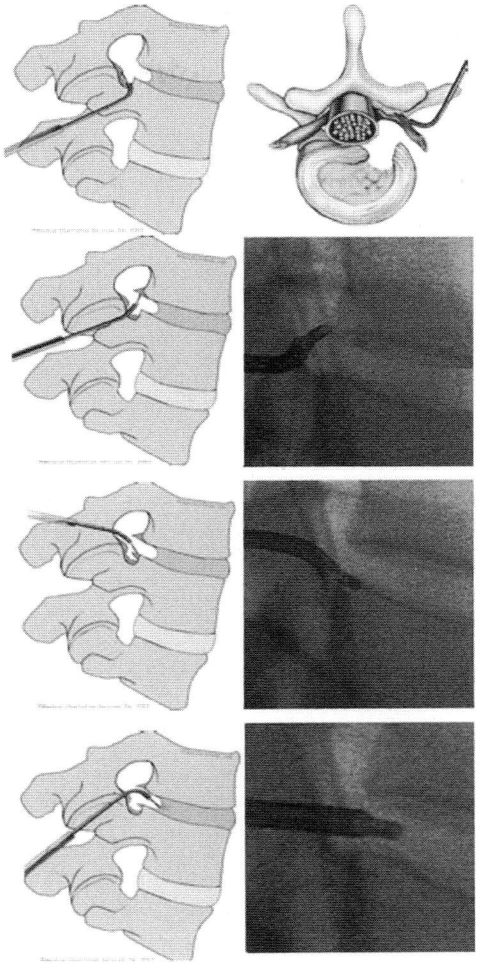

Fig. 6. Drawing and X-ray appearance of Steerable Spinoscope with bendable tip *in situ.*

the sciatic nerve or its large branches. Reflex sympathetic dystrophy may occur following minor trauma to the neural structures that accompanies fractures, soft-tissue injuries, and surgical incisions. Clinical characteristics include burning, poorly localized dermatomal distribution of stabbing pain, hyperesthesia, vasomotor alterations leading to trophic changes, changes in skin temperature, alteration of sweating patterns, piloerection, and swelling. Other conditions complicated by sympathetic dysfunction are amputation stump pain, circulatory insufficiency in the legs, arteriosclerotic disease of the lower limbs, intermittent claudication, and arterial embolism.

Lumbar disc surgery, including percutaneous endoscopic discectomy, may cause mechanical trauma to the somatic nerves, and a certain percentage of patients do complain of burning pain, lower-extremity swelling, and color changes and hypersensitivity of the skin. Diagnostic lumbar sympathetic blocks can identify sympathetic nervous system involvement as the causative factor. The sympathetic nervous system becomes involved owing to damage to A delta and C fibers that develop hypersensitivity to circulating norepinephrine, pressure, and movement. Spontaneous firing causes the typical pain of sympathetic origin. Shortly afterward, small neuromas form that sprout small myelinated and unmyelinated fibers. Normally silent fibers then generate, even in the absence of stimulation, an ongoing barrage of impulses that traverse the afferent fibers to the spinal cord.

In the past, permanent interruption of the lumbar sympathetic chain has been accomplished by open surgery or phenol or alcohol injection *(43)*. Subsequently, percutaneous lumbar sympathectomy by radiofrequency lesions involved less morbidity. The Ho:YAG laser has now been found to be even more effective and longer lasting than radiofrequency.

Anatomically, the lumbar sympathetic chain lies at the anterolateral border of the vertebral bodies. The aorta is positioned anteriorly and slightly medial to the chain on the left side. The inferior vena cava is more closely approximated to the chain on the right in an anterior plane. Many other small lumbar arteries and veins are positioned near the sympathetic chain. The psoas muscle is situated posteriorly. Blockade of the sympathetic nerves can also be performed with spinal, epidural, or peripheral nerve blocks, but relief of pain after lumbar sympathetic block will most clearly confirm the painful etiology as sympathetically mediated. Most fibers headed for the lower extremity pass through the second and third lumbar ganglia, so that a sympathetic block placed at this level provides almost complete sympathetic denervation to the lower extremity. The pain relief obtained is usually immediate and can be long-lasting, outlasting the duration of action of the local anesthetic.

Sites for needle placement for the sympathetic chain at the L2, L3, and L4 vertebral levels are identified on projection fluoroscopy (Fig. 7). Small skin incisions are made with a scalpel blade, and a 20-gage, 15-cm radiofrequency needle with a 10-mm active tip is advanced to the anterolateral aspect of the vertebral column. Aspiration for blood and cerebrospinal fluid is performed to make certain that the needle is not in a blood vessel or the intrathecal space. Further confirmation is provided by injecting radiocontrast dye to outline the sympathetic chain. Stimulation is then performed with 50 Hz at 0.8–1.0 V of radiofequency stimulation to ensure that no somatic nerve is involved. The stylet of the needle is removed, and a guide wire inserted through the needle. The needle is removed, and a 12-gage,10-cm cannula is advanced until it makes contact with the anterolateral aspect of the vertebra at the contrast site outlining the sympathetic chain. A side-firing Ho:YAG laser probe is passed through the cannula, and laser heat is applied at 5 Hz, 10 W for a total of 90–100 J. The laser probe is rotated superiorly, medially, inferiorly, and laterally to thermocoagulate the sympathetic chain at all three levels.

Application of Ho:YAG laser heat or radiofrequency heat is more precise and has fewer complications than the use of a neurolytic solution for chemical sympathectomy. There is no spread to the psoas muscle, somatic nerves, or subarachnoid space; no ureteral strictures occur; hypotension is less frequent; postsympathectomy sympathalgia is virtually absent; and impotence is rare. Potential complications include puncture of major blood vessels or the renal pelvis, genitofemoral neuralgia, perforation of the disc, and puncture of the ureter. Fewer postoperative thromboembolic phenomena occur in the elderly, because an operation and bed rest are avoided. The procedure can be repeated with minimal morbidity, and anatomical landmarks are not altered if a repeat procedure

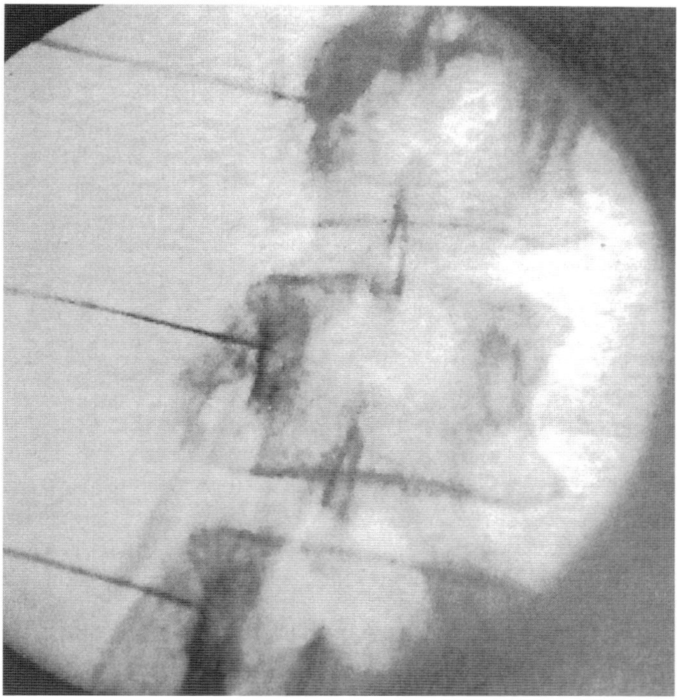

Fig. 7. Fluoroscopic view of multiple needle placements at L2, L3, and L4 levels for laser sympathectomy.

is needed. By comparison, surgical or chemical sympathectomy induces an extensive fibrous reaction and obliterates the potential space in which the sympathetic chain lies, making the space impossible to identify during a subsequent procedure.

REFERENCES

1. Townes CH and Schawlow AI. Microwave Spectroscopy. Dover, NY:1975.
2. Hecht J. Laser Pioneers. Academic, NY:1992.
3. Ascher PW. Status quo and new horizons of laser therapy in neurosurgery. Lasers Surg Med 1985;5:499–506.
4. Yonezawa T, Onomura T, Kosaka R. The system and procedures of percutaneous intradiscal laser nucleotomy. Spine 1990;15:1175–1185.
5. Davis JK. Early experience with laser disc decompression: a percutaneous method. J Fla Med Assoc 1992;79:37–39.
6. Onik G, Mooney V, Maroon JC, et al. Automated percutaneous discectomy: a pro-spective multi-institutional study. Neurosurgery 1990;26:228–232.
7. Choy DS, Case RB, Fielding W, et al. Percutaneous laser nucleolysis of lumbar disks. N Engl J Med 1987;317:771, 772.
8. Kambin P. Arthroscopic Microdiscectomy, Urban & Schwarzenberg, Baltimore, 1991.
9. Sherk HH, Black J, Rhodes A. Laser discectomy. Clin Sports Med 1993;12:569–577.
10. Hellinger J. Technical aspects of the percutaneous cervical and lumbar laser disc decompression and nucleotomy. Neurol Res 1999;21:99–102.

11. Hendler N, Raja SN. Reflex sympathetic dystrophy and causalgia, in Handbook of Pain Management (Tollison CD, Satterthwaite JR, Tollison JW, eds.), Williams & Wilkins, Baltimore: 1994, pp. 484–496.
12. Choy DSJ. Percutaneous laser disc decompression (PLDD): 12 years' experience with 752 procedures in 518 patients. J Clin Laser Med Surg 1998;16:325–331.
13. Ohnmeiss DD, Guyer RD, Hochschuler SH. Laser disc decompression: the importance of proper patient selection. Spine 1994;19:2054–2058.
14. Simons P, Lensker E, von Wild K. Percutaneous nucleus pulposus denaturation in treatment of lumbar disc protrusions. Eur Spine J 1994;3:219–221.
15. Schatz SW, Talalla A. Preliminary experience with percutaneous laser disc decompression in the treatment of sciatica. Can J Surg 1995;38:432–436.
16. Liebler WA. Percutaneous laser disc nucleotomy. Clin Orthop 1995;310:58–66.
17. Siebert WE, Barendsen BT, Tollgard J. Percutaneous laser disc decompression. Experience since 1989. *Orthopade* 1996;25:42–48.
18. Casper GD, Hartman VL, Mullins LL. Results of a clinical trial of holmium:YAG laser in disc decompression utilizing a side-firing fiber: a two-year follow-up. Lasers Surg Med 1996;19:90–96.
19. Nerubay J, Caspi I, Levinkopf M. Pecutaneous carbon dioxide laser nucleolysis with 2 to 5 year follow-up. Clin Orthop 1997;312:45-48.
20. Pedachenko EG, Khizhniak MV, Tanaseichuk AF, et al. Laser puncture diskectomy in discogenic lumbosacral radiculitis. Lik Sprava 1998;1:143–145.
21. Hellinger J. Erfahrungen mit der perkutanen laserkoagulation des discus intervertebralis. Orthop Mitteilungen 1991;3:157.
22. Hellinger J. Ein neuer Weg der Bandscheibenchirurgie. Arztliche Praxis 1992;44:21 22.
23. Hellinger J. Percutaneous laser disc decompression, in: Lasers at the Dawn of the 3rd Millennium, Antypas G, ed. Monduzzi, Bologna, 1996, pp. 201–205.
24. Hellinger J. Die Laserosteotomie als Zugangsmöglichkeit zur lumbalen und zervikalen perkutanen Nukleotomie. Lasermedizin 1992;8:105.
25. Hellinger J, Kornelli H, Einenkel RN. Der computerisierte spine-motion-Test mit integriertem Rücken-Muskel-EMG zur Quantifizierung lokaler vertebragener Befunde, in Wirbelsäulendiagnostik, Schmitt E, Lorenz R, eds. Enke, Stuttgart, 1998, pp. 32–36.
26. Craig F. Vertebral body biopsy. J Bone Joint Surg 1956;38:93–102.
27. Castro WHM, Halm H, Schinkel V. Neodymium-YAG 1064 nm Laservaporisation von lumbalen Bandscheibenvorfällen: Klinische Frühergebnisse, Laser 92, Shaker, Aachen 1992, pp. 187–189.
28. Chiu J. Endoscopic lumbar foraminoplasty. In: Kim D, Fessler R, Regan J, eds, Endoscopic Spine Surgery and Instrumentation. Thieme Medical, NY:2004; pp.212–229.
29. Choy DS, Ascher PW, Ranu HS, et al. Percutaneous laser disc decompression: a new therapeutic modality. Spine 1992;17:949–956.
30. Choy DS, Case RB, Fielding W, et al. Percutaneous laser nucleolysis of lumbar disks. N Engl J Med 1987;317:771, 772.
31. Savitz MH. Same-day microsurgical arthroscopic lateral-approach laser-assisted (SMALL) fluoroscopic discectomy. J Neurosurg 1994;80:1039–1045.
32. Stöhr M. In Iatrogene Nervenläsionen, Thieme, Stuttgart, 1996, pp. 47–52.
33. Suseki K, Takahashi Y, Takahashi K. Innervation of the lumbar facet joints: origins and functions. Spine 1975;22:477–485.
34. Bough B, Thakore J, Davies A. Degeneration of the lumbar facet joints: arthropathy and pathology. J Bone Joint Surg 1999;72A:275, 276.
35. Kantha S. Laser lumbar facet rhizotomy. J Minim Invasive Technol 2001;1:31, 32.
36. Katzman S. Arthroscopic laser assisted facet joint denervation. J Minim Invasive Technol 2003;3:48–50.

37. Chiu JC, Clifford TI, Negrer F, et al. Microdecompressive percutaneous discectomy: spinal discectomy with new laser thermodiskoplasty for nonextruded herniated nucleus pulposus. Surg Technol Int 1999;VIll:343–351.
38. Knight M, Goswami A, Patko J, Buxton N. Endoscopic foraminoplasty: an independent prospective evaluation, in Laser in the Musculoskeletal System (Gerber BE, Knight M, Seibert WE, eds.), Springer-Verlag, Berlin, 2001, pp. 320–329.
39. Haag M. Transforaminal endoscopic microdiscectomy: indications and short-term to intermediate-term results. Orthopade 1999;7:615–621.
40. Clifford T, Chiu JC, Rogers G. Neurophysiological monitoring of peripheral nerve function during endoscopic laser discectomy. J Minim Invasive Spinal Technol 2001;1:54–57.
41. Chiu J, Clifford T. Microdecompressive percutaneous discectomy: spinal discectomy with new laser thermodiskoplasty for non extruded herniated nucleus pulposus. Surg Technol Int 1999;VIII:343–351.
42. Chiu J. Anterior endoscopic cervical microdiscectomy. In:Kim D, Fessler R, Regan J, eds, Endoscopic Spine Surgery and Instrumentation. Thieme Medical, New York: 2004; pp 48–58.
43. Ewing M. The history of lumbar sympathectomy. Surgery 1971;70:790–796.

14
Minimally Invasive Techniques in Pain Management

James Reynolds, MD and Garrett Kine, MD

INTRODUCTION

Epidurals were the first minimally invasive technique for the relief of lumbosacral pain. This spurred the development of the subspecialty of pain management in anesthesia, which has evolved and added many techniques to alleviate or reduce lumbosacral pain. Specialists including physiatrists, orthopedic surgeons, and neurosurgeons also perform these procedures. This chapter discusses the proven techniques used to relieve lumbosacral pain, and the clinical presentation of herniated discs, spinal stenosis, facet syndrome, and pain arising from the sacroiliac joint and coccyx. Pain may arise from one or all the structures in the lumbosacral spine, complicating treatment. The technique for injections or other proven pain-relieving methods are described. Newer techniques for the treatment of the painful disc are in the early stages of development and have not completely evolved. The therapeutic benefits have not been proven by randomized blinded studies. These techniques are discussed but not described in detail.

THE FACET JOINT

The facet joint is a synovial joint between the articular processes of the laminae. The joint has an intracapsular superior recess and an extra-articular inferior recess. The facet joint will accept 1 to 2 mL and excess will extravasate into the epidural space, not into the paraspinal muscle *(1)*. Problems in the facet joint account for 15% of patients with low-back pain *(2)*. The patient with low-back pain arising from the facet joint does not have clinical features that discriminate the facet joint from other causes of low-back pain *(3)*. There are no findings on clinical examination that consistently identify the facet as the cause of pain. Classic teaching saying that low-back pain with extension or with extension and rotation is caused by the facet was not confirmed with zygoapophyseal joint block *(4)*. Patients with pain arising from the facet do not have pain in the midline. The pain arising from the facet joint is always lateral to the midline and may radiate to the buttocks and distally to the toes. Anesthetizing the medial branch of the zygoapophysial joint will relieve pain arising from this joint *(5)*. The medial branch can be anesthetized by injecting anesthetic solution at the base of the transverse process just above the midpoint.

From: *Arthroscopic and Endoscopic Spinal Surgery: Text and Atlas: Second Edition*
Edited by: P. Kambin © Humana Press Inc., Totowa, NJ

Contrast must be used to avoid an intravascular injection, a complication that occurs 8% of the time *(5,6)*. Degenerative changes identified on computed tomography (CT) do not correlate with the presence or absence of pain arising from the zygoapophyseal joint *(2)*. Discogenic pain and pain arising from the zygoapophyseal joint do not usually occur in the same patient *(7)*. Disc degeneration always occurs before facet degeneration *(8)*. Facet joint injections do not show good long-term relief of low-back pain *(9)*. Randomized, placebo-controlled trials have not shown a significant difference between corticosteroid injections and placebo *(10)*. However, there are a small number of patients who respond very well to facet injections and benefit from injections every 3–6 mo.

RADIOFREQUENCY MEDIAL BRANCH ABLATION

Patients with short-term relief of low-back pain from facet injections may be given longer relief by radiofrequency medial branch ablation. Pain arising from the facet joint should be proven by two injections using anesthetic agents with different durations of action. Lidocaine has a rapid onset and brief duration of action. A confirmatory injection with bupivacaine should have a longer duration of action of at least 3 h. The patient with at least 50% relief of low-back pain from injections of both the short- and longer-lasting anesthetic agents are considered appropriate responders. The injection may be in the joint of the facet or at the medial branch *(3)*. Provocation of low-back pain by injection of contrast into the facet joint is not a good indicator of the facet joint as the source of the low-back pain. The relief of pain by anesthetic agents injected into the joint or at the medial branch to the facet is the only appropriate indicator that the facet is the source of pain in the lower back *(11)*. There is conflicting evidence that radiofrequency ablation of the medial branch to the facet in the lumbar spine relieves low-back pain *(12,13)*. When inadequate diagnostic criteria were used to select patients to undergo radiofrequency facet joint denervation, the results of facet joint denervation were not shown to be effective in the relief of low-back pain *(14)*. When a single diagnostic injection was used, radiofrequency lumbar facet denervation was shown to be more effective than a sham procedure *(15)*. When very strict diagnostic criteria were used, including two diagnostic medial branch blocks with a very high percentage of pain relief, excellent relief of low-back pain was obtained, with 87% of patients experiencing at least a 60% reduction in their visual analog scale (VAS) (16). Relief of back pain was maintained for at least 6 mo, but the majority of patients sustained relief for 12 mo. No complications occurred in the study *(16)*. Other studies have shown good relief of pain from repetition of the radiofrequency denervation of the lumbar facet joint *(17)*. The patient undergoing radiofrequency denervation of the lumbar facet joint experiences an increase in low-back pain for 2–4 wk after the procedure. Therefore, it is best to wait until the low-back pain has returned to significant levels before recommending a repeat radiofrequency neurotomy of the lumbar facet. Patients experiencing satisfactory relief from the injection of corticosteroids in the facet joint for 3 mo can be managed with quarterly injections until the relief from the facet injection no longer lasts 3 mo.

EPIDURAL STEROID INJECTION INTO LUMBAR SPINE

There are three portals to deliver steroids to the epidural space in the lumbar spine: interlaminar, caudal, and transforaminal. Blind placement of epidural steroids into the epidural space in the lumbar spine through the caudal or interlaminar route results in misplacement of the corticosteroid in 14–38% of lumbar epidural corticosteroid injections. The use of contrast during the epidural procedure assists in visualizing the proper placement of the corticosteroid solution and prevents intravascular injection of the solution *(18–20)*. Transforaminal lumbar epidural injection is the most precise technique for delivery of the corticosteroid into the lumbar epidural space *(21)*. Selective nerve root block and transforaminal epidural lumbar injection differ in the amount and placement of the solution into the lumbar epidural space. Selective nerve root block is only 1 to 2 mL of volume and is meant to be diagnostic as well as therapeutic. The bevel of the needle faces distally and is placed within the epiradicular membrane. Diagnostic selective nerve root injection results in a minimal increase in the risk of neural injury and reduces the chance of a false negative *(22)*.

The efficacy of therapeutic epidural injections for significant long-term improvement has been questioned, but in such studies fluoroscopic imaging and contrast were not used to ensure that the corticosteroid reached the pathology *(23,24)*. Studies that showed epidural steroids to be effective all were reformed with fluoroscopic guidance through a transforaminal approach. The use of a single injection through a periradicular corticosteroid injection of a lumbar nerve root showed short-term improvement compared with an injection without corticosteroids *(25)*. Studies that allowed one to four injections had a favorable long-term outcome. Seventy-five percent of patients had a 50% or greater reduction in pain and a return to normal or near-normal activity *(26)*. Other studies showed similar relief of sciatica, with 77% of patients avoiding surgery *(27)*. A single periradicular membrane injection of the L4, L5, or S1 nerve roots containing corticosteroid was superior to the same injection without corticosteroid for patients with a contained herniated nucleus pulposus. Fewer than half of the patients with the contained herniated disc who received injections with corticosteroids chose to undergo surgery compared with the control subjects. The result was a cost savings of $12,666 per patient. Patients with an extruded herniation did not experience statistically significant improvement compared with the control subjects *(28)*. A randomized double-blind study showed that selective nerve root injections reduced the number of patients electing to undergo decompression in the lumbar spine for spinal stenosis. The patients received selective nerve root injections with anesthetic agent with or without corticosteroid. They could elect to receive as many as three injections, but always with the same solution—either with or without corticosteroids. The group receiving injections with corticosteroids elected to undergo surgical decompression less than half as frequently as the control group *(29)*.

Infiltration of a lumbosacral nerve root was shown to be predictive of a successful surgical procedure when the patient had reproduction by needle placement and relief of symptoms with infiltration of an anesthetic agent *(30)*. Injection of anesthetic agents and corticosteroid in the perineural membrane of a lumbar nerve root was shown to be useful in predicting the response to surgical procedures in patients with radicular symptoms in the lumbar spine present for more than 1 yr. For those patients who experienced relief of radicular pain during the anesthetic phase and relief for 1 wk from the corticosteroids, 85% had a successful surgical outcome. Those patients without relief from the corticosteroid phase had an unsuccessful outcome 95% of the time *(31)*.

The International Spinal Injection Society has specific recommendations for the frequency and number of spinal injections. Injections should be 7–14 d apart, and no more than four in a 6 mo period *(31,32)*. The potential side effects and possible complications include vasovagal reactions, facial flushing, insomnia, and bleeding *(32)*. These effects are reactions to medication rather than true complications. Other procedure-related complications are dural puncture and associated headaches, infection within the epidural space, nerve injury, bleeding, transient weakness or numbness, and paraplegia *(32)*. Adverse reactions can include reaction to the contrast and fluid retention with associated peripheral swelling. Contraindications are known hypersensitivity to medications used in the injection, malignancy, infection, bleeding diathesis or anticoagulation, congestive heart failure, or uncontrolled diabetes *(32)*. Celestone™ is a corticosteroid containing betamethasone, and the flare resolves faster than prednisolone or triamcinolone acetate, thus making Celestone the preferred corticosteroid for epidural injections.

SACROILIAC INJECTIONS

The sacroiliac joint is the great imitator. It can produce groin pain that mimics the pain of a degenerative hip joint, back pain similar to discogenic pain, and pain radiating on the posterior portion of the leg even below the knee that is similar to sciatica *(33)*. In 14% of patients, pain from the sacroiliac joint was referred to the foot *(34)*. Anatomical studies of innervation of the sacroiliac joint using special staining techniques have been conducted in animals. The sensory nerve fibers to the dorsal side of the sacroiliac joint arise from L4 to S2 and from the ventral side from L1 to S2 *(34,35)*. The L4 and L5 nerve roots converge to begin the formation of the lumbosacral trunk. As this portion of the lumbosacral trunk reaches the pelvic brim, the combined roots of L4 and L5 are within 5 mm of the sacroiliac joint *(36)*. No study has determined whether the cause of the pain is referred pain, direct irritation of the lumbosacral plexus, or another source.

Physical examination does not correlate or always lead to the diagnosis of sacroiliac joint pain. Classic physical examination of the sacroiliac joint includes the Patrick test, also known as the FABER test or figure 4 test; Gaenslen's test; and the posterior shear test *(37–39)*. CT showed abnormal joints in 57.5% of patients with pain arising from the sacroiliac joint and 31% of matched control subjects *(40)*. In the intact pelvis, the degree of motion of the sacroiliac joint was $<2°$ *(41)*. Even in patients with postpartum sacroiliac pain, no more than 2° of motion on any axis could be demonstrated *(42)*. The only symptom that correlated with sacroiliac pain proven by diagnostic blocks was groin pain *(33)*. Others have found the sacroiliac as the source of persistent pain after a lumbosacral fusion. In a group of patients undergoing diagnostic injection to determine the source of persistent lumbosacral pain after lumbosacral fusion, 32% of patients were diagnosed with sacroiliac pain as the cause of persistent pain after lumbosacral fusion. Seventy-five percent relief of pain was the criterion used to determine that the sacroiliac joint was the remaining cause of pain that persisted after a lumbosacral fusion *(43)*.

Injection of the sacroiliac joint is difficult without image guidance. Injection into the sacroiliac joint was successful in only 22% of attempts done without image guidance. CT performed immediately after blind sacroiliac injection showed that in 24% of patients the dye entered the epidural space *(44)*. Injection of the sacroiliac joint of patients with inflammatory spondyloarthropathy has been shown to be effective for short-term relief of 1–3 mo for symptoms arising from the sacroiliac joint, but it did not provide significant relief at 6 mo *(45)*. In patients without spondyloarthropathy, injection of a corticosteroid was shown to be effective for relief of pain arising from the sacroiliac joint when compared with an injection of saline *(46)*. Injection of the painful sacroiliac joint resulted in an improvement in function for more than 1 yr. The number of injections per patient was 2.1 *(47)*. The use of radiofrequency for denervation of the sacroiliac joint is being explored. Of patients undergoing such a procedure, 36.4% reported at least a 50% reduction in pain for at least 6 mo, with an average duration of relief of 12 mo *(48)*. Many details must be considered when performing such a procedure, and the efficacy is still to be determined.

THE COCCYX

Coccydynia historically has been viewed as having a psychological origin, but a very comprehensive study showed "no evidence of neurosis" *(49)*. One of the factors that contribute to this myth is the common association of an additional source of pain. Studies have shown that as high as 77% of patients with coccydynia have associated conditions causing back pain. These conditions include painful degenerative discs, herniated discs, and sacroiliac dysfunction *(50)*. The symptoms of coccydynia are classic and localized to the "tail bone." Palpation of the coccyx is always painful. Injections of the sacrococcygeal joint should give good relief of pain arising from the coccyx. The patient will be able to distinguish pain arising from another source as being a different pain from coccydynia. Between 60 and 75% of patients with coccydynia will get significant relief of pain from sacrococcygeal joint injections *(49,50)*.

TECHNIQUES OF LUMBAR SPINAL BLOCKADE

Introduction

Intent

Injection in and around the spine may be performed with both diagnostic and therapeutic intent. As in any diagnostic test, there exists the possibility of both true positive and false positive responses as well as true negative and false negative responses. Injections may be used as a "rule-out" procedure. In this instance, if a properly performed procedure in an awake, cooperative patient does not produce relief of the regionalized pain, then, more than likely, it is a true negative response. That particular structure is not a significant pain generator in this individual. A false negative response may occur in an individual with multiple pain generators. In addition, there exists the possibility of multiple behavior and psychological issues that predispose a patient to perceive that he or she is actually not feeling better.

Interpretation of positive responses carries with it inherent difficulties as well. False positive responses may occur owing to placebo response, anesthetizing of structures other than the target, and other considerations. The use of concomitant intravenous medications is controversial during the performance of diagnostic blocks and adds yet another complex factor to interpretation of the results. All this having been said, true positive responses can be very rewarding to both the patient and the medical practitioner. These true positive responses lead to a diagnosis; lend credence to the patient's pain complaint; and may lead the patient down the path to cointerventions with the ultimate goal of recovery, or at least a higher functioning and more satisfying standard of living.

Scientific inquiry is based on the notion of quantifying data, introducing a single variable, then carefully observing the resultant change. In the case of diagnostic injection procedures, careful preblock condition of the patient should be assessed with provocative maneuvers, the block should be performed accurately with proper fluoroscopic visualization, and then the results should be evaluated and quantified through the same provocative maneuvers. Independent assessment of the individual by a qualified person should yield more accurate data.

The therapeutic intent of injection procedures has been the mainstay of their existence for many decades. The duration of the perceived benefit is variable. Often, injections give a window of relief where cointerventions may be administered. Injections are also often used in conjunction with physical therapy. In addition, injections may help people over very difficult times of flare, and they may be employed as a maintenance therapy when all other available options have been exhausted.

Disclaimer

The techniques described as follows are those of the authors. Certainly, other techniques exist that are safe and sound. These techniques are generally consistent with those offered by the guidelines of the International Spinal Injection Society.

This chapter is not a substitute for proper training. Any individual performing these injections should be fully cognizant of the medications being used, be aware of their potential side effects, and be prepared for any potential adverse reactions. Resuscitative mediations and equipment should at all times be immediately available.

Lumbar Transforaminal Epidurals

Background

Transforaminal epidurals have also been called selective epidurals or selective nerve root blocks. The transforaminal route has emerged in the last couple of decades as a generally superior technique compared to the interlaminar and caudal routes for administration of medications to the spinal canal. It has the advantage of enabling the physician to deliver the injectate to the ventral epidural space, in closer proximity to disc pathology. The availability and increasing quality of fluoroscopy equipment have certainly also led to this emergence. Although interlaminar and caudal epidurals may certainly be attempted without radiological guidance, fluoroscopy has enabled verification of placement of medication and minimized several safety concerns.

Positioning

The patient is generally placed prone on the fluoroscopy table. A pillow under the abdomen may help open the foramen and contribute to patient comfort. Although the patient could be placed in an oblique position, a C-arm fluoroscopy machine negates the need for this. Prone positioning also allows for bilateral procedures without the need to reposition.

Imaging

In the standard subpedicular technique, the target point is the "safe" triangle. A needle placed here is just inferior to the pedicle, lateral to the dural sleeve, and medial to an imaginary line dropped from the most lateral aspect of the pedicle. The pedicle is often described as a clock and the optimal needle position would then be 6:00. It is better to err on the safer side, and this is sometimes described as being at the 5:30 position on the right of the spine and the 6:30 position on the left.

The C-arm should be adjusted in a cephalocaudal angulation so that the inferior edge of the pedicle is a sharp line. This should correspond to also having the X-ray beams parallel to the inferior and superior end plates of the vertebral body. The C-arm can then be moved through slight obliquity to see if this target area can be reached without any

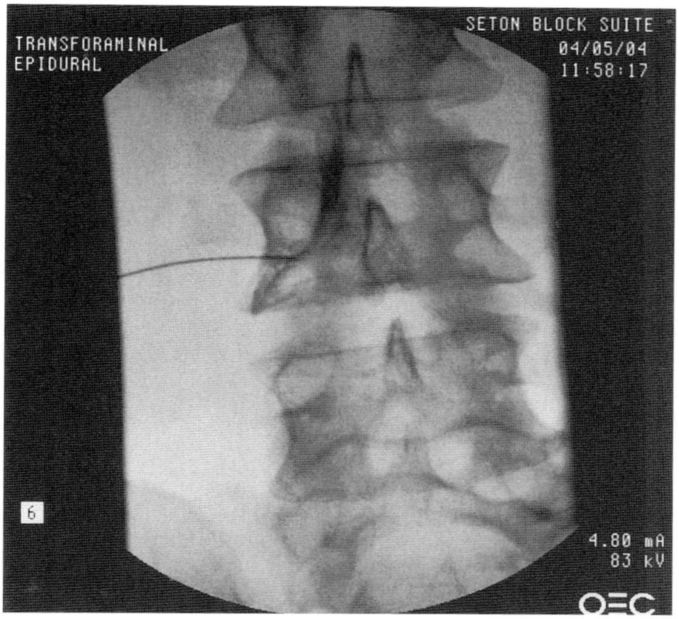

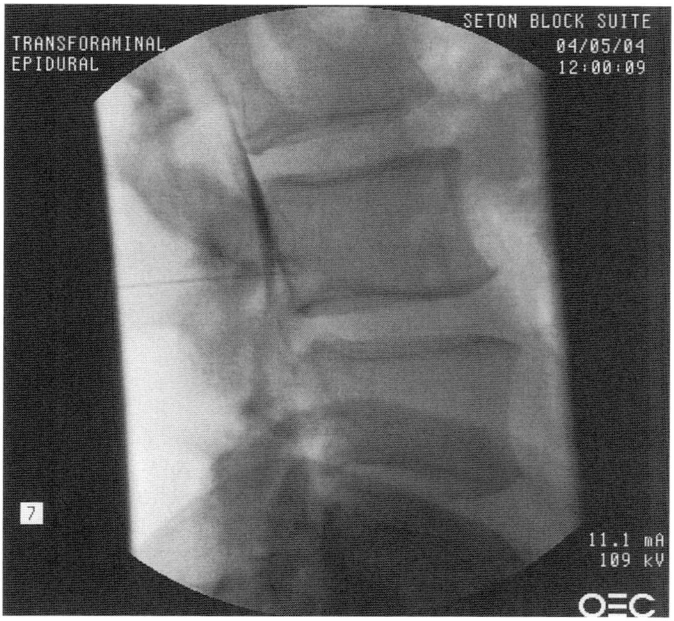

Fig. 1. **(A)** Anteropostenor (AP) view of left L4 transforaminal epidural utilizing single-needle technique. **(B)** Lateral view of L4 transforaminal epidural. Contrast is seen to travel in ventral epidural space more in a cephalad than a caudad direction. A filling defect at L4-L5 suggests a protrusion. **(C)** AP view of left L5 transforaminal epidural with double-needle technique.

bony interference. Sometimes the inferior edge of the transverse process, the lamina, or the superior articular process of the facet may interfere with a direct shot at the "safe" triangle. Slight C-arm adjustments will evaluate this. A single straight-needle technique

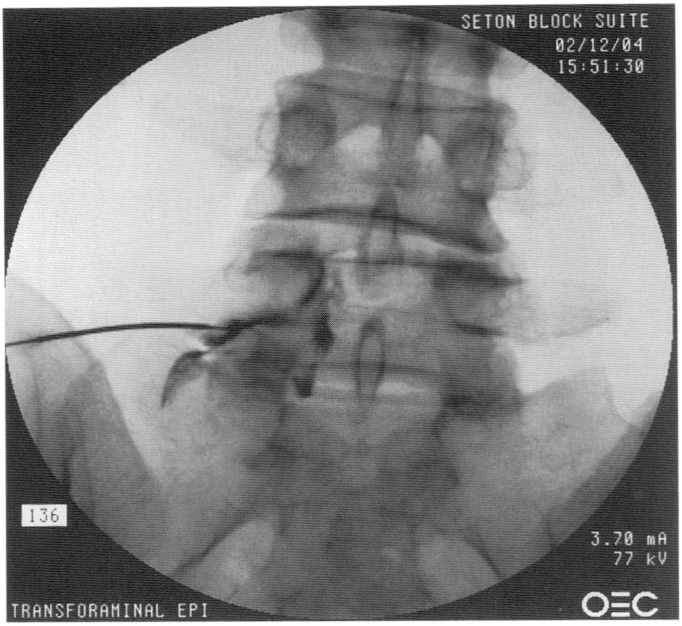

Fig. 1. *(Continued)*

can be used if there is no osseous encroachment (Figs. 1A,B). Otherwise, a double-needle technique can be used to direct a curved needle through an introducer to go around any bony obstacles (Fig. 1C).

Once the needle is placed at the target point, the initial injection should be under real-time fluoroscopy with a nonionic hypoallergenic contrast agent. An extension tube can be used to keep the operator's hands out of the direct X-ray beam. Care should be taken to ensure that there is no sign of intrathecal spread as well as no indication of intra-articular injection in a radicular artery.

Needle Techniques

Generally, one should strive to use the thinnest needle possible for any blocking procedure. With transforaminal epidurals, usually a 25- to 22-gage needle should suffice. It becomes difficult to inject through a 27-gage needle with particulate steroids.

As mentioned under Imaging, if an unobstructed view of the target area can be seen with a fluoroscopy machine, then a single straight needle should be sufficient. Placing the needle accurately and using the bevel for slight adjustments is all that is typically necessary. However, if the aforementioned lateral border of the lamina, inferior edge of the transverse process, or superior articular process of the zygapophyseal joint is in the way of a direct shot to the "safe" triangle, then a double-needle technique can be employed. This would also be useful if there has been surgical modification of the spine such as an intertransverse fusion mass. A 6-in., 25-gage needle fits through a 31/2-in., 20-gage introducer. In a larger individual, or in a situation in which one really has to maintain a strong curve of the longer needle, a 6-in., 22-gage needle fits through a 31/2-in., 18-gage introducer. This latter combination is useful, e.g., in an intertransverse fusion mass, where it helps keep the needle from going too ventral into the body.

Injectate

After needle placement, initial injection should be of contrast only under real-time fluoroscopy. This initial injection of 0.5–1 mL will give an indication of the spread of the medication. The majority of medicine should be traveling centrally into the epidural space. If the majority of medicine remains external to the neural foramina, then attempts should be made to reposition the needle to achieve better spread of medication.

The choice of anesthetic should be based on multiple considerations. In the case of transforaminal injections, there is the possibility of a significant motor blockade. This is especially the case when multiple levels are being injected simultaneously. Therefore, medications such as lidocaine would often be preferred over a longer-acting agent such as bupivacaine. It is generally recognized that optimal medical care would dictate that an individual be kept under medical observation while any significant motor, sensory, or hemodynamic events are possible. Therefore, with the use of lidocaine, an individual can be recovered in <1 h. Obviously, all anesthetics should be preservative free, because there is always the potential risk of an unintentional dural puncture.

A more concentrated anesthetic may be diluted with a contrast agent to achieve a solution of lesser concentration that can be visualized. An example of this would be diluting 2% preservative-free lidocaine in a 50/50 mixture with the contrast agent. A glucocorticoid can then be added to the solution and the total mixture injected under fluoroscopic observation to help judge the extent of spread of the medication. The volumes used will vary from individual to individual. If there is diagnostic intent, such as trying to predict the clinical effect of a single-level foraminotomy, then one would choose to use a more concentrated anesthetic with less contrast and far smaller volumes.

Other Considerations

An S1 transforaminal injection is basically the same as the subpedicular approach in the lumbar region. The big difference is that access is achieved through the dorsal foramen. Typically, the dorsal foramen is located approx 15° oblique to the easier seen ventral foramen. Consequently, lateralizing the C-arm 15° oblique often provides better visualization. A straight single needle is usually all that is necessary. A slight caudocephalad angulation regarding the sacrum allows for more cephalad spread of medicine reaching toward and above the L5-S1 disc space. The volumes necessary to reach this disc space may be somewhat greater than are typically found in the lumbar region.

If at any time a nerve is touched, the needle should be immediately repositioned. Often the paresthesia is very transient and there should be no continued pain. If the pain does continue, one should consider discontinuing the procedure. Furthermore, if an unintentional dural puncture occurs or injectate in a radicular artery is noticed, one should consider abandoning the procedure at that point and possibly returning after the artery or dural sleeve has had adequate time to heal.

Lumbar Interlaminar Epidural

Background

Lumbar interlaminar epidurals have also been called translaminar epidurals. This is the traditional approach that has been used for many decades for surgical levels of anesthesia or for labor and delivery. Most of the initial studies regarding epidural steroid injections were performed without fluoroscopy and were mostly uncontrolled.

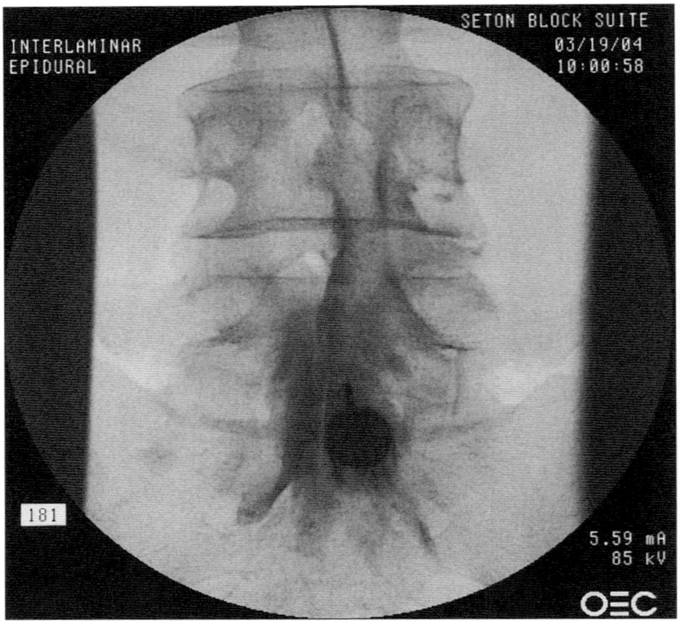

Fig. 2. AP view of L5-S1 interlaminar epidural with right paravertebral approach using Crawford needle.

More recently, controlled studies have questioned the efficacy of the interlaminar route. Logic dictates that there may be a subset population for whom the interlaminar route is more efficacious. An example of this is the aging population in whom neurogenic claudication becomes symptomatic owing to central canal stenosis. A interlaminar route should theoretically deliver 100% of the medication into the neuraxis. Controlled studies of this patient population are still forthcoming.

Positioning

The patient is placed prone on the fluoroscopy table. Generally, a pillow or bolster is placed under the abdomen to induce a gentle flexion. If a patient is unable to lie prone, the procedure can be performed in the lateral position with the more dominant painful side down. It is believed that gravity may help lateralize the medication toward the site of pathology.

Imaging

The interlaminar space is visualized in the AP projection so that the spinal processes appear end on. Some cephalocaudal angulation may be used to better visualize the interlaminar spaces. If necessary, lateral fluoroscopic imaging can show the depth of the needle; however, it is generally advised to visualize needle movement in the AP direction to ensure that the needle tip is close to the midline.

After the needle is properly placed, the first injection should be nonionic contrast under real-time fluoroscopy (Fig. 2). Visual inspection should include possible venous uptake as well as possible intrathecal spread of the contrast. If an inadvertent intrathecal spread is suspected, a lateral fluoroscopic image can confirm or deny this suspicion.

The classic myelogram type of pattern should be easily recognized if it is present in the lateral imaging. The contrast materials are relatively hyperbaric compared to the cerebrospinal fluid and, therefore, slight table tilting can confirm or deny the presence of a dural puncture.

Needle Techniques

The procedure may be performed with a midline approach or a paravertebral approach. The paravertebral approach has the advantage of not going through the supraspinous and interspinous ligaments. Going through these ligaments can sometimes lead to a false feeling of loss of resistance when, in actuality, the needle is too shallow. Additionally, these ligaments are supporting structures in the posterior compartment.

An entry point is made perpendicular to the lamina just inferior to the interlaminar space. After anesthetizing the skin with a small bore needle, often a longer needle, such as a 22-gage, 31/2-in. spinal needle, is used to anesthetize the deeper structures and is brought in direct contact with the lamina. This gives the physician direct knowledge of the expected depth of the interlaminar space.

Several specially designed needles are used for the actual epidural injection. If a single injection is desired without the use of a catheter, a Crawford-type needle should be considered. It is specifically designed for this purpose. The shallow bevel of the needle is placed so that it is parallel to the fibers of the ligamentum flavum. The needle is directed from slightly paravertebral toward the midline of the interlaminar space. The stylette is kept within the needle so as not to allow any organic material to potentially clog the hollow bore of the needle. With a paravertebral approach, the first real resistance that should be met at the appropriate depth is the ligamentum flavum. At this point, the stylette is removed. Most interventional specialists prefer a loss-of-resistance-to-fluid technique. This technique involves placing 1 to 2 cc of either normal saline or 1% preservative-free lidocaine in a standard 5-cc syringe or a specialty syringe designed for this purpose. With the needle tip engaged in the ligamentum flavum, there is a great deal of difficulty injecting any fluid. As the needle is slowly advanced, there will be an immediate loss of resistance to injection of the fluid. At this point, all additional needle movements should be curtailed. Care should be taken so that one hand holding the needle additionally contacts the patient. That way, there is less risk of sudden advancement of the needle should the patient move. At this point, the loss-of-resistance syringe should with replaced with an injection of contrast material under real-time fluoroscopy. Extension tubing that has been purged of air with the contrast is helpful in keeping the operator's hands out of the direct fluoroscopic beam.

At times, it is desirable to thread a catheter. Radiopaque catheters are available for this purpose. For this procedure, a blunt curved-tip needle, such as a Tuohy needle, is used. The loss-of-resistance sequence is the same as with the Crawford needle. If unilateral depositing of medicine is desired, one should consider performing the paravertebral approach from the contralateral side. The point of entry is then at the midline, and typically the catheter will then thread to the desired side without difficulty. Catheters are generally threaded in a cephalad direction; however, experienced hands can thread the catheter in a caudad direction as well. Catheters can often be directed toward the neural foramina if this is the site of pathology.

Injectate

Initial injections should once again be solely with contrast under real-time fluoroscopy. After confirmation of correct placement, a glucocorticoid and anesthetic mixture may be instilled. The volume used will vary with the patient's size, the amount of epidural fat and venous vasculature, and the degree of stenosis and other pathology. A total volume may range from 1 or 2 mL up to 10 mL or more. If multiple segmental pain generators are suspected, the higher volumes might be employed. On the other hand, in an elderly patient with spinal stenosis, it would be prudent to use much smaller volumes.

Other Considerations

The interlaminar technique generally deposits a greater amount of medicine in the dorsal epidural space rather than the ventral. If the patient's pathology is a disc abnormality, certainly a transforaminal approach may prove more beneficial than an interlaminar one. A transforaminal epidural can be purposely delivered toward the ventral epidural space.

If there is any suspicion of a dural puncture, it may prove prudent to abandon the procedure. An injection can occur that is subdural, but not truly subarachnoid. When this occurs, patients have a stronger than normal sensory block that is often delayed by some 5–10 min. Vasodilation can occur with subsequent hypotension. Additionally, patients with blockade are at risk of falling when they first try to ambulate. They should be kept in the recovery area until all signs of blockade have dissipated.

Caudal Epidurals

Background

The caudal approach for performing epidurals has a long history. It is still being used for administering several types of surgical levels of anesthesia as well as in the management of pain under certain circumstances.

Transforaminal epidurals have generally supplanted the use of caudal epidurals. However, there are certain clinical presentations for which a caudal may be desirable. In advanced degeneration of the spine, the interlaminar spaces may no longer be accessible. In individuals with large intertransverse fusions, the transforaminal route becomes more technically challenging. In extremely obese individuals, the caudal canal can often be reached when standard needle equipment may not be long enough to reach other avenues into the epidural space.

Positioning

The patient is generally prone on the fluoroscopy table. A meticulous prep and drape should be employed to minimize the risk of any infection.

Imaging

Generally, AP imaging is first used to ensure midline placement of the needle. Then, if necessary, lateral fluoroscopic imaging can confirm whether or not the needle has entered the sacral hiatus (Fig. 3). Again, initial injections should be with contrast because quite often there is vascular uptake with initial placement of needles. The initial volume of injectate will help determine what volume should ultimately be used. There is a fair amount of so-called dead space before any glucocorticoid would reach the L5-S1 disc space.

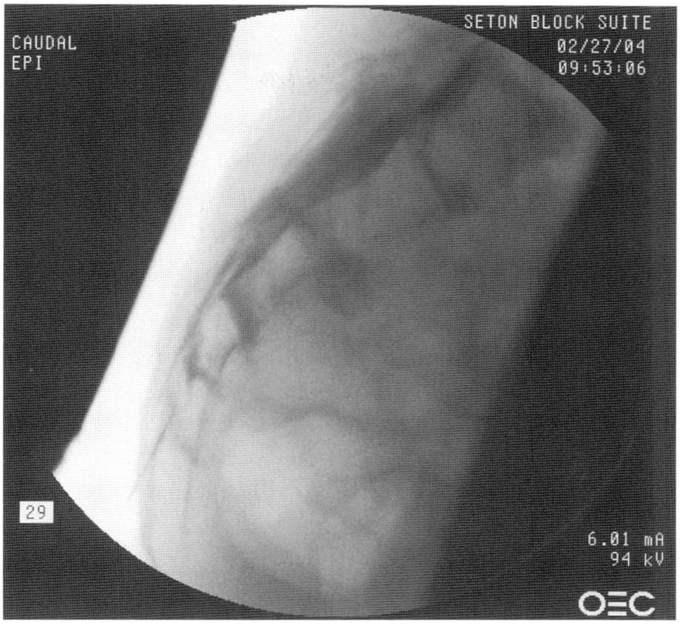

Fig. 3. Lateral view of caudal epidural with 22-gage spinal needle. Contrast is seen in the sacral caudal canal.

Needle Techniques

After the meticulous prep and drape, a 22- or 23-gage spinal needle can be used. A caudal epidural can often be performed with manual palpation of the bony structure followed by confirmation of needle placement with fluoroscopy.

The midline sacral prominences are felt with one hand. As the structures are palpated caudally, usually around S4, the sacral promontory is felt. The 22- or 23-gage needle is then placed slightly caudad to the sacral hiatus. The bevel of the needle is faced down so that it may glide more easily over the osseous structures. As the sacral hiatus is approached, the bevel of the needle is then placed face up to help guide it within the caudal canal. Contrast is injected and outlining of the sacral nerve roots is typically seen. One should carefully observe for possible vascular uptake of contrast. An inadvertent dural puncture should be highly unlikely.

Injectate

After placing the contrast-confirming caudal epidural spread, a solution of glucocorticoid with anesthetic can be placed. Mixing the glucocorticoid with a small amount of anesthetic may be considered. The anesthetic may be diluted with contrast so that it can be ascertained where the medicine travels. After this first aliquot of glucocorticoid with anesthetic and contrast (approx 5 mL) is delivered, it may then be followed by either dilute anesthetic or additional contrast. The concept is to push the glucocorticoid solution more cephalad up the epidural tree to its desired location.

Other Considerations

Caudal epidurals can also be placed with a catheter. An advantage is that one can deliver the medicine more cephalad and more likely closer to the area of pathology.

Catheters can often be steered toward the dominant site of pathology and also may be directed toward the ventral or dorsal epidural space. The disadvantage of a catheter is that it generally requires a larger-bore introducer needle. Care should be taken to minimize scraping the periosteum, because this can be painful.

Sacroiliac Joint Blocks

Background

The idea that the sacroiliac joint could be a potential source of pain has been debated throughout the last century. Over the past several decades, technology has advanced to a point where injections into the sacroiliac joints can be performed both safely and confidently. The primary reason for performing the injection is to obtain a diagnosis. It is generally believed that there is no set of clinical features or manual examinations that can accurately predict pain of sacroiliac origin. To date, there is no convincing evidence that the use of glucocorticoid will consistently produce long-term relief. However, there is anecdotal evidence that short-term relief may often occur.

Positioning

The patient is prone on the fluoroscopy table. A pillow bolster under the abdomen may make for a more comfortable experience for the patient and help to correct extreme lordosis if this is present.

Imaging

The most consistent way to enter the sacroiliac joint is at its inferior aspect. An AP view, perpendicular to the sacrum, often gives the most initial information. It should be remembered that the image is a two-dimensional interpretation of a three-dimensional (3D) joint. The more medial radiolucency represents the dorsal aspect of the joint, and the more lateral is the more ventral aspect. Often, these two joint surfaces converge 1 to 2 cm above the most inferior aspect of the joint. If this bright radiolucency occurs at the convergence of the joints, this is often an easy access to the joint (Fig. 4).

If this radiolucency at the convergence of the joint is not immediately seen, slight rotation through the C-axis may make it more prominent. Additionally, this allows the operator to study the joint to develop a 3D picture of the approximate shape of the joint. Some physicians find it beneficial to rotate through the C-axis to line up the two joint surfaces. Others find it more useful to separate out the dorsal and ventral surfaces of the joint. When rotating the C-arm contralaterally through its axis, thereby separating out the joints, often the medial cortical line of the joint silhouette becomes sharp. When this is obtained, it represents a direct straight-line access into this medial inferior part of the joint. If all of these maneuvers through the C-axis do not clearly demonstrate the inferior aspect of the joint, slow cephalocaudad angulation of the C-axis may be useful.

A typical sacroiliac joint holds about 1.5 mL of solution intra-articularly. When viewed under real-time fluoroscopy, a fully filled joint can have a "classic lightning bolt" appearance (Fig. 5). The joints often leak with capsular tears that may place additional medicine medially in close proximity to the dorsal sacral foramina, superiorly near the L5 nerve root, and ventrally in proximity to the lumbosacral plexus.

When leak of contrast is observed, the joint can be visualized in the AP to determine leaks from the superior or inferior ends. In addition, an oblique "en-face" view can be obtained to see the shape of the joint margins.

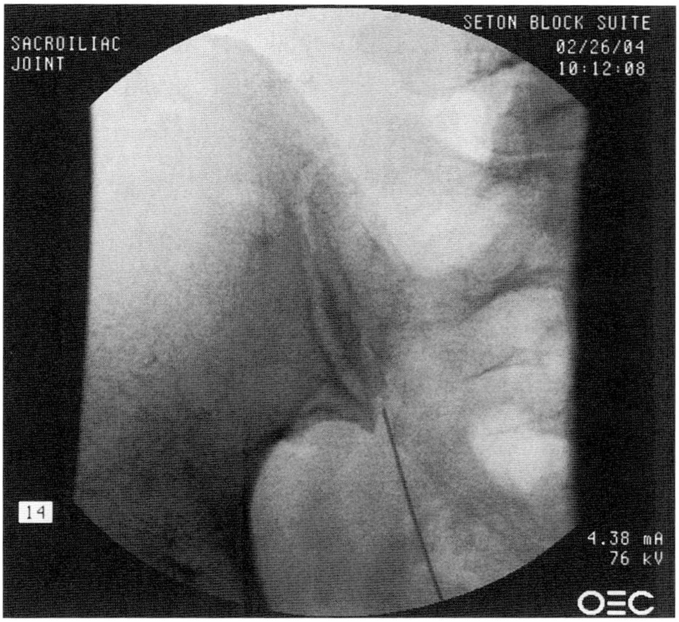

Fig. 4. Placement of 25-guge needle in radiolucency of left sacroiliac joint.

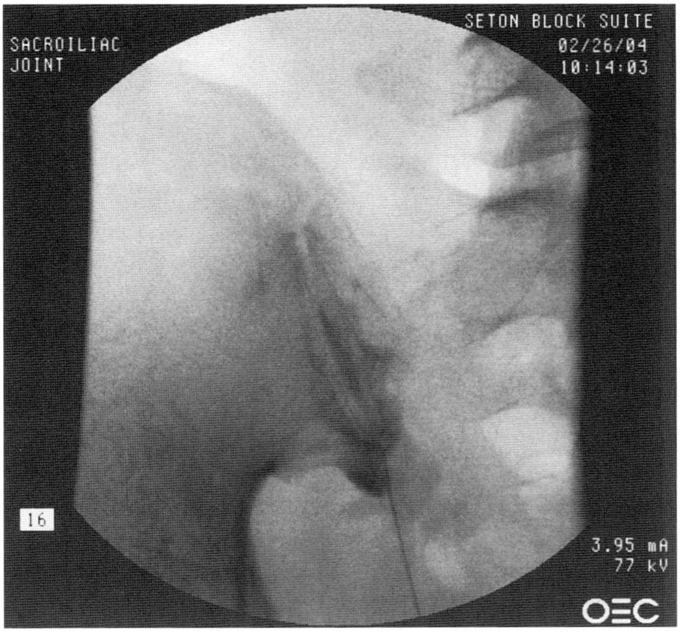

Fig. 5. Arthrogram of sacroiliac joint.

If all attempts at entering the inferior aspect of the joint 1 to 2 cm above the most inferior edge fail, injections can be attempted into the superior or inferior capsular recesses. On rare occasions, it may be necessary to try to enter the midpoint of the joint. Studying a CT axial image will help guide the practitioner in this endeavor.

Typically, the needle must traverse medially to laterally as well as somewhat inferiorly to achieve entry.

Needle Techniques

A 31/2-in., 25-gage needle should be sufficient for most needs. The depth of the inferior aspect of the joint is such that rarely more than a small percentage of the needle must penetrate the skin. Care should be taken to strike the sacrum first and then pass the needle more laterally into the joint. This prevents inadvertent passage of the needle through the sciatic notch and into the pelvic cavity.

If on first injection there is difficulty, one should try turning the bevel of the needle so that the bevel is facing cephalad toward the plane of the joint. A 3-cc syringe with a Luer-Lok should be used because this joint requires very little volume and occasionally modest pressurization is needed to inject through a small-bore needle such as a 25 gage.

Injectate

As previously mentioned, the sacroiliac joint on average holds about 1.5 cc of solution. If an optimal quality arthrogram is desired, one should consider injecting just contrast first. It is important to remember to keep the volumes low (0.5–1 cc) so as to leave room for the anesthetic. Alternatively, the contrast and anesthetic may be mixed together. A somewhat stronger anesthetic such as 2% lidocaine may be considered in the hope of creating a sufficient block. A glucocorticoid may be included in the mixture, with somewhat guarded expectations.

Other Considerations

Sacroiliac joint blocks are regarded as primarily a diagnostic tool. A diagnosis of sacroiliac dysfunction should be considered when the most intense pain is found below the L5 level, when the patient points directly to the posterior superior iliac spine, and if there is tenderness on palpation of the sacral sulcus just medial to the posterior superior iliac spine. These signs should also be considered in a patient who has had a previously successful arthrodesis of the lumbar spine that then deteriorates over time.

Medial Branch Blocks

Background

Blockade of the medial branch of the dorsal primary ramus has been advocated as the best method for determining pain of posterior element origin. It has a lesser potential for false positive response compared to true intra-articular injection of the facets. It has also been used as a screening procedure prior to radiofrequency neurotomy.

Performing the blocks on different occasions using anesthetics of different durations has been advocated to minimize the false positive rate of a single block. Although certainly this paradigm is advantageous in a scientific study, in clinical practice, it leads to a quandary. A placebo responder may have true pathology. Therefore, a potentially therapeutic procedure, such as radiofrequency neurotomy, may be denied to an individual owing to the fact that he or she simply exhibits a placebo response. Another school of thought would then say that in a known placebo responder, quite simply, to see if a neurotomy will be useful, the neurotomy should be performed. A neurotomy has been shown to be safe and reproducible in experienced hands.

Perhaps medial branch block testing has as its strongest virtue the ability to rule out a source of pain. A carefully performed, fluoroscopically controlled procedure that does not decrease the regionalized pain directs the practitioner to search for other potential sources.

The nomenclature and anatomy for the procedure should be well understood. Each joint is innervated by two medial branches. For example, to anesthetize the L4-L5 zygopophyseal joint, it is necessary to anesthetize the L3 and L4 branches. These L3 and L4 branches are found at the base of the superior articular process where it meets the transverse processes of L4 and L5. At the L5 level over the sacrum, the anatomy is somewhat different. The medial branch has not yet separated from the intermediate and lateral branches. It is generally agreed on that there is no consistent branch from the S1 neural foramina innervating the L5-S1 joint.

Positioning

The patient is prone on the fluoroscopy table. A pillow or bolster may be used to reduce the lordosis.

Imaging

The patient is visualized in the AP view with cephalocaudad angulation used to align the end plates with the fluoroscopy beam (Fig. 6). Then, slight oblique C-arm movement is used to best visualize the superior articulating process. It is also necessary to visualize the superior border of the transverse process.

A small amount of contrast should be mixed with the anesthetic (Fig. 7). Visualization of the block should occur under real-time fluoroscopy to ensure that there is no vascular uptake. If necessary, lateral imaging will ensure that the medication is sitting in the valley where the superior articulating process and transverse process meet. Occasionally the medicine is deposited dorsally, so if visualization is only in the AP or oblique modes, this can be checked by obtaining a more oblique view or a full lateral.

Needle Techniques

Generally, a very small-bore needle is all that is necessary. A 25-gage needle should be sufficient. Occasionally, in an extremely obese patient, it may be necessary to use a slightly greater-diameter needle.

Care should be taken to use minimal anesthetic to reach the target point. A 1-cc syringe with anesthetic may be used and the anesthetic administered in minute quantities as the needle is passed through the skin and tissue levels. This will ensure that too much anesthetic is not used, thereby eliminating the possibility of a false positive response. The target point is 2 to 3 mm below the superior edge of the transverse process at the junction of the superior articulating process. If the needle target point is too close to the superior edge, there is a chance that the medicine will track medially along the nerve root path toward the neural foramen. If the needle is placed too caudad along the transverse process, the chance of not properly anesthetizing the nerve becomes greater.

Injectate

Generally, 0.2–0.4 cc of total injectate is needed. Commonly used is 2% lidocaine, mixed in a 50/50 mixture with contrast or 0.75% bupivacaine diluted with contrast. There is no generally accepted use of glucocorticoid for this injection.

Other Considerations

Medial branch blocks are a diagnostic tool. Meticulous pre- and postblock evaluations are mandatory. Optimally, the patient is blinded as to the duration of the anesthetic. Pain assessment should be guided by a trained professional.

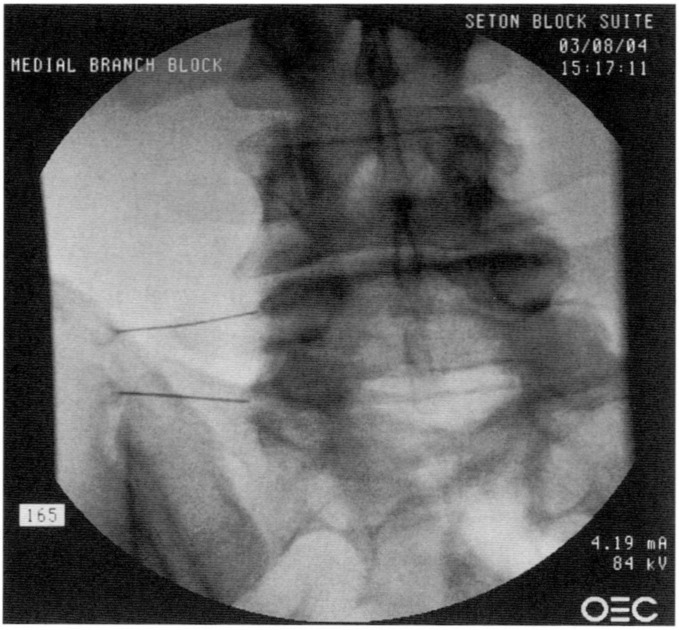

Fig. 6. AP view of needle placement for left L4 and L5 medial branch blocks.

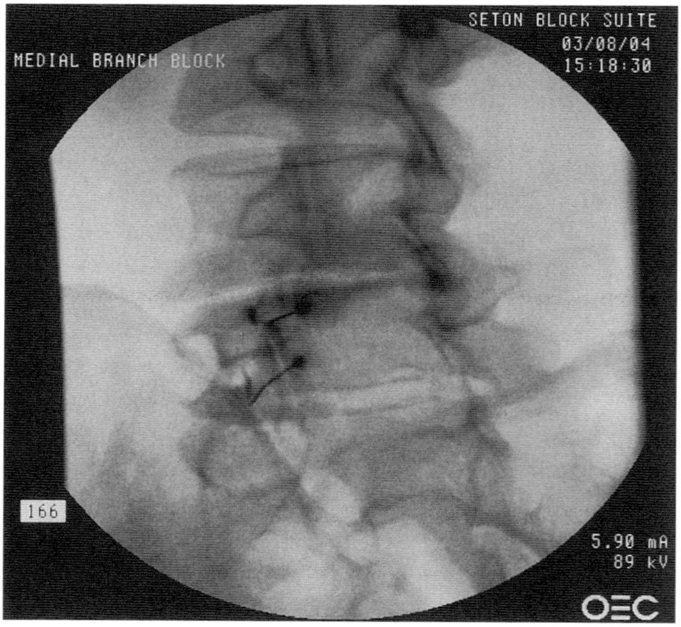

Fig. 7. Oblique view of contrast and anesthetic injected for L4 and L5 medial branch block.

Occasionally, it will be impossible to block the medial branch accurately. One example of this is in the individual who has had a previous arthrodesis. In such an individual, there may exist an intertransverse fusion mass preventing access to the expected location of the medial branch. In this instance, it may prove useful to perform an intra-articular zygopophyseal joint block at this first mobile segment. Naturally, this fusion mass would also interfere with the performance of a medial branch neurotomy.

Facet (Zygapophyseal Joint) Blocks

Background

Facet joint injections have been performed for many decades. Many clinical signs and symptoms are suggestive of posterior element pain, but none are 100% diagnostic. Currently, medial branch blockade is thought to be the better diagnostic tool as compared to intra-articular injections. There is always the chance of spillover of the joints into other structures, leading to a false positive. However, there are occasions when medial branch block testing cannot be physically performed.

Positioning

The patient is generally prone on the fluoroscopy table. However, an oblique positioning is sometimes useful, particularly if the plane of the joint is especially coronal in orientation. Additionally, with oblique positioning, it is possible to rotate the patient's shoulders back while maintaining the position of the hips, thereby partially subluxing the joints and allowing easier access.

Medicine may be deposited into the joints through either the superior or inferior recesses or by directly going to the joint itself. Of the superior and inferior recesses, typically it is the inferior that is much easier to enter. For this method of blockade, the patient is best in the prone position with several pillows under the abdomen to induce mild flexion of the spine. When the attempt is to enter the joint itself, often it is necessary to put the patient in a more oblique position.

Imaging

Studying any previously obtained axial images of the spine can prove useful. By knowing the concavity of the joint in question, it is possible to then plan the entry into each joint. When visualizing a joint under the process of fluoroscopy, cephalocaudad angulation of the C-arm is accomplished to line up the beam with the end plates of the vertebral body. The C-arm next goes through the maximum obliquity to best visualize the joint. The C-arm is then brought to a more AP view until the joint just disappears. Because of the concave nature of the surfaces of the joint, this most likely is the easiest entrance point (Fig. 8).

If access of the inferior recess of the joint is anticipated, then the patient should be prone on the fluoroscopy table (Fig. 9). The C-arm is adjusted so that the inferior border of the lamina is best visualized. Tracing this line out laterally should then help the observer appreciate the approximate location of the inferior articulating process.

With any method used, correct placement is confirmed only through the use of contrast. Extravasation of contrast can then be studied, which will lead to some degree of confidence in the selection of the intra-articular injection.

Needle Techniques

A smaller-bore needle is preferred. In most patients, a 25 gage needle should be sufficient. Additionally, with this smaller-bore needle, it is very easy to introduce the tip fully within the capsule of the joint. This smaller needle also has less chance of introducing any trauma. Occasionally, in larger patients, a somewhat larger-bore needle may be necessary.

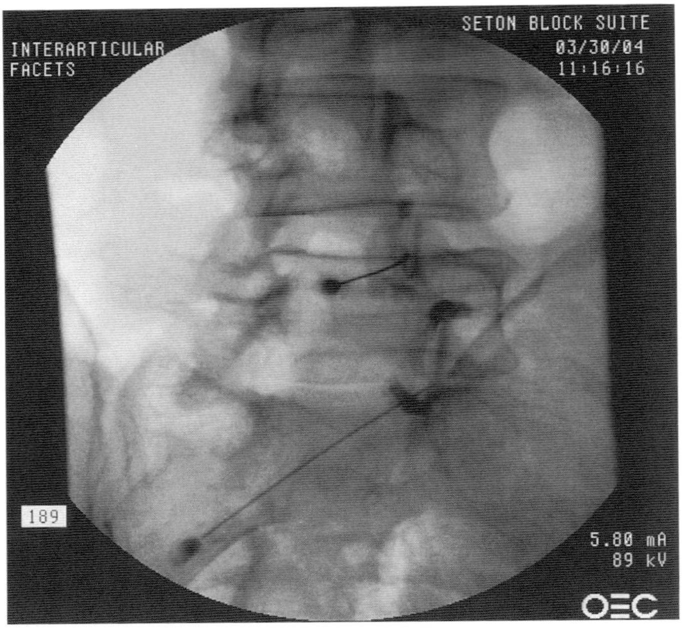

Fig. 8. Oblique view of interarticular arthrograms of right L4-L5 and L5-S1. The needle targets the midportion of the joint of L4-L5 and the inferior recess of the L5-S1 joint.

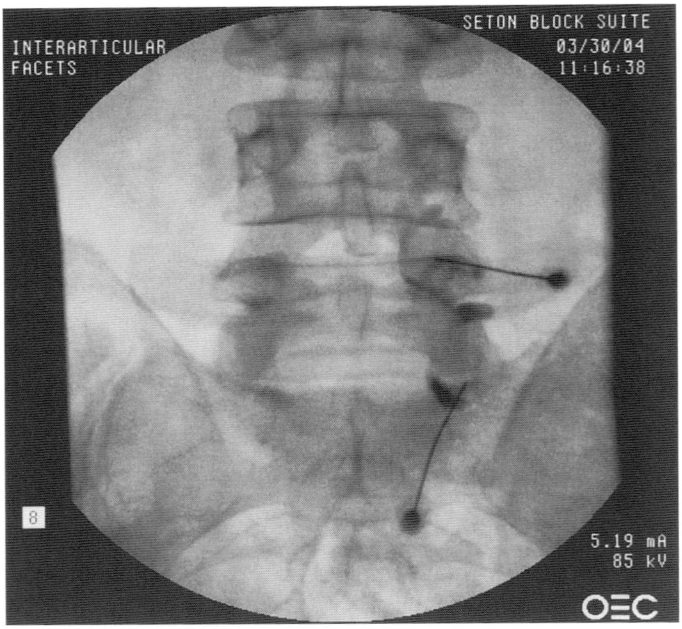

Fig. 9. AP view of arthrograms of L4-L5 and L5-S1 showing different approaches when targeting midportion of joint vs inferior recess.

As in the case with medial branch blocks, it is necessary to use minimal anesthetic to reach the target point. This minimizes the chance of a false positive response. If no anesthetic is used, increases the chance of a false negative block; the patient perceives postprocedural pain from the needling itself and cannot determine whether or not the regionalized pain has been removed.

Injectate

The injectate may consist of anesthetic, contrast, and glucocorticoid. Generally, very small volumes are necessary. A typical joint will hold approx 1.5 cc or less. A joint should not be overpressurized because this could potentially rupture the capsule.

Other Considerations

Although not scientifically validated with double-blind controlled studies, numerous observational studies and anecdotal experience suggest, in certain individuals, that glucocorticoid placed intra-articularly may reduce discomfort. The duration of this relief may be more likely on the order of weeks or months, rather than years. Although not proved with absolute scientific scrutiny, anecdotal evidence suggests that duration of relief on the order of days most likely is nondiagnostic and may be from systemic uptake of glucocorticoid or other factors. Durations of relief in excess of 2 wk, however, are suggestive, although not conclusive, of the medicine having been placed in or near the pain generator.

Sacrococcygeal Joint Injections

Background

The sacrococcygeal joint is a potential source of localized pain. Trauma to this joint may occur during a fall and is occasionally seen after childbirth. There may be damage to the joint itself or there may be a contusion to the sacrococcygeal nerves supplying the joint. Occasionally, discomfort in the area of the coccyx is a referred pain from a structure higher up.

Positioning

The patient is prone on the fluoroscopy table. The area is meticulously prepped and draped.

Imaging

Initial imaging should be in AP view. This will ensure that needle placement is in the midline, which will help prevent sliding alongside the joint into the deeper structures.

A lateral fluoroscopic image should be obtained to assess the plane of the joint (Fig. 10). Occasionally, more than one radiolucency is observed. There is sometimes complete separation of the joint, and this should be ascertained prior to placement of the needle.

Needle Techniques

A short 25- or 27-gage needle is all that is typically necessary. After the joint architecture is assessed by biplanar fluoroscopy, the needle should be placed with AP visualization. The needle generally travels only a few millimeters to reach the joint. The C-arm can then show lateral imaging to assess whether the joint can indeed be entered. Often, collimation of the image intensifier will aid in proper visualization of the joint.

Injectate

Only an extremely small volume of injectate is necessary. Usually, this is <0.5 cc. The mixture should consist of anesthetic, contrast material, and glucocorticoid. Larger volumes will also anesthetize the sacrococcygeal nerve.

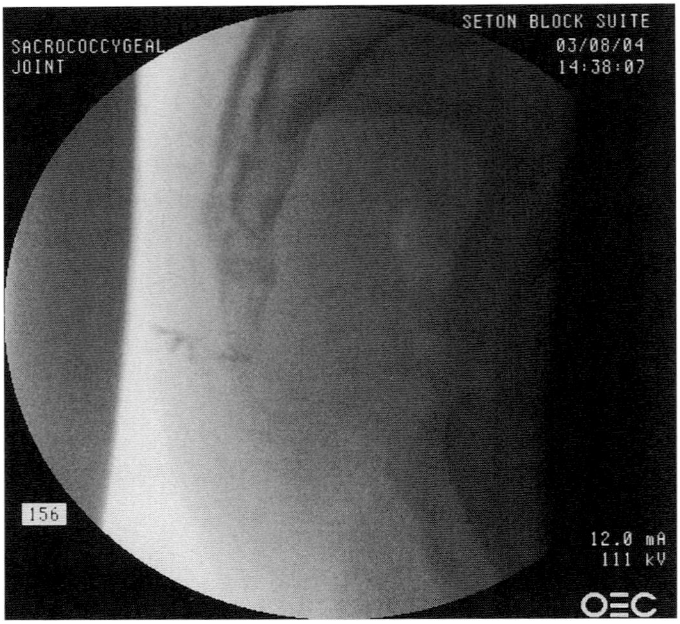

Fig. 10. Lateral image of sacrococcygeal joint injection with contrast and anesthetic.

Other Considerations

Use of glucocorticoid in the sacrococcygeal joint is based on anecdotal evidence and observational analysis. Initial relief may be on the order of weeks or months. Repeat injections have the potential to give more prolonged relief. Ultimately, surgical coccygectomy may be necessary in the most refractory and distressing cases.

REFERENCES

1. Moran R, O'Connell D, Walsh MG. The diagnostic value of facet joint injections. Spine 1988;13(12):1407–1410.
2. Schwarzer AC, Wang SC, O'Driscoll D, Harrington T, Bogduk N, Laurent R. The ability of computed tomography to identify a painful zygapophysial joint in patients with chronic low back pain. Spine 1995;20(8):907–912.
3. Schwarzer AC, Aprill CN, Derby R, Fortin J, Kine G, Bogduk N. Clinical features of patients with pain stemming from the lumbar zygapophysial joints: is the lumbar facet syndrome a clinical entity? Spine 1994;19(10):1132–1137.
4. Revel M, Poiraudeau S, Auleley GR, et al. Capacity of the clinical picture to characterize low back pain relieved by facet joint anesthesia: proposed criteria to identify patients with painful facet joints. Spine 1998;23(18):1972–1976; discussion, 1977.
5. Kaplan M, Dreyfuss P, Halbrook B, Bogduk N. The ability of lumbar medial branch blocks to anesthetize the zygapophysial joint: a physiologic challenge. Spine 1998; 23(17):1847–1852.
6. Dreyfuss P, Schwarzer AC, Lau P, Bogduk N. Specificity of lumbar medial branch and L5 dorsal ramus blocks: a computed tomography study. Spine 1997;22(8):895–902.
7. Schwarzer AC, Aprill CN, Derby R, Fortin J, Kine G, Bogduk N. The relative contributions of the disc and zygapophyseal joint in chronic low back pain. Spine 1994;19(7): 801-806.

8. Butler D, Trafimow JH, Andersson GB, Mcneill TW, Huckman MS. Discs degenerate before facets. Spine 1990;15(2):111–113.
9. Marks RC, Houston T, Thulbourne T. Facet joint injection and facet nerve block: a randomised comparison in 86 patients with chronic low back pain. Pain 1992;49(3):325–328.
10. Carette S, Marcoux S, Truchon R, et al. A controlled trial of corticosteroid injections into facet joints for chronic low back pain. N Engl J Med 1991;325(14):1002–1007.
11. Schwarzer AC, Derby R, Aprill CN, Fortin J, Kine G, Bogduk N. The value of the provocation response in lumbar zygapophyseal joint injections. Clin J Pain 1994;10(4):309–313.
12. Niemisto L, Kalso E, Malmivaara A, Seitsalo S, Hurri H. Radiofrequency denervation for neck and back pain: a systematic review within the framework of the cochrane collaboration back review group. Spine 2003;28(16):1877–1888.
13. Slipman CW, Bhat AL, Gilchrist RV, Issac Z, Chou L, Lenrow DA. A critical review of the evidence for the use of zygapophysial injections and radiofrequency denervation in the treatment of low back pain. Spine J 2003;3(4):310–316.
14. Leclaire R, Fortin L, Lambert R, Bergeron YM, Rossignol M. Radiofrequency facet joint denervation in the treatment of low back pain: a placebo-controlled clinical trial to assess efficacy. Spine 2001;26(13):1411–1416; discussion, 1417.
15. van Kleef M, Barendse GA, Kessels A, Voets HM, Weber WE, de Lange S. Randomized trial of radiofrequency lumbar facet denervation for chronic low back pain. Spine 1999; 24(18):1937–1942.
16. Dreyfuss P, Halbrook B, Pauza K, Joshi A, Mclarty J, Bogduk N. Efficacy and validity of radiofrequency neurotomy for chronic lumbar zygapophysial joint pain. Spine 2000;25(10):1270–1277.
17. Schofferman J, Kine G. The effectiveness of repeated radiofrequency neurotomy for lumbar facet pain. Spine 2004;29:2471–2473.
18. Stitz MY, Sommer HM. Accuracy of blind versus fluoroscopically guided caudal epidural injection. Spine 1999;24(13):1371–1376.
19. Renfrew DL, Moore TE, Kathol MH, el-Khoury GY, Lemke JH, Walker CW. Correct placement of epidural steroid injections: fluoroscopic guidance and contrast administration. Am J Neuroradiol 1991;12(5):1003–1007.
20. White AH, Derby R, Wynne G. Epidural injections for the diagnosis and treatment of low-back pain. Spine 1980;5(1):78–86.
21. Bogduk N, April C, Derby R. Epidural steroid injection, in Spine Care Diagnosis and Conservative Treatment White A, Schofferman J, eds. (AH W, eds.), Mosby, St. Louis, 1995, pp. 322–343.
22. Derby R, Lee SH, Chen Y. Injection therapies, nerve ablation, and intradiscal electrothermal annuloplasty for degenerative lumbar conditions. Semin Spine Surg 2003;15(4): 393–410.
23. Buchner M, Zeifang F, Brocai DR, Schiltenwolf M. Epidural corticosteroid injection in the conservative management of sciatica. Clin Orthop 2000(375):149–156.
24. Carette S, Leclaire R, Marcoux S, et al. Epidural corticosteroid injections for sciatica due to herniated nucleus pulposus. N Engl J Med 1997;336(23):1634–1640.
25. Karppinen J, Malmivaara A, Kurunlahti M, et al. Periradicular infiltration for sciatica: a randomized controlled trial. Spine 2001;26(9):1059–1067.
26. Vad VB, Bhat AL, Lutz GE, Cammisa F. Transforaminal epidural steroid injections in lumbosacral radiculopathy: a prospective randomized study. Spine 2002;27(1):11–16.
27. Wang JC, Lin E, Brodke DS, Youssef JA. Epidural injections for the treatment of symptomatic lumbar herniated discs. J Spinal Disord Tech 2002;15(4):269–272.
28. Karppinen J, Ohinmaa A, Malmivaara A, et el. Cost effectiveness of periradicular infiltration for sciatica: subgroup analysis of a randomized controlled trial. Spine 2001; 26(23):2587–2595.
29. Riew KD, Yin Y, Gilula L, et al. The effect of nerve-root injections on the need for operative treatment of lumbar radicular pain: a prospective, randomized, controlled, double-blind study. J Bone Joint Surg Am 2000;82-A(11):1589–1593.

30. Dooley JF, Mcbroom RJ, Taguchi T, Macnab I. Nerve root infiltration in the diagnosis of radicular pain. Spine 1988;13(1):79–83.
31. Derby R, Kine G, Saal JA, et al. Response to steroid and duration of radicular pain as predictors of surgical outcome. Spine 1992;17(6 Suppl):S176–S183.
32. Chen Y, Derby R, Kim BJ, Lee SH. Epidural steroid injections: past, present and future. Spineline 2003;4:9–20.
33. Schwarzer AC, Aprill CN, Bogduk N. The Sacroiliac joint in chronic low back pain. Spine 1995;20(1):31–37.
34. Slipman CW, Jackson HB, Lipetz JS, Chan KT, Lenrow D, Vresilovic EJ. Sacroiliac joint pain referral zones. Arch Phys Med Rehabil 2000;81(3):334–338.
35. Murata Y, Takahashi K, Yamagata M, Takahashi Y, Shimada Y, Moriya H. Origin and pathway of sensory nerve fibers to the ventral and dorsal sides of the sacroiliac joint in rats. J Orthop Res 2001;19(3):379–383.
36. Atlihan D, Tekdemir I, Ates Y, Elhan A. Anatomy of the anterior sacroiliac joint with reference to lumbosacral nerves. Clin Orthop 2000(376):236–241.
37. Maigne JY, Aivaliklis A, Pfefer F. Results of sacroiliac joint double block and value of sacroiliac pain provocation tests in 54 patients with low back pain. Spine 1996;21(16):1889–1892.
38. Dreyfuss P, Michaelsen M, Pauza K, Mclarty J, Bogduk N. The value of medical history and physical examination in diagnosing sacroiliac joint pain. Spine 1996;21(22):2594–2602.
39. Slipman CW, Sterenfeld EB, Chou LH, Herzog R, Vresilovic E. The predictive value of provocative sacroiliac joint stress maneuvers in the diagnosis of sacroiliac joint syndrome. Arch Phys Med Rehabil 1998;79(3):288–292.
40. Elgafy H, Semaan HB, Ebraheim NA, Coombs RJ. Computed tomography findings in patients with sacroiliac pain. Clin Orthop 2001(382):112–118.
41. Miller JA, Schultz AB, Andersson GB. Load-displacement behavior of sacroiliac joints. J Orthop Res 1987;5(1):92–101.
42. Sturesson B, Uden A, Vleeming A. A radiostereometric analysis of the movements of the sacroiliac joints in the reciprocal straddle position. Spine 2000;25(2):214–217.
43. Katz V, Schofferman J, Reynolds J. The sacroiliac joint: a potential cause of pain after lumbar fusion to the sacrum. J Spinal Disord Tech 2003;16(1):96–99.
44. Rosenberg JM, Quint TJ, De Rosayro AM. Computerized tomographic localization of clinically-guided sacroiliac joint injections. Clin J Pain 2000;16(1):18–21.
45. Hanly JG, Mitchell M, Macmillan L, Mosher D, Sutton E. Efficacy of sacroiliac corticosteroid injections in patients with inflammatory spondyloarthropathy: results of a 6 month controlled study. J Rheumatol 2000;27(3):719–722.
46. Luukkainen RK, Wennerstrand PV, Kautiainen HH, Sanila MT, Asikainen EL. Efficacy of periarticular corticosteroid treatment of the sacroiliac joint in non-spondylarthropathic patients with chronic low back pain in the region of the sacroiliac joint. Clin Exp Rheumatol 2002;20(1):52–54.
47. Slipman CW, Lipetz JS, Plastaras CT, et al. Fluoroscopically guided therapeutic sacroiliac joint injections for sacroiliac joint syndrome. Am J Phys Med Rehabil 2001;80(6):425–432.
48. Ferrante FM, King LF, Roche EA, et al. Radiofrequency sacroiliac joint denervation for sacroiliac syndrome. Reg Anesth Pain Med 2001;26(2):137–142.
49. Wray CC, Easom S, Hoskinson J. Coccydynia. Aetiology and treatment. J Bone Joint Surg Br 1991;73(2):335–338.
50. Perkins R, Schofferman J, Reynolds J. Coccygectomy for severe refractory sacrococcygeal joint pain. J Spinal Disord Tech 2003;16(1):100–103.

15
Experience With Minimally Invasive Nucleus Replacement

Michele Marcolongo, PhD, Parviz Kambin, MD, Anthony Lowman, PhD, and Andrew Karduna, PhD

BACKGROUND

Scope of the Problem

More than 5 million Americans suffer from chronic low-back pain, making it the leading cause of lost workdays in the United States and one of the most expensive health care issues today *(1)*. Although the causes of low-back pain remain unclear, it is believed that approx 75% of cases are associated with degenerative disc disease *(1)*. It is generally believed that dehydration of the degenerated nucleus pulposus (NP) leads to a reduction in hydrostatic pressure on the internal surface of the annulus, resulting in an abnormal stress state in the tissue and, consequently, a breakdown of the annular tissue seen macroscopically as fissures and tears. This manifests as chronic and debilitating pain owing to tissue impingement on nerve roots and presents as a herniated or ruptured disc. Current treatment options, such as discectomy and fusion, are fairly successful in reducing pain but do not restore normal biomechanical function to the disc. The likely outcome of these procedures is further degeneration of either the initially affected disc (for discectomy) or adjacent segments (for fusion). Degenerative disease of the spine is one of if not *the* leading musculoskeletal disorder confronting our health system. The spine provides the major structural element of the neck and trunk while protecting the spinal cord. Spinal degeneration is an irreversible process leading to loss of mechanical integrity with the potential for neurological compromise. Clinical manifestations of degenerative spine disease are variable and graded and are categorized into a variety of diseases. These diseases include mechanical cervical and lumbar pain such as internal disc disruption, acute spinal instability, herniated NP, degenerative spondylolisthesis, degenerative scoliosis, and spinal stenosis.

Spine degeneration is ubiquitous. Cadaveric examination of lumbar disc showed a 97% incidence of disc degeneration by age 50 *(2)*. Approximately one-third of the population has evidence of degenerative disease on radiographic study by age 40 *(3,4)*. Sixty to 80% of all working adults lose time from work owing to back pain *(5)*. Tremendous pain and suffering are associated with the degenerative diseases of the spine, in addition to the societal costs.

From: *Arthroscopic and Endoscopic Spinal Surgery: Text and Atlas: Second Edition*
Edited by: P. Kambin © Humana Press Inc., Totowa, NJ

Treatment of Degenerative Disc Disease

Current treatment for degenerative disc disease focuses primarily on relieving back and leg pain. The inflammatory response secondary to tissue injury and nerve root impingement are frequently observed in association with degenerative disc changes and are thought to mediate a pain response. Although the exact mechanism of pain generation is debated, >75% of low-back pain is associated with degenerative disc disease *(1)*. Moreover, sciatica has an even stronger association with disc herniation and nerve root impingement. In the absence of neurological impairment, treatment begins with conservative care, activity modification, and anti-inflammatory medication. Under this regimen, 85–90% of patients are treated successfully in 3 mo *(10,11)*. However, the remaining 10–15% of patients incur >75% of the treatment costs, often requiring highly invasive surgical interventions. The most common surgical treatments—discectomy and spinal fusion—are performed to reduce pain, not to restore disc function. Discectomy is employed when the disc has herniated and is impinging on nerve roots, causing pain. In this surgery, the impinging region of the annulus fibrosus (AF) and NP is excised, hence alleviating pressure on the nerves and eliminating pain. Pain is eliminated in 90–95% of cases *(12)*. However, as previously noted, this approach does nothing to restore normal biomechanics of the vertebral segment *(13)*: the NP is still dehydrated and the annulus fibers are still likely operating in compression. Therefore, the patient continues along the path of disc degeneration over ensuing years.

Surgical fusion—inducing bone growth across the functional spinal unit to eliminate disc loading and motion—is reserved for patients with chronic severely disabling pain. Generally, discs treated with fusion are farther along the path of degeneration. Without delineating the specific indications for fusion of the functional spinal unit (which are varied depending on the signs and symptoms of the degenerative disease), suffice it to say that approx 150,000 spinal fusions are performed per year in the United States alone. The numbers are growing exponentially. Regardless of the extent to which this procedure is performed, the results of spinal fusion vary extensively *(14)*. Failure of fusion can be common in 10–30% of patients depending on disease. More perplexing is the clinical outcome, which may not improve with increased rates of fusion. Significant long-term limitations are associated with a spinal fusion. Spinal fusion does nothing to restore the normal biomechanics of the vertebral segment. In fact, the lack of motion within the segment can lead to further degeneration of the adjacent intervertebral discs *(15)*. Lehmann et al. *(16)* pursued a long-term follow-up of lumbar fusions in patients from 21 to 52 yr of age and found that 44% of the patients were currently still experiencing low-back pain, 50% had back pain within the previous year, 53% were on medications, 5% had late sequelae secondary to surgery, and 15% had repeat lumbar surgery. This suggests the need for alternatives to fusion.

Intervertebral Disc Replacement

An alternate approach to the treatment of degenerative disc disease is to remove the diseased disc in its entirety and replace it with a synthetic implant *(17–33)*. Disc replacement may serve to eliminate pain while restoring physiological motion. This approach for total knee and hip replacement has been highly successful. However, disc replacement has not enjoyed the same clinical success. More than 56 reports on mechanical replacement have been described *(28)*, most from the standpoint of design concept, with very few clinical reports. In general, these solutions provide dynamic load bearing with passive restraint but mechanically fail in long-term application. One of the most promising designs is the LINK disc replacement developed by Buttner-Janz et al. *(30,31)* and Zippel *(32)*, which has had clinically success. This sandwich design consists of cobalt chromium alloy end plates and a polyethylene core. The results of clinical trial in 93 patients showed back pain relief in 20% of patients and leg pain relief in 40–50% of patients after an average implantation time of 1 yr *(33)*. This device is currently an investigational device in the United States.

NP Replacement

Rather than replacing the entire disc, several investigators have attempted to replace the NP alone. This is intended to provide a surgical technique that would offer a less invasive approach to pain relief while potentially restoring the functional biomechanics to the system. This approach could be most effective in patients with early diagnosis of disc disease, before the annulus has suffered significant degeneration. The concept of nucleus replacement was developed by Nachemson in the early 1960s, who attempted injection of a self-curing silicone into the disc space in cadavers *(34)*. Further research into silicone replacement of the nucleus continued into the early 1990s *(35–40)*. The silicone prostheses have been promising as far as mechanical properties and ease of insertion into the nucleus; however, silicone synovitis and its associated complications may play a significant role in limiting the clinical success of this material, as it has in other orthopedic joints *(41)*. Gan et al. *(42)* investigated nucleus tissue engineering as a way of regenerating the degenerated tissue. Although the cells clearly adhered to the glass substrate and primarily held their phenotype after 3 wk in vitro, it was not clear that the matrix was that of a healthy NP. This approach is reasonable in an era of tissue engineering solutions, but cell and molecular biologists are still struggling to determine the nature of the NP cell. Therefore, setting and meeting the requirements of regenerating the tissue, although promising, has many challenges to overcome before adaptation as a clinical treatment.

Ray and colleagues have developed and internationally commercialized a polyacrylonitrile hydrogel nucleus replacement covered with a polyethylene fiber jacket. The device, generally implanted in pairs, is intended to improve disc height, restore motion, and relieve pain owing to disc herniation *(43)*. The current surgical success rate for patients implanted from 1999 through 2001 is 88%, with the primary failure being dislocation of the implant from the nucleus. The open procedure through the annulus can allow the hydrogels (which are implanted in the hydrated state) to exit through the incision site. Although the surgical technique is still evolving to the level of having a truly satisfactory procedure, patient pain in this short-term follow-up study was reduced 86% (Oswestry and visual analog scale pain levels) and spinal flexibility increased 67%. This clinical trial has provided the first evidence of improvement in the treatment of degenerative disc disease via nucleus replacement. This nucleus replacement device is currently completing a phase I clinical investigation in the United States and is being sold commercially in Europe.

Bao and Higham *(44,45)* have also approached nucleus replacement with a hydrogel polymer. This material selection has resulted in an implant that has similar mechanical properties to those of the nucleus as well as similar physiological properties, maintaining about 70% water content under physiological loading conditions. The particular hydrogel employed by these researchess comprises semicrystalline polyvinyl alcohol

(PVA) *(44,45)*. PVA is a biocompatible polymer *(46)* that has the ability to absorb water or physiological fluid and survive mechanical loading as would exist in the nucleus region of the intervertebral disc. However, PVA is not entirely stable within the physiological environment of the body, showing degradation through the melting out of small crystallites over time, which can result in a reduction of mechanical properties and leaching of molecules into the physiological environment *(47)*.

Intervertebral Disc Mechanics

Earlier work was performed for nucleus replacement with a synthetic material in cadaveric FSUs *(48–51)* and in animals *(52,53)*. The data reported were primarily for end-plate strains *(48)* and segmental mobility in combined loading modes *(49–51)*. Parameters such as rotational displacement, disc height, and range of motion were observed before and after nucleus implantation to assess the restoration ability of the nucleus implant device used. However, in all of the cases, nucleotomy was facilitated by making a small incision through the AF. This may not be the ideal approach for assessing the effect of nucleus implant because the surrounding annulus was damaged at least partially. No human cadaver studies have reported the effect of nucleus implant replacement on the pure compressive behavior of the FSU. However, Meakin et al. *(52)* used sheep discs to assess the effect of nucleus implant on bulging direction of the annulus fibers in pure compression. They observed that a nucleus implant with a modulus in the range of 0.2–40 MPa prevented the inward bulging of the annulus, seen in the case of a denucleated specimen. However, their numerical modeling *(52)* showed that the stresses were restored to those of the intact FSU only with an implant in the modulus range of 3–5 MPa. The idea of nucleus replacement by a synthetic material was proven feasible in all of the studies just descnbed. Mechanisms of interactions between the nucleus implant and surrounding tissue have not been thoroughly explored. In addition, numerical modeling of the human lumbar FSU with a nucleus replacement has not been reported in the peer-reviewed literature.

Stable, Solid Hydrogel Polymer NP Implant

Previous work in our laboratory focused on developing and characterizing a highly chemically stable hydrogel polymer system *(54–56)*. The motivation for materials selection for a device to replace the nucleus is fourfold: (1) the individual polymers are biocompatible; (2) the polymers interact to form physical crosslinks that serve to stabilize the hydrogel material; (3) the material can be processed in a variety of ways that allow the tailoring of mechanical properties without modification of chemistry; and (4) the material displays shape memory properties with hydration level, which may facilitate minimally invasive implantation of the device. This polymer is based on PVA but incorporates a second polymer, polyvinylpyrrolidone (PVP), that serves to stabilize the hydrogel through interpolymer complexes, which serve as secondary, physical crosslinks and provide the networks with additional stability, as demonstrated in vitro *(55,56)*.

One major concern about the use of hydrogels is the potential leaching of unreacted monomers or crosslinking agents from the insoluble, chemically crosslinked structures. A significant benefit of the proposed hydrogels is that the structure of the proposed implants relies on physical crosslinking, rather than covalent chemical crosslinking, to hold polymer chains together. The gels are prepared by blending the two polymers.

The polymers proposed for use are soluble and can thus be purified easily prior to blending. Because PVA *(46)* and PVP *(57)* have been shown to be compatible in the body, the blend of the two is also likely to be compatible.

Aside from chemical considerations in hydrogel stablility in vivo, there are mechanical considerations for this structural application: (1) the hydrogel must be able to withstand the repetitive loading environment of movement; (2) the hydrogel must have a viscoelastic behavior that matches fairly closely that of the AF so that there is no excessive deformation of the device owing to creep; and (3) the hydrogel must display a modulus and Poisson's ratio that, on loading, will provide an interfacial stress with the annulus that mimics the normal intradiscal pressure to restore mechanical function to the implanted vertebral segment. Our preliminary data have demonstrated that the family of PVA/PVP hydrogels is promising in meeting these material requirements. However, if further mechanical analysis shows a limitation to the mechanical behavior of the gels, the mechanical behavior of the material may be altered through processing changes, or through variation of the polymer composition and/or polymer concentration, making this family of materials very desirable when the need arises to tailor mechanical properties.

DESIGN AND CHARACTERIZATION OF HYDROGEL

Characterization and Surgical Feasibility of PVA/PVP Hydrogel Material

Previous research in our laboratories led to the development and characterization of novel hydrogels prepared from blends of PVA and PVP *(55,56)*. As already stated, the motivation for materials selection for a device to replace the nucleus is fourfold. The goal of this prior work was to establish the in vitro stability of the gels and to determine the surface chemical changes and mechanical behavior of the gels over time of immersion in vitro. These properties were examined as a function of the composition of PVA/PVP as well as the molecular weight of PVA and PVP.

In Vitro Stability: Swelling and Dissolution Behavior

Blends containing between 0.5 and 75 wt% PVP and the balance PVA were prepared with four different molecular weight combinations. Solutions of PVA and PVP were prepared by dissolving various ratios of the polymers in deionized water at 90°C overnight. The solutions, which contained 10% by weight polymer, were homogenized for 30 min using sonication. The solutions were then cast into Plexiglas® trays and dried at 37°C for 72 h. On drying, residual water was removed from the polymer films in a vacuum oven at 35°C with an absolute pressure of 127 mmHg. The polymer blends were swollen in deionized water for 1 to 2 h to form gels. Circular discs were punched from the films and dried in an oven to evaporate deionized water introduced in swelling. After the dry mass of the circular discs ($n = 3$) was measured, the discs were swollen at 37°C in deionized water. The mass of each swollen gel was measured regularly for 120 d. Additionally, the deionized water was replaced frequently. Following 120 d of swelling, the gels were removed from solution and dried under vacuum. The dry weights of the discs were recorded in air and heptane in order to determine the volume and density. The weight swelling ratio (weight of swollen gel/weight of dry polymer) and volume swelling ratio (volume of swollen gel/volume of dry polymer) for the polymers were calculated. Additionally, the dissolution of the polymer was determined by comparing the initial preswollen weight to the final dry weight.

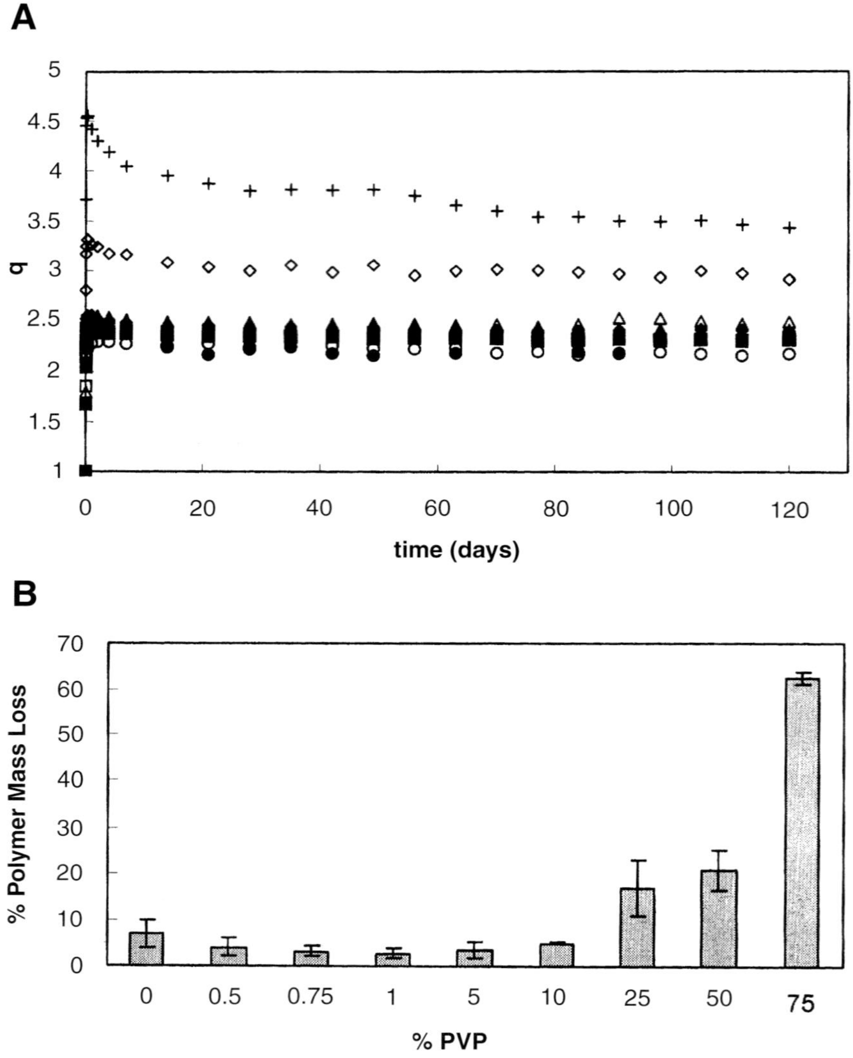

Fig. 1. (A) Mass swelling ratio over time of immersion for gels prepared with (A) 143K PVA/10K PVP molecular weight combination with (●) 0% PVP, (○) 0.5% PVP, (■) 0.75% PVP, (□) 1% PVP, (▲) 5% PVP, (Δ) 10% PVP, (◆) 25% PVP, and (✧) 50% PVP (+) 75% PVP and (**B**) 50% PVA/50% PVP hydrogel prepared with (●) 143K PVA/10K PVP (○) 143K PVA/40K PVP (■) 95K PVA/10K PVP, and (□) 95K PVA/40K PVP. (B) Polymer mass loss is minimized from that of PVA alone with the addition of 0.5–5% PVP.

The swelling and dissolution data are presented in Fig. 1 for the average molecular weight combination of 143,000 g/mol (PVA) and 10,000 g/mol (PVP), the most stable molecular weight combination tested. For all of the samples, the gels rapidly hydrated to maximum value, followed by some decrease in gel mass. The initial reduction was owing to the gels relaxing during swelling followed by some dissolution of the polymers. However, for polymers containing <25% PVP, the swelling behavior reached equilibrium within 2 d. Increasing amounts of PVP, however, led to a material that was not

Table 1
Weight Loss (%) of PVA/PVP Hydrogels From Dissolution Analysis ($n = 3$)

	Weight loss (%)				
Time (h)	100/0 PVA/PVP	95/5 PVA/PVP	90/10 PVA/PVP	75/25 PVA/PVP	50/50 PVA/PVP
1	0.67 ± 0.58	0.77 ± 0.56	4.28 ± 3.80	22.93 ± 1.82	45.46 ± 3.65
8	0.77 ± 0.33	1.91 ± 0.16	7.02 ± 2.92	23.59 ± 3.11	48.39 ± 2.89
24	1.57 ± 1.14	3.60 ± 0.15	7.92 ± 1.26	22.06 ± 2.62	47.00 ± 0.73

stable, as indicated by the declining q values over time of immersion in physiological solution. The total polymer mass loss after 120 d resulted in 7% loss for PVA alone, vs 3% for PVA with up to 1% PVP. Increasing amounts of PVP in the gel led to increased polymer mass loss, indicating reduced stability of the material in vitro.

The dissolution behavior of the gels was examined using swelling studies and attenuated total reflectance-Fourier transform infrared spectroscopy (ATR-FTIR) (Nicolet Magna-IR 560 Spectrometer; Madison, WI). For the studies, thin, flat strips of the dried polymers were mounted on a zinc-selenium ATR crystal and the IR spectra were obtained using 2048 scans and a resolution of 2 cm^{-1}. These samples were then weighed in air and heptane and placed in phosphate-buffered saline solutions at 37°C. At set times following immersion (1, 2, 4, 8, and 12 h), the strips were removed from solution and weighed. These strips were then dried under vacuum between flat plates for 72 h and the weights were recorded. The percent weight loss for the gels was calculated.

As seen in Table 1, short-term dissolution studies showed that for the gels a majority of the polymer dissolving out of the gel was lost during the first 24 h. Based on the nature of the blends, we hypothesized that the early time mass loss was owing to dissolution of the nonhydrogen bonded, amorphous PVP from the semicrystalline PVA. To demonstrate This hypothesis, ATR-FTIR spectra were obtained for the gels prior to swelling and postswelling in the same time period as the weight loss analysis. The characteristic peaks that we chose to represent the two polymers were the secondary alcohol –C-C-O stretch peak at 1075 cm^{-1} for PVA *(58)*, and a mixed mode of carbonyl group stretch and –N-C stretch at 1654 cm^{-1} for PVP *(59)*. The IR spectra of the dried blend films prior to any swelling are shown in Fig. 2. The changes in the relative peak height with changing composition are clear.

The IR spectra of dried films postswelling were obtained for each set time. A representative sample is shown in Fig. 2B. For each blend film, the carbonyl peak of PVP lost the initial height after swelling. The height of the 1075-cm^{-1} peak of PVA remained nearly constant for the entire period, indicating that most of the PVA remained in the hydrogel networks after swelling. On the other hand, for the 1654-cm^{-1} peak of PVP, the peak height decreased dramatically at the end of the first hour of swelling but remained nearly constant for the rest of the study. These changes are in agreement with the dissolution experiments and support the hypothesis that PVP initially dissolves out the gel, followed by increased gel stability.

Finally, tensile tests of thin strips of swollen hydrogels were performed after 2 d and 1, 2, 4, and 8 wk of immersion in vitro ($n = 5$). The dimensions of the strips (4.25 mm wide and 75 mm long) were in accordance with ASTM Standard Test Method for Tensile

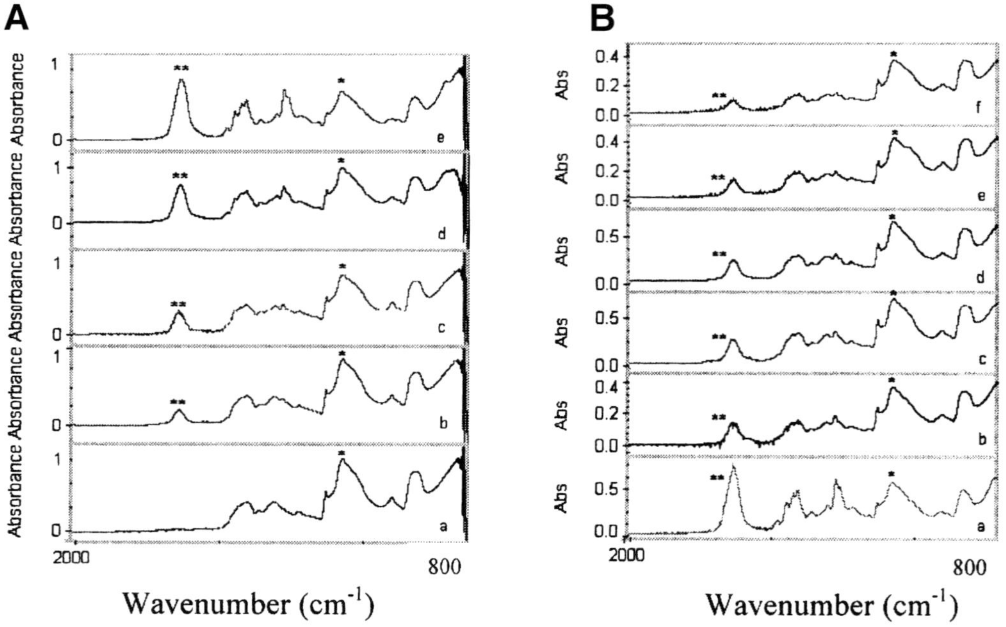

Fig. 2 **(A)** ATR-FTIR spectra prior to swelling: (*) –C-C-O stretch peak of PVA; (**) carbonyl group stretch peak of PVP; a, 100/0 (PVA/PVP); b, 95/5 (PVA/PVP); c, 90/10 (PVA/PVP); d, 75/25 (PVA/PVP); e, 50/50 (PVA/PVP). **(B)** ATR-FTIR spectra postswelling for initially 95/5 (PVA/PVP) hydrogels: (*) –C-C-O stretch peak of PVA; (**) carbonyl group stretch peak of PVP; a, prior to swelling; b, 1 h of swelling; c, 4 h of swelling; d, 8 h of swelling; e, 12 h of swelling; f, 24 h of swelling.

Properties of Thin Plastic Sheeting (D882-95A) *(60)*. Tensile modulus measurements indicated that the modulus was approx 2 MPa and that for the composition with 1% PVP, the modulus was stable over 56 d of immersion *(55)*. A statistically significant reduction in modulus was measured for PVA alone. The reduction in modulus in PVA is most likely owing to the significant mass loss, whereas the 1% PVP compositions had no statistically significant reduction in modulus and correspondingly little mass loss compared to PVA alone. The structures of the hydrogels were evaluated and characterized using rubber elasticity theory based on swelling studies and tensile experiments *(55,61)*. The values of M_c increased for the hydrogels with more PVP initially blended in the system, indicating the presence of fewer physical crosslinks (Fig. 3).

Mechanical Behavior: Stress Relaxation and Fatigue

Stress relaxation behavior of the PVA/PVP hydrogel (10 w/w% polymer, 99% PVA, 1% PVP) is important to understand because of the effect of constant deformation on the ability of this viscoelastic material to hold or dissipate stress. Pilot experiments were conducted in our laboratory in which the hydrogel was held in a compressive displacement of 15% strain in a hydrated environment at 25°C. The load was monitored and the load relaxation was examined over time. Figure 4 shows that the material reached half of its initial load after 4 h of loading and that an equilibrium load level was

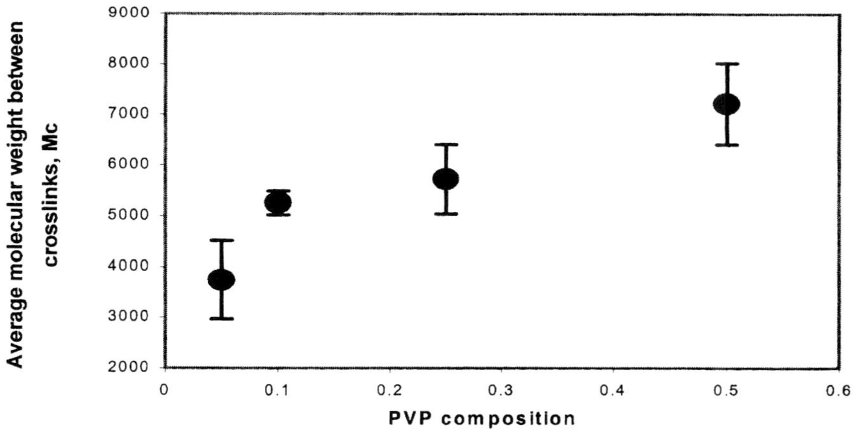

Fig. 3. The molecular weight between crosslinks increased for hydrogels with more PVP initially blended into the system, indicating the presence of fewer physical crosslinks.

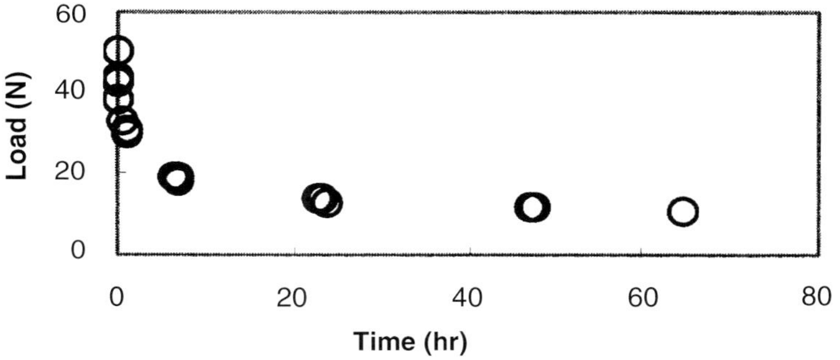

Fig. 4. Stress relaxation behavior of PVA/PVP hydrogel.

approached after 60 h. This pilot study enabled the test methodology to be developed (although temperature control at 37°C will be added) and indicates that the viscoelastic response is very typical of elastomeric polymers.

Compression–compression fatigue was used to determine the duration of the material over repeated cycling in vitro. Samples were cycled from 1 to15% strain to represent physiological strains achieved while walking *(62)* for either 10,000, 100,000, or 1,000,000 cycles in a simulated physiological solution *(63)* held at 37°C for the duration of loading (n = 3). The test was conducted at 5 Hz. A customized fixture was designed and fabricated that included grooved bearing plates so that the hydrogel would remain in a stable position for the duration of the test. Earlier work showed that the hydrogel tended to slip out of the smooth bearing plates. The load was recorded over the cycling period. After testing, the material was permitted to recover in vitro for 14 d, and then a single compression test was run to determine whether any permanent mechanical degradation had occurred to the material.

Results showed that the instantaneous compressive modulus of the hydrogel after any of the cycles up to and including 10 million cycles of fatigue was not appreciably

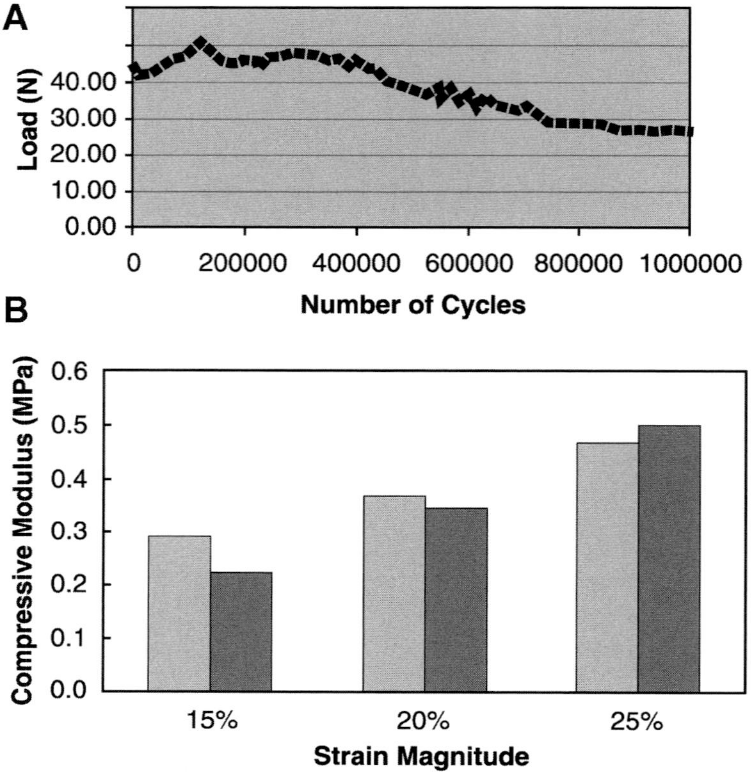

Fig. 5. **(A)** Load-carrying capability of PVA/PVP hydrogel over 1 million cycles of strain-controlled loading. **(B)** Compression-proof test after hydrogel was loaded for 10 million cycles and subsequently allowed to recover in vitro. The dark gray bars represent the compressive modulus data of control samples that did not undergo any mechanical loading, and the light gray bars represent the data from samples tested after 10 million cycles of fatigue. **(C)** Photograph of control (left) and 10 million cycle-fatigued implants.

different from that of the unfatigued samples. (Fig. 5B). In addition, there was no permanent change in dimensions of the implant up to 1 million cycles. However, after 10 million cycles in fatigue, a change in dimensions had occurred. The height was reduced by 22% and the diameter increased by 8% (Fig. 5C). An analysis of the load-VS-number-of-cycles curve (Fig. 5A) shows that the load-carrying capacity of the material was reduced as the number of cycles increased. This may be attributed in part to the stress relaxation behavior of the material, as described in Fig. 4. The 1 million-cycle test took 54 h to run; this corresponds to the point of equilibrium observed in the preliminary stress relaxation experiment, which may explain the reduced load-carrying capability of the material held at constant strain amplitude over time of cycling.

Cadaveric Endoscopic Implantation of Dehydrated Hydrogel Implant

To demonstrate the ability to remove damaged NP material and to insert the dehydrated hydrogel endoscopically, a human cadaveric model was incorporated. Using a C-arm X-ray machine and instrumentation developed by a colleague (P. Kambin, MD,

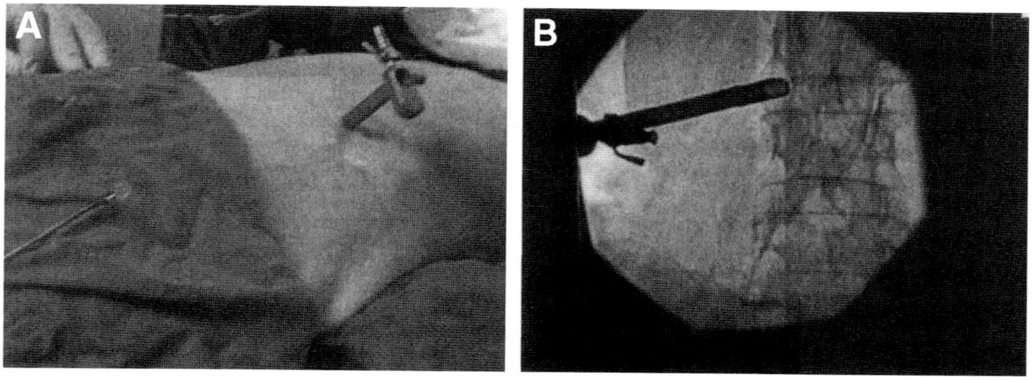

Fig. 6. Cadaveric endoscopic implantation of dehydrated hydrogel implant using annular approach.

Drexel University), we introduced an oval cannula through the triangular working zone of the annulus *(12)*. The 5 × 8 mm oval cannula provided a space for inserting forceps, which were used to resect a region of the nucleus. Once the nucleus was cleared, the dehydrated hydrogel polymer implant was inserted through the cannula into the nuclear cavity (Fig. 6). A saline drip was used to rehydrate the implanted gel *in situ*. Figure 6 shows the implant and cadaveric model as well as an X-ray of the positioning of the cannula in the nucleus region of the intervertebral disc. This exercise demonstrated the ability of the implant to be introduced endoscopically; however, details regarding the dehydration/rehydration of the implant as well as further development of the surgical technique are required.

BIOMECHANICAL CONSIDERATIONS OF NUCLEUS REPLACEMENT: COMPRESSIVE STIFFNESS OF IMPLANTED HUMAN CADAVERIC FSUs

In a separate study, we examined the compressive mechanical behavior of the human cadaveric FSU after implantation with a hydrogel nucleus replacement *(64)*. This work focused on the ability of the gel to re-create the "normal" biomechanics of the intact vertebral segment. The gel was not implanted in a dehydrated state, and the insertion method was not intended to represent the case of clinical implantation, which would require significant modification. However, the aim of this work was to establish the implant biomechanics with an intact annulus.

A 10% polymer mixture was prepared from a blend of 95% PVA/5% PVP as described previously, and the mixture was processed using six freeze-thawing processes. Hydrogel implants were mechanically tested in unconfined compression at 100% strain/min. Lumbar spines were harvested from eight cadavers (three males, five female) with an average age 65 yr. FSUs (n = 15) from L1 to L5 levels were resected and prepared by removing the facet joints and posterior elements. Two flat, parallel cuts were made in the bone to ensure alignment of the axial compression load, and the bone was stored in a freezer until the day of testing. Specimens were thawed for at least 2 h at room temperature prior to testing. Mechanical testing was performed on an Instron mechanical test machine (Model 1331). Specimens were potted in the test fixture with

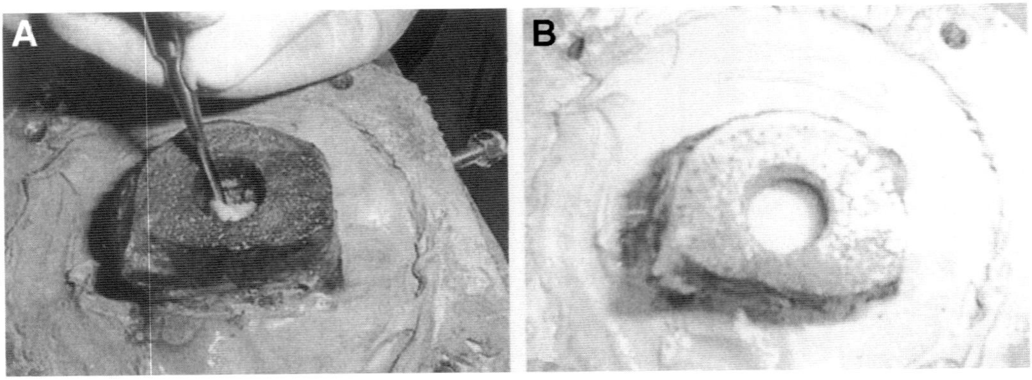

Fig. 7. Surgical preparation for cadaveric implantation of hydrogel nucleus replacement: **(A)** removal of NP, **(B)** implanted FSU.

commercially available bonding material, and all specimens were preconditioned for 50 cycles at 3% strain (commonly used for spine preconditioning) *(65–67)*. Specimens were axially compressed with a loading rate of 1 mm/s up to 15% of total height of intervertebral disc (IVD) at 0.5 Hz for 5 cycles for each condition. The data of the fifth loading cycle were taken for analysis.

The following series of axial compressive tests was completed on each specimen. The intact specimen was first tested (intact condition). Then, the upper vertebral body was drilled using, a 16-mm-diameter Cloward core drill bit. This hollow-core drill was positioned over the NP on the upper cut surface of the vertebral body and drilled perpendicular to this surface. The vertebral body was penetrated to the top of the IVD, and the cylindrical bone plug above the IVD was removed (Fig. 7). The bone plug was reinserted and the specimen was tested with the bone plug placed in its original position on the FSU (BI condition). Then, the bone plug was again removed and the NP was incised in line with the core drill and the central portion of the NP was removed using standard surgical instruments. This procedure allowed the AF to remain intact and the FSU was again tested (DN-1 denucleated condition). Next, a hydrogel implant with a 16-mm diameter and a height equal to the IVD height was implanted in the cavity (formed by excision of the NP). The cylindrical bone plug was again placed in its position as before, and the specimen was tested (implanted condition). Finally, the implant was removed, and the specimen was tested again in "denucleated" condition (DN-2 condition).

Figure 8B shows the typical nonlinear nature of the load-displacement curve for one of the specimens, in axial compression. In all the specimens, curves for DN-1 condition and for DN-2 condition superimposed, indicating return of the specimen to its original denucleated state after removal of the implant. Drilling into the vertebrae (BI) reduced the stiffness compared to the intact condition and was significantly different ($p < 0.05$). A more dramatic reduction in the stiffness was observed for denucleated specimens (stiffness value of 48% of BI at 15% strain, $p < 0.05$). Insertion of the hydrogel implant restored the stiffness of the FSU to a value of 89% of BI at 15% strain and was significantly different at higher deformations ($p < 0.05$).

Calculated stiffness values agreed well with those previously reported in the literature *(68,69)*. Restoration of the stiffness to the denucleated FSU after implantation with a

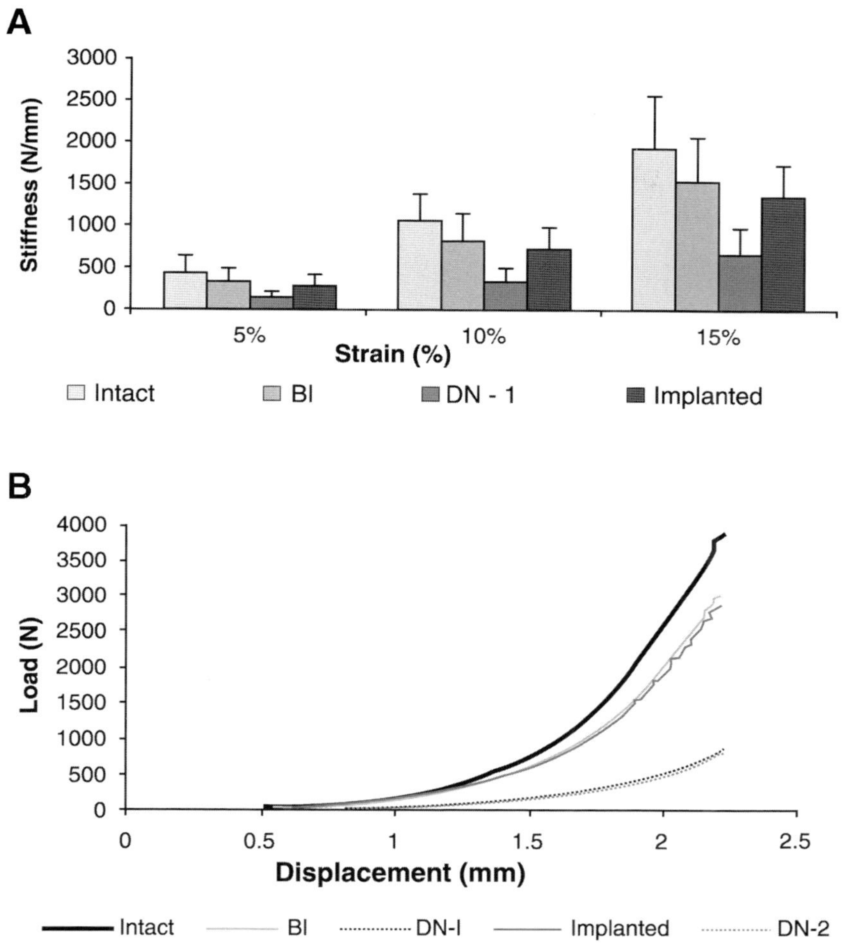

Fig. 8. **(A)** Stiffness vs strain for FSU under different conditions ($n = 15$) and **(B)** typical load deformation curve for FSU under different conditions.

polymeric hydrogel is evident from Fig. 8. The general premise that the spinal biomechanics results from a synergistic effect between the implanted hydrogel and the surrounding annulus has been shown through this experimentation. A linear summation of the stiffness of the denucleated FSU (776.0 N/mm at 15% strain) and that of only hydrogel (2.0 N/mm at 15% strain) does not equal the stiffness of the implanted FSU (1433.0 N/mm at 15% strain). We hypothesize that this nonlinear increase in stiffness after hydrogel implantation is the result of a mechanical interaction between the annulus and the implant, in which the Poisson effect of the implant results in tension developing in the fibers of the annulus as the disc is loaded in compression.

Axisymmetric Finite Element Modeling of Human FSU

To understand better the stress state of the annulus with respect to the normal, intact human lumbar intervertebral disc and the effect of incorporating nucleus replacements of different mechanical properties, we incorporated finite element modeling *(64)*. The FSU was assumed to be an axisymmetric object with respect to the sagittal plane, with

Table 2
Input Material Properties to Axisymmetric Finite Element Model

	Young's modulus (MPa)	Poisson's ratio (ν)
Bone	12,000	0.30
AF	Hyperelastic	0.45
NP	1	0.49

simplified geometry. To simulate the experimental condition, posterior elements were not modeled for this analysis because the anterior region provides a major load-bearing area in axial compression *(70)*. The FSU was modeled as a cylindrical object with three main components—NP, AF, and vertebrae—with the cartilage end plates neglected for this preliminary analysis (as demonstrated in our modeling).

The axisymmetric FE model (ABAQUS) contained 14,702 nodes and 10,775 elements. NP and bone were modeled as elastic materials. The AF was modeled as a hyperelastic material. Material properties for the AF were assumed isotropic for this preliminary study (a limitation of the analysis, in that the actual tissue properties are anisotropic), and bone was assumed to be entirely trabecular. Values were obtained from the literature *(71)*. Mooney-Rivlin strain energy potential of first order was used to characterize the properties of the AF. The material properties used are presented in Table 2. Four-node axisymmetric elements were used. The total number of variables in the model was 32,241.

The FE Model was validated against the experimental results obtained in our laboratory. The validation criterion was matching of the load-displacement curve of the intact FSU. Using the geometry described and the properties noted in Table 2, we adjusted the Mooney-Rivlan constants for the AF until the solution converged on the load-displacement curve best representing that of the experimentally determined curve for the intact FSU (Fig. 9).

In this study, we were interested in determining the mechanism responsible for the restoration of near-intact compressive stiffness values by the implanted cadaver FSU experiment. We investigated radial displacements of the annulus in the region of the nucleus interface, and the calculations revealed that the radial displacements of the intact and implanted conditions were quite similar, showing tensile displacements in the annulus near the nucleus interface, whereas those of the denucleated condition revealed marked differences in that compressive displacements were calculated in the interface between the annulus and the nuclear cavity.

To test the effect of nucleus implant modulus on the stiffness of the FSU using the validated model, we examined a range of moduli for the nucleus implant ranging from 0.01 to 100 MPa. The results, shown in Fig. 10, demonstrated that the implant modulus did affect compressive stiffness of the FSU and that those moduli in the range of 0.01–1 MPa resulted in the closest matching of the implanted to the intact condition. In addition, calculated intradiscal stresses (at the interface between the implant and the annulus) also changed with implant material modulus.

This analysis does correlate with our experimental observations and shows that there is a relationship among intradiscal pressure, FSU compressive stiffness, and modulus of the nucleus implant. The relationship between modulus and annulus radial displacements has also been observed in a cadaveric sheep experimental model *(52)*.

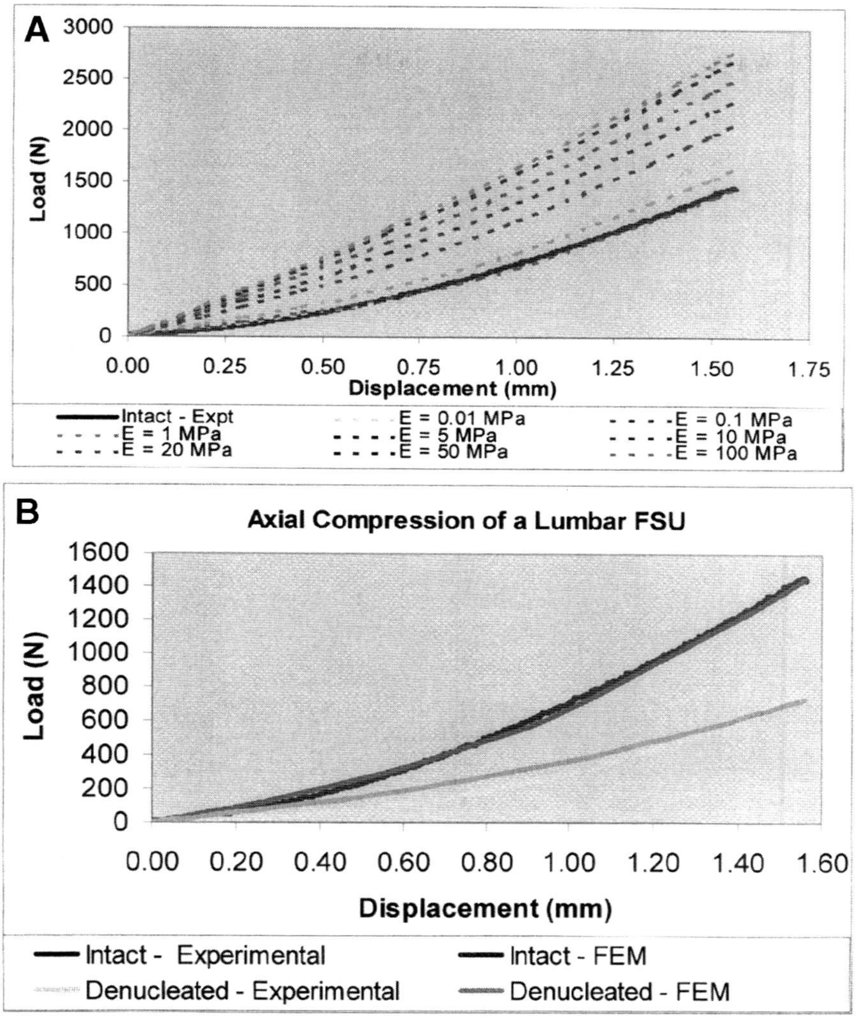

Fig. 9. (**A**) Validation of the FE Model (FEM) to the compressive load-displacement curve of the modeled intact condition to the experimental intact condition also resulted in close matching of the denucleated modeled and experimental conditions. (**B**) Effect of implant material modulus on load-displacement curves of implanted FSU model. Implant moduli between 0.01 and 1 MPa showed closest matching to the load-displacement curve of the intact experimental FSU.

CONCLUSION

We have developed and characterized a PVA/PVP hydrogel polymer as a candidate for nucleus replacement of the intervertebral disc. The material was shown to be highly stable in vitro and demonstrated mechanical integrity over 10 million cycles of compression–compression fatigue under physiological strain levels. When used as a nucleus implant, the PVA/PVP material was able to interact with the annulus in a synergistic fashion to restore the compressive stiffness of the vertebral segment to 89% of that of the BI condition. Likely, this is a result of the nucleus implant providing a stress

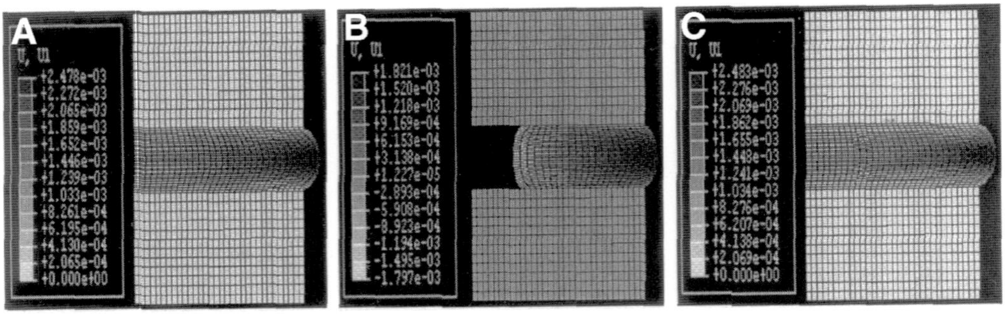

Fig. 10. Finite element predictions for radial displacements in **(A)** intact, **(B)** denucleated, and **(C)** PVA/PVP-implanted human lumbar FSU. The radial displacements of the intact and implanted conditions were quite similar, showing tensile displacements in the annulus near the nucleus interface, whereas those of the denucleated condition showed marked differences in that compressive displacements were calculated in the interface between the annulus and the nuclear cavity.

to the annulus that mimics the intradiscal pressure of the normal NP. Although our preliminary data support the premise that treatment of degenerative disc disease with a hydrogel nuclear implant may reproduce intact FSU biomechanics from the compressive loading perspective, important questions still need to be answered, including static implant biomechanics in order in order under different loading regimes as well as time-dependent implant biomechanics, in order to begin to address viscoelastic considerations. In addition, a critical design challenge to the success of such a device will be the ability of the implant to be inserted in a minimally invasive fashion and to maintain its position within the nucleus cavity without expulsing through the defect created on insertion or through any preexisting tears in the AF. Although the data thus far are promising for this technique, on going studies are necessary in order to achieve clinical success in incorporating nucleus replacement.

REFERENCES

1. MedPro, Month, 1998;VIII(1).
2. Miller JAA, Schmatz C, Schultz, AB. Lumbar disc degeneration: correlation with age, sex, and spine level in 600 autopsy specimens. Spine 1988;13(2):173.
3. Boden SD, Davis DO, Dina TS, Patronas NJ, Wiesel SW. Abnormal magnetic-resonance scans of the lumbar spine in asymptomatic subjects. J Bone Joint Surg 1990;72A:403–408.
4. Wiesel SA, Tsournas N, Feffer HL, Citrin CM, Patronas NJ. Incidence of positive CAT scans in an asymptomatic group of patients. Spine 1984;9:549–551.
5. Deyo RA, Tsui-Wu YJ. Descriptive epidemiology of low back pain and its related medical care in the United States. Spine 1987;12:264–268.
6. Frymoyer JW. Back pain and sciatica. N Eng J Med 1988;318:291–300.
7. Snook SH, Jensen RC. Cost, in Occupational Low Back Pain, (Pope MH, Frymoyer JW, Andersson C et al.), Praeger, New York 1984, pp. 115–121.
8. Biering-Sorensen F. Physical measurements as risk indicators for low back trouble over a one-year period. Spine 1984;9:106–119.
9. Holbrook TL, Grazier KL, Kelsey JL, Stauffer RN (eds.). The Frequency of Occurence, Impact, and Cost of Musculoskeletal Conditions in the United States American Academy of Orthopaedic Surgeons, Chicago, 1984.
10. Bush K, Cowan N, Katz DE, Gishen P. The natural history of sciatica associated with disc pathology. Spine 1992;17:1205–1212.

11. Ahn S-H. Comparison of clinical outcomes and natural morphologic changes between sequestered and large central extruded disc herniations. Yonsei Med 2002;43(3):283–290.
12. Kambin P, Savitz MH. Arthroscopic microdicectomy: an alternative to open disc surgery. M Sinai J Med 2000;67(4):283–287.
13. Weber H. Lumbar disc herniation: a controlled prospective study with ten years of observation. Spine 1993;8:131–140.
14. Lee C, Langrana NA, Parsons JR, Zimmerman MC Development of a prosthetic intervertebral disc. Spine 1991;16(6 Suppl): S253-S255.
15. Leong JC, Chun SY, Grange WJ, Fang D. Long-term results of lumbar intervertebral disc prolapse. Spine 1983:793–799.
16. Lehmann TR, Spratt KF, Tozzi JE, et al. Long-term follow-up of lower lumbar fusion patients. Spine 1987; 12:97–104.
17. Salib RM, Pettine KA. Intervertebral disk arthroplasty. 1993: US Patent 5258031.
18. Patil A. Artificial intervertebral disc. 1982: US Patent 4309777.
19. Baumgartner W. Intervertebral disk prosthesis. 1994: US patent 5320644.
20. Hedman TP, Koastiuk JP, Fernie GR, Hellier WG Artificial spinal disc. 1988: US Patent 529548.
21. Monson GL. Synthetic intervertebral disc prosthesis. 1969: US.
22. Fischer H. Support chamber for holding two adjacent vertebrae. 1987: West Germany patent.
23. Edeland HG. Some additional suggestions for an intervertebral disc prosthesis. J Biomed Mater Res: Appl Biomater 1989;23:189–194.
24. Lee CK, et al. Functional and biocompatible intervertebral disc spacer. 1990: US Patent.
25. Parsons JR, et al. Functional and biocompatible intervertebral disc spacer containing elastomeric material of varying hardness. 1992: US Patent.
26. Steffon AD. Artificial disc. 1991: US Patent.
27. Enker P, Steffee A, McMillin C, Keppler L, Biscup R, Miller S. Artificial disc replacement. Spine 1993;18:1067–1070.
28. McMillin CR, Steffee AD. Artificial spinal disc with up to five years follow-up, in Transactions of the 20th Annual Society for Biomaterials, 1994, p. 89.
29. Steffee AD. The Steffee artificial disc, in Clinical Efficacy and Outcome in the Diagnosis and Treatment of Low Back Pain (Weinstein JN, ed.) Raven, New York: 1992, pp. 245-257.
30. Buttner-Janz K, et al. Intervertebral disc endoprosthesis. 1988: US Patent.
31. Buttner-Janz K, Schellmack R, Zippel H. Biomechanics of the SB Charite lumbar intervertebral disc endoprosthesis. Int Orthop 1989;13:173–176.
32. Zipple H. Charite modular: concept, experience, and results, in The Artificial Disc, (Brock M, Myer HM, Weigel K, ed.) Springer, Berlin: 1991; pp. 69–77.
33. Griffith SL, Shelukov AP, Buttner-Janz K. A multicenter retrospective study of the clinical results of the LINK SB Charite intervertebral prosthesis. Spine 1994;19:842–1849.
34. Nachemson A. Some mechanical properties of the lumbar intervertebral disc. Bull Hosp Joint Dis 1962;23:130–132.
35. Schneider PG, Oven R. Intervertebral disc replacement: experimental studies, clinical consequences. Z Othop 1974;112:791–792.
36. Schneider PG, Oven R. Plastic surgery on intervertebral disc. Part 1: Intervertebral disc replacement in the lumbar region with silicone rubber: theoretical and experimental studies. Z Othop 1974;112:1078–1086.
37. Camille RG, Sailani R. Livaste, Experimental study of lumar disc replacement. Rev Chir Othop Appar Mat 1978; 64(Suppl III):106–107.
38. Fassie B, Ginestle JF. Disc prosthesis made of silicone: experimental study and first clinical cases. Nouvelle Presse Med, 1978;21:207.
39. Bost M. Mechanical loading of the vertebral body cover plate: measurement of the direct stress distribution at the interface between intervertebral disc and vertebral body, in Die Wirbelsuule in Forschung, Praxis, Junulanns H, ed. Hippokrates, Stuttgart, 1982.

40. Ashida H, Yolurnvaniva K, Okumulu A. An attempt to develop artificial nuclei pulposi in lumbar intervertebral discs. I. Jpn Orthop Assoc 1990;64:S947.
41. Chan M, Chowchuen P, Workman T, Eilenberg S, Schweitzer M, Resnick D. Silicone synovitis: MR imaging in five patients. Skeletal Radiol 1998;27(1):13–17.
42. Gan JC, Ducheyne P, Vresilovic E, Shapiro IM. Bioactive glass serves as a substrates as a substrate for maintenance of phenotype of nucleus pulposus cells of the intervertebral disc. J Biomed Mater Res 2000;51(4):596–604.
43. Bertagnoli R, Schonmayr R. Surgical and clinical results with the PDN prosthetic disc-nucleus device. Eur Spine J 2002;11(Suppl 2):S143–S148.
44. Bao QB. Higham PA. Hydrogel intervertebral disc nucleus. 1991: US Patent.
45. Bao QB, Higham PA. Hydrogel intervertebral disc nucleus. 1993: US. Patent
46. Hara Y, Matsuura T, Taketani F. Biocompatibility of polyvinylalcohol gel as a vitreous substitute. Nippon Ganka Gakkai Zasshi 1998;102(4):247–255.
47. Peppas NA, Merrill EW. Development of semicrystalline PVA networks for biomedical applications. J Biomed Mater Res. 1977;11:423–434.
48. Frei H, Oxland T, Rathonyi G. The effect of nucleus prosthetic device on a lumbar spine mechanics, in Transactions of the 47th Annual Meeting of the Orthopaedic Research Society, 2001.
49. Dooris A, Hudgins G, Goel VK. Biomechanics of a multisegmental lumbar spine with a prosthetic nucleus. Spine 2002;2:3S–44S.
50. Bain AC, Sherman T, Norton BK, Hutton WC. A comparison of the viscoelastic behavior of the lumbar intervertebral disc before and after the implantation of a prosthetic disc nucleus. BED 2000;48:203–204.
51. Eysel P, Rompe JD, Schoemayr R. Biomechanical behavior of a prosthetic lumbar nucleus. Acta Neurochir (Wien) 1999;141:1083–1087.
52. Meakin JR, Reid JE, Hukins DW. Replacing the nucleus pulposus of the intervertebral disc. Clin Biomech 2001;16:560–565.
53. Ledet E, Dirisio D, Tymeson M. The Raymedica PDN prosthetic disc nucleus device in the baboon lumbar spine. Spine 2002;2:47S–128S.
54. Thomas J, Gomes K, Lowman A, Marcolongo M. Novel associated hydrogels for nucleus pulposus replacement. J Appl Biomater, in press.
55. Thomas J, Lowman A, Marcolongo M. Novel associated hydrogels for nucleus pulposus replacement. J Biomed Mater Res 2003;67A:1329–1337.
56. Liu X, Marcolongo M, Lowman A. Short term in vitro response of associating hydrogels. Polymers, submitted.
57. Risbud MV, Bhat SV. Properties of polyvinyl pyrrolidone / beta-chitosan hydrogel membranes and their biocompatibility evaluation by haemorheological method. J Mater Sci: Mater Med 2001;12:75–79.
58. Lin-Vien D, Colthup NB, Fateley WG, Grasselli J. Alcohols and phenols, in The Handbook of Infrared and Raman Characteristic Frequencies of Organic Molecules, Academic, San Diego: 1991.
59. Hu Y, et al. In Macromolecular Chemistry and Physics, 200. pp. 705–714.
60. American society for Testing and Materials. Standard Test Method for Tensile Properties of Thin Plastic Sheeting (D882-95a), ASTM in Annual Book of ASTM Standards, New York, 1995: pp. 182–187.
61. Melrose J, et al. R D A longitudinal study of the matrix changes induced in the intervertebral disc by surgical damage to the annulus fibrosis. J Orthop Res: Off Publ Orthop Res Soc, 1992. 10(5): p. 665–676.
62. Bagga CS, Williams P, Higham PA, Bao QB. Development of fatigue test model for a spinal nucleus prosthesis with preliminary results for a hydrogel spinal prosthetic nucleus. BED 1997;35: p. 441–442.

63. Marcolongo M, Ducheyne P, Lacourse W. Surface reaction layer formation in vitro on a bioactive glass fiber/polymeric composite. J Biomed Mater Res, 1997;37: 440–448.
64. Joshi A, Karduna A, Marcolongo M. A non-linear finite element model of the lumbar functional spinal unit to determine the ideal material properties of a hydrogel nucleus implant. in 29th Annual Proceedings of the Society for Biomaterials, 2003; p. 672.
65. Glazer PA, et al. In vivo evaluation of calcium sulfate as a graft substitute for lumbar spinal fusion. Spine 2001;1:395–401.
66. Goel VK, Weinstein JN. Biomechanics of intact ligamentous spine, in Biomechanics of the Spine: Clinical and Surgical Perspective, CRC Press, Boca Raton FL: 1990; p. 116.
67. Suh JK, et al. Viscoelastic behavior of human cervical FSU in torsion, in NASS 11th Annual Meeting, 1996.
68. Langrana NA, Edwards T, Sharma M. Biomechanical Analyses of Loads on the Lumbar Spine. In The Lumbar Spine (Wiesel SW, Weinstein J, Herkowitz H, Dvorak J, Bell G, eds) W. B. Saunders, Philadelphia: 1996; pp. 163–171.
69. White AA, Panjabi MM. Clinical Biomechanics of the Spine, 2nd ed. Lippincott, Philadelphia, 1990.
70. Frankel V, Nordin M. Basic Biomechanics of the Skeletal System. Lea & Febinger, Philadelphia: 1980.
71. Goel A. combined finite element and optimization investigation of lumbar spine mechanics with and without muscles. Spine 1993;18(11):1531–1541.

16

Interspinous Process Implant for Treatment of Lateral and Central Spinal Stenosis

Operative Technique and Results

Douglas Wardlaw, ChM, FRCSEd

INTRODUCTION

The clinical syndrome of spinal stenosis is usually seen in middle-aged or elderly individuals who complain of leg pain, weakness, paresthesia, or sensory changes that generally develop on standing or walking and are relieved, typically, by sitting and lying down. Often patients stoop forward to ease the symptoms when standing or walking. The condition can be extremely disabling, making the sufferer, in many cases, housebound.

The earliest description of spinal stenosis in the English literature was in 1899 by Sachs and Frankl, who described patients with lumbar or lower-extremity pain who walked bent forward and whose symptoms were relieved by laminectomy *(1)*. In 1927, there was a similar description by Putti *(2)*, and he and Hirsch, in 1948 *(3)*, described foraminal compression. Both recommended facetectomy as treatment. Harris and MacNab *(4)* described the basic pathology of disc degeneration and its consequent effects on other spinal structures and pathological anatomy. MacNab *(5)* described lateral recess stenosis, foraminal encroachment by the posterior articular process, and foraminal and lateral disc herniation. Verbiest from Holland is generally accredited with recognizing the clinical syndrome and relating it to spinal stenosis. The story typically told is that he noted that patients had difficulty walking, but less or no difficulty cycling, which could be accounted for by the fact that the patients' lumbar spines are in the flexed position while cycling but in the erect position while walking. His treatment was by wide laminectomy *(6–9)*.

PATHOLOGICAL ANATOMY

The syndrome of adult spinal stenosis is almost certainly brought about by a combination of factors. Verbiest, in his early work, demonstrated in his patients with spinal stenosis that the interpedicular distance of the lumbar spine vertebrae was close to the expected normal range, but that the anteroposterior (AP) distance was significantly less

From: *Arthroscopic and Endoscopic Spinal Surgery: Text and Atlas: Second Edition*
Edited by: P. Kambin © Humana Press Inc., Totowa, NJ

than expected *(6)*. He suggested that the narrowing was owing to encroachment on the spinal canal by the articular processes.

The size and shape of the spinal canal vary enormously from a relatively open rounded triangular configuration to a trefoil shape *(10)*. Eisenstein *(11)* studied the morphometry and pathological anatomy of the lumbar spine in South African Negro and Caucasoid skeletons with specific reference to spinal stenosis, He measured the interpedicular and AP diameter and found the canals narrowest from L2 to L4, and the trefoil configuration was usually at L5, making L4/L5 potentially the narrowest level. Bony degenerative changes increased in the lower level and tended to be in a situation likely to cause foraminal impingement of a nerve root *(11)*.

Porter used ultrasound to measure the oblique diameter of the spinal canal in young men and women to assess the degree and extent of bony stenosis and showed that there was a wide range representing a Gaussian curve *(12)*. Kadziolka et al. *(13)* confirmed his findings in a cadaver study. He subsequently went on to show that patients who subsequently developed symptomatic disc lesions all had canals within the narrow range, strongly suggesting that available space in the spinal canal is significant in the symptomatology of cauda equina and nerve root entrapment syndromes and in the response to treatment *(14)*. He and Eisenstein surveyed the lumbar spines of skeletons and showed that the interpedicular distance at L5 is the narrowest point in the lumbar spine canal. Poor nutrition in early childhood may be a factor *(15)*. Papp et al. *(16)* demonstrated that the trefoil configuration occurs in about 25% of the population but that shape is not generally apparent until adulthood and that the midsagittal diameter of trefoil canals was significantly smaller than in the unaffected canals. The AP diameter is affected by the length of the pedicles *(17–19)*. Postacchini showed that loss of disc height leads to reduction in foraminal height but not AP distance, which is affected by pedicle length *(20,21)*. In addition, degenerative spondylolisthesis is most common at the L4/L5 level. It is not surprising, therefore, that L4/L5 is the level most commonly affected in spinal and foraminal stenosis *(22–25)*.

The main risk factors, therefore, for the development of symptoms of spinal stenosis are undoubtedly hereditary and developmental. The subsequent development of symptoms will ultimately depend on the degree of herniation or degenerative change that develops in the discs and segments of the lumbar spine throughout life.

As degenerative changes develop, the general structure of the nucleus of the disc breaks down with narrowing of the disc space and bulging outward of the annulus. At the same time, the root canals narrow because of overriding of the facet joints *(4,5,17,26)*. This in itself narrows the spinal canal, but also the subsequent bulging and hypertrophy of the facet joint capsule and infolding of the ligamentum flavum narrow the spinal canal and nerve root exit foramen further *(26–29)*. Degenerative spinal stenosis narrows the spinal and root canals even further because as the cephalad vertebra moves forward, its lamina and the inferior facet move closer to the posterosuperior edge of the vertebral body below, continuing to narrow the spinal and nerve root exit canal. Degenerative scoliosis occurs when there is asymmetrical collapse of a disc in the process of disc degeneration and can affect several segments in the lumbar spine. Postacchini suggested classification of degenerative spinal stenosis as follows: central degenerative spinal stenosis alone, spinal stenosis owing to or in association with degenerative spondylolisthesis, and spinal stenosis in association with degenerative scoliosis *(30)*.

The symptoms produced do not seem to have any direct relationship to the degree of apparent stenosis seen on radiological, computed tomography (CT), or magnetic resonance imaging (MRI) images *(31)*. It would appear that a process like this happening slowly in adult life does allow the neural tissue to accommodate to the changing environment because often when patients become symptomatic, the actual degree of stenosis seen on MRI and CT scan is surprisingly severe and a point comes at which the blood supply to the nerve roots cannot accommodate for increased demand on walking. The leg pain produced is neurogenic pain and not muscle ischemia *(32)*. Whether the symptoms are owing primarily to reduced arterial flow or venous obstruction or a combination of both needs to be ascertained *(14,33,34)*. Of course, these symptoms are often associated with a feeling of weakness in the leg, as well as paresthesia and other sensory changes. Positional changes occur in the normal spine resulting in variations in the sizes of the spinal and root canals *(27,28,35)*. Classically, these symptoms occur on standing, when the upright posture brings about relative extension of the lumbar spine compared to the sitting position, compressing the neural tissues and narrowing the root canals. The pain then increases with exercise, when there is increased demand on the neural tissues, and is relieved at rest, particularly by sitting down. In the sitting position, the lumbar spine is relatively flexed compared with the standing position and, therefore, the spinal canal and nerve root exit foramena are opened up, allowing improved blood supply to neural tissue and relief of symptoms *(6,14,36–41)*. Patients often stand or walk stooped forward to relieve symptoms *(42)*.

TREATMENT

When symptoms are mild, conservative treatment has been shown to be successful in approximately half of patients *(22)*. When conservative treatment fails, surgery is always a subsequent option. If surgical treatment is the treatment of choice, this may consist of unilateral or bilateral laminectomy, medial or undercutting facetectomy, limited laminotomy procedures with partial or undercutting facetectomy, or removal of disc herniations and osteophytes from the vertebral margins or from the facets. Traditionally, the thick or "hypertrophic" ligamenta flava are removed *(43–57)*. There is evidence of bone regrowth following decompression procedures, which may lead to a recurrence of symptoms *(30,58)*. Spinal fusion is often performed, particularly if back pain is a dominant feature of the symptom complex or if bony decompression is likely to result in an unstable situation such as degenerative spondylolisthesis, when posterolateral or cage fusion combined with pedicle screw fixation is often advocated *(46)*. Spinal fusion has been shown to alter the biomechanics of the segment above or adjacent to the fusion *(59–66)* and potentially carries the risk of future degenerative change in that segment *(67–80)*.

My own surgical treatment of choice has been mobilization of the ligamentum flavum from bone, leaving it attached medially; preservation of the flavum; and bony decompression followed by reposition of the flavum. Preserving the ligamentum flavum until the bony decompression has been carried out significantly reduces the complication rate in terms of root injury and dural tears, and the ligamentum flavum can continue to perform its normal function in protecting and separating the dura from the more superficial musculature. It is certainly true that the ligamentum flavum may be thickened and hypertrophied, tending to get in the way. It has two layers. The outer interlaminar layer is the one that becomes thickened, and it can be separated from the inner layer and removed if necessary, leaving the inner protective layer. The results from this procedure compare very favorably with those of other published series of decompression *(81)*.

Lumbar decompression is a major operative procedure, particularly for elderly people, many of whom have comorbidities and are poor risks for general anesthesia *(82)*. Consequently, although they may have severe symptoms, they may be deemed poor operative risks and not offered surgical decompression. Following surgery, patients require a significant period of in-hospital stay followed by a rehabilitative process of recovery from a fairly long general anesthetic, and appropriate support in the community if they are elderly. Furthermore, it is estimated that in the United States the population over the age of 60 will almost double by the year 2025 *(82)*. The development of less invasive procedures to treat this disabling condition in such individuals is therefore important.

Percutaneous endoscopic decompression by means of rongeurs, burrs, and laser cannot adequately deal with lateral recess or central canal stenosis. It can deal with foraminal stenosis, but there is a significant incidence of flaring up of root pain owing to manipulation or heating of the nerve root. Fortunately, this usually dissipates after a few weeks.

A novel approach to deal with this problem is the X-Stop interspinous process distraction device (Fig. 1A). The instrumentation is very simple and effective (Fig. 1B). Many other similar devices are now coming on the market. In addition, other devices that could be used to have a similar effect are on the market. However, for their insertion, they require excision of the supra- and interspinous ligaments, which are essential to ensure that overdistraction cannot occur and, in my opinion, are essential to maintain stability of the motion segment. Furthermore, some devices cut into the base of the spinous process, which must inevitably induce a stress riser, risking stress fracture of the process.

RESULTS OF INTERSPINOUS PROCESS DISTRACTION DEVICE

The X-Stop has been trialed in a prospective randomized study comparing surgical treatment by insertion of the device to nonoperative, conservative management *(83)*. Two hundred patients were initially enrolled in the study, and 100 were treated by the X-Stop and 91 by nonoperative therapy as the control group. The Zurich Claudication Questionnaire (ZCQ), validated for lumbar spinal stenosis, was the primary outcome measure. It measures physical function, symptom severity, and patient satisfaction. Insertion of the X-Stop has quite clearly shown a significant difference from conservative treatment in terms of clinical improvement, satisfaction rate, and success rate. Two of the X-Stop patients had the implants removed at 1 yr, three withdrew from the study, and three went on to have a laminectomy. In the nonoperative group, 12 patients withdrew from the study and 17 went on to have a laminectomy. There was no significant difference in the ZCQ between the groups preoperatively. At 6 wk, the success rate was 52% for the X-Stop group, and 10% for the control group. At 6 mo, the success rates were 52 and 9%, and at 1 yr, 59 and 12%, respectively. The success rate is comparable with that for other published series for surgical decompression, but with considerably lower morbidity.

In vitro biomechanical testing in cadaver spines has demonstrated that insertion of the interspinous process distraction device increased the dimensions of the spinal and

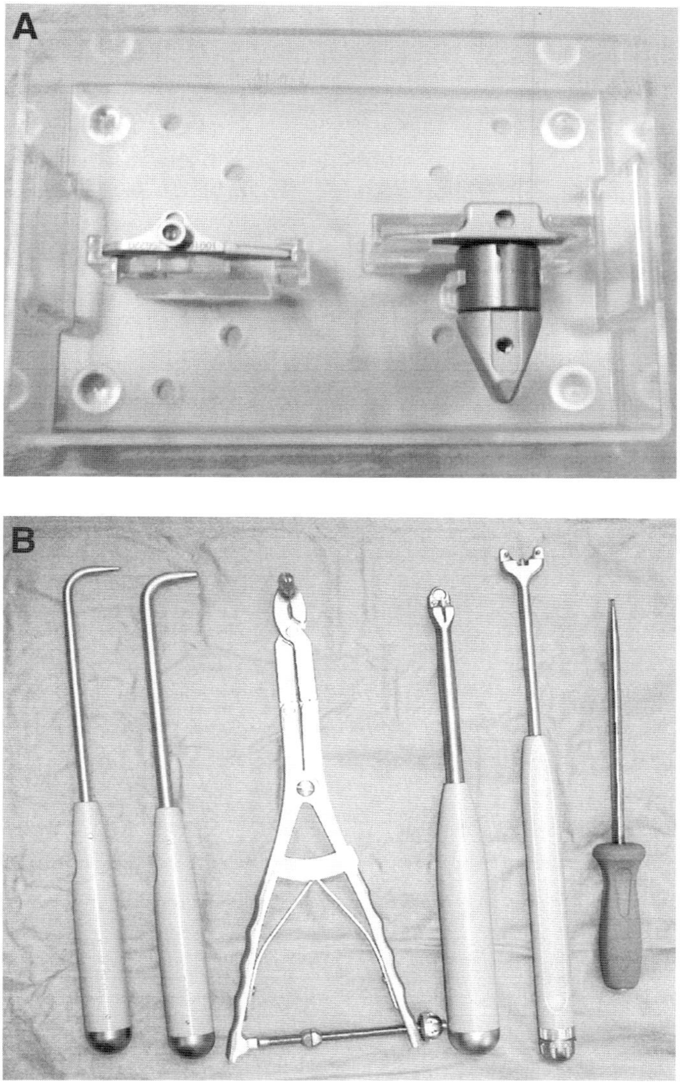

Fig. 1. (A) X-Stop device; **(B)** instrumentation for the device (from left to right): small dilator, intermediate dilator, distraction and measuring instrument, holder for main body of device, holder for wing, torque screwdriver.

neural canal at the implanted level and tended to hold the segment in flexion *(84)*. It did not alter the dimensions of the adjacent intact levels. Distraction also brought about a reduction in pressure on the posterior annulus and nucleus at the implanted levels without altering the pressures at adjacent level. In effect, the device places the segment in the sitting position, which is the position in which patients typically obtain relief of symptoms, by increasing the space within the spinal and nerve root canals.

Radiological studies of the sagittal alignment have demonstrated subtle changes of $<1°$ in patients implanted at one level and a change of just over $1°$ in patients implanted at two levels *(85)*.

OPERATIVE TECHNIQUE

It is my experience that all one-level and many two-level implantation procedures can be carried out under local anesthetic block. Sedation or light general anesthetic may be given in addition. The limiting factor is the safe amount of local anesthetic one can give to individual patients. The procedures are carried out with an anesthetist present and quite often some sedation is added. In obese patients, in whom it is very difficult to obtain adequate anesthesia with local anesthetic, and for three-level procedures, generally a light general anesthetic is used in addition.

Following local anesthetic or light general anesthetics, a few hours after the procedure patients are allowed to go to the toilet or are taken for a short walk. If back pain is a significant component of patients' symptoms prior to the procedure, then it tends to be a problem in the immediate postoperative period but generally rapidly subsides. Patients are given appropriate analgesia and reassured that being mobile is the best thing to do. In the first few weeks, sitting for short periods is permitted, but generally patients are advised to rest lying down, rather than sitting, and otherwise to be up and about and to go for walks.

For the implantation procedure, the patient is placed in the right lateral position. The level to be operated on is checked by an image intensifier. Local anesthetic is used in the form of 1% lignocaine or Xylocaine® in 1:200,000 adrenaline. This is used to anesthetize the skin, the superficial tissues, and the muscles and midline structures. In addition, 0.5% bupivacaine in 1:200,000 adrenaline is used to anesthetize the muscles and deeper structures. This is best done by injecting local anesthetic directly into the muscle bulk and then adjacent to the facet joint below the pars at the level of, and the facet joints above, the level for surgery. It generally takes the local anesthetic 5–10 min to work effectively, and the long-acting bupivacaine provides good postoperative pain relief for up to 8 h.

The procedure is then performed by centering the skin incision over the interspinous process space. The lumbar fascia is incised longitudinally on either side of the supraspinous ligament, leaving the supraspinous ligament and interspinous ligaments completely intact. The muscles are separated from the spinous processes down to the laminae on either side. A small dilator is then inserted through the interspinous ligament at the base of the spinous processes and the hole dilated. An intermediate dilator is inserted followed by the distraction device. The distraction device is then employed, with the surgeon using his or her hand to feel the tension developing. Initially, distraction is continued until the tissues become tight. The distraction device is then locked in that position and left for a few minutes. At the same time, the supraspinous ligament is palpated with the index finger of the surgeon's other hand to feel the tension in it. Usually after a few minutes, owing to the creep in the tissues, the surgeon finds that further distraction is possible and continues distraction until he or she can feel that the tissues are completely distracted and taut. It is recommended that in patients who are perhaps slightly osteoporotic, such distraction be carried out very carefully.

At this point, it is possible to read off from the distraction device the size of the X-Stop device to be inserted (Fig. 2). The largest possible size should be inserted. The two parts of the device are then attached to their introducers (Fig. 3), and then the patient is asked to curl up in the fully flexed position, bending knees up to the chest and head and chin over the top of the knees. In a patient relaxed by a general anesthetic, this is not necessary. This position opens up the interspace to the optimum while the distraction

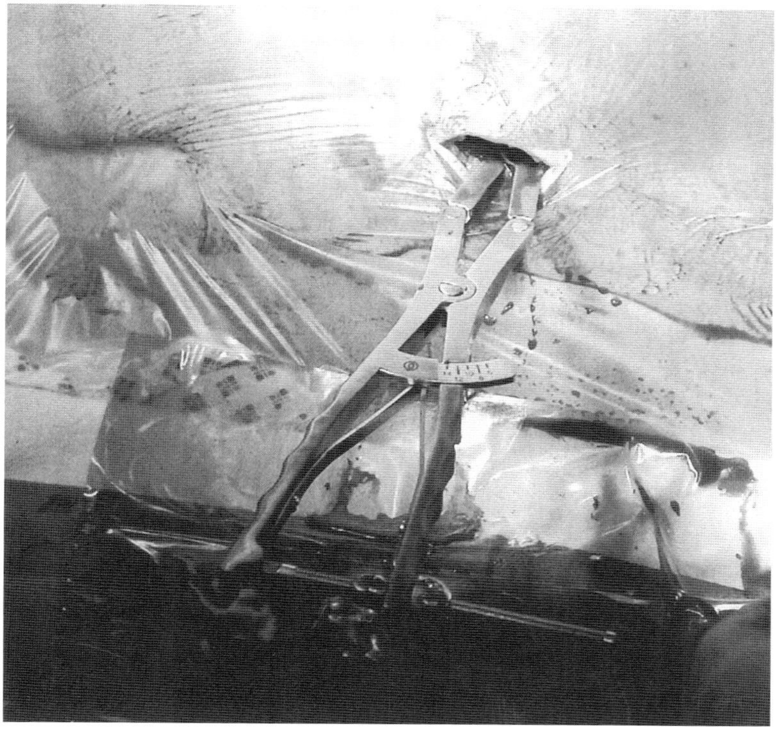

Fig. 2. Distraction and measuring instrument showing size 14.

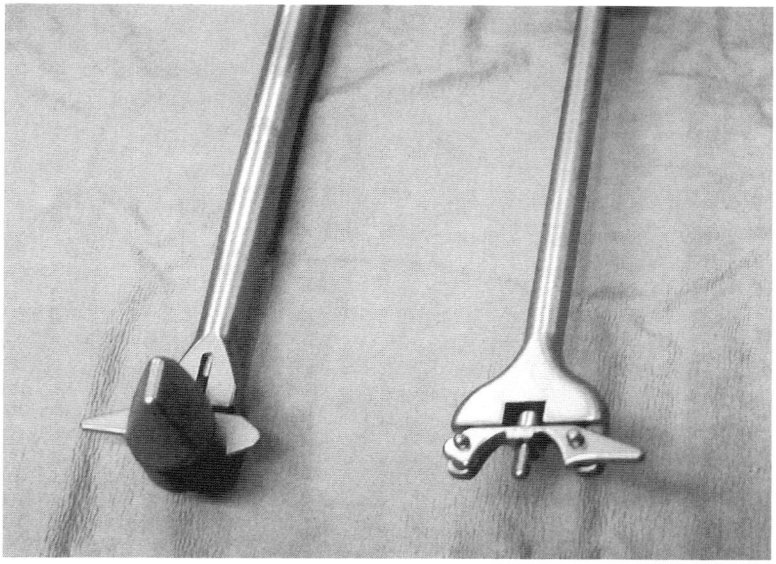

Fig. 3. X-Stop device attached to introducers.

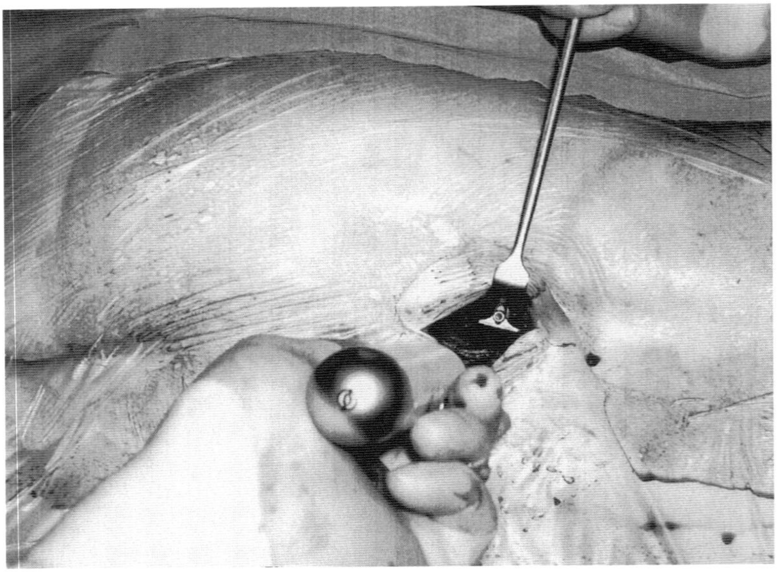

Fig. 4. Main body of X-Stop device inserted.

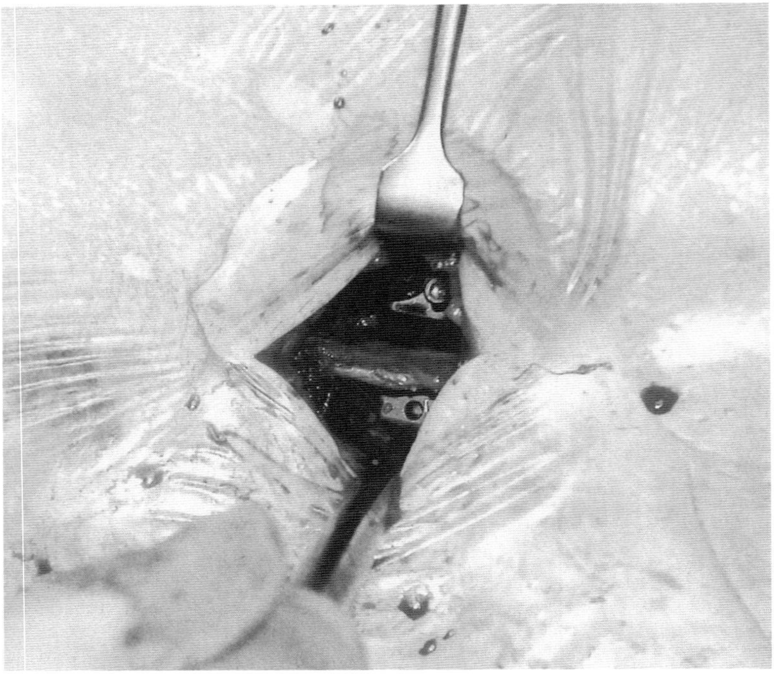

Fig. 5. X-Stop device in position.

device is removed and the x-stop device inserted. It is usually a little difficult to insert the device in the first instance, but it will slip into place with gentle, persistent pressure (Fig. 4). The retaining wing is then screwed onto the device and tightened off with the torque screwdriver (Fig. 5).

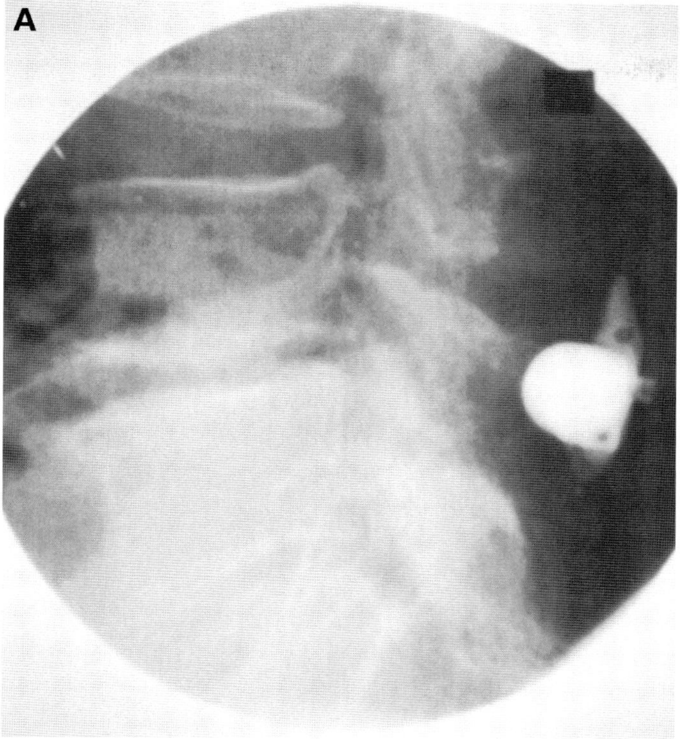

Fig. 6. **(A)** Lateral X-ray of device at L4/L5; **(B)** AP X-ray of device at L4/L5.

Owing to the use of local anesthetic in 1:200,000 adrenaline, there is very little bleeding. The wound is then closed by resuturing the lumbar fascia to the supraspinous ligaments on either side with one or two sutures, as necessary. The skin is then closed. To date, 30 patients have been operated on, many of whom had significant comorbidities, without significant perioperative complications.

X-ray image intensification is used throughout the procedure to ensure that a correct level is inserted. It is also reassuring to the surgeon to be able to view the distraction being obtained prior to inserting the device. X-rays are taken to demonstrate the final position of the device (Fig. 6A,B).

MOST RECENT STUDIES

In Aberdeen, Scotland, we are carrying out studies using the Fonar positional MRI scan to measure a range of parameters before and after insertion of the device. These are total flexion and extension of the lumbar spine (Fig. 7A,B), the AP distance and cross-sectional area of the spinal canal (Fig. 8), the cross-sectional area of the nerve root foramen (Fig. 9), and the effect on the flexion and extension movement of the segments above and below the treated segment. There also appears to be an effect on the coronal alignment in patients who have degenerative scoliosis in that insertion of the device seems to reduce the degree of lateral bend at the treated level.

The number of postoperative measurements made is small; however, there is a clear trend showing that there is no significant difference in the total range of flexion and

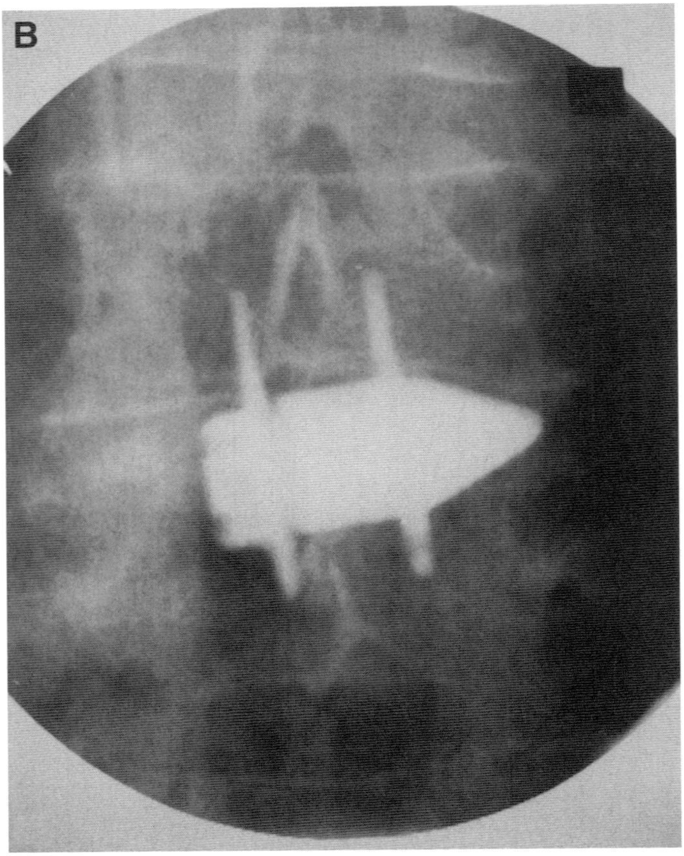

Fig. 6. *(Continued)*

extension of the lumbar spine. There is a highly significant increase in the AP distance and cross-sectional area of the spinal canal and the cross-sectional area of the nerve root exit foramen at the treated level. There is no evidence of any difference in flexion and extension movement at the levels above and below the treated level. For the positional MRI scan study, the plan is to treat some 45 patients who have been treated at one, two, and three levels.

Figure 7A,B shows MRIs of a patient (patient 1) with two-level disease in flexion and extension prior to insertion of the device. The patient was a 75-yr-old female with a history of bilateral leg pain, worse on the right side, of increasing severity over an 18-mo period unrelieved by conservative therapies including nonsteroidal anti-inflammatory and analgesic therapy, physiotherapy, and sacral epidural injection. She had no pain on sitting and lying on her side but had some pain lying on her back. Pain occurred immediately on standing, and she preferred to stand and walk stooped forward using a walking stick. Her walking distance was 20 yd maximum, and she developed weakness and paresthesia in her lower legs and feet. She had surgery under local anesthesia and a light sedation. Six hours afterward, she was up walking without pain and able to stand upright. At 6-mo follow up, there was no restriction in her walking distance; she was able to shop, do gardening, and play golf; and her positional MRI scan in the vertical

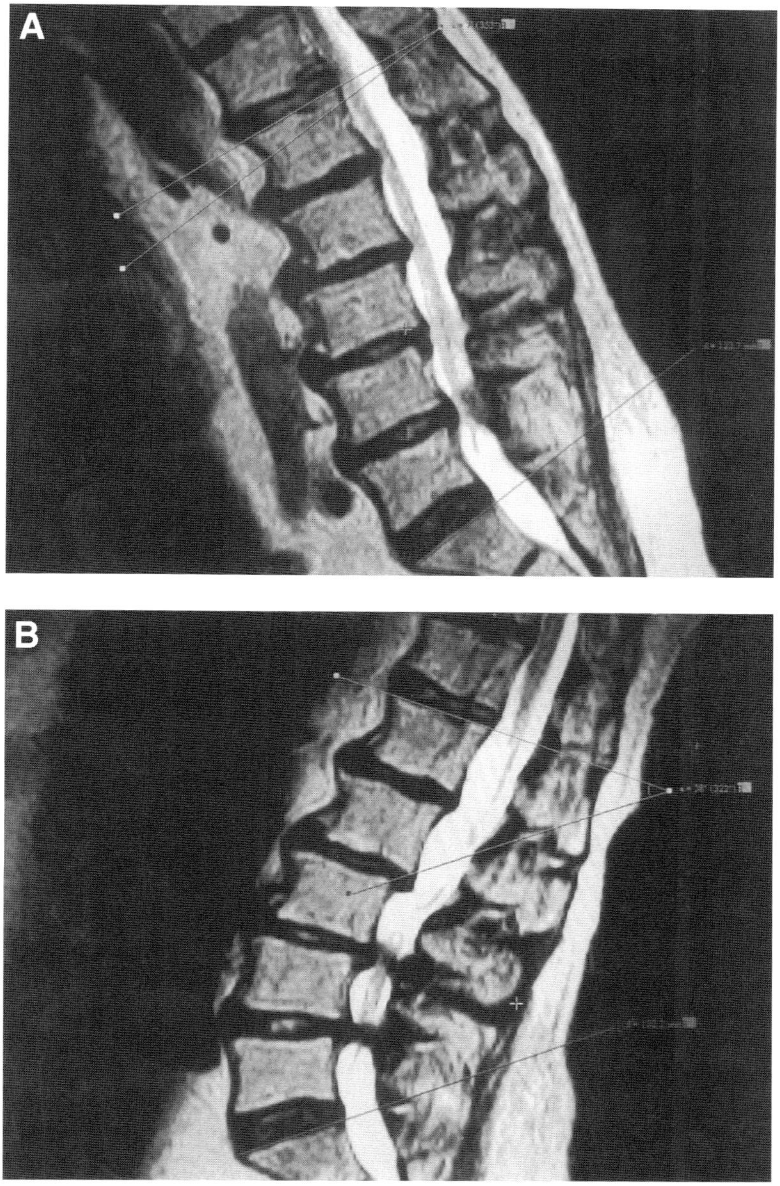

Fig. 7. **(A)** Positional MRI scan of patient 1 in flexion; **(B)** positional MRI scan of patient 1 in extension.

position (Fig. 10) demonstrated the X-Stop in position and its effect on the spinal canal. The midsagittal AP distance at L3/L4 and L4/L5 were clearly improved with relief of the stenosis.

Patient (patient 2) is an extremely fit 85-yr-old man who was unable to walk more than 50 yards owing to left leg pain radiating from the buttock down the posterolateral thigh to the foot. X-ray demonstrated a degenerative spondylolisthesis at L4/L5, and positional MRI scans confirmed stenosis (Fig. 11A,B). The treatment options were

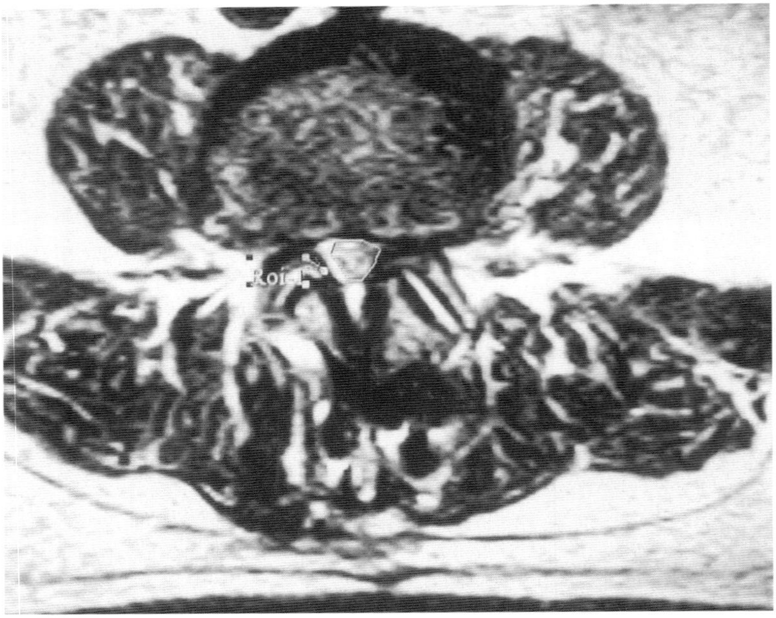

Fig. 8. Spinal canal measurement.

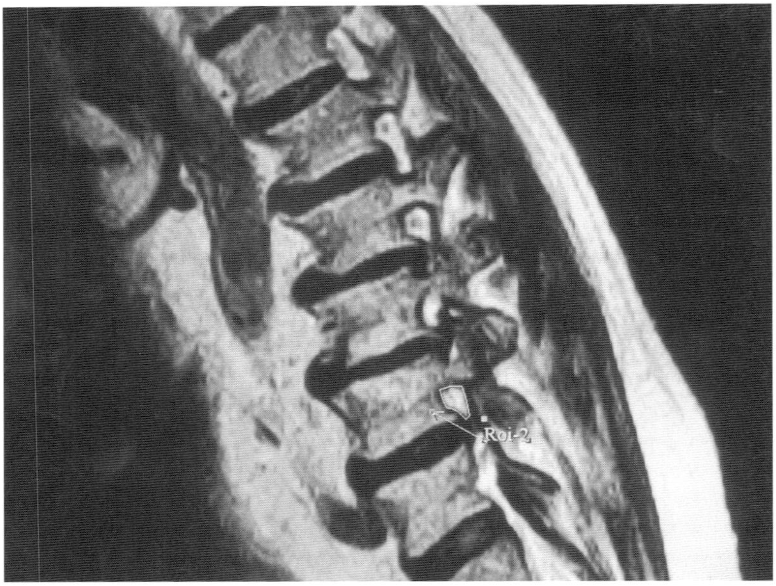

Fig. 9. Foraminal measurement.

discussed with him and he preferred to pursue nonoperative treatments. He was offered an epidural injection, with the option of an X-Stop if it failed to relieve his symptoms. He chose to seek a second opinion. He was offered and treated with a left L5 nerve root infiltration, which relieved pain for only 2 wk, again with the option of an X-Stop if it

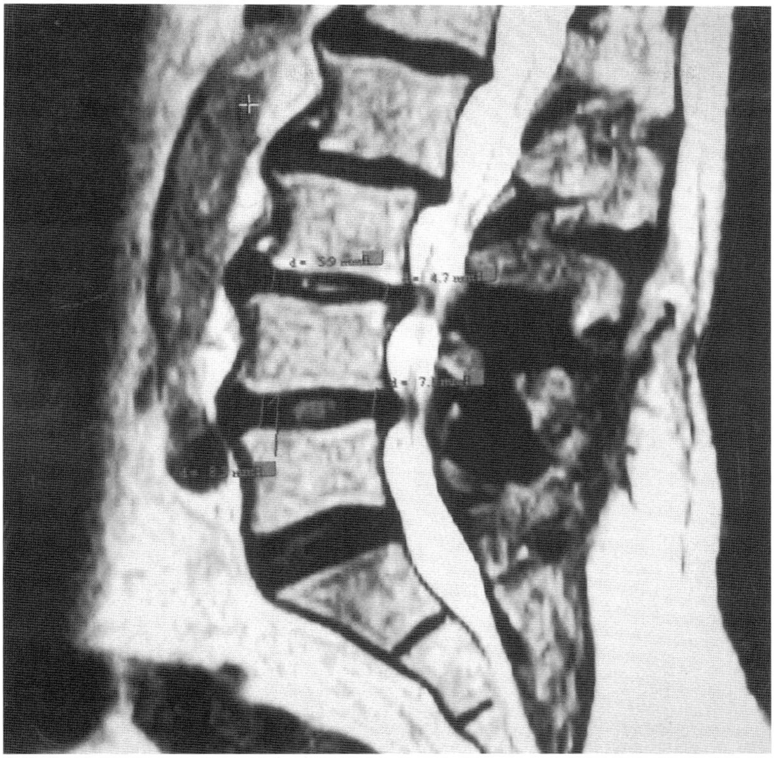

Fig. 10. Positional MRI scan of patient no. 1 with X-Stop in position at L3/L4 and L4/L5 at 6-mo follow-up.

failed to relieve his symptoms. He decided to opt for the X-Stop treatment, which immediately relieved his symptoms. At 6 wk, he was walking 3 mi/d, and at 6 mo, 5 mi/d, enjoying fishing and shooting, his favorite pastimes. His positional MRI scan at 6 mo demonstrates the current position (Fig. 12A,B).

So far, I have treated 30 patients. Clinical improvement has taken place in all of these patients. Perhaps the most striking effect in most patients is the immediate pain relief and ability to stand up straight, rather than stooped forward. Walking distance is also improved immediately. There have been no significant complications. However, follow-up is short at the present time, with 10 patients followed to 6 mo, and the long-term results will be published in due course.

CONCLUSION

Treatment of spinal stenosis by means of an interspinous process distraction device such as the X-Stop appears to be a significant improvement in the treatment of this condition. The procedure can be carried out under local anesthetic as a day case or, in elderly patients, with one overnight stay. Mobilization is quick and patients do not require any specific postoperative rehabilitation or extra social support after discharge home. A small number of patients do have increased back pain, but this does dissipate within a few days, or certainly within a few weeks. The procedure is extremely safe and, so far, no significant complications have been encountered. It is accepted that if the

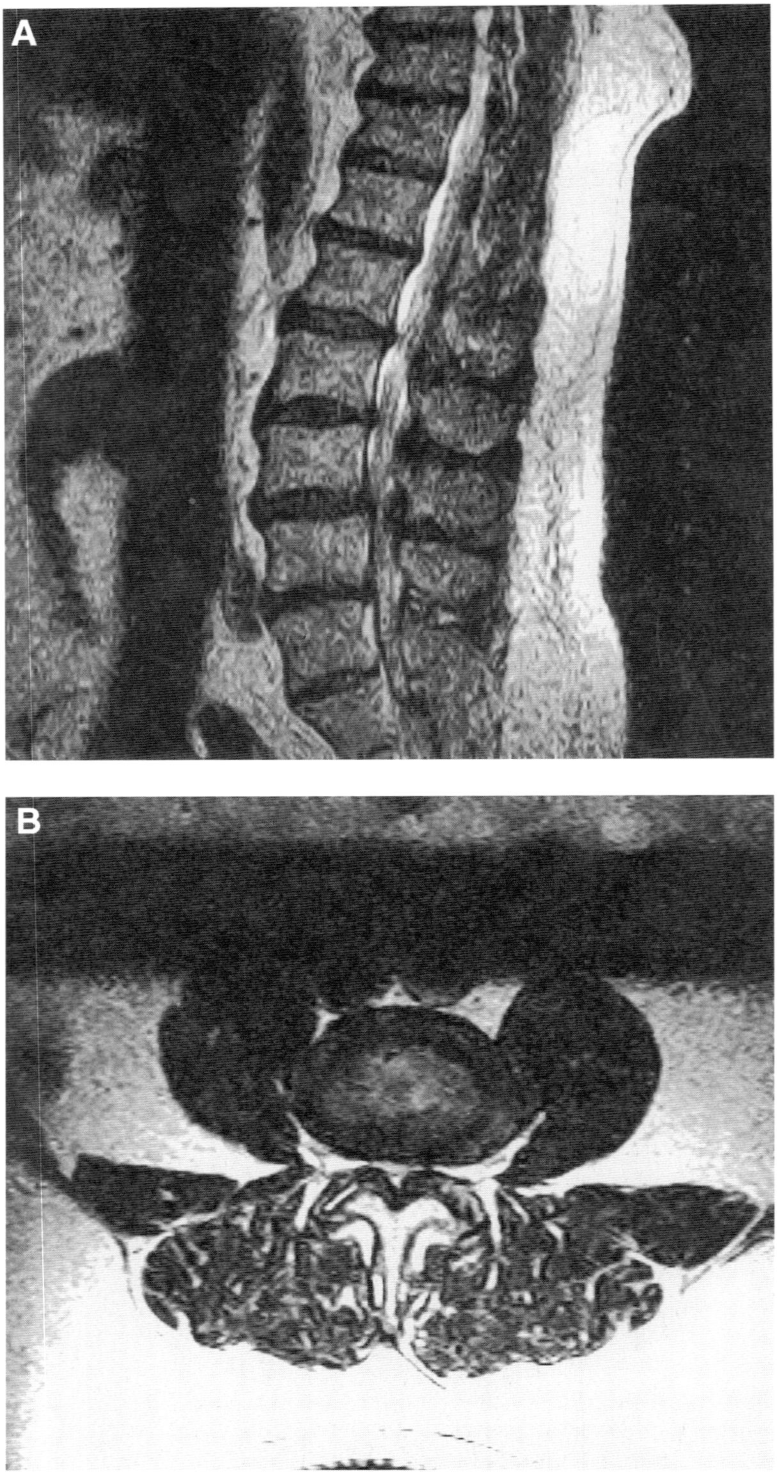

Fig. 11. (**A**) Positional MRI scan of patient 2 showing stenosis at L4/L5; (**B**) positional MRI scan of patient 2 showing stenosis at L4/L5 axial view.

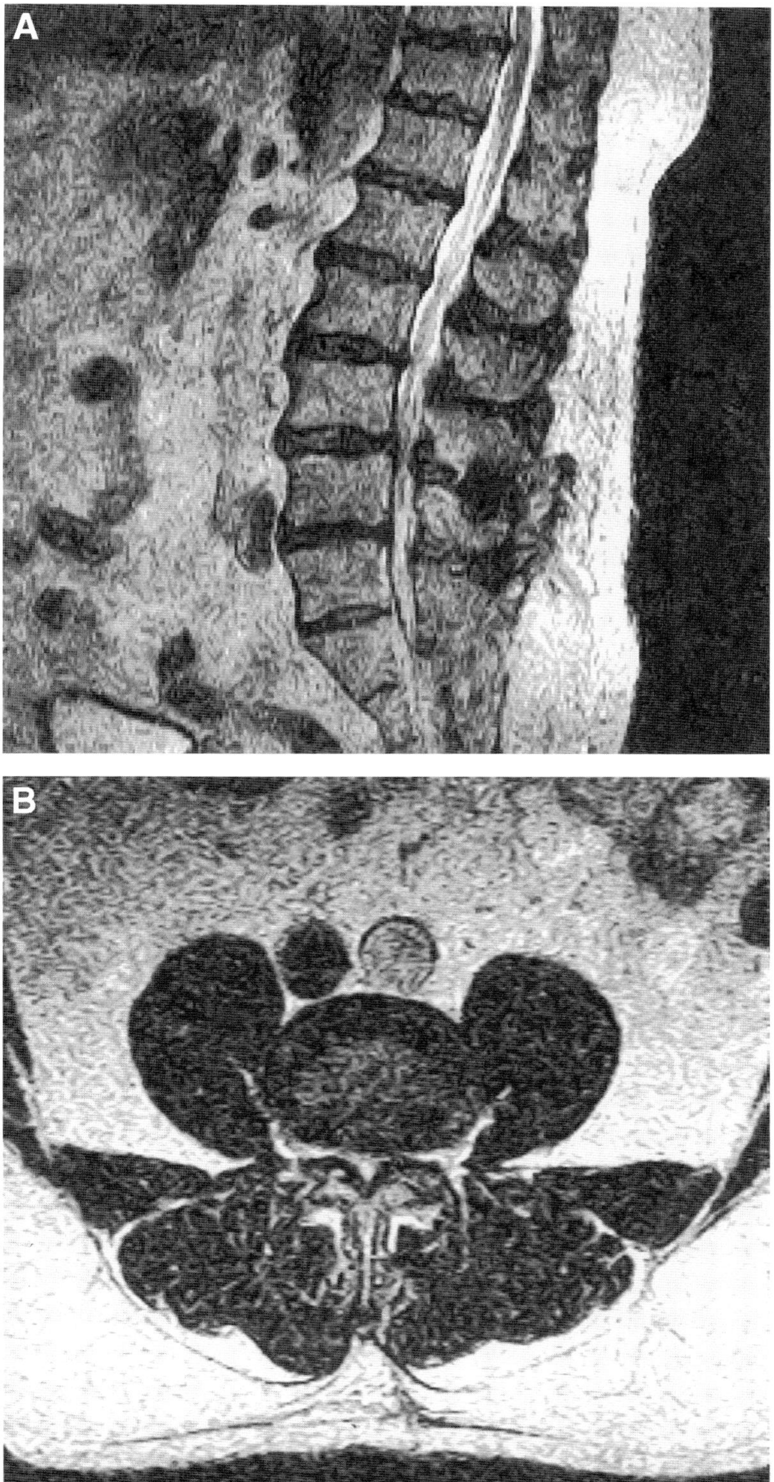

Fig. 12. (**A**) Positional MRI scan of patient 2 showing X-Stop at L4/L5 at 6 mo; (**B**) postional MRI scan of patient 2 following X-Stop at L4/L5 at 6 mo.

device fails, the patient still has the option of surgical decompression in the traditional manner. The long-term results of the original prospective study demonstrate that there is no deterioration in symptoms over time. This is clearly a minimal intervention procedure that is safe and effective, particularly for elderly patients who are otherwise infirm and unfit for a full general anesthetic. They can quickly return home and resume normal activities with an immediate improvement in symptoms.

REFERENCES

1. Sachs B, Frankel V. Progressive and kyphotic rigidity of the spine. J Nerv Ment Dis 1900;27:l.
2. Putti V. Lady Jones lecture: on new concepts on the pathogenesis of sciatic pain. Lancet 1927;210:(5491)53–60.
3. Hirsch C. On lumbar pacetectomies. Acta Orthop Scand 1948;17:240–252.
4. Harris RI, MacNab I. Structural changes in the lumbar intervertebral discs: their relationship to low back pain and sciatica. J Bone Joint Surg 1954;386:304–322.
5. MacNab I. Negative disc exploration. J Bone Joint Surg 1971;53A:891–903.
6. Verbiest H. Neurogenic intermittent claudication in cases with absolute and relative stenosis of the lumbar vertebral canal (ASLC and RSLC), in cases with narrow lumbar intervertebral foramina, and in cases with both entities. Clin Neurosurg 1973;20:204–214.
7. Verbiest H. Results of surgical treatment of idiopathic developmental stenosis of the lumbar vertebral canal: a review of twenty-seven years' experience. J Bone Joint Surg 1977;59B(2).
8. Verbiest H. Stenosis of the lumbar vertebral canal and sciatica. Neurosurg Rev 1980;3:75–89.
9. Verbiest H. The treatment of lumbar spondyloptosis or impending lumbar spondyloptosis accompanied by neurologic deficit and/or neurogenic intermittent claudication. Spine 1979;4:68–77.
10. Porter RW. Variations in shape and size of the lumbar spinal canal. Paleopathol Newsle 1980;32:9–11.
11. Eisenstein S. The morphometry and pathological anatomy of the lumbar spine in South African Negroes and Caucasoids with special reference to spinal stenosis. J Bone Joint Surg 1977;59B:172–180.
12. Porter RW, Wicks M, Ottwell D. Measurement of the spinal canal by diagnostic ultrasound. J Bone Joint Surg (Br) 1978;60B(4):481–484.
13. Kadziolka R, Asztely M, Hanai K, Hansson T, Nachemson A. Ultrasonic measurement of the lumbar spinal canal: the origin and precision of the recorded echoes. J Bone Joint Surg 1981;63B(4):504–507.
14. Porter RW, Hibbert CS, Wicks M. The spinal canal in symptomatic lumbar disc lesions. J Bone Joint Surg (Br) 1978;60B(4):485–487.
15. Papp T, Porter RW, Aspden RM. The growth of the lumbar vertebral canal. Spine 1994;19(24):2770–2773.
16. Papp T, Porter RW, Aspden RM. Trefoil configuration and developmental stenosis of the lumbar vertebral canal. J Bone Joint Surg (Br) 1995;77B:469–472.
17. Arnoldi CC, Brodsky AE, Cauchoix J, et al. Lumbar spinal stenosis and nerve root entrapment syndromes: definition and classification. Clin Orthop 1976; (115):4–5.
18. Hawkes CH, Roberts GM. Neurogenic and vascular claudication. J Neurol Sci 1978;38:337–345.
19. Salibi BS. Neurogenic intermittent claudication and stenosis of the lumbar spinal canal. Surg Neurol 1976;5:269–272.
20. Cinotti, G, De Santis P, Nofroni I, Postacchini F. Stenosis of lumbar intervertebral foramen: anatomic study on predisposing factors. Spine 2002;27(3):223–229.
21. Panjabi MM, Takata K, Goel VK. Kinematics of lumbar intervertebral foramen. Spine 1983;8:348–357.

22. Araksinen O, Herno A, Turunen V, Saari T, Suomlainen O. Degenerative spondylolisthesis: surgical outcome of 438 patients treated surgically for lumbar spinal stenosis. Spine 1997; 22:2278–2282.
23. Amundsen T, Weber H, Nordal HJ, Hele J, Magnaes B, Adelnoor MMPH, Lilleas F. Lumbar spinal stenosis: conservative or surgical management? a prospective 10 year study. Spine 2000;25:1424–1436.
24. Herkowitz HN, Kurz LT. Degenerative lumbar spondylolisthesis with spinal stenosis. J Bone Joint Surg (Am) 1991;73:802–807.
25. Mardjetko SM, Connolly PJ, Short S. Degenerative lumbar spondylolisthesis: a meta-analysis of literature 1970–1993. Spine 1994;19:2257S–2265S.
26. Crock HV. Normal and pathological anatomy of the lumbar spinal nerve root canals. J Bone Joint Surg (Br) 1981;63:487–490.
27. Adams MA, May S, Freeman BJ, et al. Effects of backward bending on lumbar intervertebral discs: relevance to physical therapy treatments for low back pain. Spine 2000;25:431–437: discussion, 438.
28. Chung SS, Lee CS, Kim SH, et al. Effect of low back posture on the morphology of the spinal canal. Skeletal Radiol 2000;29:217–223.
29. Rauschning W. Normal and pathologic anatomy of the lumbar root canals. Spine 1987;12:1008–1019.
30. Postacchini F, Cinotti G. Bone regrowth after surgical decompression for lumbar spinal stenosis. J Bone Joint Surg (Br) 1992;74:862–869.
31. Amundsen T, Weber H, Lilleas F, et al. Lumbar spinal stenosis: clinical and radiologic features. Spine 1995;20:1178–1186.
32. Keenan GF, Ashcroft GP, Roditi GH, et al. Measurement of lower limb blood flow in patients with neurogenic claudication using positron emission tomography. Spine 1995;20(4):408–411.
33. Naylor A. Factors in the development of the spinal stenosis syndrome. J Bone Joint Surg (Br) 1979;61B(3):306–309.
34. Porter RW. Spinal stenosis and neurogenic claudication. Spine 1996;21:2046–2052.
35. Schmid MR, Stucki G, Duewell S, et al. Changes in cross-sectional measurements of the spinal canal and intervertebral foramina as a function of body position: in vivo studies on an open-configuration MR system. Am J Roentgenol 1999;172:1095–1102.
36. Fujiwara A, An HS, Lim TH, et al. Morphologic changes in the lumbar intervertebral foramen due to flexion-extension, lateral bending, and axial rotation an in vitro anatomic and biomechanical study. Spine 2001;26:876–882.
37. Inufusa A, An HS, Lim TH, et al. Anatomic changes of the spinal canal and intervertebral foramen associated with flexion-extension movement. Spine 1996;21:2412–2420.
38. Penning L, Wilmink JT. Posture-dependent bilateral compression of L4 or L5 nerve roots in facet hypertrophy: a dynamic CT-myelographic study. Spine 1987;12:488–500.
39. Rothman SL. Dynamic effect on the lumbar spinal canal. Spine 1998;23:1506, 1507.
40. Vitzthum HE, Konig A, Seifert V. Dynamic examination of the lumbar spine by using vertical, open magnetic resonance imaging. J Neurosurg 2000;93:58–64.
41. Wildermuth S, Zanetti M, Duewell S, et al. Lumbar spine: quantitative and qualitative assessment of positional (upright flexion and extension) MR imaging and myelography. Radiology 1998;207:391–398.
42. Dyck P. The Stoop test in lumbar entrapment radiculopathy. Spine 1979;4:89–92.
43. Aryanpur J, Ducker T. Multilevel lumbar laminotomies: an alternative to laminectomy in the treatment of lumbar stenosis. Neurosurgery 1990;26:429–433.
44. Cinotti G, Postacchini F, Weinstein JN. Lumbar spinal, stenosis and diabetes: outcome of surgical decompression. J Bone Joint Surg (Br) 1994;76:215–219.
45. Getty CJM. Lumbar spinal stenosis: the clinical spectrum and results of operations. J Bone Joint Surg (Br) 1980;62:481–485.

46. Grob D, Humke T, Dvorak J. Degenerative lumbar spinal stenosis: decompression with and without arthrodesis. J Bone Joint Surg (Am) 1995;77:1036–1041.
47. Herno A, Airaksinen O, Saari T. Long-term results of surgical treatment of lumbar spinal stenosis. Spine 1993;18:1471–1474.
48. Herron LD, Mangelsdorf C. Lumbar spinal stenosis. J Spinal Disord 1991;4:26–33.
49. Hilibrand AS, Rand N. Degenerative lumbar stenosis: diagnosis and management. J Am Acad Orthop Surg 1999;7:239–249.
50. Jonsson B, Annertz M, Sioberg C, et al. A prospective and consecutive study of surgically treated lumbar spinal stenosis. Part II: five-year follow-up by an independent observer. Spine 1997;22:2938–2944.
51. Jonsson B, Stromqvist B, Decompression for lateral lumbar stenosis: results and impact on sick leave and working conditions. Spine 1994;19:2381–2386.
52. Katz JN, Lipson SJ, Chang LC, et al. Seven- to 10-year outcome of decompressive surgery for degenerative lumbar spinal stenosis. Spine 1996;21:92–98.
53. Katz JN, Lipson SJ, Larson MG, et al. The outcome of decompressive laminectomy for degenerative lumbar stenosis. J Bone Joint Surg (Am) 1991;73:809–816.
54. Katz JN, Lipson SJ, Larson MG, Mclnnes JM, Fossel AH, Liang MH. The outcome of decompressive laminectomy for degenerative lumbar spinal stenosis. J Bone Joint Surg (Am) 1991;73:809–813.
55. Postacchini F, Cinotti G, Gumina S, et al. Long-term results of surgery in lumbar stenosis: 8-year review of 64 patients. Acta Orthop Scand 1993;64 78–80.
56. Postacchini F, Cinotti G, Perugia D, et al. The surgical treatment of central lumbar stenosis: multiple laminotomy compared with total laminectomy. J Bone Joint Surg (Br) 1993;75: 386–392.
57. Postacchini F. Surgical management of lumbar spinal stenosis. Spine 1999;24:1043–1047.
58. Chen O, Baba H, Kamitani K, et al. Postoperative bone re-growth in lumbar spinal stenosis: a multivariate analysis of 48 patients. Spine 1994;19:2144–2149.
59. Chow DH, Luk KD, Evans JH, et al. Effects of short anterior lumbar interbody fusion on biomechanics of neighboring unfused segments. Spine 1996;21:549–555.
60. Cunningham BW, Kotani Y, McNulty PS, et al. The effect of spinal destabilization and instrumentation on lumbar intradiscal pressure: an in vitro biomechanical analysis. Spine 1997;22:2655–2663.
61. Ha KY, Schendel MJ, Lewis JL, et al. Effect of immobilization and configuration on lumbar adjacent-segment biomechanics. J Spinal Disord 1993;6:99–105.
62. Kim YE, Goel VK, Weinstein JN, et al. Effect of disc degeneration at one level on the adjacent level in axial mode. Spine 1991;16:331–335.
63. Marchesi DG, Aebi M. Pedicle fixation devices in the treatment of adult lumbar scoliosis. Spine 1992;17:S304–S309.
64. Rohlmann A, Calisse J, Bergmann G, et al. Internal spinal fixator stiffness has only a minor influence on stresses in the adjacent discs. Spine 1999;24:1192–1195.
65. Rohlmann A, Neller S, Bergmann G, et al. Effect of an internal fixator and a bone graft on intersegmental spinal motion and intradiscal pressure in the adjacent regions. Eur Spine J 2001;10:301–308.
66. Weinhoffer SL, Guyer RD, Herbert M, et al. Intradiscal pressure measurements above an instrumented fusion: a cadaveric study. Spine 1995;20:526–531.
67. Aota Y, Kumano K, Hirabayashi S. Postfusion instability at the adjacent segments after rigid pedicle screw fixation for degenerative lumbar spinal disorders. J Spinal Disord 1995;8:464–473.
68. Etebar S, Cahill DW. Risk factors for adjacent-segment failure following lumbar fixation with rigid instrumentation for degenerative instability. J Neurosurg 1999;90:163–169.
69. Frymoyer JW, Hanley EN Jr, Howe J, et al. A comparison of radiographic findings in fusion and nonfusion patients ten or more years following lumbar disc surgery. Spine 1979;4:435–440.

70. Guigui P, Lambert P, Lassale B, et al. Long-term outcome at adjacent levels of lumbar arthrodesis. Rev Chir Orthop Reparatrice Appar Mot 1997;83:685–696.
71. Kumar MN, Baklanov A, Chopin D, Correlation between sagittal plane changes and adjacent segment degeneration following lumbar spine fusion. Eur Spine J 2001;10:314–319.
72. Kumar MN, Jacquot F, Hall H. Long-term follow-up of functional outcomes and radiographic changes at adjacent levels following lumbar spine fusion for degenerative disc disease. Eur Spine J 2001;10:309–313.
73. Lee CK. Accelerated degeneration of the segment adjacent to a lumbar fusion. Spine 1988;13:375–377.
74. Lehmann TR, Spratt KF, Tozzi JE, et al. Long-term follow-up of lower lumbar fusion patients. Spine 1987;12:97–104.
75. Miyakoshi N, Abe E, Shimada Y, et al. Outcome of one-level posterior lumbar interbody fusion for spondylolisthesis and postoperative intervertebral disc degeneration adjacent to the fusion. Spine 2000;25:1837–1842.
76. Nagata H, Schendel MJ, Transfeldt EE, et al. The effects of immobilization of long segments of the spine on the adjacent and distal facet force and lumbosacral motion. Spine 1993;18:2471–2479.
77. Schlegel JD, Smith JA, Schleusener RL. Lumbar motion segment pathology adjacent to thoracolumbar, lumbar, and lumbosacral fusions. Spine 1996;21:970–981.
78. Shono Y, Kaneda K, Abumi K, et al. Stability of posterior spinal instrumentation and its effects on adjacent motion segments in the lumbosacral spine. Spine 1998;23:1550–1558.
79. Van Horn JR, Bohnen LM. The development of discopathy in lumbar discs adjacent to a lumbar anterior interbody spondylodesis: a retrospective matched-pair study with a postoperative follow-up of 16 years. Acta Orthop Belg 1992;58:280–286.
80. Whitecloud TS III, Davis JM, Olive PM. Operative treatment of the degenerated segment adjacent to a lumbar fusion. Spine 1994;19:531–536.
81. Askar Z, Wardlaw D, Choudhary S, Rege A. A ligamentum flavum-preserving approach to the lumbar spinal canal. Spine 2003;28(19):E385–E390.
82. Reeg SE. A review of comorbidities and spinal surgery. Clin Orthop 2001;384:101–109.
83. Zucherman JF, Hsu KY, Hartjen CA, et al. A prospective randomized multi-center study for the treatment of lumbar spinal stenosis with the X STOP interspinous implant: 1 year results. Eur Spine J 2004;13:22–31.
84. Swanson KE, Lindsey DP, Hsu KY, Zucherman JF, Yerby SA. The effects of an interspinous implant on intervertebral disc pressure. Spine 2003;28(l):26–32.
85. Lindsey DP, Swanson KF, Fuchs P, Hsu KY, Zucherman JF, Yerby SA. (2003) The effects of an interspinous implant on the kinematics of the instrumented and adjacent levels in the lumbar spine. Spine 28:2192–2197.

17

Frameless Stereotactic Imaging Techniques in Minimally Invasive Spinal Surgery

Kern Singh, MD, **Laurence N. Fitzhenry**, MD, and **Alexander R. Vaccaro**, MD

INTRODUCTION

Frameless stereotactic imaging is widely used in intracranial neurosurgical procedures to locate pathology precisely and decrease the morbidity of traditional open exploratory procedures. However, the clinical application of computer-assisted image-guided spinal surgery has not been widely accepted owing to the time-consuming and arduous nature of maintaining accurate registration coordinates. Frameless spinal stereotaxy is an evolving adjunct to the surgeon's anatomical knowledge and skill. Newer technology involving intraoperative real-time image acquisition and user-friendly instruments will undoubtedly improve the popularity of this technology in complex spinal procedures. Currently, computer image-guided spinal surgery is used for the placement of pedicle screws; transarticular C1-C2 fixation; transoral odontoid resection; anterior cervical corpectomies; and, most recently, in endoscopic spinal surgery.

STEREOTAXIS

Computer-assisted navigation systems are based on the principle of stereotaxis. The basic components of the original "frame-based" stereotaxis included the surgical object (e.g., the cervical spine), the virtual object (an image of the cervical spine obtained from computed tomography (CT) or magnetic resonance imaging (MRI) and a frame (navigator) fixed to the surgical object (cervical spine) for guidance of the surgical instruments according to the coordinates extrapolated from the preoperative images. "Frameless" sterotaxis is possible now owing to further development in medical imaging and computer science. The exact coordinates of the surgical object can be defined in a three-dimensional (3D) data set (CT or MRI) of the region of interest. The surgeon navigates, the instruments via a motion analysis system without any mechanical frame. Optical (infrared light), magnetic, or acoustic (ultrasound) signals are utilized to localize the position of the instrument or implant in space.

A major problem in applying frameless stereotaxy to the spine is the relative mobility between adjacent vertebrae and the overlying soft-tissue structures. As a result, frameless stereotaxy in the spine requires registration that is based on the exposed anatomy of

From: *Arthroscopic and Endoscopic Spinal Surgery: Text and Atlas: Second Edition*
Edited by: P. Kambin © Humana Press Inc., Totowa, NJ

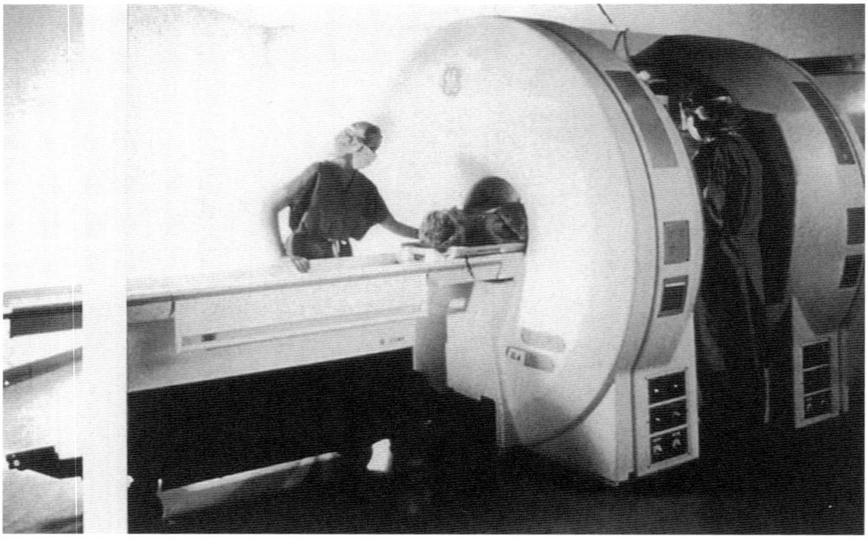

Fig. 1. Photograph of open-configuration intraoperative magnetic resonance imager. The magnet is constructed with two interconnected cryostats with a 56-cm vertical opening permitting access to the patient during imaging. (Courtesy of General Electric, Milwaukee, WI.)

the vertebrae. Navigation is then reliable only on that registered anatomical structure. To navigate on adjacent vertebrae, the registration process has to be repeated. As one can see, the process can become time-consuming, especially when the registration process is not proceeding fluidly.

IMAGE ACQUISITION

Image-guided spinal surgery typically begins with preoperative acquisition of 3D images using CT or MRI. A CT scanner is an effective tool for collecting preoperative images with thin-slice (approx 1 mm) imaging. The image data are then transmitted via DICOM interfaces to the picture archiving and communication system (PACS) and into the image-guided spinal surgery local area network. The connectivity of the scanners and the PACS interfaces are the most important aspects of successfully orchestrating image-guided therapy. Alternatively, a surgery-dedicated server can be used, in conjunction with the existing PACS system, for presurgical planning and delivery of postprocessed images to the operating room.

The main limitation in existing stereotactic systems is that images are acquired before surgery and are not updated to reflect intraoperative changes. In addition, existing frameless stereotactic systems for spinal surgery do not provide localization of the spinal segment, typically obtained using a lateral radiograph, and necessitate manual registration of fiducial landmarks in the operative field to the image data set acquired before surgery. However, recently, Woodward et al. *(1)* have described the use of intraoperative MRI (IMRI) as an adjunct in minimally invasive spinal surgery.

The IMRI involves a novel, open-configuration, cryogenless superconducting magnet with a vertical gap between the two magnetic components that allows direct access to the patient during imaging (Fig. 1). IMRI provides all the advantages of conventional

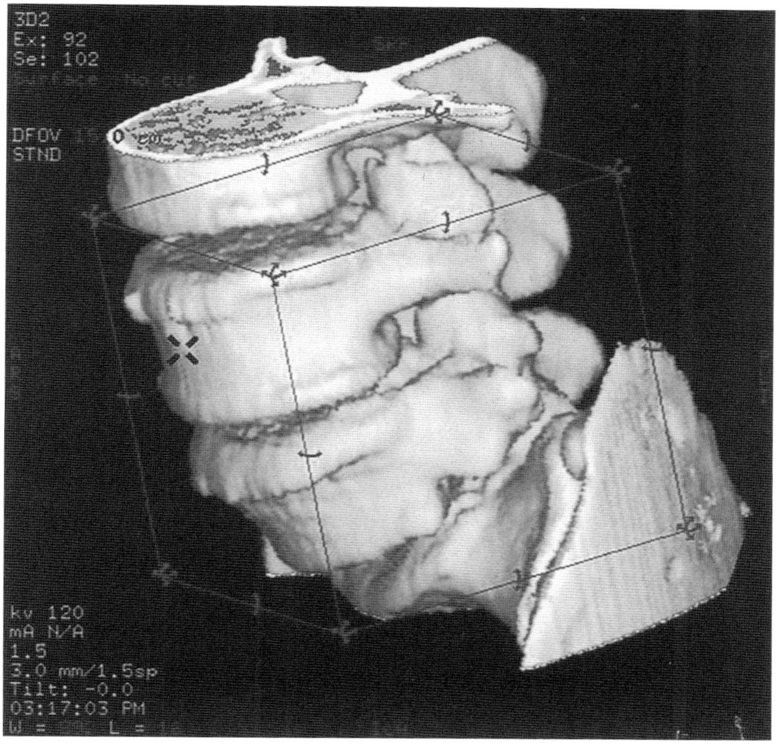

Fig. 2. Typical 3D reconstruction image obtained from thin-slice (1-mm) CT of lumbosacral junction.

MRI including multiplanar image acquisition and excellent definition of soft-tissue anatomy. Using IMRI, 12 patients underwent successful spinal surgery involving three lumbar discectomies, three anterior cervical discectomies and fusions, three cervical vertebrectomies with allograft fusions, two cervical foraminotomies, and one decompressive cervical laminectomy. The primary advantage of IMRI is that it provides accurate real-time imaging that can be used in surgical planning and assessment. However, as with conventional MRI, IMRI affords limited depiction of osseous anatomy, which may limit its role in spinal surgery. Nevertheless, the improved real-time imaging afforded by IMRI makes this an attractive intraoperative adjunct to spinal surgery in the future.

PRESURGICAL PLANNING

Preparation for the use of computer-assisted image guidance depends on the specific requirements of the surgical procedure. All procedures, however, require special software tools to manipulate the acquired images in order to create a graphic model of the surgical anatomy. Prior to surgery, CT or MRI images of the spine are obtained using a 3D imaging protocol. The scan is transferred to the computer workstation via a dedicated imaging network. A 3D image of the spine is segmented from the slice images obtained prior to surgery (Fig. 2). Morphological operations, such as thresholding and voxel connectivity, can be used on the images to create a 3D image of the bony surface of the spine. In addition, 3D CT images can be used for standard orthogonal views as well as oblique

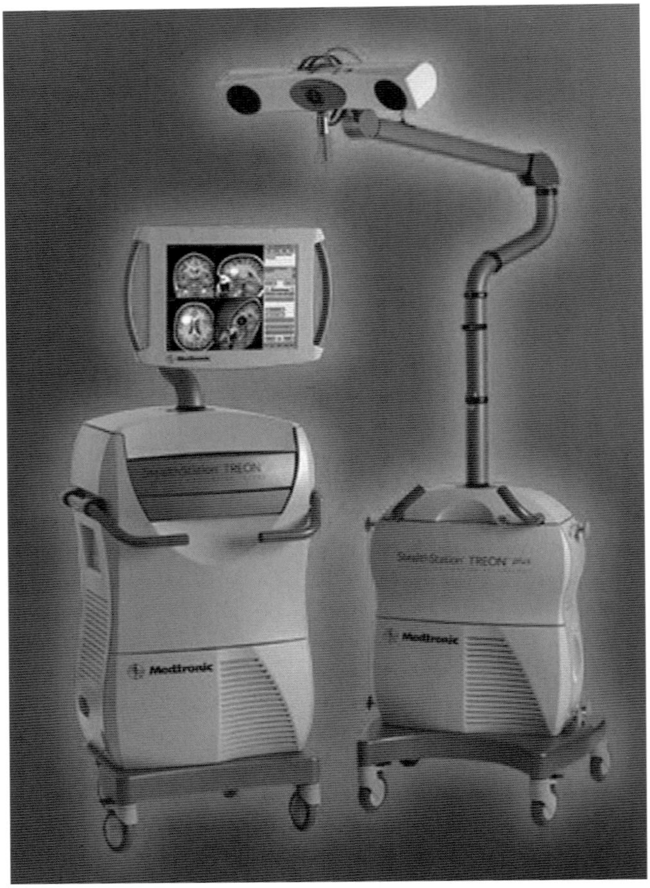

Fig. 3. Typical optoelectric navigational system. The Stealth system (courtesy of Medtronic Sofamor Danek, Memphis, TN) is depicted with the optical tracking apparatus and the intraoperative computer imaging display.

cuts that display the planned trajectory of the surgical probe. For example, in a lumbar pedicle screw case, these visualizations can help in determining the trajectory and diameter of a pedicle screw that is needed, as well as the depths of screw insertion. Surgical planning is done in the virtual space of the 3D image model, and relationships to soft tissues, such as spinal cord and critical arteries, can be defined during presurgical planning.

SURGICAL NAVIGATION

Components of a surgical navigation system include a computer workstation with a network interface, surgical instruments that may be tracked via light-emitting diodes, a reference arc or other method for tracking patient anatomy, and an optical camera that tracks the reference arc and the surgical probes (Figs. 3 and 4). The technical requirements for performing image-guided surgery may vary among different systems, but conceptually the methods are very similar.

The surgical navigation system enables free-hand navigation of the surgical space and frameless stereotactic surgery through image guidance. It allows a surgeon to track both patient anatomy and instruments in three dimensions with improved accuracy. Error in

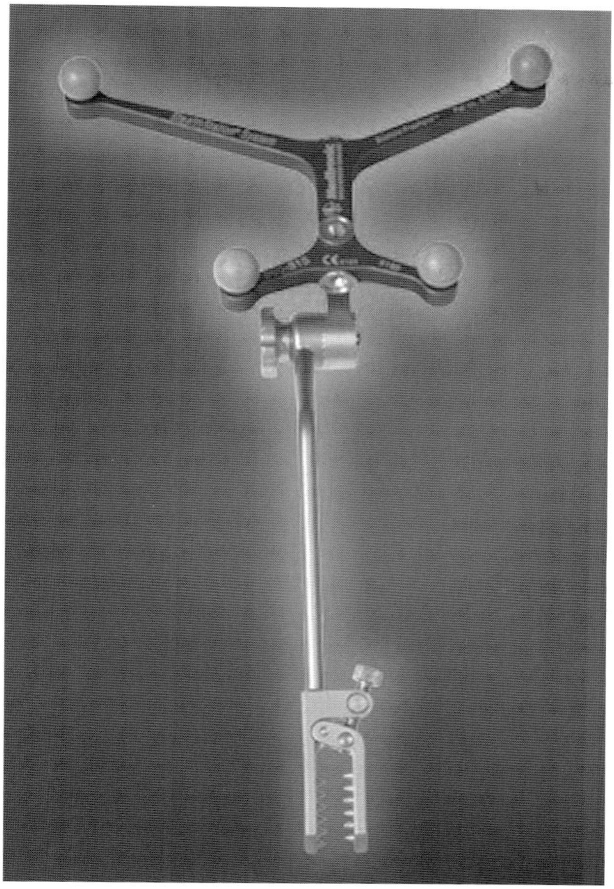

Fig. 4. Photograph showing close-up of wireless dynamic reference frame with attached clamp that connects to StealthStation. (Courtesy of Medtronic Sofamor Danek, Memphis, TN.)

localizing the target in a phantom is typically 2.5 mm or less. Real-time manipulation of the computer model allows a surgeon to localize surgical position on preoperative images. The optical tracking technology permits real-time, dynamically referenced localization of patient anatomy and surgical instrumentation. By equipping standard surgical instruments with this technology, a surgeon can operate with familiar instrumentation that is coupled with the patient's diagnostic images.

Typically the reference arc is attached to the spinous process of the involved vertebra (Fig. 5). Without the reference frame, even slight movement by the patient would adversely affect navigational accuracy. Therefore, the patient's anatomy must be defined in conjunction with the position of the reference frame. It is logical to assume that rigid fixation of the reference frame must be performed for each vertebral segment requiring surgical intervention. The smallest movement of the reference frame in relationship to the spinous process may result in drastic changes in navigational accuracy. The frame is attached to the patient's spine via either a clamp or pin. The bony landmarks of the spine are exposed and identified by touching the surgical probe to identifiable points on the surface anatomy. The camera array dynamically tracks the reference arc and motion of the vertebral segments to which the arc is attached.

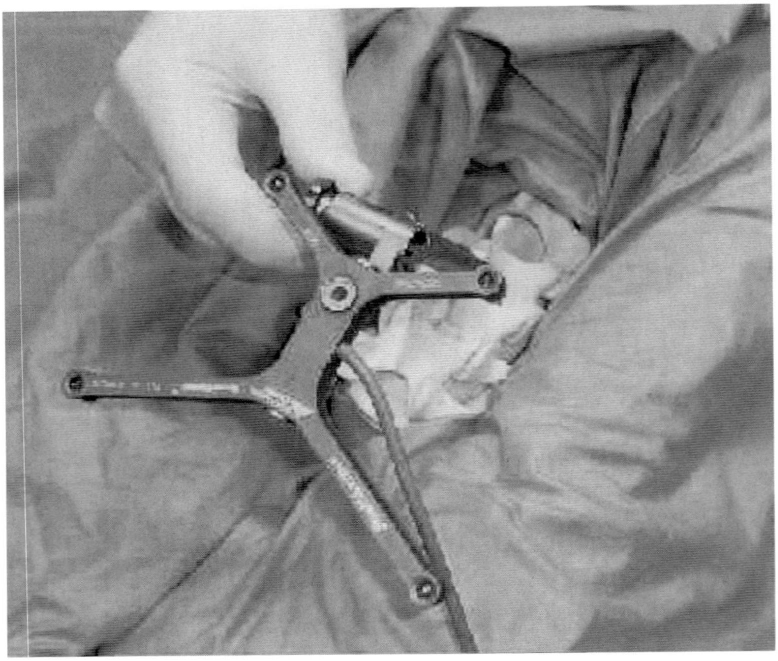

Fig. 5. Photograph showing close-up of dynamic reference frame rigidly attached to spinous process of a cadaveric spine. (Courtesy of Medtronic Sofamor Danek, Memphis, TN.)

Registration accuracy is a critical variable in the use of image-guided spinal surgery. Accurate and reliable identification of anatomical landmarks in the spine is relatively difficult. Misregistration of anatomical landmarks with preacquired imaging landmarks is a major factor in potential inaccuracy of these systems. Although alternative methods using internal fiducial markers have been tested *(2–9)*, the reliance on the identification of anatomical landmarks remains the most widely used technique for coregistration of image and patient coordinate spaces. Minimizing registration error involves centering the target over the anatomical landmark and increasing the number of and distance between anatomical landmarks.

The average misalignment, or gap, between corresponding landmarks may be reported by the surgical navigation workstation as the mean fiduciary error. The mean fiduciary error describes how closely points in the image correspond to points on the anatomy of the patient. The surgeon should note that the mean fiduciary error is not a true estimate of the accuracy of the system and that a perfect registration of points may still not define precisely the anatomical space. For example, equally spaced points identified on a sphere could be perfectly registered to equidistant points on an image of the sphere, yet the two spheres (the actual sphere and its virtual image) could be rotated 180° relative to each other. For this reason, noncollinear landmarks that are widely spaced around the target anatomy are recommended. It should be emphasized that the surgeon should always perform a global assessment of the registration accuracy by identifying independent surface points and by visually confirming how well the image space and surgical space correlate.

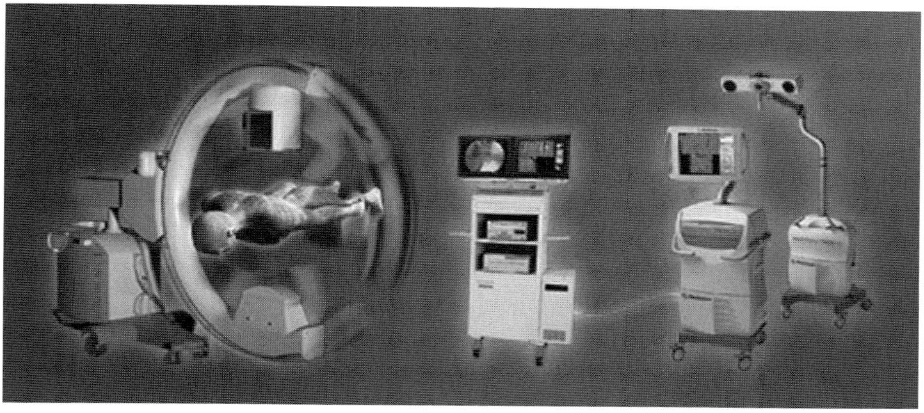

Fig. 6. Photograph of FluoroNav system including StealthStation, C-arm with imaging target, and dual-lens camera. (Courtesy of Medtronic Sofamor Danek, Memphis, TN.)

ALTERNATIVE IMAGING MODALITIES: REAL-TIME FLUOROSCOPY

Compared with current 3D computer image-guided surgery systems, virtual fluoroscopy is readily applicable to a wide variety of spinal procedures such as pedicle screw insertion, anterior odontoid screw fixation, and interbody cage placement *(10–15)*. Virtual fluoroscopy offers several distinct advantages over computer-assisted imaging, such as avoiding the time and cost of obtaining specially formatted preoperative CT or MRI images. The often time-consuming and frustrating step of image-to-patient registration is unnecessary. The image calibration process for virtual fluoroscopy is fully automated. In addition, real-time image updating for positional changes of the patient after manipulation of a given spinal segment is easily achieved during surgery by simply acquiring a new fluoroscopic image. Likewise, real-time intraoperative fluoroscopic validation of the virtually displayed instrument position can be obtained at any time, providing a "safety check" (Figs. 6 and 7).

Despite these many advantages, virtual fluoroscopy is a two-dimensional (2D) navigational system (Figs. 8 and 9). It does not provide the detailed multiplanar imaging generated by 3D systems. Errors in the clinical interpretation of 2D images and the extrapolation of 2D information to 3D anatomy are still dependent on the expertise of the spine surgeon. Additionally, virtual fluoroscopy cannot compensate for factors resulting in poor image quality such as obesity, the presence of bowel contrast after trauma assessment, or the inadvertent positioning of radioopaque structures. The effects of parallax also must be considered when using a virtual fluoroscopy system. Despite these limitations, computer enhancement of fluoroscopically assisted procedures provides a broad-based and practical application of surgical navigational technology.

CURRENT APPLICATIONS OF IMAGE-GUIDED SURGERY

Because of the complex and varied nature of cervical spine anatomy, instrumentation in the spine can be extremely challenging, even in very experienced hands. Placement of C2-C1 transarticular screws exemplifies the deficiencies in current techniques for spinal navigation. Up to 15–20% of patients lack the required bony volume in the region of the C2 isthmus to accept safely a screw with a 3.5 mm diameter. Although

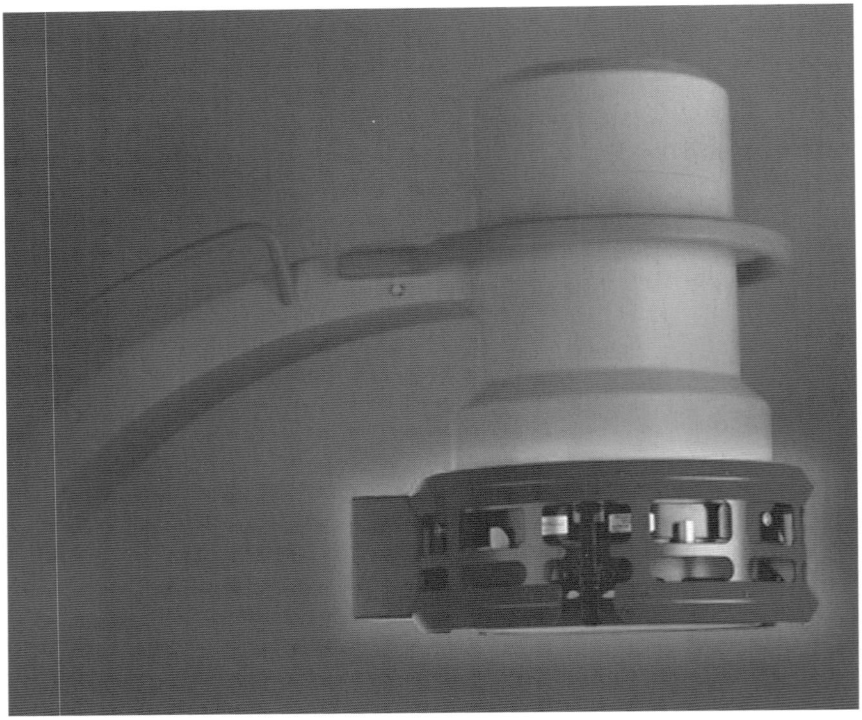

Fig. 7. Photograph showing close-up of C-arm with target guide mounted on image intensifier. (Courtesy of Medtronic Sofamor Danek, Memphis, TN.)

cervical lateral mass screw placement has been considered extremely safe regarding potential injury to the vertebral artery or spinal cord, Heller et al. *(16,17)*, in a cadaveric study, noted a 7.3% rate of cervical root injury using the Magerl technique for lateral mass screw placement. They also reported on a clinical series of 78 patients of whom four developed a symptomatic radiculopathy owing to misplaced screws (5%) *(16,17)*. Clearly, these studies indicate the potential benefit of better intraoperative neurovascular surveillance and guidance when spinal implants are placed.

The value of spinal imaging becomes more obvious when one realizes the difficulty associated with so-called hidden spinal structures. Accurate knowledge of spinal anatomy is totally dependent on the surgeon's experience and the ability to visualize anatomical structures three dimensionally *(18–22)*. Weinstein et al. *(18)* reported that 21% of instrumented thoracolumbar pedicles placed using standard fluoroscopy showed evidence of cortical perforation. Even more shocking was that 92% of these failures occurred medially within the spinal canal. Clearly, the potential for serious neurological sequelae exists as a result of misdirected spinal implants using current conventional imaging techniques.

Several researchers have detailed their experiences with computer-assisted imaging in the cervical spine. Welch et al. *(23)* performed 11 upper cervical spine procedures including transoral odontoid resection, posterior atlantoaxial fusion with transarticular C2-C1 screw fixation, and spinal tumor resection utilizing CT-guided stereotaxis. In each case, frameless stereotaxy was used to plan the incision, delineate the resection margins, and determine the appropriate trajection of implant placement. They noted no

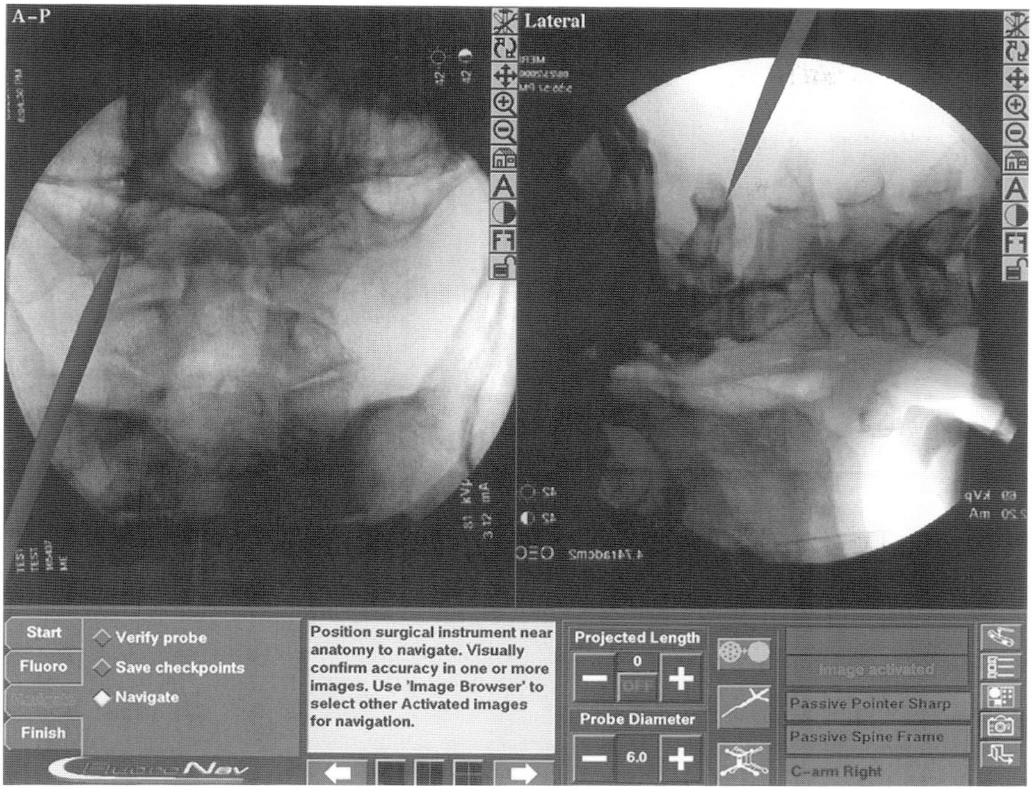

Fig. 8. Anteropasterior (AP) (open-mouth odontoid)/lateral virtual fluoroscopic image of C1 lateral mass and spinous process. (Courtesy of Medtronic Sofamor Danek, Memphis, TN.)

intraoperative complications, and each patient successfully underwent adequate resection of the pathological lesion and satisfactory placement of cervical instrumentation.

Bolger and Wigfield *(24,25)* retrospectively reviewed 120 cases in which imaged-guided surgery involving the cervical and thoracic spine was utilized. Of these, 34 cases involved transarticular atlantoaxial screw placement, 22 cases involved cervical lateral mass plating, 40 cases involved anterior cervical decompressions, and 18 cases involved vertebrectomies. The authors concluded that the use of image-guided technology provided an enormous amount of anatomical information, particularly in aberrant anatomical cases, and that it was easier to determine the best screw trajectory on an individual basis rather then having to rely on population-based, predetermined implant placement recommendations.

More recently, Richter et al. *(26)* evaluated whether C2–C1 transarticular anatomical screws as well as transpedicular screws in C3 and C4 could be applied safely with computer-assisted surgery. Hole positions were evaluated by palpation, CT, and dissections. The investigators noted that 48 (92%) of the 52 drilled pedicles were correctly positioned. The vertebral artery was not injured in any specimen. Finally, all of the 26 C2–C1 transarticular k-wires were placed properly with no injury to the vascular structures noted. Richter et al. *(26)* concluded that image guidance greatly improved the accuracy of implant placement and reduced potential complications.

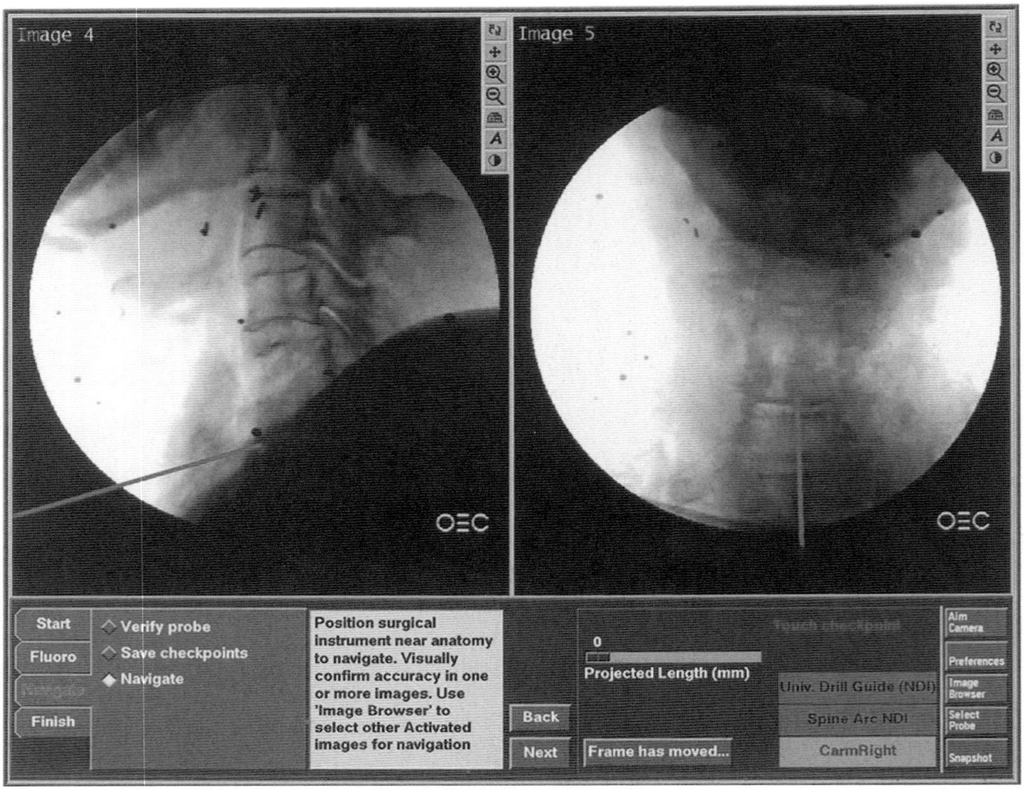

Fig. 9. AP/lateral C-spine fluoroscopic image with image marker indicating midline of C5 vertebral body. (Courtesy of Medtronic Sofamor Danek, Memphis, TN.)

Laine et al. *(27)* prospectively evaluated 30 adult patients who had undergone placement of 174 thoracolumbar pedicle screws. Of those screws, 139 were placed using a CT-guided imaging system, and the remaining 35 were placed without computer assistance. The investigators noted a significantly higher rate of cortical wall perforation without the use of image-guided assistance (14.3 vs 4.3%). In fact, of the screws placed conventionally, three perforated the medial wall of the pedicle, with one screw requiring repositioning secondary to nerve root irritation (Fig. 10).

Foley and colleagues presented their experience with the FluoroNav (Medtronic Surgical Navigation Technologies, Louisville, CO) image guidance system in the cervical spine (10,11,28,29). The FluoroNav system was used for three separate cervical spine applications: odontoid screw placement, lateral mass screw placement, and anterior cervical corpectomy and plate placement. By using (virtual) preacquired AP, open-mouth, and lateral views, the investigators were able to successfully place all three odontoid screws, as well as match the intended midsagittal plane screw angulation in the 24 cervical lateral mass screws placed. The intended angle of projection was 30∞ in the sagittal plane. The actual measured screw placement measured approx 30.5∞, with a range of 27–35∞. All corpectomy troughs had a symmetric boundary regarding the midline, with an average trough diameter of 16.8 mm, which was 0.8 mm larger than the intended diameter of 16 mm. All cervical plates were placed in the correct midline orientation.

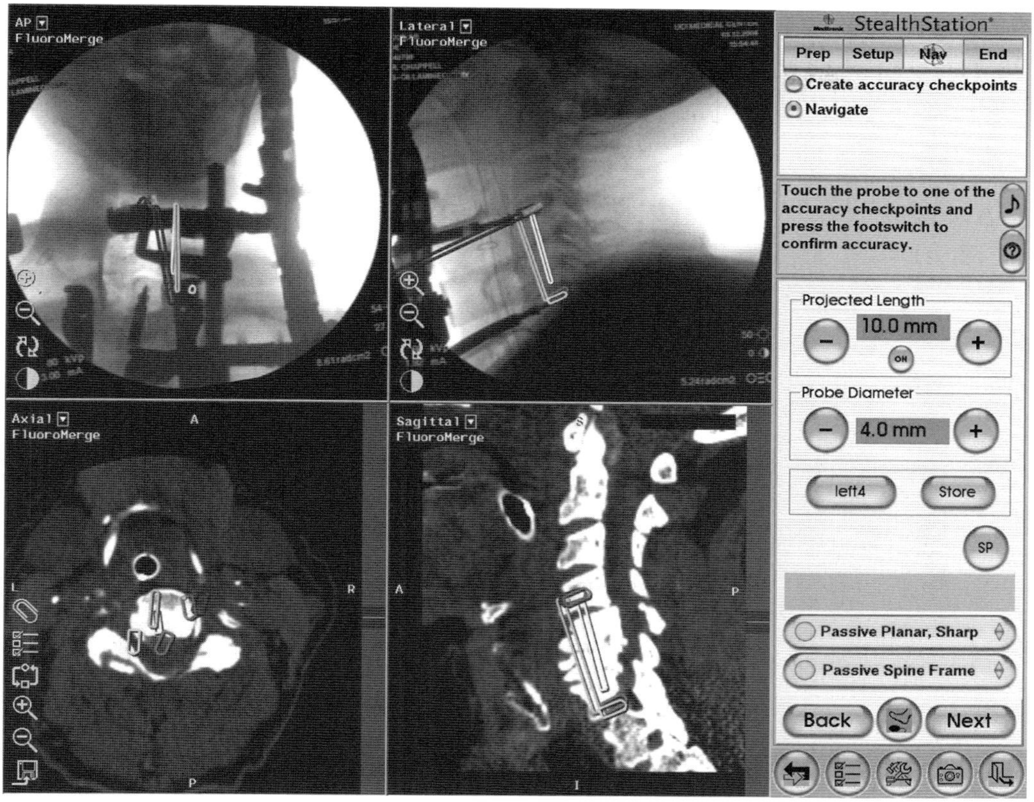

Fig. 10. Intraoperative depiction of pedicle screw placement utilizing an image-guided CT navigational system. (Courtesy of Medtronic Sofamor Danek, Memphis, TN.)

FUTURE APPLICATIONS

Successful applications of image-guided spinal surgery have been reported to achieve complex spinal procedures such as pedicle screw placement, transarticular C1–C2 fixation, transoral odontoid resection, and anterior vertebral corpectomies. The future undoubtedly will fuse the precision of computer assisted image technology with the celebrated techniques of minimally invasive spinal applications. The greatest challenge for this merger are the difficulties encountered with accurate percutaneous registration of the spine using standard endoscopy techniques. The registration process at this time requires the physical exposure of a part of the vertebra, whereas percutaneous endoscopic exposures avoid unncessary soft-tissue dissections. Unfortunately, at this time, external landmarks cannot be reliably used as fiducials for registration because of tissue deformation.

A potential solution to this problem is the development of a percutaneously placed reference frame recently described by Assaker et al *(30)*. They confirmed the efficacy of this strategy in a cadaveric feasibility study and then reported successful clinical results in two patients treated endoscopically with image-guided assistance.

Assaker et al. *(30)* utilized the Stealth computer-assisted image-guided system (Medtronic). The reference frame was designed to be inserted percutaneously into the pedicle of the affected vertebra under CT guidance with local sedation (Fig. 11). An

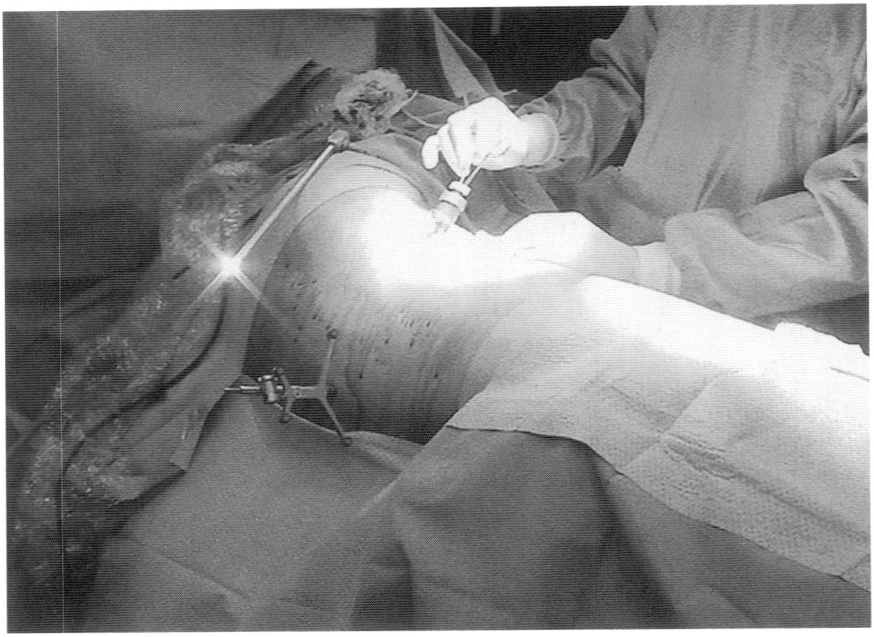

Fig. 11. Patient positioned in lateral decubitus position for thoracoscopic surgical approach. The reference frame has been percutaneously placed under CT guidance into the pedicle of the T9 vertebra.

additional antirotational tube locked the pedicle implant to the spine, creating a single rigid body for subsequent image acquisition.

The purpose of using an external reference frame in endoscopic surgery is twofold. First, the frame acts as a reference system (fiducial) necessary to assimilate the image data with the surgical space. Second, the frame is a dynamic 3D localizer. As mentioned previously, fiducials are necessary for registration. For endoscopic use, fiducials have to be independent of the vertebrae. To resolve this problem, six points were chosen on the CT images of a frame (Figs. 12 and 13). The corresponding points were identified on the frame and touched with the calibrated pointer for registration. This enabled a frame-based registration and navigation with image guidance. Two patients were subsequently treated using this computer-assisted endoscopic spinal technology (Fig. 14). One patient, a 70-yr-old male, underwent a thoracoscopic decompression of a calcified central disc herniation at T8-T9. The second patient, a 32-yr-old man, underwent an endoscopic decompression of a sacroiliac osteophyte causing intermittent low-back pain. Both patients had postoperative CT scans that showed complete decompression of the offending pathology, which resulted in complete resolution of symptoms.

The combination of endoscopic surgery and computer-assisted imaging should be a revolutionary advancement for both sciences in their quest to become more broadly accepted by the spine community. The benefits of endoscopic surgery, such as limited soft-tissue dissection, faster postoperative recovery period, and decreased hospitalization costs, may be safely balanced by the improved visualization afforded by frameless stereotaxy.

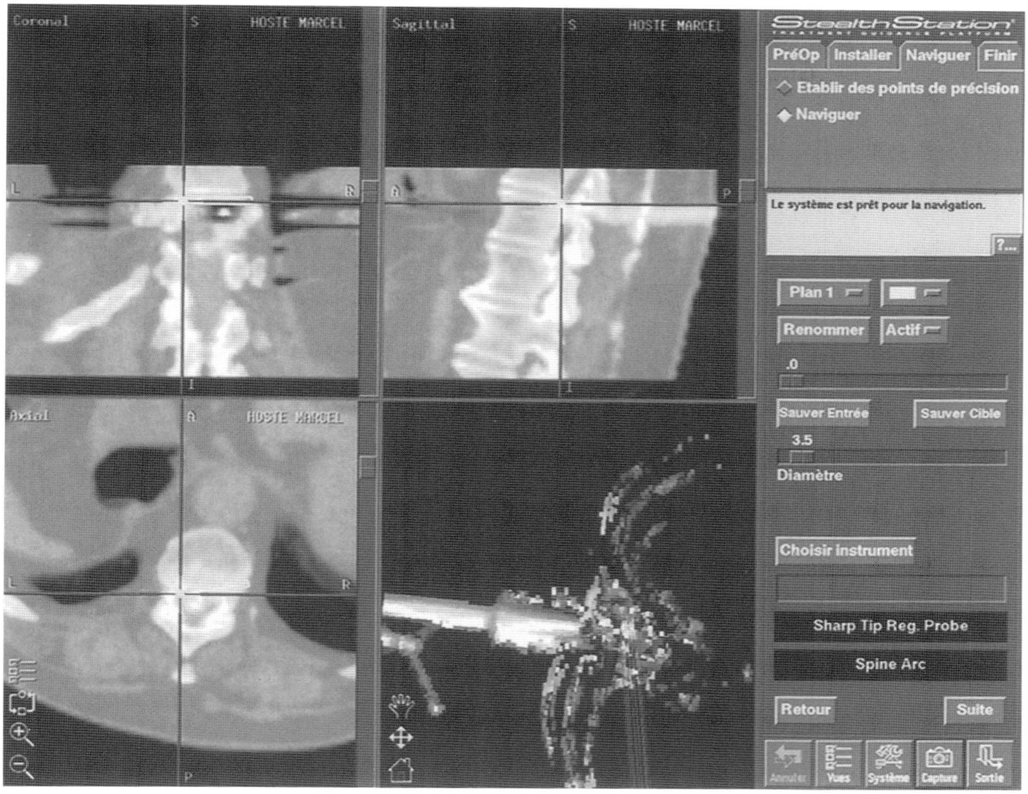

Fig. 12. View of monitor during endoscopic navigation showing tip of pointer on preplanned target.

CONCLUSION

Despite the advances made in spinal imaging and computer-assisted spinal surgery, many limitations still exist impeding its widespread acceptance. This includes primarily its lack of user-friendly applications and its cost. The current cost of computer-guided systems and their lack of documented efficacy at this time in terms of cost savings and reduced patient morbidity limits their acceptance at many spine centers. However, dismissing computer image-guided surgery as too expensive to be practical is by far premature. A cost–benefit analysis should take into account the infancy of the technology and the enormous potential of the synergy of frameless stereotaxis and minimally invasive spinal techniques.

The technological limitations of image-assisted surgery are clearly evident. The lack of real-time image acquisition, the difficulties with optical apprecation of light-emitting diode (LED) sensors, and the time-consuming nature of preoperative image acquisition limit the current application of frameless stereotaxy in general spinal applications.

In an elegantly performed study by Rampersaud et al. *(31)*, a geometric model was developed relating spinal pedicle anatomy to accuracy requirements for image-guided surgery. The investigators noted a very small maximum permissible translational error of <1 mm and rotational error of <5° at the midcervical spine, midthoracic spine, and

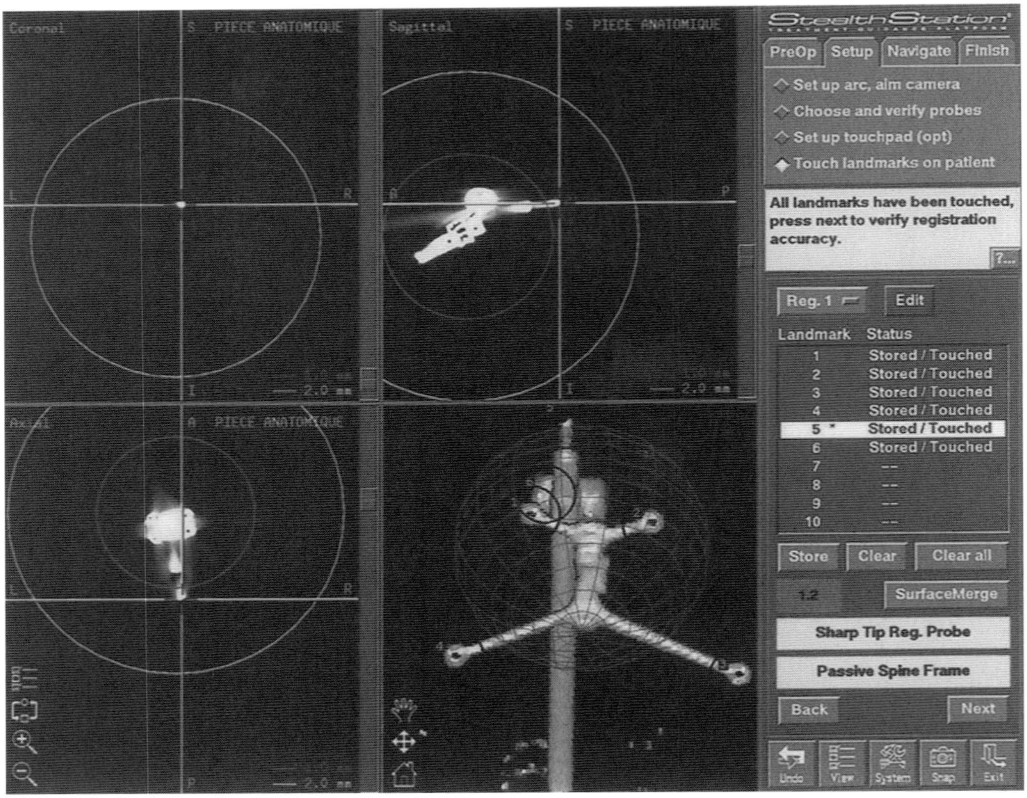

Fig. 13. CT image of geometry of frame used as a fiducial for registration. Paired point matching and surface mapping are systematically performed.

thoracolumbar junction *(31)*. These accuracy requirements far exceeded the overall clinical utility error of current image-guided systems. This raises the question, Why do image-guidance systems improve the clinical accuracy of pedicle screw placement? What may actually happen intraoperatively is that the image-guided system may bring the surgeon much closer to the actual starting point and trajectory. Further refinements of the screw path result from the surgeon's appropriate response to visual and tactile feedback, and the self-centering, mechanical constraint provided by the pedicle wall. Thus, an image-guided surgical system functions as a synergistic tool along with the surgeon's judgment of the intraoperative anatomy.

Accordingly, users of image-guided surgery systems must be cognizant of the limitations of these current systems. The progressive development of real-time imaging technology, coupled with refinements in minimally invasive spinal techniques, appears to be very promising in improving patient outcomes and reducing the morbidity of invasive spinal procedures. In conclusion, image-guided surgical systems can aid the surgeon in navigating complex spinal anatomy; however, these systems are only tools that must be combined with good surgical judgment and skill to achieve successful surgical outcomes.

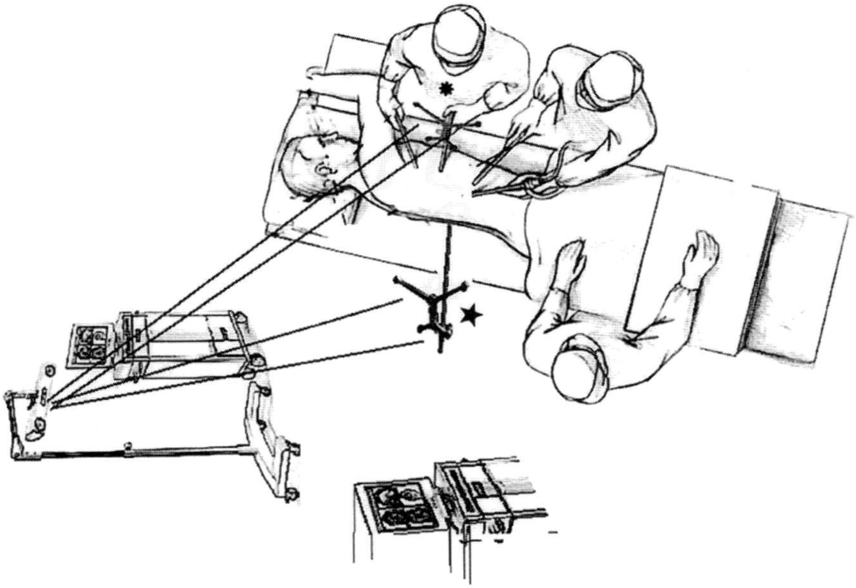

Fig. 14. Schematic of typical operative setup for image-guided thoracoscopy.

REFERENCES

1. Woodward E, Leon S, Moriarty T, et al. Initial experience with intraoperative magnetic resonance imaging in spine surgery. Spine 2001;26(4):410–407.
2. Salehi SA, Ondra SL. Use of internal fiducial markers in frameless stereotactic navigational systems during spinal surgery: technical note. Neurosurgery 2000;47(6):1460–1462.
3. Albert T, Klein G, Vaccaro A. Image-guided anterior cervical corpectomy: a feasibility study. Spine 1999;24:826–830.
4. Dyer P, Patel N, Pell G. The ISG viewing wand: an application to altanto-axial cervical surgery using the LeFort I maxillary osteotomy. Br J Oral Maxillofac Surg 1995;33:370–374.
5. Glossop ND, Hu RW, Randle JA. Computer-aided pedicle screw placement using frameless stereotaxis. Spine 1996;21:2026–2034.
6. Kalfas I, Kormos D, Murphy M. Application of frameless stereotaxy to pedicle screw fixation of the spine. J Neurosurg 1995;83:641–647.
7. Kamimura M, Ebara S, Itoh H, et al. Accurate pedicle screw insertion under the control of a computer assisted image guiding system: laboratory test and clinical study. J Orthop Sci 1999;4:197–206.
8. Kato A, Yoshimine T, Hayakawa T. A frameless, armless navigational system for computer-assisted neurosurgery. J Neurosurg 1991;74:845–849.
9. Kramer DL, Ludwig SC, Balderston RA, Vaccaro AR, Foley KT, Albert TJ. Placement of pedicle screws in the cervical spine: comparative accuracy of three techniques. Spine 2000;25:1655–1667.
10. Foley K, Silveri C, Vaccaro AR, et al. Atlantoaxial transarticular screw fixation: risk assessment and bone morphology using an image guidance system. J Bone Joint Sury (Br) 1998;80:245.
11. Foley K, Smith M. Image-guided spine surgery. Neurosurg Clin North Am 1996;7:171–186.
12. Ludwig SC, Klein GR, Vaccaro AR, Rushton SA, Lazar RD, Albert TJ. The efficacy of using an image-guided Kerrison in performing an anterior cervical foraminotomy: an anatomic analysis of the spine. Spine 1999;24:1358–1362.

13. Ludwig SC, Kramer DL, Balderston RA, Vaccaro AR, Foley KT, Albert TJ. Placement of pedicle screws in the human cadaveric cervical spine: comparative accuracy of three techniques. Spine 2000;25(13):1665–1667.
14. Notle L, Slomczykowski M, Berlemann U, et al. A new approach to computer aided spine surgery: fluoroscopy-based surgical navigation. Eur Spine J 2000;9(Suppl 1):S78–S88.
15. Pollack I, Welch W, Jacobs G. A frameless stereotactic guidance: an intraoperative adjunct in the transoral approach for ventral cervicomedullary junction decompression. Spine 1995;20:216–220.
16. Heller JG, Carlson GD, Abitbol JJ, et al. Anatomic comparison of the Roy-Camille and Magerl techniques for screw placement in the lower cervical spine. Spine 1991;16:S552–S557.
17. Heller JG, Silcox H, Sutterlin C. Complications of posterior cervical plating. Spine 1995;20(22):2442–2448.
18. Weinstein JN, Spratt KF, Spengler D, et al. Spinal pedicle fixation: reliability and validity of roentgenogram-based assessment and surgical factors on successful screw placement. Spine 1988;13:1012–1018.
19. Roessler K, Ungerboeck K, Dietrich E. Frameless stereotactic guided neurosurgery: clinical experience with an infrared based pointer device navigational system. Acta Neurochir 1997;139:551–559.
20. Sandeman D, Gill S. The impact of interactive image guided surgery: the Bristol experience with the ISG/Elekta viewing wand. Acta Neurochir Suppl 1995;64:54–58.
21. Silveri CP, Foley KT, Vaccaro AR, Shah S, Garfin SR. Atlantoaxial transarticular screw fixation: risk assessment and bone morphology using an image guidance system. Annual meeting, 25th CSRS, Dec. 7–7, 1997, Rancho Mirage, CA.
22. Smith K, Frank K, Bucholz R. The neurostation—a highly accurate, minimally invasive solution to frameless stereotactic neurosurgery. Comput Med Imaging Graph 1994;18:247–256.
23. Welch E, Sunach B, Pollack I, et al. Frameless stereotactic guidance for surgery of the upper cervical spine. Neurosurgery 1997;40:958–964.
24. Bolger C, Wigfield C. Frameless stereotaxy and anterior cervical surgery. Computer Aided Surg 1999;4:322–327.
25. Bolger C, Wigfield C. Image-guided surgery: applications to the cervical and thoracic spine and review of the first 120 procedures. J Neurosurg (Spine 2) 2000;92:175–180.
26. Richter M, Amiot LP, Neller S, Kluger P, Puhl W. Computer assisted surgery in posterior instrumentation of the cervical spine: an in-vitro feasibility study. Eur Spine J 2000;(Suppl 1):S65–S70.
27. Laine T, Schlenzka D, Makitalo K, et al. Improved accuracy of pedicle screw insertion with computer-assisted surgery: a prospective clinical trial of 30 patients. Spine 1997;22:1254–1258.
28. Foley K, Rampersaud Y. Frameless spinal stereotaxis. Curr Orthop 1998;12:104–110.
29. Foley K, Rampersaud YR, Simone DA, Jansen TH. Virtual fluoroscopy for cervical spine surgery, annual meeting, 27th CSRS, Dec 16–18, 1999, Seattle, WA.
30. Assaker R, Cinquin P, Cotton A, Lejeune J. Image-guided endoscopic spine surgery: part I and II. Spine 2001;26(15):1705–1718.
31. Rampersaud Y, Simon D, Foley KT. Accuracy requirements for image-guided spinal pedicle screw placement. Spine 2001;26(4):352–359.

18
The Rise and Fall of Chemonucleolysis

James W. Simmons, Jr., MD and Robert D. Fraser, MD

INTRODUCTION

The past four decades have witnessed the arrival of numerous interventional procedures for the treatment of sciatica and back pain. Some have failed to gain general acceptance and have simply faded away, and others continue to be used without evidence of efficacy. What is unique about chymopapain is that it has fallen out of favor despite convincing evidence of its utility and efficacy in the treatment of sciatica from lumbar disc protrusion. It has been shown to be superior to placebo in no less than three double-blind, randomized controlled trials *(1,2)*, and to be cost-effective with low morbidity when compared with open surgery *(3)*.

This chapter describes the circumstances and events leading to the rise and fall of chymopapain, exploring how commercial interests and emotional influences have overridden substantial scientific evidence of efficacy and safety *(4–7)*. Much of this account describes information that has already been published extensively, but some of it emphasizes details not well known but considered important in the overall context, particularly from a historical perspective.

The attraction for the use of chymopapain as a proteolytic agent for the treatment of herniated nucleus pulposus (NP), is readily understandable and its introduction and rise to prominence are covered in some detail in this chapter. On the other hand, the factors leading to the demise of chemonucleolysis are less well documented in the literature but are equally apparent in light of events to be described.

The use of chymopapain B in the treatment of problems related to the disc is probably one of the most critically appraised invasive procedures involving a pharmaceutical drug that we as clinicians have dealt with. However, in spite of extensive evidence that supported safety and efficacy leading to worldwide use, the product suffered a demise that occurred without a satisfactory official explanation. What follows is an account of the history of chymopapain followed by an assessment of the factors leading to its removal from clinical use.

Eugene Jansen and Arnold Balls isolated chymopapain in 1941 from the crude latex derived from the fruit of carica papaya by "milking" the green papaya fruit while on the plant prior to harvest *(8)*.

From: *Arthroscopic and Endoscopic Spinal Surgery: Text and Atlas: Second Edition*
Edited by: P. Kambin © Humana Press Inc., Totowa, NJ

Lewis Thomas was seeking an enzyme that would reduce circulating protein in blood that clogged the renal tubules resulting in renal shutdown, as enzymatic activity cannot be produced by known chemical methods and has to be obtained by way of naturally occurring biologicals. In 1956, he injected rabbits intravenously with crude papain and noticed that their ears drooped. Forty-eight hours later, the rabbits' ears resumed their erect posture. This indicated a reversible action on the chondral intracellular substance of the ears. It was also noted that the trachea softened, but there was no effect on any other tissue in the rabbit. It was particularly of interest that

> apart from the unusual cosmetic effect, the animals exhibited no evidence of systemic illness or discomfort. The ears had replenished their basophilic chondroid matrix allowing them to regain their original shape. Larger doses of papain were injected and had an impact on joint cartilage, epiphyseal growth plates, and tracheal and bronchial cartilage; however, no systemic problems were found to be present *(9)*.

Lyman Smith first thought that could papain might be of value in treating chondroblastic tumors. Although this did not prove worthy, he found that intradiscal injections in rabbits removed the NP, leaving the annulus largely intact *(10)*.

Prior to this, Carl Hirsch had the concept of injecting a specific enzyme into the intervertebral disc but not specifically for the treatment of disc herniation *(11)*. He reasoned that an intradiscal injection of a chondrolytic enzyme would cause the disc to become stable and asymptomatic by accelerating the process of disc degeneration. He had envisioned an enzyme similar to that produced by bacteria as is seen in infectious processes. Other proteolytic enzymes were investigated and found to have a similar effect on the disc tissue, but toxicological studies revealed chymopapain to be the least toxic and to have the most specific action on the mucopolysaccharide of the intervertebral disc. Other proteolytic enzymes such as collagenase were advocated *(12)*. Extensive research with collagenases proved it not to be "safe and effective."

Subsequently, Smith sold the patent for chymopapain to Baxter-Travenol for $1. The company then formulated a product called Discase, which was a combination of chymopapain B, cysteine sodium sulfite, and EDTA in lyophilized form. During the period of the first phase of investigation, it was used in 10 patients in Switzerland in 1963, and by 1975, 35 of us as investigators in a phase 3 trial had injected approx 17,000 patients.

A controversial study done at Walter Reed Army Medical Center in 1975 triggered the withdrawal of the New Drug Application that had been filed with the Food and Drug Administration (FDA) for the use and treatment of intervertebral disc disease with Discase *(13)*. The study reported no statistical difference in instance or quality of improvement between the placebo group (29% success rate) and the group treated with Discase (58% success rate). Baxter-Travenol voluntarily withdrew the drug, rather than take the chance of rejection by the FDA. Although Brown and Daroff *(14)* criticized the Walter Reed Army Medical Center study because of the early code break, the lack of inert placebo, the insufficient dose of Discase, and the lack of technical experience, the drug continued to be unavailable for use in indicated patients. Physicians in the United States who had been using the drug with excellent results were disheartened that no effort appeared to be being made toward an FDA approval. Investigational use continued throughout most of the world, particularly in Australia and in England. Yugoslavia had produced a product (Lekopain) that was basically a chymopapain B and was widely used in the Eastern bloc countries and, to a lesser extent, in France and Italy with favorable results.

On October 15, 1975, Baxter-Travenol withdrew its new drug application for chymopapain from the FDA, effectively removing the drug from use in the United States *(15)*. Patients desiring chemonucleolysis with chymopapain were forced to seek treatment in Canada, where the drug was commercially available. In early 1977, a coalition of American physicians interested in making chymopapain available to patients was formed and chartered the Committee Advocating the Development and Use of Chymopapain to Eliminate Unnecessary Surgery (CADUCEUS). This group pursued legislative approaches to reactivate the withdrawn new drug application and even considered submitting its own application. For several years, the group worked diligently to gain national approval. However, in the late 1970s, other groups seeing little progress in the national trust began to explore state legislative approval to allow the production and use of chymopapain at the suggestions of CADUCEUS. Illinois, Indiana, and Texas all had legal vehicles to allow such interstate use, but of these states only Texas had the environment that would support growth of the raw materials. This was of critical importance, because according to FDA regulations all materials had to be available within the state and not cross-state boundaries. Subsequently, the State of Texas was granted approval for local manufacture of chymopapain preparation under the Food, Drug & Cosmetic Act. The product Chemolase produced in Texas was used from January 1980 until approval by the FDA of Chymodiactin® in 1982. Although the Texas group attempted to get FDA approval of Chemolase, it was apparent that only Chymodiactin would be approved. Without FDA approval for national distribution, the production of Chemolase was discontinued.

During the use of Chemolase *(16,17)*, orthopedic surgeons and neurosurgeons and 919 patients participated in an open-label uncontrolled clinical trial involving the use of chymopapain (Chemolase) in Texas from 1980 to 1982. Patients admitted to the study had persistent low-back pain or sciatica owing to protrusion, extrusion, or degeneration of the lumbar intervertebral disc that was not responsive to conservative management. Although the study was not specifically designated to assess safety and efficacy, it did allow retrospective analysis of these entities following intradiscal administration of chymopapain. Patients were considered candidates for the study if a myelogram or computed tomography scan suggested lumbar disc disease and specific clinical signs of lumbar disc disease were present. The dose of chymopapain most frequently used ranged from 3000 to 4000 U/disc. Responses to chemonucleolysis were assessed at 1, 3, or 6 mo after injection, depending on patient and physician adherence to the protocol. Patients' responses were assessed by point reduction systems that were deducted from an initial patient score of 10, based on the presence of various levels of discomfort or limitations of daily activities. Based on the point scores, patients' responses were categorized as poor, fair, good, or excellent. Fair, good, and excellent responses were considered treatment successes. Of the 919 patients who underwent chemonucleolysis with chemolase (chymopapain B), 408 were evaluated 1, 3, or 6 mo after injection by a physician. An independent biostatistician reviewed all of the data and performed the statistical analysis. Fifty-five percent of patients received injections in a single intervertebral disc, and the remainder in two to four discs. Success rates were 93% 1 mo after injection, 92% at 3 mo, and 93% at 6 mo. An unusual finding was observed when the effect of different variables on treatment efficacy was analyzed. Significantly lower response rates were found for Hispanics, blue-collar workers, and patients covered by workers' compensation insurance in the categories of race, occupation, and type of insurance coverage, respectively. In the other 511 patients, either the patient did not report for follow-up examinations or the follow-up evaluation was not recorded appropriately for evaluation of efficacy. For the 919 patients who received chymopapain by intradiscal injection, 70 adverse reactions were noted in 46 patients (5.0%). Erythema was the most common side effect, occurring in 1.8% of patients. The most serious reaction was anaphylaxis, which occurred in 1.1% of patients; however, based on the individual physician assessment, severe anaphylactic reactions were reported in only 0.54% of patients. All patients were managed medically without lasting effects. Giant urticaria, hypotension, and paraspinal muscle spasm occurred at similar frequency. Back pain was reported in only 0.4% of the treated patients. No deaths occurred. Although more sophisticated studies have since been done, the Texas study provides additional support for the safety and efficacy of chymopapain chemonucleolysis in the treatment of low-back pain and sciatica of discogenic origin that do not respond to more conservative management.

In 1979, Baxter-Travenol began a blinded study of chymopapain vs cysteine-edetate-iothalamate (CEI) or saline control, which allowed patients to have a laminectomy in the United States or go to Canada as a control. Patients during that period had a choice of having a laminectomy in the United States, going to Canada for chemonucleolysis, or going to Canada for chemonucleolysis if they had a placebo failure. It was apparent that significant difficulty was encountered in accumulating adequate numbers of trial participants. The results were finally published in 1998. One hundred seventy three participants at 25 locations reported 71% success with Discase compared with 45% with CEI *(13)*. More sophisticated studies were being done in Australia. Immunological, vascular, and neurological complications as well as discitis have all been discussed scientifically in detail, along with the risk of mortality *(18)*.

Was the fall from favor of chymopapain simply the result of adverse reports about complications, even though as reported in this chapter such reports were not well founded? If the answer to this question is "yes" it is a sad misconception on the part of the treating physicians as well as the patient population. Could it have been an administrative decision? We know that the FDA license to produce and sell Chymodiactin went from Smith to Baxter-Travenol and was separated off later into a company called Omnis. Boots Pharmaceutical acquired Omnis, thereby obtaining the license from Baxter-Travenol, and the next step in this procession was for Knoll Pharmaceuticals to purchase the license from Boots *(19)*. The license to manufacture and sell chymodiactin was subsequently sold to Abbott along with other pharmaceutical products. It was Abbott' decision, in about 1999, to discontinue the manufacture of Chymodiactin, thereby making it unavailable for use.

The official explanation for the discontinuation of the manufacture of Chymodiactin has yet to be obtained. However, the factors influencing the downfall can be summarized as follows:

- *Income*: Chemonucleolysis with chymopapain competed with discectomy, a surgical procedure that was the main source of income for many surgeons. This led, unfortunately, to biased and unfavorable comments being made by those with a vested interest in its demise.
- *Inappropriate patient selection*: It is apparent that chymopapain was being used to treat patients who were not good candidates for discectomy. To quote Ian Macnab (*personal communication, 1977*), a leading authority on the treatment of lumbar disc disease in the

1970s, "If a surgeon cannot get good results with chymopapain he should not be operating on the spine!"

- *Poor technique leading to complications*: In 1984, during the first few months following the release of Chymodiactin in the United States, approx 8000 orthopedic surgeons and neurosurgeons attended 1-d training courses. It is apparent that this alone was inadequate training for a percutaneous interventional technique that demanded precision for its safety and efficacy.
- *Fear of litigation*: This was generated to a large degree by the much-publicized complications that resulted in part from poor training in technique.
- *Competition from the introduction of the automated nucleotome*: This is a device that allowed removal of disc tissue; hence, the procedure achieved greater initial acceptance by surgeons.
- *Change in attitude to early rehabilitation following disc surgery*: The practice of early ambulation and early hospital discharge after disc surgery, first introduced in the early 1990s, reduced the advantage in cost-effectiveness of chemonucleolysis.
- *Use of targeted epidural steroids*: Posterior epidural steroids were of lesser therapeutic value in the treatment of lumbar disc prolapse and did not greatly compete with chemonucleolysis. The increased success of foraminal epidural steroids *(20)*, whereby the solution was delivered to the affected root canal with image intensifier guidance, greatly lessened the number of patients being considered for chemonucleolysis.

In all probability these factors combined to reduce dramatically the use of Chymodiactin to the point where the manufacturer made a commercial decision to remove the product from the market.

Dr. Lyman Smith addressed most of the questions and doubts regarding the use, safety, and efficacy in the following three personal communications:

In April 1987, a report on chemonucleolysis was aired on the ABC program *20/20*. Timothy Johnson, MD, ABC News medical editor, conducted this report, and the following is quoted from a letter written to Dr. Johnson by Lyman Smith, MD, dated August 27, 1990, in response to his report.

> Chemonucleolysis is widely used in Europe. The explanation for this is that surgeons in Europe are commonly on salaries and contingency fees for plaintiff lawyers are illegal. Clearly, the health care crisis in this country today has reached extraordinary proportions. We cannot afford to overlook effective alternatives to dangerous and costly invasive surgery.
>
> Your report on Chemonucleolysis, which aired on the "20/20" program, in April 1987, condemned thousands of individuals suffering from disc disease in the United States to unnecessary major surgery. Due to your blasted and inaccurate report, very little of which was substantiated by facts, use of Chymopapain fell precipitously (40% in the two months following the program!).
>
> The result was that either more invasive laminectomy or the percutaneous automated discectomy procedure, touted on the program (and since proven a therapeutic failure), were utilized far more often than the less dangerous and less costly Chemonucleolysis.
>
> Further, your reference to Chemonucleolysis causing acute transverse myelitis (ATM) has been proven to be unfounded. The appearance of these reported six cases of alleged acute transverse myelitis was devastating. As with other severe conditions following any procedure in the United States, the patient records were sealed and access to them denied. Rumors were the natural consequences. Symptoms in all but one of the cases appeared two to three weeks after apparently successful treatments with Chymopapain. In that one case, symptoms appeared shortly after treatment and got worse as time went on. All had flaccid paralysis and none developed signs of spastic paralysis, a characteristic of transverse myelitis. At the time

of diagnosis, one patient had a suggestive history of multiple sclerosis and another later developed clear evidence of this disease. One had a history of viral infection before treatment and another was diabetic. The other, Mr. Devletsah, who appeared on "20/20", only developed paralysis after laminectomy following Chemonucleolysis. This, the causes of paralysis in these six patients are far from certain. Some could have been due to inept injections and others to causes other than the enzyme or the procedure. Finally, it may interest you to know the ATM has been reported in Australia after intradiscal injection of saline and another, in this country, following removal of an intramedullary nail. Other causative agents were sought in these and other comparable cases. Why should this not have been done in the case of a useful and effective therapeutic agent such as Chymopapain?

Statistics show that Chemonucleolysis is a valid and effective alternative to surgery. I would be delighted to review these data with you. These findings are certainly newsworthy and something your audience will be interested in."

On August 27, 1990, a telephone conversation was held between Dr. Lyman Smith and Dr. Helene M. Cole, senior editor of *JAMA*. After their conversation, Dr. Smith sent Dr. Cole his rebuttal to the Diagnostic and Therapeutic Technology Assessment (D.A.T.T.A.) *(21)* on chemonucleolysis, published in *Clinical Orthopaedics and Related Research.*

D.A.T.T.A. Statement #3: "Even small intrathecal leaks of Chymopapain have a potential for damage to the central nervous system."

REBUTTAL: Chymopapain will cause bleeding from the capillaries of the pia arachnoid, which are not protected by collagen, as are larger blood vessels. Large doses will cause enough bleeding to raise C.S.F. pressure to unacceptable levels and the animal will die. The toxic effect is purely a pressure phenomenon. If a spinal tap is done early to relieve the pressure, the animal will survive without a following neurological deficit. Small amounts do not damage the central nervous system. The L.D. 50 in Rhesus monkeys, for example, is 1000 units per kilogram. Fifty units are therapeutic. *(22)*

The following is a quote from a letter dated September 4, 1990, to Prof. Alf Nachemson, Department of Orthopaedics, Gothenburg University, Sweden, from Dr. Lyman Smith, in response to statements made by Prof. Nachemson during a symposium published in *Contemporary Orthopaedics (23).*

I have just been saddled with a sever diagnosis leaving a poor prognosis; so I wish to clear the air with you. You are basically a great scientist, however, some of your biased statements on Chemonucleolysis throughout the years have bordered on the ridiculous.

In 1961, I began work with Baxter Laboratories on the ceramics and after awhile, I told the Director of Research about the rabbits. He was interested and we formed a research team—the million-dollar question to be pursued: "Was papain the best enzyme and was it safe?" You know the rest of the story!

In the British Journal of Bone and Joint Surgery, February 1959, Carl Hirsch theorized as follows: "Sooner or later a substance may be found by which a degenerated disc could be transformed. It might be possible to create a chemolytic enzyme that, injected into a disc, would cause a connective tissue reaction." As you know, Chymopapain does not act in that sclerosing fashion. Carl came to my hospital in Elgin on November 6, 1968, with Jorge Galante and we examined some patients and viewed the x-rays of the first 80 patients I had injected. The only other investigators at the time were Lee Ford and Leon Wiltse. Carl seemed favourably impressed; it's a shame that impression did not wash off upon you!

You continue to quote your poor results with Chymopapain obtained with partially inactivated DISCASE, "Surgery versus Chemonucleolysis for Herniated Lumbar Discs," Clinical Orthopaedics, No. 174, April 1983. I pointed out to you then that the Chymopapain had been shipped to you from the United States without being refrigerated. DISCASE, unlike the present version, CHYMODIACTIN, was sensitive to heat. Mulholland

> of Nottingham received the same shipment and complained that laminectomies on the failed patients showed little or no action of the enzyme. Active enzyme would have led to an accurate study!
>
> Chemonucleolysis is neater, quicker, safer, cheaper, and if performed on an ideal patient, as effective as any invasive mechanical procedure. Prove me wrong!"

A citizens' petition was made to the FDA February 8, 2002, to determine whether the drug was withdrawn from sale for reasons of safety and effectiveness. A response to the citizens' petition was received January 27, 2003, stating that

> the FDA has reviewed its records and has determined that Chymopapain 10,000 units/vial injections (Chymodiactin), NDA 18-663, was not withdrawn from sale for reasons of safety or effectiveness. FDA will maintain Chymopapain 10,000 units/vial injections in the "discontinued drug product list" of approved drug products with therapeutic equivalence evaluations (the orange book). *(24)*

Whatever the reasons for discontinuation of the manufacture of Chymodiactin, it was not for safety and effectiveness. "The results of Chemonucleolysis depend not only on the enzyme, but more importantly on the diagnostic acumen of clinician. If you can't get a good result from Chemonucleolysis you shouldn't really be allowed to operate on backs." Chymopapain continues to be unavailable for use in the United States *(25)*.

REFERENCES

1. Fraser RD. Chymopapain for the treatment of intervertebral disc herniation: a preliminary report of a double-blind study. Spine 1982;7:608–612.
2. Javid MD, Norby EJ, Ford LT, et al. Safety and efficacy of chymopapain (Chymodiactin®) in herniated nucleus pulposus with sciatica: results of a randomized, double-blind study. JAMA 1983;249:2489–2494.
3. Nordby EJ, Wright PH, Schofield SR. Safety of chemonucleolysis: adverse effects reported in the USA 1982 to 1989. Clin Orthop 1993;(293):122–134.
4. Bradford DS, Oegema TR Jr, Cooper M, et al. Chymopapain, chemonucleolysis and nucleus pulposus regeneration: biological and biochemical study. Spine 1984;9:135–147.
5. Brown M, Daroff RB. The double-blind study comparing disease to placebo: an editorial comment Spine 1977;2:33.
6. Darakjian HE, Wiltse LL. Low-dose chymopapain as a safe alternative to laminectomy, paper presented at the 3rd annual meeting of the International Intradiscal Therapy Society (IITS), Marbella, Spain. March 1990;7–11.
7. Garvin PG, Jennings RB, Smith L, Gesler RM. Chymopapain: a pharmacologic and toxicologic evaluation in experimental animals. Clin Orthop 1965;41:204–223.
8. Jansen EF, Balls AK. Chymopapain: a new crystalline proteinase from papaya latex. J Biol Chem 1941;137:459–460.
9. Thomas LB. Reversible collapse of rabbit ears after intravenous papain, and prevention of recovery by cortisone. J Exp Med 1956;104:245–251.
10. Smith L, Garvin PJ, Jennings RB, Gesler RM. Enzyme dissolution of the nucleus pulposus. Nature 1963;198:1311–1312.
11. Hirsch C. Studies on the pathology of low back pain. J Bone Joint Surg 1959;41B:237–243.
12. Brown M. Intradiscal Therapy: Chymopapain or Collagenase. Year Book Medical, Chicago, 1983, pp. 120–127.
13. Schwetschenau PR, Ramirez A, Johnston J, Wiggs C, Martins AN. Double-blind evaluation of intradiscal chymopapain for herniated lumbar discs. J Neurosurg 1976;45:622–627.

14. Brown MD, Daroff RB. The double blind study comparing discase to placebo: an editorial comment. Spine 1977;2:233–236.
15. FDA Drug Bull 1984;14(2).
16. Simmons JW, Stavinoha WB, Knodel LC. Update and review of chemonucleolysis. Clin Orthop 1964;183:51–60.
17. Simmons JW, Upman PJ, Stavinoha WB. Pharmacologic and toxicologic profile of chymopapain B (chemolase). Drug Chem Toxicol 1984;7:299–314.
18. Nordby EJ, Fraser RD. Chemonucleolysis, in The Adult Spine, Principals and Practices, 2nd ed, 1997.
19. Data on file, Boots Pharmaceuticals, Lincolnshire, IL.
20. Weiner B, Fraser RD. Foraminal injection for lateral lumbar disc herniation. J Bone Joint Surg (Br) 1997;79-B:804–807.
21. Cole HM. A Diagnostic and Therapeutic Technology Assessment (D.A.T.T.A). JAMA 1989;262(7).
22. Gesler RM. Pharmacologic properties of chymopapain. CORR 1969;67:47–51.
23. Mooney V, Brown A, Nachemson JA, McCulloch, Schroeder FW, Simmons JW. Symposium: chemonucleolysis in the management of herniated lumbar disc. Contemp Orthop. 1984;9(5):97–124.
24. Simmons JW Jr. Citizen petition (docket no. 02P-0068/CP1). Federal Register Vol. 68, No. 17, Monday, January 27, 2003, Notices.
25. Macnab I. Chemonucleolysis Seminar, Montreal, Quebec, November 1977.

19
Lumbar Microendoscopic Discectomy

Trent L. Tredway, MD and Richard G. Fessler, MD, PhD

INTRODUCTION

Low-back pain is one of the most common complaints that lead patients to seek medical attention. It is estimated that there are nearly 15 million physician office visits each year for low-back pain *(1)*. Additionally, back pain causes nearly 80% of workers to miss at least 8 wk of work following a back injury *(2)*. Estimates of lifetime prevalence and annual incidence has been reported to be 60–90 and 5%, respectively *(3)*. With this prevalence, it has been estimated that the total health care expenditures incurred by individuals with back pain in the United States reached $90.7 billion. The total incremental expenditures attributable to back pain among these individuals are estimated to be approx $23.6 billion. On average, individuals with back pain encumbered health care expenditures about 60% higher than individuals without back pain *(4)*.

Although many individuals present with the common complaint of low-back pain, the etiology is often multifactorial. One cause of back pain is related to soft-tissue injury secondary to back strain. This type of injury involves musculoskeletal and ligamentous injury, is usually self-limiting, and resolves with nonoperative management. Other causes of back pain may include varying degrees of arthritic changes of the lumbosacral spine; compression fractures secondary to trauma or osteoporosis; and, less commonly, metastases. However, one of the more common causes of back pain is related to the changes that occur within the intervertebral disc. Herniated discs, bulging discs, ruptured discs, and radial tears in the annulus have all been used to describe the pathological alterations of the intervertebral disc.

Vesalius *(5)* first described anatomically the intervertebral disc in 1555. Since then, the intervertebral disc has been eloquently studied and determined to be composed of an outer annulus consisting of dense connective tissue and an inner nucleus pulposus (NP) that is largely composed of collagen and glycosaminoglycans *(6–8)*. This functional design contributes to the dynamic properties of the disc that permit flexion, extension, lateral bending, and rotation to occur along the spinal axis. However, as a patient ages, the NP, a remnant of the notochord, gradually loses its water content as well as its elastic properties, leading to degeneration of the functional disc unit. These changes may best be exemplified on magnetic resonance imaging (MRI), with the degenerative disc appearing dark compared with nondegenerative discs (Fig. 1).

From: *Arthroscopic and Endoscopic Spinal Surgery: Text and Atlas: Second Edition*
Edited by: P. Kambin © Humana Press Inc., Totowa, NJ

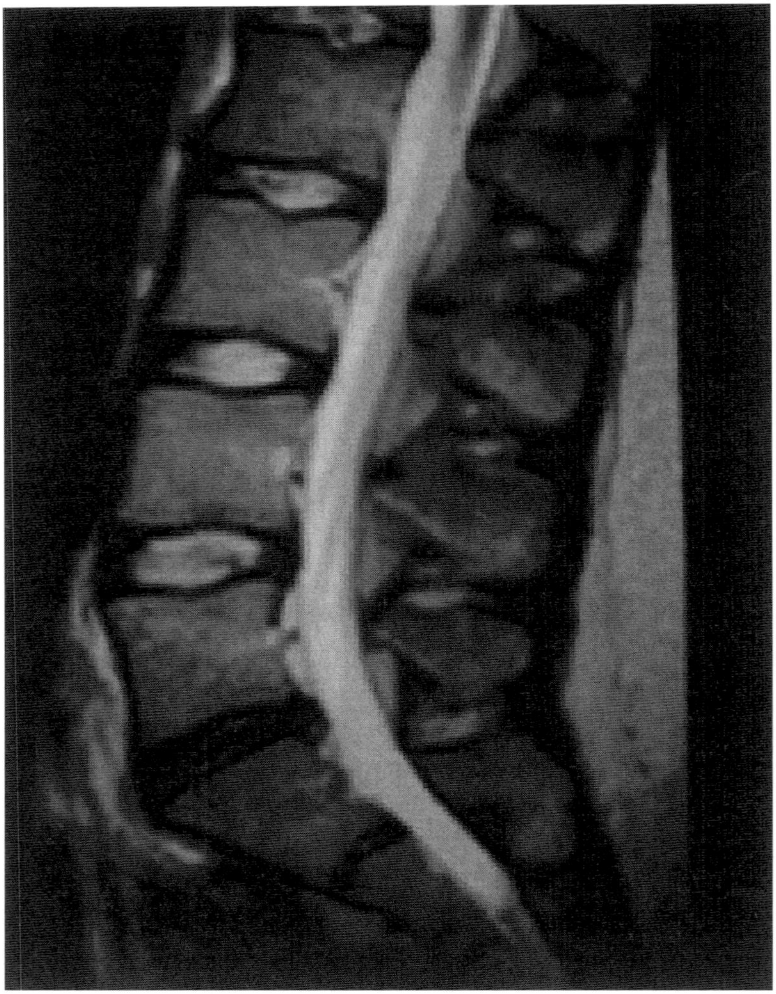

Fig. 1. Sagittal T2WI MRI of patient with degenerative disc disease at L5/S1 level. The signal intensity is decreased compared with the normal levels.

CLINICAL PRESENTATION

Patients with herniated disc fragments often present with radicular pain, back pain, or both (Fig. 2). The exact nature of the pain associated with a lumbar herniated disc is controversial. It is thought that direct compression of the neural elements at or near the level of the foramen contributes to the radicular pattern of pain often experienced. Therefore, removal of the offending fragment and inspection of the neural foramen to ensure decompression may alleviate the radicular pain. However, patients may present with tremendous radicular pain and radiological imaging that does not substantiate a compressive syndrome. It has been surmised that the composition of the disc itself may induce an inflammatory response after herniation. The release of local substances derived from the inflammatory response may be perceived as a painful stimulus. For example, increased levels of glutamate are purported to be involved in the perception of pain secondary to intervertebral disc herniation *(9)*.

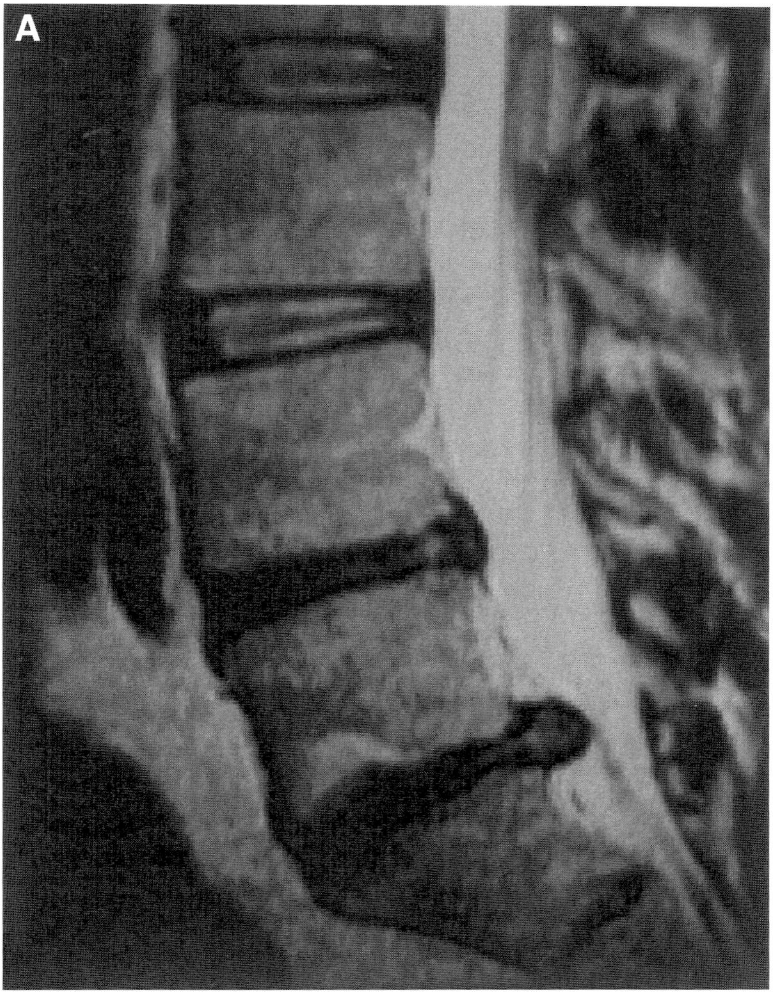

Fig. 2. **(A)** Sagittal T2WI MRI of patient with herniated NP at L4/L5 disc level; **(B)** axial T2WI MRI of same patient with herniated fragment located to right of midline and causing compression of right exiting nerve root.

Compressive syndromes secondary to disc herniation without associated pain may occur. Rarely, a patient may present with an acute neurological deficit that is attributable to neural compression secondary to disc herniation. This may best be exemplified in patients with L4 or L5 nerve root involvement that notice weakness in dorsiflexion (tibialis anterior) and extension of the great toe (extensor hallicus longus), respectively. The neurological deficit may be so pronounced on presentation that the patient may demonstrate a "foot drop" on examination. By contrast, some patients may present only with sensory loss along a dermatomal pattern. Finally, patients with large, centrally located lumbar disc herniations may present with cauda equina syndrome. In this syndrome, bowel, bladder, and even sexual dysfunction can occur and should be considered a neurosurgical urgency. In review of patients presenting with a cauda equina syndrome secondary to a herniated disc, patients undergoing decompression early in the time course (less than 24 h after onset of bladder paralysis) have an excellent

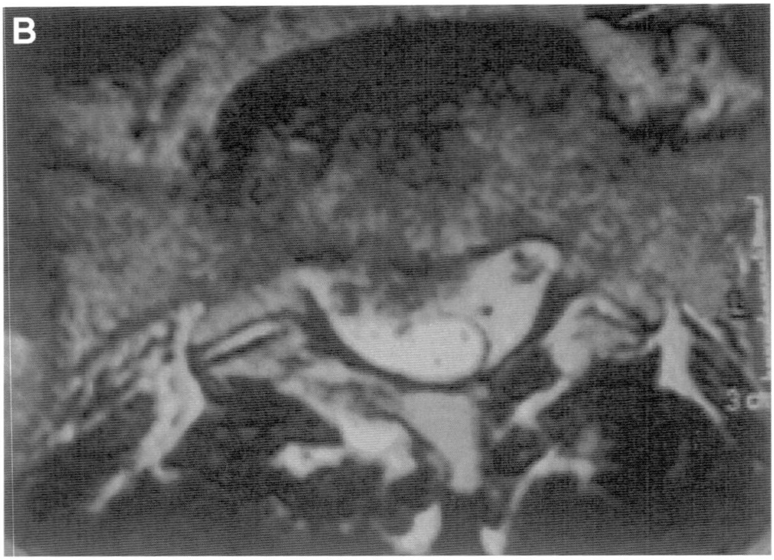

Fig. 2. *(Continued)*

chance of recovery compared with patients undergoing surgery after 24 h of symptoms *(10)*. Therefore, a careful history and physical examination should always be performed at the earliest possible time in order to improve functional outcome.

PATIENT EVALUATION

Examination of a patient presenting with symptoms relating to a herniated lumbar disc should include a complete history focusing on the exact location and pattern of the pain; onset and duration of the complaint, factors that aggravate or relieve the symptoms; and, of course, any changes in bowel, bladder, or sexual function. Many of these individuals will report coinciding activities including lifting, straining, twisting, or bending at the time of the acute onset. Other risk factors for disc herniation include smoking; having a sedentary occupation; driving a motor vehicle for prolonged periods; and operating heavy, vibrating machinery *(11–14)*.

After a history of the symptoms is elicited, a complete physical examination is performed focusing on the area involved. A thorough neurological examination includes testing the strength and tone of isolated muscle groups. The affected side is compared with the contralateral muscle groups and any existing discrepancies are carefully documented. A thorough sensory examination including testing all modalities including light touch, two-point discrimination, pinprick, and vibratory sensation is also performed. With this organized approach to sensory evaluation, differences in a dermatomal pattern may be observed. In addition, deep tendon reflex testing may also provide the physician with information concerning which nerve root or roots are involved. Furthermore, the straight leg raise test (also known as Lasègue's sign) should always be performed in patients suspected of having a radiculopathy secondary to an intervertebral disc herniation. This maneuver, which comprises raising the supine patient's straightened leg with pain elicited at <60°, is present in approx 83% of patients with nerve root compression secondary to disc herniation *(15)*. Finally, a thorough neurological examination is not complete unless evaluation of the perineal region is conducted. Sensory examination of the sacral and genital regions may demonstrate a cauda equina syndrome. If any neurological deficit exists, correlation with radiographic imaging is recommended.

In general, radiographs of the lumbar spine are obtained and the osseous anatomy is evaluated. Fractures, scoliotic changes, congenital abnormalities, degenerative changes, as well as pathological processes may be revealed with careful review of the images. The etiology of the complaint may be evident on these routine radiographs. If there is no evidence of pathology on the radiographs of the lumbar spine, further evaluation may be necessary. An MRI of the lumbar spine, if possible, is the imaging modality of choice. This will enable the physician to evaluate the intervertebral discs as well as demonstrate other pathological features of the spine. The only limitation to MRI is that it will not clearly demonstrate osseous pathology. If significant osseous pathology is suspected, a computed tomography (CT) examination of the lumbar spine may prove more diagnostic. However, the findings on imaging should be cautiously interpreted because many asymptomatic individuals will have an abnormality on routine MRI *(16)*. For this reason, the results of the MRI should be correlated with a thorough history and physical examination. If the symptoms and radiographic results are congruent, then treatment outcome results are improved *(17)*.

TREATMENT OPTIONS

We routinely recommend conservative, nonoperative treatment for at least 6–8 wk after initial onset of symptoms secondary to an intervertebral disc herniation. Therapy generally consists of the use of nonsteroidal anti-inflammatory drugs, muscle relaxants, physical therapy, and occasionally epidural steroid injections for acute exacerbations. It has been reported that approx 85% of patients with acute disc herniation will improve without surgical intervention in an average of 6 wk *(18)*. Therefore, only patients that do not respond to a trial of nonoperative therapy are considered for surgical intervention. However, if a neurological deficit is present, as may be observed in a patient with a foot drop, early intervention may be entertained. Once again, if a cauda equina syndrome exists, urgent surgical intervention is recommended.

Virchow noted pathological changes related to the intervertebral disc when he described traumatic disc disease in 1857; however, surgical intervention for treatment of degenerative disc disease did not occur until the early twentieth century. Oppenheim *(19)* first described a posterior lumbar surgical approach for removal of an "enchondroma" in 1909, and 4 yr later, Elsberg *(20)* described a laminectomy for removal of a "chondroma." Dandy *(21)* also described removal of a "disc," which he described as mimicking a tumor. However, it was not until 1934, when Mixter and Barr *(22)* compiled numerous case reports from the literature, that a relationship between disc herniation and sciatica was finally established. Since then, the surgical treatment of degenerative disc disease has been well established as well as controversial.

Traditional discectomies involved performing a laminectomy and removal of the offending disc fragment through an intradural approach. Later, through improvements in surgical technique, the discectomy procedure evolved into a hemilaminotomy and microdiscectomy after Caspar *(23)* and Yasargil *(24)* introduced the operating microscope into the spine surgeon's armamentarium. This technological advancement allowed surgeons to perform arguably a more complete discectomy with better visualization and set the "gold standard" for clinical outcomes in which other surgical interventions for disc disease are compared.

Although lumbar microdiscectomy is the most common surgical intervention for the treatment of lumbar herniated discs, a variety of treatment options have been performed as an alternative. One alternative treatment for herniated lumbar discs is chemonucleolysis. This procedure, first performed by Chicago orthopedic surgeon Lyman Smith, consists of percutaneously injecting chymopapain into the symptomatic intervertebral disc. The enzymatic activity of the chymopapain hydrolyzes the mucoprotein of the NP *(25)*. More than 75,000 patients underwent chemonucleolysis treatment in a 12-mo period after Chymodiactin® (Boots Pharmaceuticals, Nottingham, UK), a new formulation of chymopapain, was introduced in 1983 *(26)*. Despite its safety performance in clinical trials, complications occurred, including fatal anaphylactic reactions, cauda equina syndromes, and acute transverse myelitis, from inadvertent intradural injections *(27,28)*. With these reports, the use of Chymodiactin decreased and is no longer manufactured or distributed in the United States.

Another alternative to surgical intervention for disc disease is intradiscal electrothermal coagulation (IDET). This therapeutic option is designed to treat internal disc disruption in which the disc is painful secondary to the development of radial fissures extending into the outer region of the annulus fibrosus. IDET consists of introducing a heating electrode into the NP percutaneously. A recent study has demonstrated that IDET may provide relief in a small subset of patients with intractable back pain; however, the results cannot be generalized to patients who did not fit the strict inclusion criteria for the study *(29)*. Furthermore, IDET is not recommended for large, free-fragment disc herniations observed on radiographic imaging.

Despite the popularity, low morbidity, and clinical outcomes of microsurgical discectomy, many surgeons continued to develop innovative ways to treat lumbar herniated discs. In 1975, Hijikata et al. *(30)* introduced the "percutaneous nucleotomy," which was performed through a cannula placed percutaneously using fluoroscopic guidance. Similarly, Kambin and Gellman *(31)* reported their technique of percutaneous posterolateral discectomy via a 6.4-mm–outer diameter cannula. Kambin advocated intraoperative visualization and introduced the concept of arthroscopic microdiscectomy. Furthermore, he outlined the advantages of posterolateral access *(32)* (*see* Chapters 1 and 4).

Smith and Foley were instrumental in the development of the microendoscopic discectomy (MED) procedure, in which specially designed microendoscopic instruments are used through a working channel with a 30° endoscope attached to a MetRx™ tubular retractor system (Medtronics, Memphis, TN). The purported advantages of this technique include less iatrogenic soft-tissue injury, improved visualization, less blood loss, less postoperative pain, and earlier hospital discharge *(33,34)*. This surgical procedure is technically challenging at first, with a steep learning curve. However, after experience and mastery, this technique is an extremely attractive alternative to traditional lumbar microdiscectomy.

THE MED PROCEDURE

Anesthesia

General endotracheal intubation with adequate intravenous access is obtained prior to positioning for an MED procedure. An induction dose of Anectine® (succinylcholine

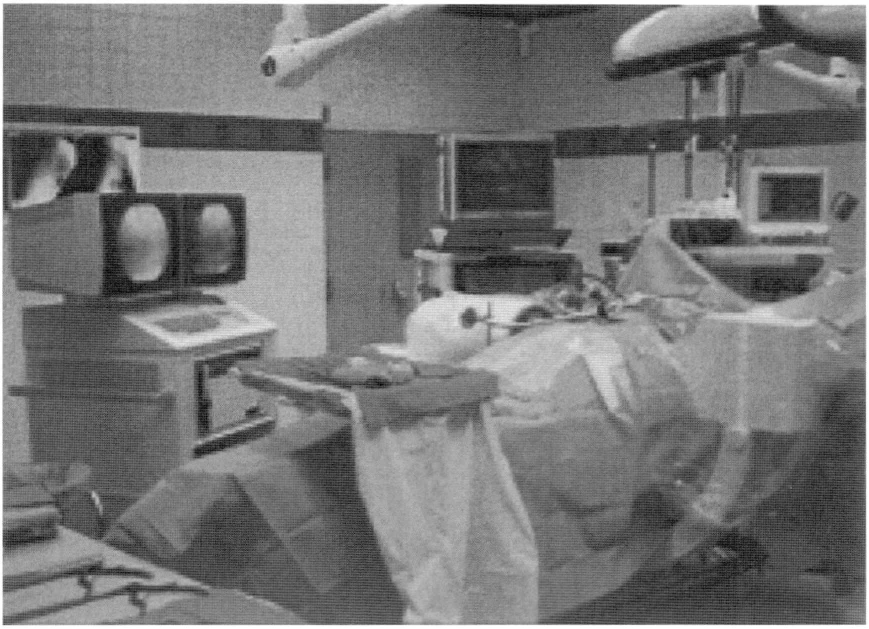

Fig. 3. Operative room setup for MED procedure. The patient is prone on a Wilson frame and Jackson table. The video tower and fluoroscopic unit is placed on the opposite side of the surgical approach and surgeon.

chloride; GlaxoSmithKline, Research Triangle Park, NC) is used for intubation purposes; however, no other paralytic agent, muscle relaxant, or nitrous oxide is administered throughout the rest of the procedure. This enables the surgeon to have direct feedback if the nerve root is irritated during the procedure. We do not routinely employ the use of intraoperative somatosensory evoked potentials and electromyography during MED because visualization of the neural elements with the 30° endoscope is excellent. Finally, because a routine MED procedure lasts approx 45–90 min, we do not place a Foley catheter.

Positioning

The MED procedure is performed with the patient in the prone position and utilizes a Wilson frame (O.S.I., Union City, CA) on a Jackson table (O.S.I.). This setup will allow a fluoroscopic unit (C-arm) to be draped into the field and is less cumbersome during the surgery (Fig. 3). The arms are positioned with the elbows at right angles to lessen traction on the brachial plexus. Care is taken to ensure that all osseous prominences are well padded, especially with respect to the ulnar and peroneal nerves. Accordingly, pillows are placed under the lower extremities to reduce traction on the sciatic nerves. Sequential compression devices are also placed on the lower extremities to reduce the incidence of deep venous thromboses. Finally, the endotracheal tube is checked after positioning to ensure that there is no compression or obstruction.

Surgical Approach

The use of fluoroscopic guidance is pertinent in the preoperative setup. An indelible marker is used to mark the skin after a lateral radiograph has identified the correct sur-

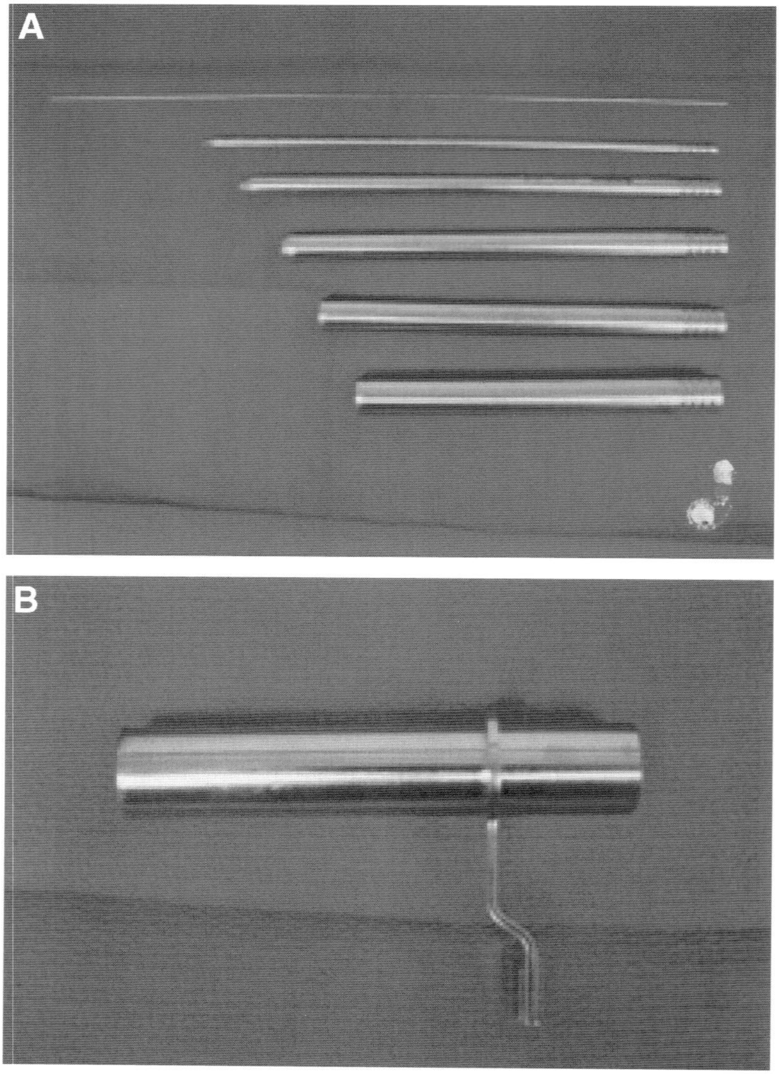

Fig. 4. **(A)** $MetR_x$ dilators for access to surgical site; **(B)** $MetR_x$ 18-mm tubular retractor working channel; **(C)** $MetR_x$ table clamp and flexible arm; **(D)** 30° endoscope utilized for MED procedure.

gical level. The incision is approx 1.5 cm paramedian to the symptomatic side. This distance will enable access to the intervertebral disc space and nerve root.

The skin is cleansed with a three-step technique. We routinely employ a povidine/iodine scrub, a 70% isopropyl alcohol wash, and a final Duraprep™ (3M, St. Paul, MN) paint. The skin and subcutaneous tissue is infiltrated with 10 cc of Marcaine® (0.5% bupivacaine and 1:200,000 epinephrine solution; Sanofi Winthrop, New York, NY). An approx 2-cm incision is then carried down through the skin and soft tissue. A stab incision is made in the lumbosacral fascia, and attention is then turned toward the placement of the $MetR_x$™ dilator and tubular retractor system (Medtronics) (Fig. 4). With fluoro-

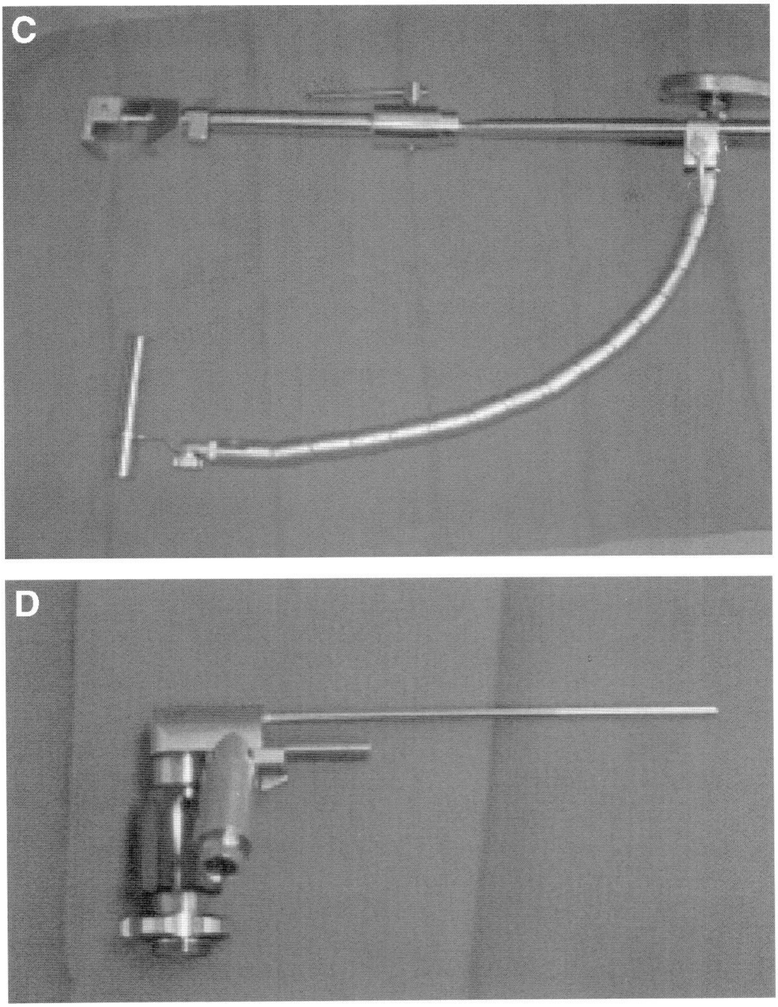

Fig. 4. *(Continued)*

scopic guidance, a Steinman pin is docked on the ipsilateral laminofacet junction. Serial fluoroscopic images are obtained while the dilators are used to spread the muscle fibers apart and advance the dilators to rest on the laminofacet junction. Once the largest dilator is placed, the 18-mm working channel is placed over the dilator. The working channel should be docked on the laminofacet region overlying the surgical disc space. After correct positioning is obtained, the working channel is locked into place using the flexible arm attached firmly to the table clamp (Fig. 5).

Removal of Soft Tissue

The soft tissue overlying the facet and lamina is removed with the use of Bovie electrocauterization (Fig. 6A). After identification of the facet and lamina, a straight or angled curette is used to define the sublaminar space from the ligamentum flavum (Fig. 6B). Next, a 45° angled Kerrison rongeur facilitates removal of the laminofacet junc-

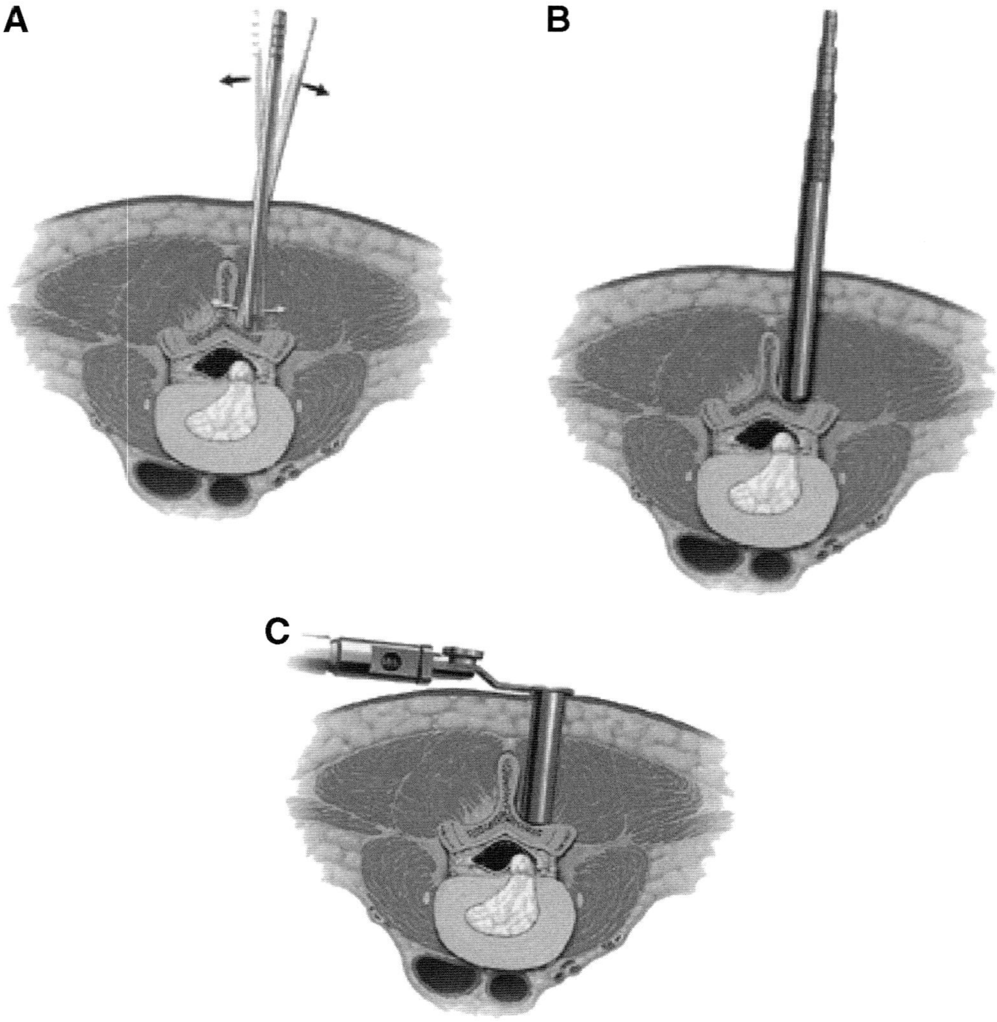

Fig. 5. **(A)** After placement of the first dilator, a gentle sweeping motion over the lamina will clear soft tissue and allow for easier docking of the subsequent dilators. This maneuver should be performed carefully because the dilator can inadvertently traverse the interlaminar space (image courtesy of Medtronics). **(B)** Image depicting $MetR_x$ dilators docked on laminofacet junction (image courtesy of Medtronics); **(C)** image depicting 18-mm working channel attached to flexible arm (image courtesy of Medtronics); **(D)** intraoperative image of MED setup showing 30° endoscope attached to working channel.

tion (Fig. 6C). The laminotomy is continued cephalad to the point of attachment of the ligamentum flavum. With this degree of osseous removal, an angled curette can easily be placed in the subligamentous/epidural space. Using a gentle sweeping motion with the angled curette, the ligamentum flavum can be removed safely with a Kerrison rongeur (Fig. 6D). The ligamentum flavum is removed to identify adequately the lateral edge of the thecal sac as well as the nerve root (Fig. 6E). Often, a partial medial facetectomy is performed to enable access to the disc space and prevent significant

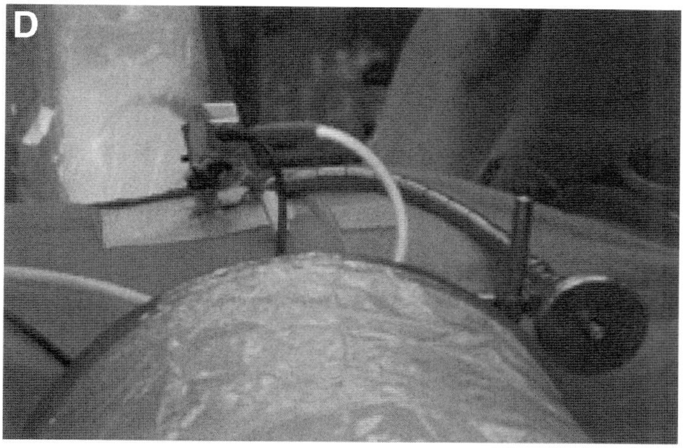

Fig. 5. *(Continued)*

retraction of the nerve root. Care must be taken to avoid removal of more than half of the facet because this could lead to iatrogenic destabilization of the spine at the surgical level. The complication of an overaggressive facetectomy could inevitably require a fusion procedure for stabilization.

Discectomy

Once the lateral edge of the dura and nerve root has been identified, a Love nerve root retractor is placed into the working channel, and the nerve root and thecal sac are gently retracted. Often, the epidural venous plexus will need to be coagulated with a bipolar electrocautery in order to decrease blood loss and improve visualization while performing the discectomy (Fig. 7A). The disc space is identified and an angled dissector is employed to separate the anterior aspect of the thecal sac from the posterior annulus of the disc. Once free, the retractor can be placed in a secure position enabling access to the herniated disc fragment. An annulotomy is performed with a retractable scalpel (Fig. 7B). A straight curette is placed within the disc space and the fragment is loosened (Fig. 7C). A down-angled curette may also be helpful in dislodging the herniated fragment. A pituitary rongeur facilitates removal of the offending disc fragment (Fig. 7D). This technique is repeated until the fragment is removed and the nerve root appears to be decompressed (Fig. 7E). It is imperative to review the MRI or CT scan prior to closure because oftentimes the radiological imaging will demonstrate the exact location of the herniated fragment. It is also critical to explore the disc space laterally because the disc may be sequestered within the foramen. Once hemostasis is achieved with a combination of bipolar electrocautery and thrombin-soaked Gelfoam® (Pharmacia, Kalamazoo, MI), the wound is irrigated with an antibiotic-containing irrigation solution.

Wound Closure

The working channel is removed under endoscopic visualization, and the wound is irrigated again with an antibiotic-containing irrigation solution. Attention is then turned toward closure of the incision. A 2-0 absorbable suture is used to reapproximate the lumbosacral fascia if possible. The subcutaneous and dermal layers are closed with a 3-0 absorbable

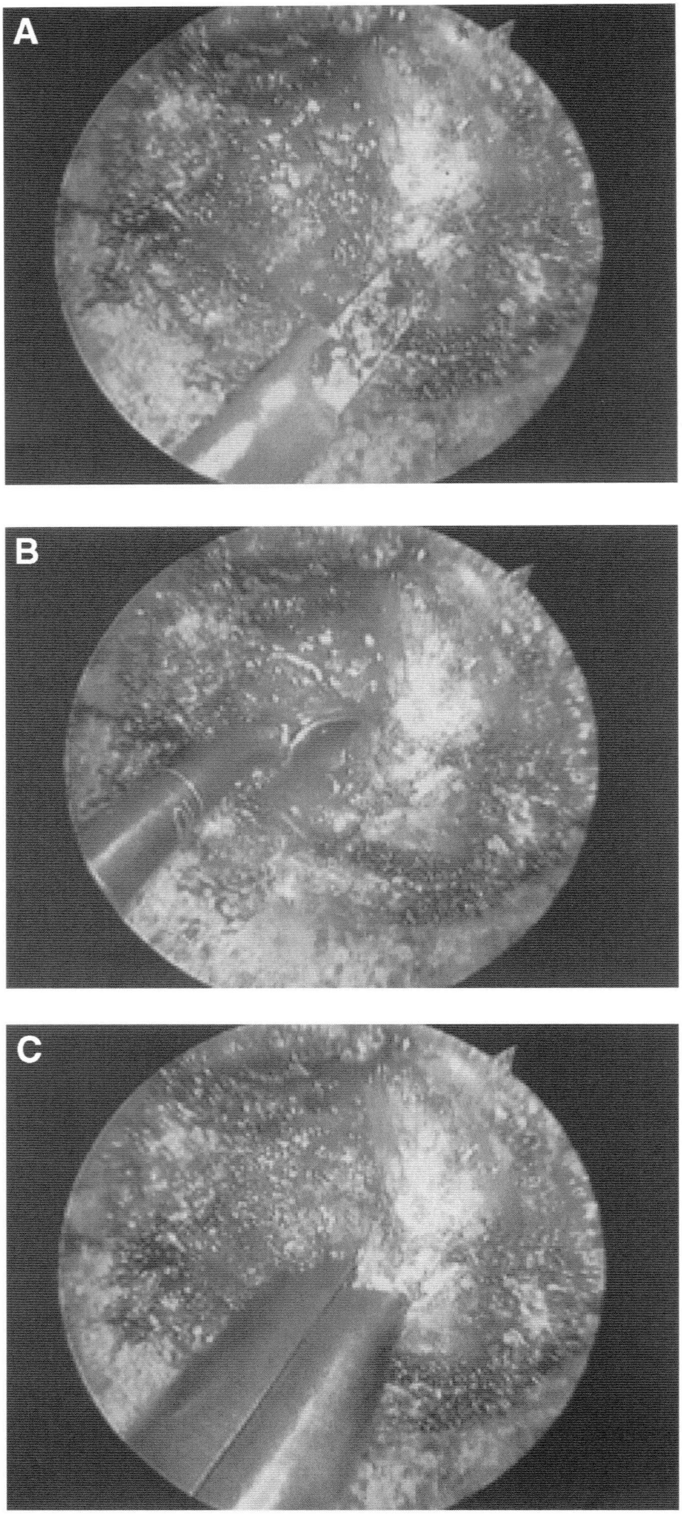
A
B
C

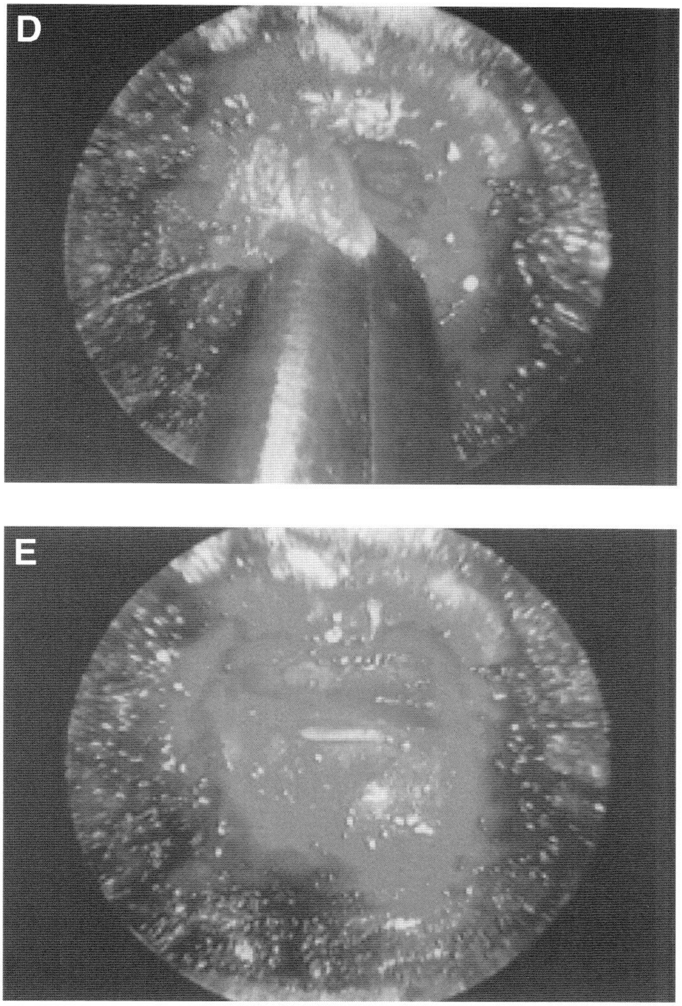

Fig. 6. Intraopertive endoscopic image demonstrating **(A)** removal of soft tissue overlying lamina with Bovie electrocauteriztion, **(B)** angle curette defining sublaminar space, **(C)** removal of lamina with a Kerrison punch, **(D)** removal of ligamentum flavum with a Kerrison punch, and **(E)** lateral edge of dural and nerve root after removal of ligament.

suture. The skin is closed with a 4-0 absorbable suture in a subcuticular fashion and then covered with Dermabond® (2-octyl cyanoacrylate; Ethicon, Somerville, NJ) (Fig. 8).

Avoidance of Complications

The complications of MED are similar to those observed in lumbar microdiscectomy. The overall mortality in lumbar microdiscectomy has been reported to be 0.06% and is usually owing to septicemia, myocardial infarction, or pulmonary embolus.(35,36). To our knowledge, no deaths have been reported utilizing the MED technique, but other risks include infection, unintended durotomy with leakage of cerebrospinal fluid (CSF), injury to the nerve root, and recurrent disc herniation. Superficial wound infections have been

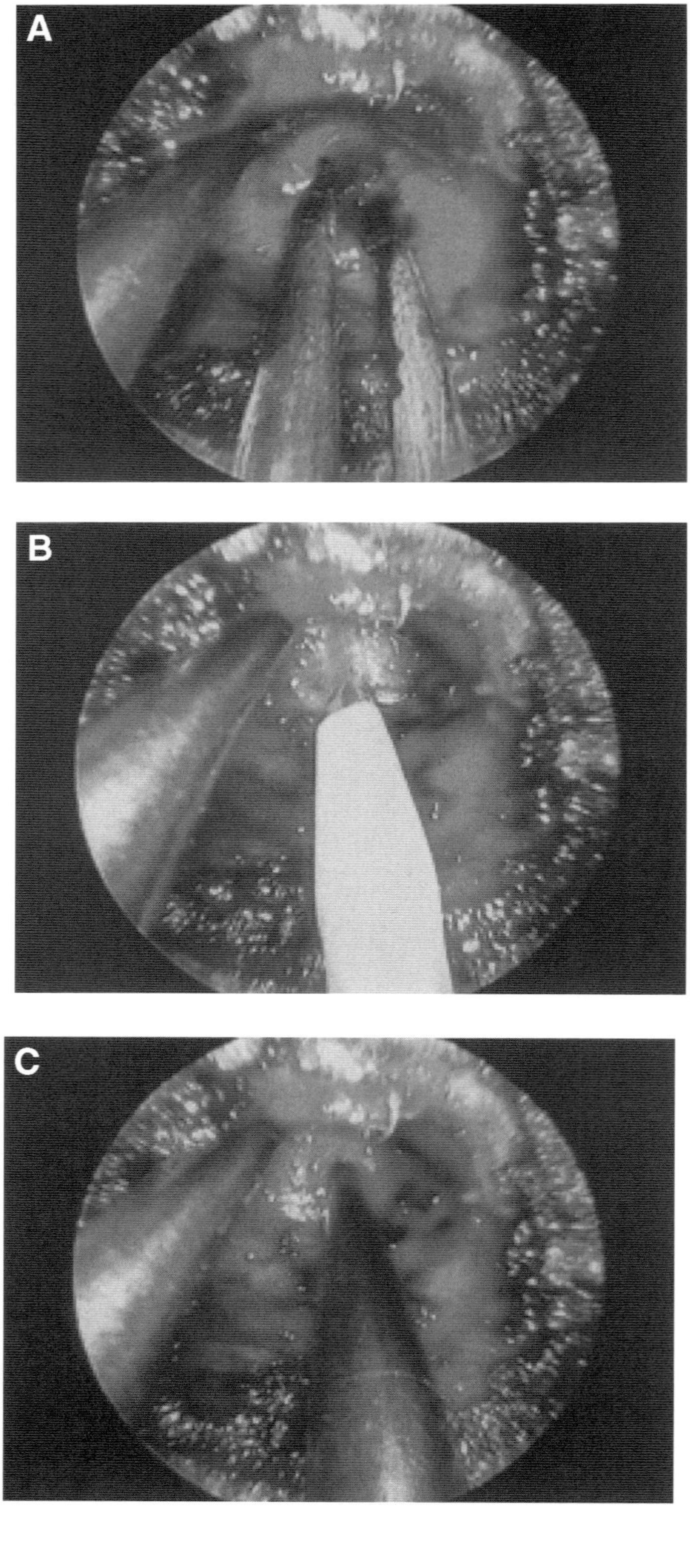
A
B
C

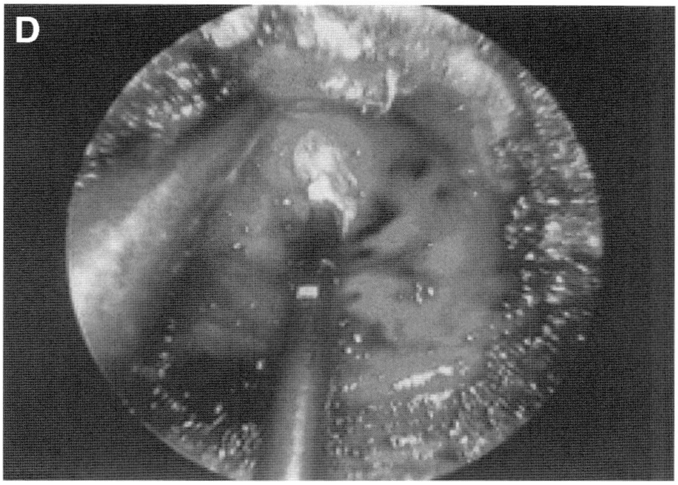

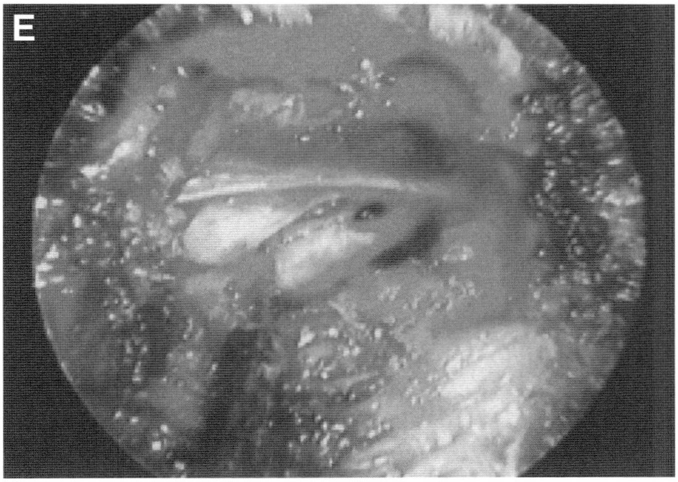

Fig. 7. Intraoperative endoscopic image demonstrating **(A)** bipolar electrocauterization of epidural plexus overlying disc space, **(B)** opening of annulus with a retractable scalpel, **(C)** loosening of NP with a straight curette, **(D)** removal of offending disc fragment with a pituitary rongeur, and **(E)** nerve roots after disc removal (note the conjoined roots in this particular case).

reported to occur in 0.9–5% of microdiscectomy cases, with a <1% occurrence of deep infections. In a retrospective series of patients undergoing the MED procedure, Perez-Cruet et al. (34) reported only one superficial wound infection in 150 patients. Theoretically, the MED procedure provides a smaller portal for entry of infectious agents in comparison to open microdiscectomy. The incidence of durotomy has been reported to be 0.3–13% and has been reported to be higher (18%) in reoperative microdiscectomies (37). Interestingly, leakage of CSF was observed in 8 of the 150 patients undergoing the MED procedure (34). This complication is usually treated by placing Dura-Gen® dural graft matrix (Integra NeuroSciences, Plainsboro, N J) over the durotomy and carefully reinforcing with a layer of fibrin glue. Lumbar drainage for 48 h is also recommended in

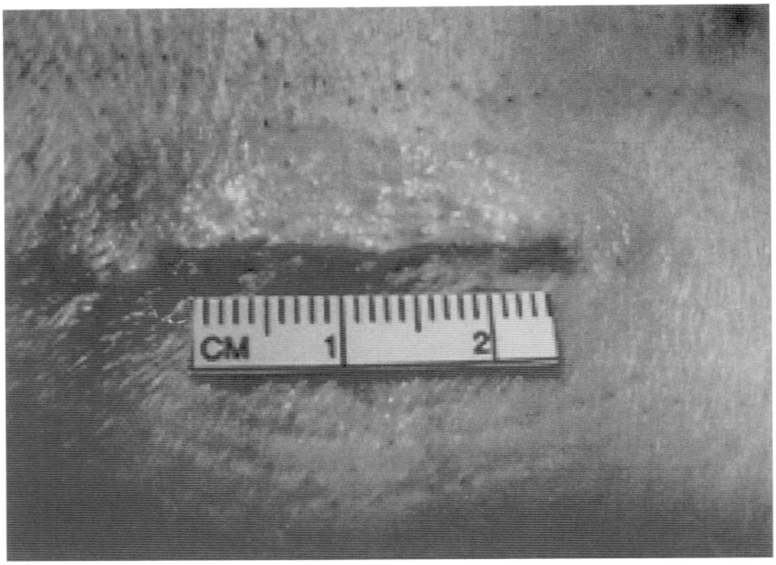

Fig. 8. MED incision with Dermabond skin closure.

larger dural tears. Nerve root injuries or cauda equina syndrome was not observed in the small series of 150 patients reported by Perez-Cruet et al. (34). Finally, recurrent disc herniation has been reported to be 4% with microdiscectomy (38). Similarly, recurrent disc herniation observed in patients undergoing the MED procedure was approx 2.7% (4 of 150). These 4 patients were subsequently treated with repeat MED (34).

Results

No randomized, prospective study has been performed comparing MED to microdiscectomy. The largest retrospective series reported in the literature to date involved 150 patients ranging in age from 18 to 76 yr *(34)*. In this series, a mean operative time of 97 min (110 min for the first 30 cases compared with 75 min for the last 30 cases), a mean hospital stay of 7.7 h, and a mean time to return to work of 17 d were reported. Clinical outcome as determined by the modified McNabb criteria, with an average follow-up of 12 mo (range: 3–24 mo), demonstrated a 77% excellent outcome, 17% good outcome, 3% fair outcome, and 3% poor outcome. These data support the claim that MED is a safe, effective alternative to traditional lumbar microdiscectomy.

CONCLUSION

The treatment of herniated lumbar discs continues to provide intellectual and technical challenges for the spine surgeon. Although recent advancements in the area of optics, microendoscopic instruments, and minimally invasive access has allowed the surgeon to perform the MED with less iatrogenic injury to surrounding soft tissue, patient selection remains one of the most critical factors in achieving excellent clinical outcomes. Therefore, with a concerted effort to train young spine surgeons in patient selection as well as this technique, perhaps one day MED will supplant microdiscectomy and become the preferred procedure for herniated lumbar discs refractory to conservative nonoperative management.

REFERENCES

1. Hart LG, Deyo RA, Cherkin DC. Physician office visits for low-back pain: frequency, clinical evaluation, and treatment patterns from a U.S. national survey. Spine 1995;20(1):11–19.
2. Mayer TG, et al. A prospective two-year study of functional restoration in industrial low-back injury: an objective assessment procedure. JAMA 1987;258(13):1763–1767.
3. Frymoyer J. Back Pain and sciatica. N Engl J Med 1988;318:291–300.
4. Luo X, et al. Estimates and patterns of direct health care expenditures among individuals with back pain in the United States. Spine 2004;29(1):79–86.
5. Vesalius A. De Humani Corporis Fabrica Libri Septem, 1555, pp. 71–73.
6. Kitano T, et al. Biochemical changes associated with the symptomatic human intervertebral disk. Clin Orthop 1993(293):372–377.
7. Inerot S, Axelsson I. Structure and composition of proteoglycans from human annulus fibrosus. Connect Tissue Res 1991;26(1-2):47–63.
8. Olczyk K. Age-related changes in proteoglycans of human intervertebral discs. Z Rheumatol 1994;53(1):19–25.
9. Harrington JF, et al. Herniated lumbar disc material as a source of free glutamate available to affect pain signals through the dorsal root ganglion. Spine 2000;25(8):929–936.
10. Dinning TA, Schaeffer HR. Discogenic compression of the cauda equina: a surgical emergency. Aust NZ J Surg 1993;63(12):927–934.
11. Damkot DK, PM, Lord J, Frymoyer JA. The relationship between work history, work environment and low-back pain in men. Spine 1984;9(4):395–399.
12. Kelsey JL. An epidemiological study of the relationship between occupations and acute herniated lumbar intervertebral discs. Int J Epidemiol 1975;4(3):197–205.
13. Kelsey JL. An epidemiological study of acute herniated lumbar intervertebral discs. Rheumatol Rehabil 1975;14(3):144–159.
14. Kelsey JL, Hardy RJ. Driving of motor vehicles as a risk factor for acute herniated lumbar intervertebral disc. Am J Epidemiol 1975;102(1):63–73.
15. Lewis PJ, et al. Long-term prospective study of lumbosacral discectomy. J Neurosurg 1987;67(1):49–53.
16. Jensen MC, et al. Magnetic resonance imaging of the lumbar spine in people without back pain. N Engl J Med 1994;331(2):69–73.
17. Fager CA, Freidberg SR. Analysis of failures and poor results of lumbar spine surgery. Spine 1980;5(1):87–94.
18. Fager CA. Observations on spontaneous recovery from intervertebral disc herniation. Surg Neurol 1994;42(4):282–286.
19. Oppenheim H, KF. Uber Einklemmung bzw: strangulation der cauda equina. Dtsch Med Wochenschr 1909;35:697–700.
20. Elsberg C. Experiences in spinal surgery: observations upon 60 laminectomies for spinal disease. Surg Gynecol Obstet 1913;16:117–120.
21. Dandy W. Loose cartilage from intervertebral disk simulating tumor of the spinal cord. Arch Surg 1929;19:660–672.
22. Mixter WJ, Barr JS. Rupture of intervertebral disc with involvement of the spinal canal. N Engl J Med 1934;211:210–215.
23. Caspar W. A new surgical procedure for lumbar disc herniation causing less tissue damage through a microsurgical approach, in Advances in Neurosurgery (Wullenweber R, Brock M, Hamer J, Klinger M, Spoerri O, eds.), Springer-Verlag: Berlin, 1977, pp. 74–77.
24. Yasargil M. Microsurgical operation for herniated disc, in Advances in Neurosurgery (Wullenweber R, Brock M, Hamer J, Klinger M, Spoerri O, eds.), Springer-Verlag: Berlin, 1977 p. 81.
25. Smith L. Enzyme dissolution of the nucleus pulposus in humans. JAMA 1964;187: 137–140.

26. Agre K, et al. Chymodiactin postmarketing surveillance; demographic and adverse experience data in 29,075 patients. Spine 1984;9(5):479–485.
27. Dubuc FL, et al. Four brief reports on long-term results of intradiscal chymopapain. Clin Orthop 1986(206):42–44.
28. Javid MJ, Nordby EJ. Current status of chymopapain for herniated nucleus pulposus. Neursurg Q 1994;4:92–101.
29. Pauza KJ, et al. A randomized, placebo-controlled trial of intradiscal electrothermal therapy for the treatment of discogenic low-back pain. Spine J 2004;4(1):27–35.
30. Hijikata SA, Yamagishi M, Nakayama T, Oomori K. Percutaneous discectomy: a new treatment method for lumbar disc herniation. J Toden Hosp 1975;5:5–13.
31. Kambin P, Gellman H. Percutaneous posterolateral discectomy of the lumbar spine. Clin Orthop 1983;174:127–132.
32. Kambin P, Savitz MH. Arthroscopic microdiscectomy: an alternative to open disc surgery. Mt Sinai J Med, 2000;67(4):283–287.
33. Smith MW, FK. MED: The first 100 cases. Paper presented at the Annual Meeting of the Congress of Neurological Surgeons; Seattle, WA, 1998.
34. Perez-Cruet MJ, et al. Microendoscopic lumbar discectomy: technical note. Neurosurgery 2002. 51(5 Suppl):129–136.
35. Ramirez LF, Thisted R. Complications and demographic characteristics of patients undergoing lumbar discectomy in community hospitals. Neurosurgery 1989;25(2):226–230; discussion, 230, 231.
36. Deyo RA, et al. Morbidity and mortality in association with operations on the lumbar spine: the influence of age, diagnosis, and procedure. J Bone Joint Surg Am 1992; 74(4):536–543.
37. Goodkin R, Laska LL. Unintended "incidental" durotomy during surgery of the lumbar spine: medicolegal implications. Surg Neurol 1995;43(1):4–12; discussion 12–14.
38. Davis RA. A long-term outcome analysis of 984 surgically treated herniated lumbar discs. J Neurosurg 1994;80(3):415–421.

Index

K,L

M

N

O

P

Q–S

T